Hearing Loss: Clinical Diagnosis and Management

Hearing Loss: Clinical Diagnosis and Management

Editor: Peter Barry

AMERICAN
MEDICAL PUBLISHERS
www.americanmedicalpublishers.com

AMERICAN
MEDICAL PUBLISHERS
www.americanmedicalpublishers.com

Cataloging-in-Publication Data

Hearing loss : clinical diagnosis and management / edited by Peter Barry.
p. cm.
Includes bibliographical references and index.
ISBN 979-8-88740-172-0
1. Deafness. 2. Deafness--Diagnosis. 3. Deafness--Treatment. 4. Hearing disorders. I. Barry, Peter.
RF290 .H43 2023
617.8--dc23

American Medical Publishers,
41 Flatbush Avenue,
1st Floor, New York,
NY 11217, USA

ISBN 979-8-88740-172-0 (Hardback)

Contents

Preface

This book has been an outcome of determined endeavour from a group of educationists in the field. The primary objective was to involve a broad spectrum of professionals from diverse cultural background involved in the field for developing new researches. The book not only targets students but also scholars pursuing higher research for further enhancement of the theoretical and practical applications of the subject.

Hearing loss refers to the impairment in perceiving or processing auditory information. Hearing impairment can be partial or complete, and may occur in one or both ears. The impairment in hearing may be acquired, inherited or caused due to perinatal problems and aging. Tinnitus, hyperacusis and presbycusis, endaural phenomena, and auditory processing disorder are a few hearing disorders. A common cause of hearing loss is chronic ear infection. During pregnancy, infections like rubella and syphilis can lead to hearing loss in the offspring. Hearing loss interferes with spoken language acquisition and causes cognitive decline. Certain cases of hearing loss can be examined medically, while others are irreversible and therefore, permanent. The usage of hearing aids, cochlear implants, sign language and subtitles are principal management tools to aid individuals suffering with this condition. The use of stem cell transplant and gene therapy for the regrowth of cochlear cells and nerve cells will prove highly beneficial in the treatment of hearing loss. This book includes some of the vital pieces of work being conducted across the world, on the various topics related to hearing loss. It will serve as a valuable source of reference on its clinical diagnosis and management for graduate and post graduate students.

It was an honour to edit such a profound book and also a challenging task to compile and examine all the relevant data for accuracy and originality. I wish to acknowledge the efforts of the contributors for submitting such brilliant and diverse chapters in the field and for endlessly working for the completion of the book. Last, but not the least; I thank my family for being a constant source of support in all my research endeavours.

Editor

1

Opa1 Prevents Apoptosis and Cisplatin-Induced Ototoxicity in Murine Cochleae

Tingting Dong[1†], Xuejie Zhang[1†], Yiqing Liu[2], Shan Xu[3], Haishuang Chang[3], Fengqiu Chen[1], Lulu Pan[1], Shaoru Hu[1], Min Wang[1] and Min Lu[4*]*

[1] Biobank of Ninth People's Hospital, Shanghai Jiao Tong University School of Medicine, Shanghai, China, [2] Shanghai Ninth People's Hospital, Shanghai Jiao Tong University School of Medicine, Shanghai, China, [3] Shanghai Ninth People's Hospital, Shanghai Institute of Precision Medicine, Shanghai Jiao Tong University School of Medicine, Shanghai, China, [4] Shanghai Key Laboratory for Prevention and Treatment of Bone and Joint Diseases, Department of Orthopaedics, Ruijin Hospital, Shanghai Institute of Traumatology and Orthopaedics, Shanghai Jiao Tong University School of Medicine, Shanghai, China

***Correspondence:**
Tingting Dong
dtt623@foxmail.com
Min Lu
luminsjtu@163.com

†These authors have contributed equally to this work

Optic atrophy1 (OPA1) is crucial for inner mitochondrial membrane (IMM) fusion and essential for maintaining crista structure and mitochondrial morphology. Optic atrophy and hearing impairment are the most prevalent clinical features associated with mutations in the *OPA1* gene, but the function of OPA1 in hearing is still unknown. In this study, we examined the ability of Opa1 to protect against cisplatin-induced cochlear cell death *in vitro* and *in vivo*. Our results revealed that knockdown of *Opa1* affects mitochondrial function in HEI-OC1 and Neuro 2a cells, as evidenced by an elevated reactive oxygen species (ROS) level and reduced mitochondrial membrane potential. The dysfunctional mitochondria release cytochrome c, which triggers apoptosis. *Opa1* expression was found to be significantly reduced after cell exposed to cisplatin in HEI-OC1 and Neuro 2a cells. Loss of Opa1 aggravated the apoptosis and mitochondrial dysfunction induced by cisplatin treatment, whereas overexpression of *Opa1* alleviated cisplatin-induced cochlear cell death *in vitro* and *in explant*. Our results demonstrate that overexpression of *Opa1* prevented cisplatin-induced ototoxicity, suggesting that Opa1 may play a vital role in ototoxicity and/or mitochondria-associated cochlear damage.

Keywords: OPA1, mitochondria, cisplatin, apoptosis, ototoxicity

INTRODUCTION

Mitochondria are responsible for numerous vital cell functions, such as respiration, oxidative phosphorylation (OXPHOS), calcium homeostasis, and apoptotic signaling. These highly dynamic organelles continually modify their shape and undergo fusion and fission in order to maintain their morphology and activity (Hoppins et al., 2007; Rogers et al., 2017). Mitofusin 1 and 2 (Mfn1 and Mfn2) are crucial for outer mitochondrial membrane (OMM) fusion (Santel and Fuller, 2001; Chen et al., 2003), and the dynamin-related GTPase, OPA1, is essential for IMM fusion (Olichon et al., 2002). Dynamin-related protein 1 (Drp1) is a cytosolic protein that is required for mitochondrial fission. The recruitment of Drp1 is regulated by the OMM proteins, mitochondrial fission factor (Mff), mitochondrial division (Mid) 49, Mid51, and mitochondrial fission protein (Fis1) (Loson et al., 2013; Palmer et al., 2013). Mitochondrial fusion and fission are vital processes for cellular functions. Numerous studies have drawn connections between abnormal mitochondrial morphology and various diseases, including neurodegenerative diseases, cardiovascular diseases, and cancers (Mishra and Chan, 2014; Liu L. et al., 2016; He et al., 2017; Li A. et al., 2018; Gao et al., 2019; Zhang et al., 2019; Zhong et al., 2020; Fu et al., 2021b).

OPA1, which is localized at chromosome 3q28, has been identified as the causative gene of Dominant Optic Atrophy (DOA) (Alexander et al., 2000; Delettre et al., 2000). The *OPA1* mRNA has eight alternatively spliced isoforms (Delettre et al., 2001), while the OPA1 protein exists in two forms, the membrane-bound long-OPA1 (L-OPA1) and the soluble short-OPA1 (S-OPA1). Both are required for mitochondrial fusion (Olichon et al., 2002; Ishihara et al., 2006). In addition to its function in IMM fusion, OPA1 is crucial for the maintenance of crista structure and mitochondrial morphology (Frezza et al., 2006; Patten et al., 2014). Opa1 depletion was associated with mitochondrial fragmentation, crista disorganization, and cytochrome c redistribution (Frezza et al., 2006). In contrast, *Opa1* overexpression was associated with: normally shaped cristae; alterations in the responses of multiple tissues to apoptotic, necrotic, and atrophic stimuli; and phenotypic rescue of mitochondrial diseases in mice (Civiletto et al., 2015; Varanita et al., 2015). Opa1 also contributes to safeguarding mtDNA integrity, preserving mtDNA function in the face of mutations (Chen et al., 2010), and supporting cellular adaptation to metabolic demand (Patten et al., 2014). Opa1 dysfunction has been linked to ROS overproduction and unbalanced redox homeostasis (Yarosh et al., 2008; Chen et al., 2012).

In the clinic, about 60–70% of DOA cases are associated with pathogenic mutations of *OPA1* (Alexander et al., 2000; Delettre et al., 2000). DOA is characterized by destruction of retinal ganglion cells (RGCs) and the optic nerve (Kjer, 1959), deafness, and chronic progressive external ophthalmoplegia (Treft et al., 1984; Meire et al., 1985). Hearing loss usually follows the onset of visual symptoms (Leruez et al., 2013). Although OPA1 is highly expressed in the retina, it is broadly expressed in multiple tissues. In cochlear tissue, OPA1 is expressed in both hair cells and ganglion cells. Unlike ganglion cells, which express OPA1 at birth, OPA1 expression in the organ of Corti increases after birth and approaches the mature expression level during the onset of hearing (Bette et al., 2007). This suggests that OPA1 is crucial for the function of hair cells and ganglion cells in the inner ear.

In this study, we investigated the potential effect of Opa1 to protect against cisplatin-induced apoptosis *in vitro* and *in vivo*. Our results indicated that loss of Opa1 caused mitochondrial dysfunction and thereby triggered apoptosis in HEI-OC1 and Neuro 2a cells, an auditory hair cell line and a neural cell line. Cisplatin treatment markedly reduced *Opa1* expression in HEI-OC1 and Neuro 2a cells. In the two tested cell lines, Opa1 depletion aggravated the cisplatin-induced apoptosis and mitochondrial dysfunction, whereas *Opa1* overexpression partially prevented cisplatin-induced apoptosis. Histological analyses were performed using cisplatin-treated organotypic cochlear cultures, and our results showed that Opa1 overexpression decreased cisplatin-induced cell death, indicating Opa1 is a potential therapeutics gene in cisplatin induced auditory impairment.

MATERIALS AND METHODS

Cell Culture

Murine HEI-OC1 cells were grown in DMEM supplemented with 10% heat-inactivated FBS and maintained at 33°C with 10% CO2. Murine Neuro 2a cells were grown in the same medium at 37°C with 5% CO2. HEI-OC1 and Neuro 2a cells were incubated in 96-well plates for cell viability assessment or 6-well plates for flow cytometry, transmission electron microscopy, and immunostaining. siRNA or plasmids were transfected after cells were grown to 60% confluence. siRNA was transfected using LipoRNAiMax (Invitrogen). Plasmids were transfected into Neuro 2a cells using Lipo2000 (Invitrogen, 11668-019) and into HEI-OC1 cells using Lipo3000 (Invitrogen, L30000015), with the relevant reagents diluted in Opti-MEM (Gibco). The cells were then treated with or without cisplatin for 24 h. For cell viability detection, HEI-OC1 or Neuro 2a cells were transfected with siRNA or plasmids, and then treated with or without cisplatin for 24 h, unless indicated the timepoint in the picture. For qRT-PCR analyses, HEI-OC1 or Neuro 2a cells were grown in a 6-well plate to 70–80% confluence, treated with siRNA, plasmids or cisplatin for 24 h. For Western blot, HEI-OC1 or Neuro 2a cells were grown in a 6-well plate to 70–80% confluence, treated with siRNA, plasmids or cisplatin for 48 h. For flow cytometry, transmission electron microscopy, and immunostaining, cells were transfected with siRNA or treated with or without cisplatin for 24 h. For almost all the experiments both HEI-OC1 and Neuro 2a cells were used. Several experiments (Mitochondria morphology detection after Opa1 knockdown and cisplatin treatment; Cytochrome C release analysis; TEM; Bcl-2 protein expression; and DCF level after cisplatin treatment) were only used HEI-OC1 cells.

Cell Viability Assessment

HEI-OC1 and Neuro 2a cells were plated in 96-well plates (1×10^5 cells/well) and incubated with 100 μL drug-supplemented DMEM. After 24, 48, or 72 h, cell viability was measured using a Cell Counting Kit-8 (CCK-8; Dojindo) according to the manufacturer's instructions. The optical density at 450 nm (OD450 nm) was measured using a Tecan Spark multimode microplate reader.

Flow Cytometry

To test the ROS level and mitochondrial membrane potential (MMP), cells were collected, washed thrice with PBS, and stained using DCFH-A (Sigma, D6883; 10 mM in DMSO, 1:1,000) or TMRM (Invitrogen, 134361; 1:1,000) at 37°C for 30 min, and then counterstained with DAPI (Invitrogen,D357; 1:1,000). Apoptosis was assessed with apoptosis detection kit (BioLegend, San Diego, CA, United States). Briefly, cells were collected, washed thrice with PBS, suspended with 500 μL binding buffer, and stained with Annexin V-FITC and propidium iodide following the manufacturer's instructions. Stained cells were analyzed using a flow cytometer and data were processed with the FlowJo software (FlowJo, LLC, Ashland, OR, United States).

Western Blot Analysis

Collected cells were lysed with RIPA buffer (Thermo Fisher Scientific, 89900) containing a complete protease inhibitor cocktail (Roche) at 4°C for 20 min with shaking, and then centrifuged at 4°C for 20 min at 13,000 rpm. The supernatant was collected, the total proteins were quantified, and 10 μg of total protein from each sample was boiled for 10 min in sample buffer (BioRad, #161-0737), resolved by SDS-PAGE, and transferred to a PVDF membrane. The membrane was blocked with TBST containing 5% skim milk, incubated with primary antibodies in TBST containing 5% skim milk, and incubated with HRP-conjugated secondary antibodies. The results were visualized with ECL reagents. The following primary antibodies were used: mouse anti-Opa1 (BD 612606), rabbit anti-Hsp60 (CST, 12165), rabbit anti-Bcl2 (CST, 2498), and rabbit anti-β-actin (CST, 4967S).

Quantitative Real-Time Reverse Transcription Polymerase Chain Reaction

Total RNA was extracted from cultured cells using a commercially available kit (Qiagen, #74136) with the optional DNase digestion step. The RNA was reverse transcribed with an Evo M-MLV RT kit with gDNA Clean for qPCR (Accurate Biotechnology, China) and qRT-PCR was performed using a Roche LightCycler 480 with a SYBR Green Premix Pro Taq HS qPCR kit (Accurate Biotechnology) and the following cycling conditions: 95℃ for 5 min followed by 45 cycles of 95℃ for 10 s, 60℃ for 10 s, and 72℃ for 10 s. The relative level of each target gene was normalized to that of endogenous *Rpl19* and calculated using the comparative Ct ($\Delta\Delta$Ct) method. The sequences of the utilized primers were as follows: 5′- TGGAAAATGGTTCGAGAGTCAG-3′ (forward) and 5′- CATTCCGTCTCTAGGTTAAAGCG-3′ (reverse) for *Opa1*; 5′-ACGGAGGCTGGGATGCCTTTG-3′ (forward) and 5′-AGTGATGCAGGCCCCGACCA-3′ (reverse) for *Bcl2*; and 5′-ACCTGGATGAGAAGGATGAG-3′ (forward) and 5′-ACCTTCAGGTACAGGCTGTG-3′ (reverse) for *Rpl19*.

Transmission Electron Microscopy

HEI-OC1 cells were collected, placed in 2.5% glutaraldehyde, and incubated at room temperature for 20 min and then at 4℃ for 1 h. The cells were post-fixed with 1% osmium tetroxide for 2 h at room temperature, dehydrated in a graded alcohol series, and infiltrated in a graded alcohol series containing eopn812. The samples were double-stained with uranyl acetate followed by lead citrate and examined with a 120 kV transmission electron microscope (FEI Talos L120C).

Organotypic Cochlear Cultures

Organotypic cochlear cultures were generated from the cochlea of postnatal day 1–2 (P1–P2) mouse pups of both sexes. Briefly, mouse pups were sacrificed by decapitation and dissected in HBSS supplemented with HEPES. The basal membrane was isolated, plated in a glass-bottom dish with DMEM/F12 medium containing 1 × N2 (Sigma, A1370701) and 1 × B27 (Sigma, 17504044), and incubated overnight at 37°C with 5% CO2. For immunostaining, the basal membrane cells were simultaneously transfected with *Opa1* plasmid (p*Opa1*) or siRNA and treated with 60 μM cisplatin for 24 h. Control cultures were treated with cisplatin alone for 24 h or left untreated.

Immunofluorescence Assay

HEI-OC1 and Neuro 2a cells were collected and rinsed thrice in phosphate-buffered saline (PBS) for 10 min per wash. The cells were fixed in 4% paraformaldehyde (PFA) for 30 min and incubated overnight at 4℃ with anti-cleaved caspase-3 (CST, 9661; rabbit, 1:400). The cells were rinsed thrice with PBS, incubated with Alexa Fluor 488 donkey anti-rabbit IgG antibody (Invitrogen, 1:400) for 60 min at room temperature, rinsed thrice in PBS, and stained with DAPI (YEASEN, 36308ES20). Alternatively, cells were incubated with MitoTracker (Invitrogen; M7510, 1:10,000) at 37℃ for 30 min, rinsed thrice in PBS, fixed in 4% PFA for 30 min, and then either directly sealed with DAPI or incubated overnight at 4℃ with anti-cytochrome c (CST, 11940; rabbit, 1:100), rinsed thrice in PBS, incubated with Alexa Fluor 488 donkey anti-rabbit IgG antibody (Invitrogen; 1:400) for 60 min at room temperature, rinsed thrice in PBS, and then sealed with DAPI.

The basal membrane cells were collected, rinsed thrice in PBS for 10 min per rinse, fixed in 4% PFA for 30 min, incubated overnight at 4℃ with MYO 7A (proteus biosciences; 1:500), rinsed thrice in PBS, incubated with Alexa Fluor 488 donkey anti-rabbit IgG antibody (Invitrogen; 1:400) for 60 min at room temperature, rinsed thrice in PBS, and sealed with DAPI.

Statistical Analysis

Data are presented as mean ± standard errors of the mean (SEM). Experiments were performed in triplicate and repeated three times. Statistical significance was assessed with *t*-test, one-way ANOVA, or two-way ANOVA, as applied using the GraphPad Prism 9.0 software (GraphPad Software). A value of $p < 0.05$ was considered statistically significant.

RESULTS

Knockdown of *Opa1* in HEI-OC1 and Neuro 2a Cells by siRNA

To study the role of Opa1 in the inner ear, we used siRNA transfection to assess the effect of *Opa1* knockdown in HEI-OC1 and Neuro 2a cells, which were chosen to represent two important cell types of the inner ear: hair cells and spiral ganglion neurons. In the latter case, we selected the most common used neuronal cell line because there was no specific cell line available for spiral ganglion neurons. The transfection efficiency was monitored by transfecting cells with fluorescence-tagged sham siRNA. Almost all HEI-OC1 and Neuro 2a cells were fluorescence-positive at 24 h post-transfection (**Figure 1A**). We designed three different mouse *Opa1* siRNA (si*Opa1*-260, si*Opa1*-1681, si*Opa1*-2361) and analyzed their effects in HEI-OC1 and Neuro 2a cells compared to those of a control scramble siRNA (Ctrl-siRNA).

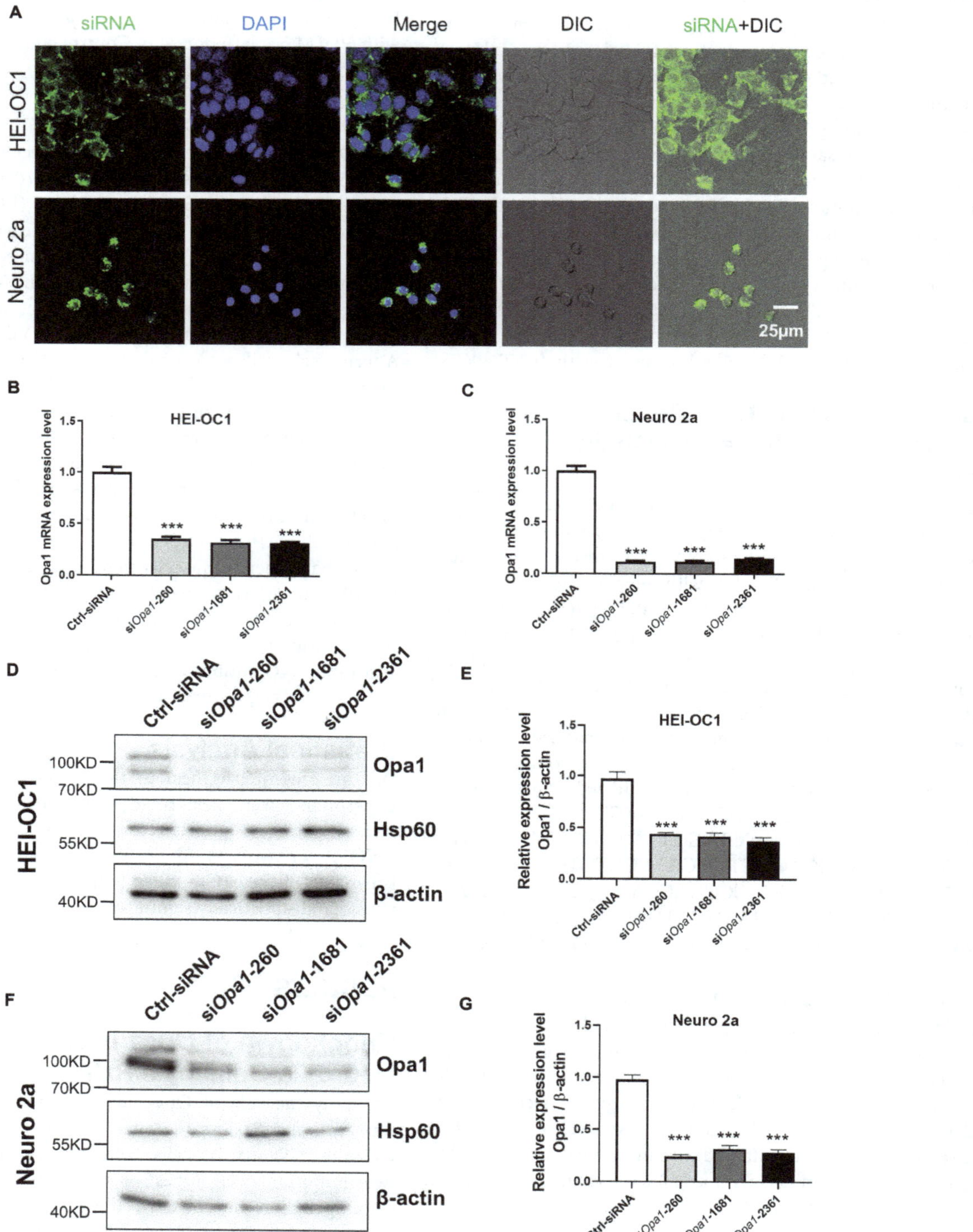

FIGURE 1 | Depletion of Opa1 in HEI-OC1 and Neuro 2a cells. **(A)** Representative confocal images of HEI-OC1 and Neuro 2a cells after siRNA transfection for 24 h, showing transfection efficiency. DIC: Differential interference contrast. Quantification of *Opa1* mRNA expression levels in HEI-OC1 **(B)** and Neuro 2a **(C)** cells transfected with si*Opa1* for 24 h. In this and all following graphs: the levels of *Opa1* mRNA were normalized to that of mouse rpl19; error bars represent standard error of the mean (SEM); and experiments were performed in triplicate and repeated three times. ***$p < 0.001$ (one-way ANOVA with Dunnett's multiple comparisons test). Representative Western blot images **(D)** and quantification **(E)** of *Opa1* expression in HEI-OC1 cells transfected with si*Opa1* for 48 h. In this and all following graphs, the protein levels of Opa1 are normalized to that of β-actin. ***$p < 0.001$ (one-way ANOVA with Dunnett's multiple comparisons test). Representative Western blot images **(F)** and quantification **(G)** of *Opa1* expression in Neuro 2a cells transfected with si*Opa1* for 48 h. ***$p < 0.001$ (one-way ANOVA with Dunnett's multiple comparisons test).

At 24 h after si*Opa1* transfection, *Opa1* mRNA expression was reduced by 70% in HEI-OC1 cells (**Figure 1B**) and by 90% in Neuro 2a cells (**Figure 1C**). To test whether there was a corresponding reduction in the protein expression of Opa1, we performed Western blot analysis at 48 h after si*Opa1* transfection. All three of the *Opa1* siRNA were found to significantly decrease the Opa1 protein levels in the two cell lines (**Figures 1D,F**). Quantification revealed that Neuro 2a cells displayed less Opa1 protein expression than HEI-OC1 cells (**Figures 1E,G**), which was consistent with the trends in their mRNA expression levels (**Figures 1B,C**). These results indicate that Opa1 could be successfully suppressed by the designed siRNA in HEI-OC1 and Neuro 2a cells. For the following experiments, si*Opa1*-260 was used for *Opa1* knockdown subsequently.

Knockdown of *Opa1* Impairs Mitochondrial Function

To study the cellular function of Opa1 in HEI-OC1 and Neuro 2a cells, we first monitored mitochondrial morphology by electron microscope and MitoTracker staining. MitoTracker staining and Electron microscopic analysis of HEI-OC1 cells transfected with Ctrl-siRNA revealed mainly elongated mitochondria (**Figure 2A**), with some tubular mitochondria (**Figure 2B**). HEI-OC1 cells transfected with *Opa1* siRNA for 24 h exhibited highly fragmented, dot-like mitochondria, as assessed by MitoTracker staining (**Figure 2A**) and electron microscopy (**Figure 2B**). In contrast, mitochondria of Neuro 2a cells displayed fragmented shapes prior to siRNA transfection (data not shown), and there was no further difference of mitochondria shape between Ctrl-siRNA- and si*Opa1*-transfected Neuro 2a cells under MitoTracker staining (data not shown). To assess whether Opa1 depletion affected mitochondrial function, we transfected the cells with siRNA for 24 h and measured the ROS level and mitochondrial membrane potential (MMP, $\Delta\Psi_m$) using DCFH-DA and TMRM, respectively. HEI-OC1 cells lacking Opa1 exhibited an increased ROS level (**Figures 2C,D**) and reduced MMP (**Figures 2G,H**) compared with control cells. Despite displaying no alteration of mitochondrial shape, *Opa1*-silenced Neuro 2a cells displayed a higher ROS level (**Figures 2E,F**) and lower MMP (**Figures 2I,J**) compared with control cells. These findings indicate that Opa1 depletion affects mitochondrial function in HEI-OC1 and Neuro 2a cells, independent of its contribution to mitochondrial formation.

Silencing of *Opa1* Increases Vulnerable to Apoptosis

Next we sought to identify the cellular changes that arise from *Opa1* silencing. At 24 h post-transfection, the cell numbers were comparable between si*Opa1*- and Ctrl-siRNA-transfected HEI-OC1 and Neuro 2a cells (**Figures 3A,B**, left). At 48 h post-transfection, Opa1-depleted Neuro 2a cells displayed a significant increase in cell death, whereas Opa1-depleted HEI-OC1 cells did not (**Figures 3A,B**, middle). At 72 h post-transfection, Opa1-depleted Neuro 2a and HEI-OC1 cells both exhibited significant increases in cell death (**Figures 3A,B**, right). To assess whether cells underwent apoptosis upon *Opa1* knockdown, we stained siRNA-transfected cells for cleaved caspase-3. Cleaved caspase-3 staining was evident in HEI-OC1 and Neuro 2a cells transfected with si*Opa1* (**Figure 3C**), indicating that apoptosis was activated upon Opa1 depletion. In agreement with this increased caspase-3 activation, transmission electron microscopy revealed the presence of apoptotic cells in cultures of Opa1-depleted HEI-OC1 cells (**Figure 3C**). We postulated that loss of Opa1 decreased the MMP (**Figures 2E,I**) and led to cytochrome c leakage, thereby increasing caspase-3 activation. In support of this proposal, staining experiments revealed that cytochrome c and mitochondria were colocalized in HEI-OC1 cells transfected with Ctrl-siRNA, as reflected by an orange color representing the merging of green (cytochrome c) and red (MitoTracker) fluorescence signals (**Figure 3D**). In *Opa1*-knockdown cells, in contrast, we observed largely non-overlapping green and red signals that suggested the cytochrome c had been released from the mitochondria (**Figure 3D**). To further confirm that cells underwent apoptosis following si*Opa1* transfection, we preformed Annexin V/PI staining and flow cytometric analysis. Annexin V staining showed that knockdown of *Opa1* induced more early apoptotic cells in HEI-OC1 cultures (**Figures 3E,F**) and more late apoptotic cells in Neuro 2a cultures (**Figures 3G,H**). This finding is consistent with our observation that Opa1 depletion led to earlier cell death in Neuro 2a cells than in HEI-OC1 cells (**Figures 3A,B**). Bcl family proteins, such as Bcl-2, regulate the release of cytochrome c through the OMM (Adams and Cory, 2007). To assess whether Bcl2 was involved in the apoptosis induced by *Opa1* knockdown, we detected Bcl2 expression in cells transfected with siRNA for 24 h. After Opa1 depletion, the mRNA level of Bcl2 was markedly reduced in both HEI-OC1 and Neuro 2a cells (**Figures 3I,J**), and the protein level of Bcl2 was reduced in Neuro 2a cells (**Figure 3K**).

Knockdown of *Opa1* Aggravates Cisplatin-Induced Mitochondrial Dysfunction and Apoptosis

Serious side effects, such as ototoxicity, are associated with the use of cisplatin. Several studies demonstrated that cisplatin-induced cytotoxicity is closely related to mitochondrial dysfunction such as that signaled by ROS generation (van Gisbergen et al., 2015; de Sa Junior et al., 2017). Increased ROS alters the MMP and induces damage in the respiratory chain, thereby triggering apoptosis. To identify a suitable concentration of cisplatin that could induce cellular damage in our system, we exposed HEI-OC1 and Neuro 2a cells to various concentrations of cisplatin. After incubation with 60 μM cisplatin for 24 h, cell death was observed in 60% of HEI-OC1 cells and 50% of Neuro 2a cells (**Figures 4A,B**). Interestingly, *Opa1* mRNA expression was reduced in HEI-OC1 and Neuro 2a cells exposed to cisplatin for 24 h (**Figure 4C**). Consistent with mRNA level, Opa1 protein level also decreased after cisplatin treatment in the two cell lines (**Figure 4D**). According to MitoTracker staining, HEI-OC1 cells

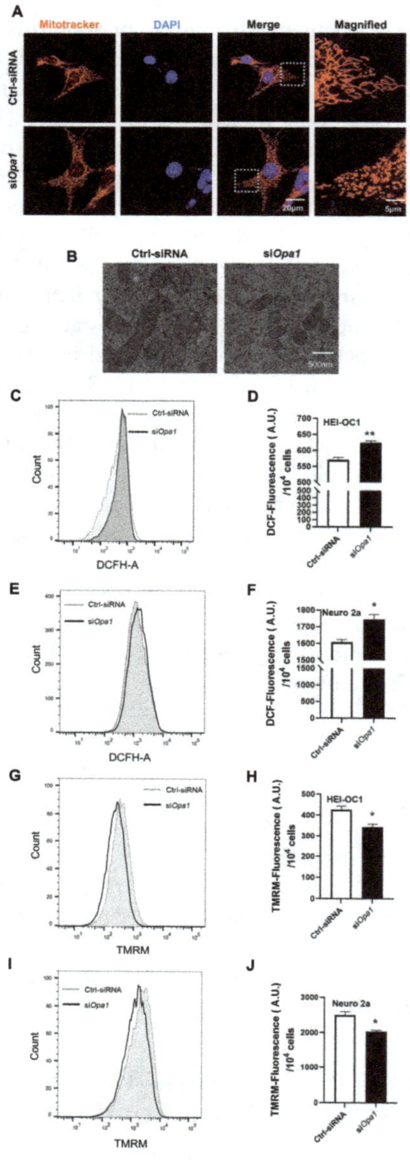

FIGURE 2 | Loss of Opa1 leads to mitochondrial dysfunction in HEI-OC1 and Neuro 2a cells. **(A)** Representative confocal microscopic images of MitoTracker staining at 24 h after siRNA transfection of HEI-OC1 cells. Right panels show magnified views of the areas marked in the left panels. **(B)** HEI-OC1 cells were transfected with scramble (Ctrl) siRNA or si*Opa1* for 24 h and fixed, and thin sections of cells were visualized by transmission electron microscopy. **(C)** Intracellular ROS level was measured by flow cytometric analysis using DCFH-DA in HEI-OC1 cells transfected with siRNA for 24 h. **(D)** Quantitative histograms of the mean fluorescence intensity of DCFH-DA in HEI-OC1 cells. $^{**}p < 0.01$ (non-parametric Mann-Whitney *t*-test). **(E,F)** Representative flow cytometric plot **(E)** and quantitative histograms **(F)** of the mean fluorescence intensity of DCFH-DA in Neuro 2a cells transfected with siRNA for 24 h. $^{*}p < 0.05$ (non-parametric Mann-Whitney *t*-test). **(G)** The mitochondrial membrane potential of HEI-OC1 cells was measured by flow cytometric analysis using TMRM fluorescence at 24 h after siRNA transfection. **(H)** Bar graph shows the relative TMRM mean intensity in HEI-OC1 cells. $^{*}p < 0.05$ (non-parametric Mann-Whitney *t*-test). Representative flow cytometric plot **(I)** and quantitative histograms **(J)** of the relative TMRM mean intensity in Neuro 2a cells. $^{*}p < 0.05$ (non-parametric Mann-Whitney *t*-test).

treated with cisplatin for 24 h exhibited highly fragmented, dot-like mitochondria (**Figure 4E**), which is similar to the morphology of mitochondrion in HEI-OC1 cells with *Opa1* knockdown (**Figure 2A**). Treatment with si*Opa1* for 24 h did not cause cell death in HEI-OC1 or Neuro 2a cells, but loss of Opa1 significantly worsened cell survival upon cisplatin treatment (**Figures 4F,G**). To confirm these cell viability results, we performed Annexin V/PI staining followed by flow cytometric analysis. Annexin V staining showed that cisplatin treatment for 24 h induced ~12% late apoptotic cells in HEI-OC1 cells and ~3.5% late apoptotic cells in Neuro 2a cells (**Figures 4H–K**). Silencing of *Opa1* additively enhanced the proportions of late apoptotic cells in cisplatin-treated HEI-OC1 and Neuro 2a cell cultures (**Figures 4I,K**). Moreover, the mitochondrial dysfunction caused by cisplatin treatment was worsened by Opa1 depletion, as evidenced by increased ROS generation in HEI-OC1 cells (**Figures 4L,M**). These results indicate that Opa1 depletion exacerbates the mitochondrial dysfunction and apoptosis induced by cisplatin in both HEI-OC1 and Neuro 2a cells.

Opa1 Upregulation Suppresses Cisplatin-Induced Apoptosis

To determine if the overexpression of *Opa1* suppresses the apoptosis induced by cisplatin, we first transiently transfected HEI-OC1 and Neuro 2a cells with *Opa1* and examined *Opa1* mRNA and protein expression levels. At 24 h after *Opa1* transfected to HEI-OC1 and Neuro 2a cells, the expression levels of the *Opa1* mRNA (**Figures 5A,C**) and protein (**Figures 5B,D**) were significantly elevated. Treatment of both cell lines with 60 μM cisplatin for 24 h caused almost half of the cells to die (**Figures 5E,F**), but these death rates were diminished significantly in cells transfected with *Opa1* (**Figures 5E,F**). Furthermore, flow cytometric analysis showed that upregulation of *Opa1* reduced the number of early and late apoptotic cells in HEI-OC1 cells (**Figures 5G,H**). Opa1 was also found to protect Neuro 2a cells from cisplatin-induced apoptosis (**Figures 5I,J**).

Opa1 Protects Against Cisplatin-Induced Hair Cell Death

Next, we tested the otoprotective potential of Opa1 *in vivo*. Organotypic cochlear cultures were treated with 60 μM cisplatin for 24 h, and hair cell damage was observed in whole-organ inner ear explants. Hair cell morphology and structure were evaluated by immunolabeling of the hair cell marker, myosin 7a. As shown in the **Figure 6A**, knockdown or overexpressed *Opa1* didn't affect cochlea morphology. Under cisplatin treatment, the numbers of OHCs were significantly reduced in the apical, middle, and basal turns of the cochlea, but there was no change in the number of IHCs (**Figures 6B,C**). *Opa1* knockdown followed by cisplatin treatment resulted in more severe cochlear lesions: There were 30% fewer OHCs and 20% fewer IHCs compared to the cisplatin treatment groups (**Figures 6B,C**). On the contrary, the overexpression of *Opa1* was modestly effective in preventing OHCs death in the middle turn of explants exposed to cisplatin (**Figures 6B,C**).

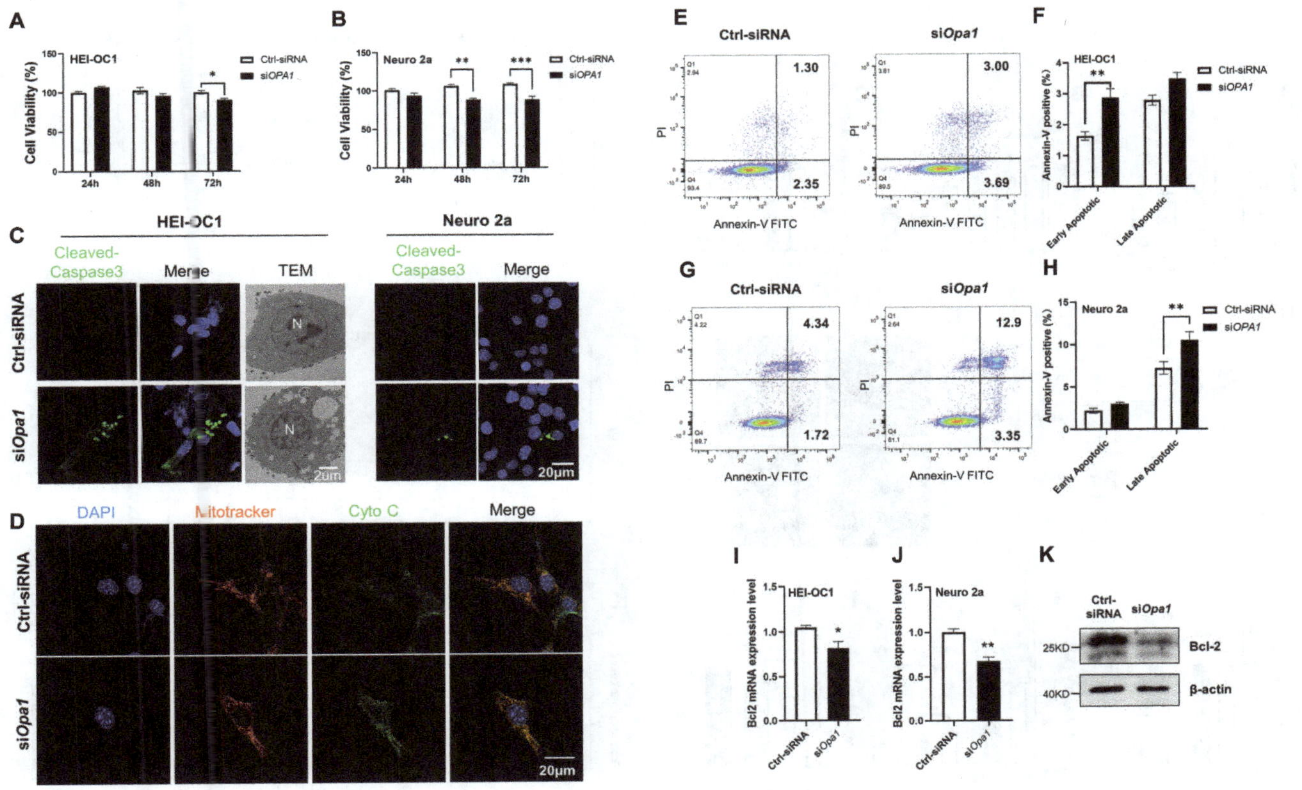

FIGURE 3 | Lacking Opa1 triggers apoptosis in HEI-OC1 and Neuro 2a cells. **(A,B)** CCK-8 was used to assess the cell viability of HEI-OC1 **(A)** and Neuro 2a **(B)** cells cultured for 24, 48, and 72 h after transfection with scramble siRNA (Ctrl) or si*Opa1*. $^{*}p < 0.05$, $^{**}p < 0.01$, $^{***}p < 0.001$ (two-way ANOVA). **(C)** Representative confocal microscopic images of cleaved caspase-3 staining at 24 h after siRNA transfection of HEI-OC1 and Neuro 2a cells. Representative transmission electron microscopic images of HEI-OC1 cells at 24 h after siRNA transfection. **(D)** Representative confocal images of HEI-OC1 cells co-stained for mitochondria (MitoTracker) and cytochrome c at 24 h after siRNA transfection. **(E)** Representative flow cytometric plots generated from HEI-OC1 cells stained with Annexin V-FITC/PI to detect apoptosis at 24 h after transfection with scramble siRNA (Ctrl) or si*Opa1*. **(F)** The percentages of early and late apoptotic cells were compared between Ctrl-siRNA- and si*OPA1*-transfected HEI-OC1 cells. $^{**}p < 0.01$ (two-way ANOVA). FITC, fluorescein isothiocyanate; PI, propidium iodide.
(G) Representative flow cytometric plots generated from Neuro 2a cells stained with Annexin V-FITC/PI to detect apoptosis at 24 h after transfection with scramble siRNA (Ctrl) or si*Opa1*. **(H)** The percentages of early and late apoptotic cells were compared between Ctrl-siRNA- and si*OPA1*-transfected Neuro 2a cells. $^{**}p < 0.01$ (two-way ANOVA). **(I,J)** Quantification of Bcl2 mRNA expression levels in HEI-OC1 (I) and Neuro 2a **(J)** cells transfected with siRNA for 24 h. $^{*}p < 0.05$, $^{**}p < 0.01$ (non-parametric Mann-Whitney *t*-test). **(K)** Representative Western blot images showing Bcl2 protein levels in Neuro 2a cells transfected with siRNA for 48 h.

DISCUSSION

Mitochondrial fission and fusion are counterbalancing mechanisms that control the shape, size, and number of organelles. These dynamic processes are also critical in regulating cell death, mitophagy, and organelle distribution (Itoh et al., 2013). In many adherent cell types, such as Hela cells, mitochondria form elongated tubules that continually divide and fuse to form a dynamic interconnecting network (Suen et al., 2008). As shown in **Figures 2A,B**, we observed elongated and tubular mitochondria in HEI-OC1 cells, then they became highly fragmented upon the loss of Opa1. In Neuro 2a cells, in contrast, fragmented mitochondria were observed by MitoTracker staining even in untreated control cells (data not shown), which is consistent with a previous report that only 30% of mitochondria in this cell line had a length at least twice their width when observed by transmission electron microscopy (Qiao et al., 2017). Because of this, we were unable to observe a change in mitochondrial shape following *Opa1* knockdown in Neuro 2a cells, as assessed by MitoTracker staining. In addition to this difference in mitochondrial shape in the effect of *Opa1* knockdown, HEI-OC1 cells and Neuro 2a cells exhibited differences in the progression of cell death following *Opa1* knockdown: *Opa1* downregulation was associated with significant cell death at 48 h in Neuro 2a cells and at 72 h in HEI-OC1 cells (**Figures 3A,B**). Moreover, at 24 h after Opa1 depletion, more early apoptotic cells were seen in HEI-OC1 cells, whereas more late apoptotic cells were found in Neuro 2a cells (**Figures 3G,H**). This difference appeared to reflect the knockdown efficiencies of the two cell lines, indicating that *Opa1* knockdown level is correlated to apoptosis.

Cisplatin is an effective chemotherapeutic agent that is widely used to treat a variety of malignant tumors. In recent years, cisplatin has been reported to affect many different pathways, including cell cycle arrest, apoptosis, proliferation, DNA repair, the TCA cycle, and glycolysis (Pabla and Dong, 2008;

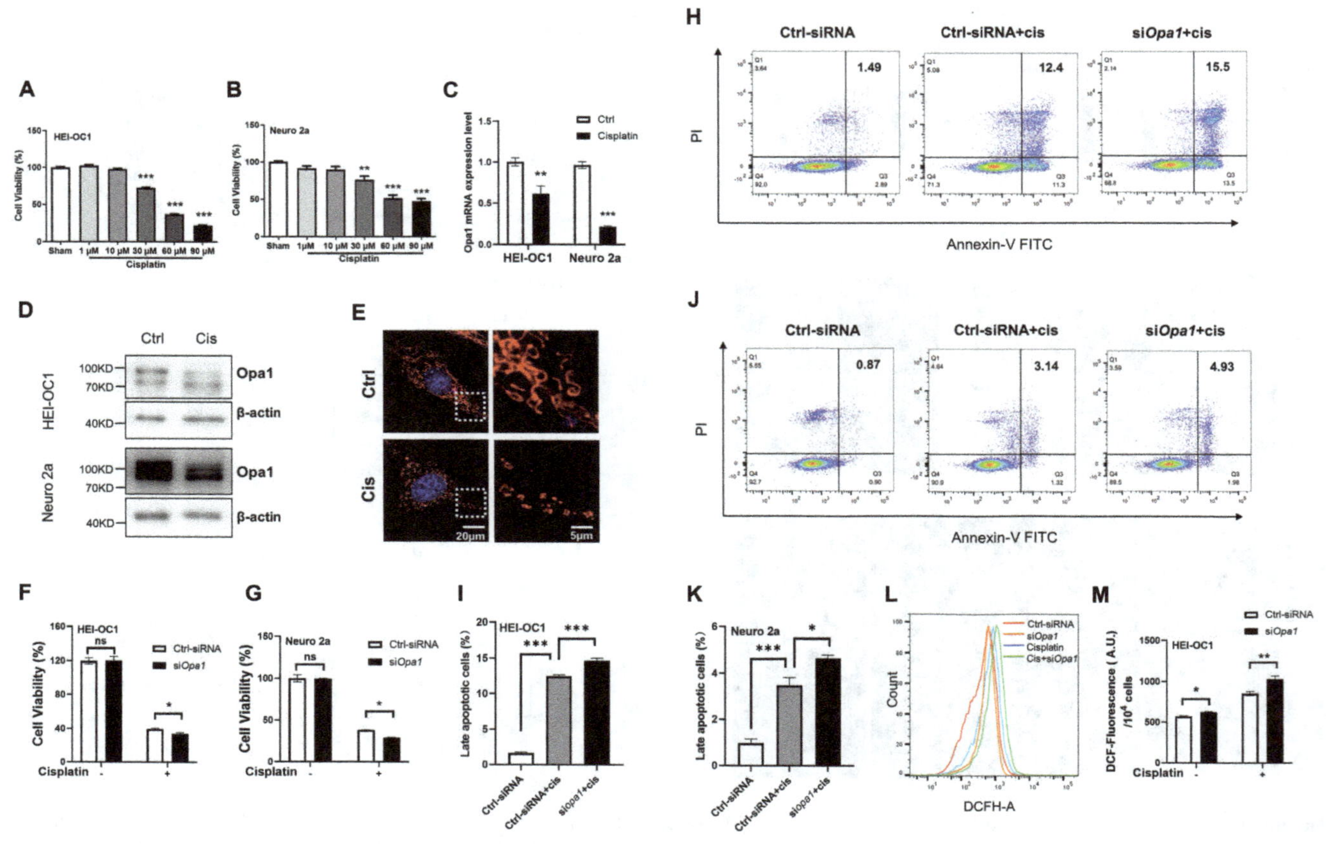

FIGURE 4 | Knockdown of *Opa1* aggravates cisplatin-induced apoptosis and mitochondrial dysfunction in HEI-OC1 and Neuro 2a cells **(A,B)** CCK-8 was used to assess cell viability in HEI-OC1 **(A)** and Neuro 2a **(B)** cells treated with the indicated doses of cisplatin for 24 h. $^{**}p < 0.01$, $^{***}p < 0.001$ (one-way ANOVA with Dunnett's multiple comparisons test). **(C)** Quantification of Opa1 mRNA expression levels in HEI-OC1 and Neuro 2a cells treated with cisplatin for 24 h. $^{**}p < 0.01$, $^{***}p < 0.001$ (two-way ANOVA). **(D)** Representative Western blot images of *Opa1* expression in HEI-OC1 and Neuro 2a cells treated with cisplatin for 24 h. **(E)** Representative confocal microscopic images of MitoTracker staining at 24 h after cisplatin treatment of HEI-OC1 cells. Right panels show magnified views of the areas marked in the left panels. **(F,G)** CCK-8 was used to assess cell viability in HEI-OC1 **(F)** and Neuro 2a **(G)** cells at 24 h after siRNA transfection with or without cisplatin treatment. N.S., non-significant, $^{*}p < 0.05$ (two-way ANOVA). **(H)** Representative flow cytometric plots were generated from HEI-OC1 cells stained with Annexin V-FITC/PI to detect apoptosis at 24 h after siRNA transfection with or without cisplatin treatment. **(I)** The percentage of late apoptotic cells in each group. $^{***}p < 0.001$ (one-way ANOVA with Dunnett's multiple comparisons test). **(J)** Representative flow cytometric plots were generated from Neuro 2a cells stained with Annexin V-FITC/PI to detect apoptosis at 24 h after siRNA transfection with or without cisplatin treatment. **(K)** The percentage of late apoptotic cells in each group. $^{*}p < 0.05$, $^{***}p < 0.001$ (one-way ANOVA with Dunnett's multiple comparisons test). **(L)** Intracellular ROS levels were measured by flow cytometric analysis of HEI-OC1 cells stained with DCFH-DA at 24 h after siRNA transfection with or without cisplatin treatment. **(M)** Quantitative histograms of the mean fluorescence intensity of DCFH-DA in HEI-OC1 cells. $^{*}p < 0.05$, $^{**}p < 0.01$ (two-way ANOVA).

Li et al., 2016; Li H. et al., 2018; Gentilin et al., 2019; Liu W. et al., 2019; Zhang et al., 2020; Liu et al., 2021). The anti-tumor effect of cisplatin is mainly due to its ability to interfere with tumor cell proliferation (Wang and Lippard, 2005). Soon after its administration, cisplatin binds to nuclear DNA, where it blocks transcription and induces double-strand breaks leading to cell cycle arrest (Siddik, 2003). As cells from the cochlea are not proliferative, it is thought that mtDNA damage is a more likely cause of cisplatin-induced hearing loss than nuclear DNA damage (Hutchin and Cortopassi, 2000). Hair cells, spiral ganglion neurons, and the stria vascularis have been considered the three major targets of cisplatin ototoxicity (Schacht et al., 2012; He et al., 2019, 2020, 2021; Liu Y. et al., 2019; Zhou et al., 2020; Fu et al., 2021b). Several molecular mechanisms have been proposed as mediators of cisplatin-induced ototoxicity. Cisplatin was reported to stimulate ROS, which in turn triggers inflammatory pathways in the cochlea and promotes apoptotic and necrotic cell death (Rybak et al., 2009; Mukhopadhyay et al., 2012; Qi et al., 2019; Ding et al., 2020; Cheng et al., 2021; Fu et al., 2021a; Lv et al., 2021). As shown in **Figure 2** of the present work, Opa1 deletion significantly elevated ROS generation and reduced MMP in both hair cells and neural cells. Cisplatin was reported to decrease *Opa1* mRNA expression in the HK-2 kidney cell line (Choi et al., 2015). We therefore speculated that *Opa1* expression might involve in cisplatin induced hair cell damage. Furthermore, our observation that HEI-OC1 and Neuro2a cells treated with cisplatin exhibited downregulation of *Opa1* transcription

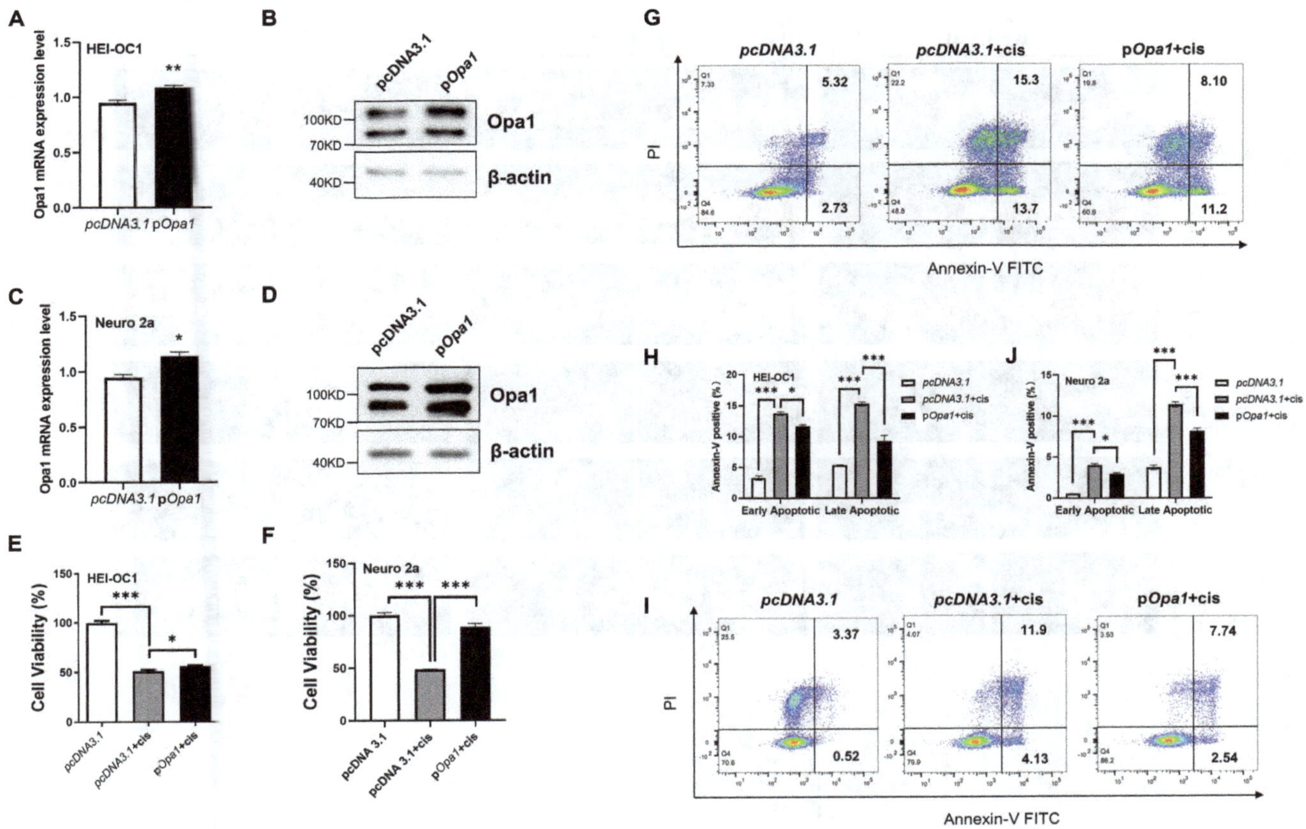

FIGURE 5 | Overexpression of *Opa1* partially restores cisplatin-induced apoptosis in HEI-OC1 and Neuro 2a cells **(A)** Quantification of *Opa1* mRNA expression in HEI-OC1 cells transfected with *Opa1* for 24 h. $^{**}p < 0.01$ (non-parametric Mann-Whitney *t*-test). **(B)** Representative Western blot images showing the Opa1 protein expression level in HEI-OC1 cells transfected with Opa1 for 48 h. **(C)** Quantification of *Opa1* mRNA expression in Neuro 2a cells transfected with Opa1 for 24 h. $^{*}p < 0.05$ (non-parametric Mann-Whitney *t*-test). **(D)** Representative Western blot images showing the Opa1 protein expression level in Neuro 2a cells transfected with *Opa1* for 48 h. **(E,F)** CCK-8 was used to assess cell viability in HEI-OC1 **(E)** and Neuro 2a **(F)** cells at 24 h after cisplatin treatment with or without *Opa1* transfection. $^{*}p < 0.05$, $^{***}p < 0.001$ (one-way ANOVA with Dunnett's multiple comparisons test). **(G)** Representative flow cytometric plots were generated from HEI-OC1 cells stained with Annexin V-FITC/PI to detect apoptosis at 24 h after cisplatin treatment with or without *Opa1* transfection. **(H)** The percentages of early and late apoptotic cells in each group. $^{*}p < 0.05$, $^{***}p < 0.001$ (two-way ANOVA). **(I)** Representative flow cytometric plots were generated from Neuro 2a cells stained with Annexin V-FITC/PI to detect apoptosis at 24 h after cisplatin treatment with or without Opa1 transfection. **(J)** The percentages of early and late apoptotic cells in each group. $^{*}p < 0.05$, $^{***}p < 0.001$ (two-way ANOVA).

and translation level (**Figures 4C,D**). Meanwhile fragmented mitochondria were observed when HEI-OC1 cells treated with cisplatin (**Figure 4E**), which may due to the reduction of Opa1. These results indicated Opa1 depletion would exacerbate cisplatin-induced damage.

OPA1 is essential for IMM fusion and plays a prominent role in maintaining the membrane ultrastructure of cristae and the function of mitochondria (Chan, 2020). OPA1 is ubiquitously expressed in all human tissue (Alexander et al., 2000; Delettre et al., 2000). The highest transcript level is found in retina, followed by the brain, testis, heart and skeletal muscle (Alexander et al., 2000).

Though OPA1 is expressed in multiple systems, OPA1 dysfunction diseases are all related to peripheric neuropathy. Furthermore, the rich expression of OPA1 is found in both white and brown adipocytes, and it's expression elevated during lipid accumulation in adipocytes (Chu et al., 2017). OPA1 has been reported as a dual-specificity A-kinase anchoring protein associated with lipid droplets (Pidoux et al., 2011). At the meantime, many studies reported that Opa1 dysfunction has been involved in muscle mass and cardiac function (Wai et al., 2015; Tezze et al., 2017). Many OPA1 disease mutations have been identified, some of which result in OPA1 haploinsufficiency (Chun and Rizzo, 2017). Mutations in OPA1, particularly truncating mutations, most often manifest as DOA (Cipolat et al., 2004). DOA is characterized by progressive bilateral vision loss, along with hearing loss, myopathy, and peripheral neuropathy (Amati-Bonneau et al., 2008; Hudson et al., 2008). Opa1 dysfunction have been known resulted in RGC neuropathy, increasing the susceptibility of RGCs to apoptosis and vulnerability to oxidative stress (Williams et al., 2010). Given the crucial functions of OPA1, many studies have sought to increase Opa1 levels *in vivo* and *in vitro* as a potential therapeutic approach (Del Dotto et al., 2018).

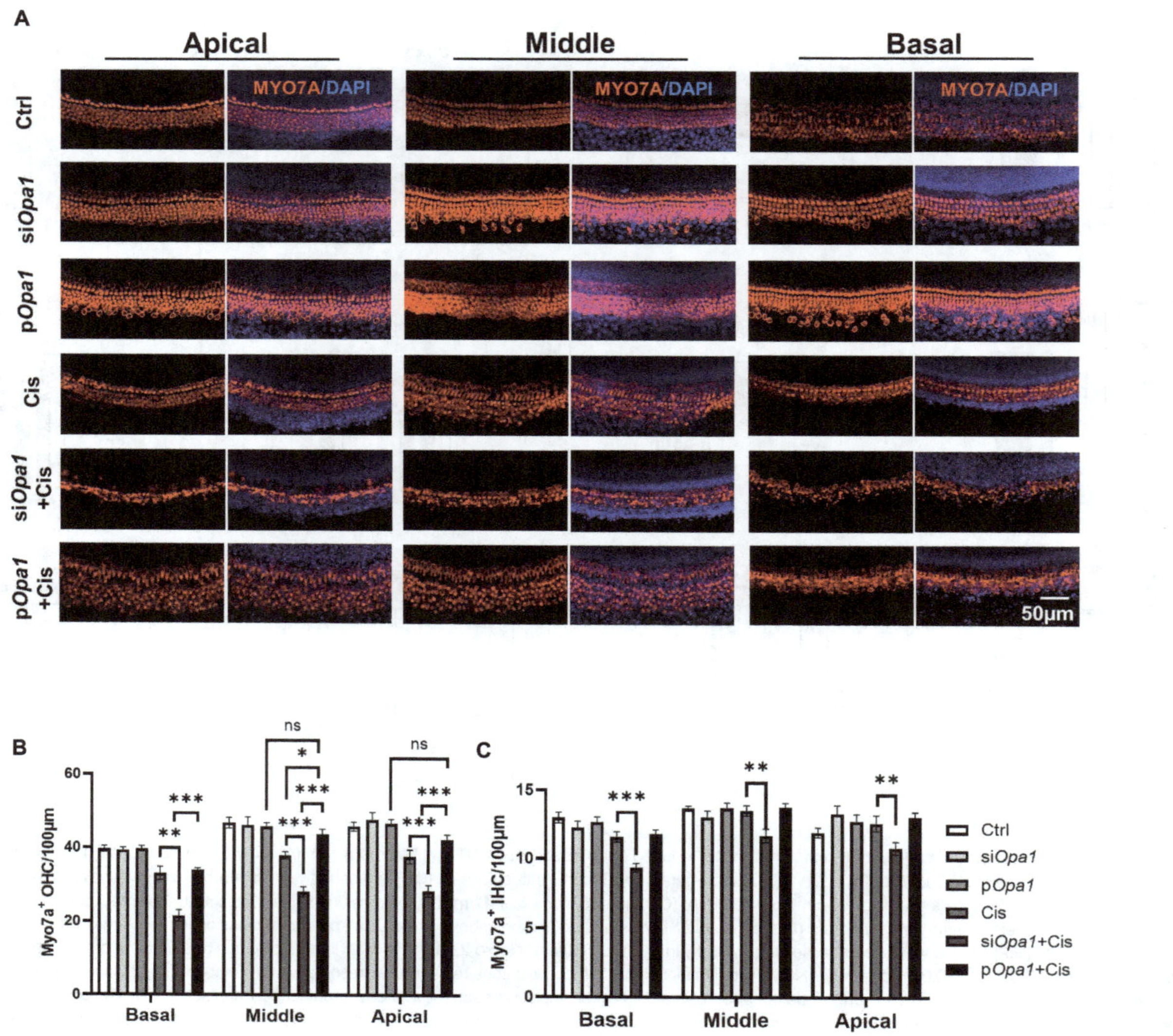

FIGURE 6 | *Opa1* knockdown or overexpression respectively aggravates or partially rescues cisplatin induced hair cell damage in organotypic cochlear cultures. **(A)** Representative confocal images of the apical, middle, and basal regions of organotypic cochlear cultures transfected with si*Opa1* or *Opa1* and treated with 60 μM cisplatin. Hair cells are indicated by MYO7A staining (red) and nuclei are indicated by DAPI staining (blue). **(B,C)** Quantification of IHCs **(B)** and OHCs **(C)** in the apical, middle, and basal turns. N = 3–5 per groups. *$p < 0.05$, **$p < 0.01$, ***$p < 0.001$ (two-way ANOVA).

In a transgenic mouse model, a mild increase of the Opa1 isoform 1 protein level was found to protect mice from denervation-induced muscular atrophy, ischemic heart and brain damage, and hepatocellular apoptosis (Varanita et al., 2015). Moreover, *Opa1* overexpression efficiently rescued the phenotypes of two mouse models of defective mitochondrial bioenergetics: Ndufs4$^{-/-}$ and Cox15$^{sm/sm}$ (Civiletto et al., 2015). Overexpression of each of the eight Opa1 isoforms or different constructs encoding isoform 1 of Opa1 in *Opa1*$^{-/-}$ MEFs revealed that any isoform could restore the crista structure, mtDNA abundance, and energetic efficiency independent of the mitochondrial network morphology (Del Dotto et al., 2017). Although it is known that mutation of *OPA1* often leads to hearing loss, it remains unclear how OPA1 is involved in cochlear dysfunction. Our present results indicate that Opa1 plays key roles in maintaining mitochondrial function and preventing apoptosis induced by cisplatin damage. Future work is warranted to assess the potential of OPA1 as a treatment target for cochlear protection and/or repair.

CONCLUSION

Our results show that depletion of Opa1 affects the mitochondrial function and cell survival of cochlear cells. We herein report that Opa1 depletion is detrimental to the survival of cisplatin-treated cochlear cells both *in vitro* and *in vivo*, and that *Opa1* overexpression protects cochlear cells against cisplatin-induced ototoxicity in cell lines and in organotypic tissue cultures. Our findings collectively suggest that Opa1 modulates mitochondrial function and is essential for the survival of cisplatin-exposed cochlear cells. In conclusion, our study provides strong cell biological evidence that Opa1 can protect against cisplatin-induced cochlear cell death by enhance mitochondrial function.

ETHICS STATEMENT

The animal study was reviewed and approved by the Ethics Committee of the Shanghai Jiao Tong University School of Medicine.

AUTHOR CONTRIBUTIONS

TD designed, supervised the research, analyzed, and interpreted the data. TD and XZ performed the research. TD and ML wrote the manuscript. All authors reviewed the manuscript and discussed the work.

ACKNOWLEDGMENTS

We thank the Electron Microscopy Center of Shanghai Institute of Precision Medicine, Shanghai Ninth People's Hospital, Shanghai Jiao Tong University School of Medicine, for their technical support and assistance in the electron microscopy. We also thank the Bioimaging Facility of Shanghai Institute of Precision Medicine, Shanghai Ninth People's Hospital, Shanghai Jiao Tong University School of Medicine, for their technical support and assistance in flow cytometry.

REFERENCES

Adams, J. M., and Cory, S. (2007). The Bcl-2 apoptotic switch in cancer development and therapy. *Oncogene* 26, 1324–1337. doi: 10.1038/sj.onc.1210220

Alexander, C., Votruba, M., Pesch, U. E., Thiselton, D. L., Mayer, S., Moore, A., et al. (2000). OPA1, encoding a dynamin-related GTPase, is mutated in autosomal dominant optic atrophy linked to chromosome 3q28. *Nat. Genet.* 26, 211–215. doi: 10.1038/79944

Amati-Bonneau, P., Valentino, M. L., Reynier, P., Gallardo, M. E., Bornstein, B., Boissiere, A., et al. (2008). OPA1 mutations induce mitochondrial DNA instability and optic atrophy 'plus' phenotypes. *Brain* 131(Pt 2), 338–351. doi: 10.1093/brain/awm298

Bette, S., Zimmermann, U., Wissinger, B., and Knipper, M. (2007). OPA1, the disease gene for optic atrophy type Kjer, is expressed in the inner ear. *Histochem. Cell Biol.* 128, 421–430. doi: 10.1007/s00418-007-0321-7

Chan, D. C. (2020). Mitochondrial dynamics and its involvement in disease. *Annu. Rev. Pathol.* 15, 235–259. doi: 10.1146/annurev-pathmechdis-012419-032711

Chen, H., Detmer, S. A., Ewald, A. J., Griffin, E. E., Fraser, S. E., and Chan, D. C. (2003). Mitofusins Mfn1 and Mfn2 coordinately regulate mitochondrial fusion and are essential for embryonic development. *J. Cell Biol.* 160, 189–200. doi: 10.1083/jcb.200211046

Chen, H., Vermulst, M., Wang, Y. E., Chomyn, A., Prolla, T. A., McCaffery, J. M., et al. (2010). Mitochondrial fusion is required for mtDNA stability in skeletal muscle and tolerance of mtDNA mutations. *Cell* 141, 280–289. doi: 10.1016/j.cell.2010.02.026

Chen, L., Liu, T., Tran, A., Lu, X., Tomilov, A. A., Davies, V., et al. (2012). OPA1 mutation and late-onset cardiomyopathy: mitochondrial dysfunction and mtDNA instability. *J. Am. Heart Assoc.* 1:e003012. doi: 10.1161/JAHA.112.003012

Cheng, C., Hou, Y., Zhang, Z., Wang, Y., Lu, L., Zhang, L., et al. (2021). Disruption of the autism-related gene Pak1 causes stereocilia disorganization, hair cell loss, and deafness in mice. *J. Genet. Genomics.* doi: 10.1016/j.jgg.2021.03.010

Choi, Y. M., Kim, H. K., Shim, W., Anwar, M. A., Kwon, J. W., Kwon, H. K., et al. (2015). Mechanism of Cisplatin-Induced cytotoxicity is correlated to impaired metabolism due to mitochondrial ROS generation. *PLoS One* 10:e0135083. doi: 10.1371/journal.pone.0135083

Chu, D.-T., Tao, Y., and Taskén, K. (2017). OPA1 in lipid metabolism: function of OPA1 in Lipolysis and Thermogenesis of Adipocytes. *Hormone Metab. Res.* 49, 276–285. doi: 10.1055/s-0043-100384

Chun, B. Y., and Rizzo, J. F. III (2017). Dominant Optic Atrophy and Leber's hereditary optic neuropathy: update on clinical features and current therapeutic approaches. *Semin. Pediatr. Neurol.* 24, 129–134. doi: 10.1016/j.spen.2017.06.001

Cipolat, S., Martins, de Brito, O., Dal Zilio, B., and Scorrano, L. (2004). OPA1 requires mitofusin 1 to promote mitochondrial fusion. *Proc. Natl. Acad. Sci. U.S.A.* 101, 15927–15932. doi: 10.1073/pnas.0407043101

Civiletto, G., Varanita, T., Cerutti, R., Gorletta, T., Barbaro, S., Marchet, S., et al. (2015). Opa1 overexpression ameliorates the phenotype of two mitochondrial disease mouse models. *Cell Metab.* 21, 845–854. doi: 10.1016/j.cmet.2015.04.016

de Sa Junior, P. L., Camara, D. A. D., Porcacchia, A. S., Fonseca, P. M. M., Jorge, S. D., Araldi, R. P., et al. (2017). The roles of ROS in cancer heterogeneity and therapy. *Oxid. Med. Cell. Longev.* 2017:2467940. doi: 10.1155/2017/2467940

Del Dotto, V., Fogazza, M., Lenaers, G., Rugolo, M., Carelli, V., and Zanna, C. (2018). OPA1: How much do we know to approach therapy? *Pharmacol. Res.* 131, 199–210. doi: 10.1016/j.phrs.2018.02.018

Del Dotto, V., Mishra, P., Vidoni, S., Fogazza, M., Maresca, A., Caporali, L., et al. (2017). OPA1 isoforms in the hierarchical organization of mitochondrial functions. *Cell Rep.* 19, 2557–2571. doi: 10.1016/j.celrep.2017.05.073

Delettre, C., Griffoin, J. M., Kaplan, J., Dollfus, H., Lorenz, B., Faivre, L., et al. (2001). Mutation spectrum and splicing variants in the OPA1 gene. *Hum. Genet.* 109, 584–591. doi: 10.1007/s00439-001-0633-y

Delettre, C., Lenaers, G., Griffoin, J. M., Gigarel, N., Lorenzo, C., Belenguer, P., et al. (2000). Nuclear gene OPA1, encoding a mitochondrial dynamin-related protein, is mutated in dominant optic atrophy. *Nat. Genet.* 26, 207–210. doi: 10.1038/79936

Ding, Y., Meng, W., Kong, W., He, Z., and Chai, R. (2020). The Role of FoxG1 in the Inner Ear. *Front. Cell Dev. Biol.* 8:614954. doi: 10.3389/fcell.2020.614954

Frezza, C., Cipolat, S., Martins, de Brito, O., Micaroni, M., Beznoussenko, G. V., et al. (2006). OPA1 controls apoptotic cristae remodeling independently from mitochondrial fusion. *Cell* 126, 177–189. doi: 10.1016/j.cell.2006.06.025

Fu, X., An, Y., Wang, H., Li, P., Lin, J., Yuan, J., et al. (2021a). Deficiency of Klc2 induces low-frequency sensorineural hearing loss in C57BL/6 J mice and human. *Mol. Neurobiol.* doi: 10.1007/s12035-021-02422-w

Fu, X., Wan, P., Li, P., Wang, J., Guo, S., Zhang, Y., et al. (2021b). Mechanism and prevention of ototoxicity induced by aminoglycosides. *Front. Cell. Neurosci.* 15:692762. doi: 10.3389/fncel.2021.692762

Gao, S., Cheng, C., Wang, M., Jiang, P., Zhang, L., Wang, Y., et al. (2019). Blebbistatin inhibits neomycin-induced apoptosis in hair cell-like HEI-OC-1 cells and in cochlear hair cells. *Front. Cell. Neurosci.* 13:590. doi: 10.3389/fncel.2019.00590

Gentilin, E., Simoni, E., Candito, M., Cazzador, D., and Astolfi, L. (2019). Cisplatin-induced ototoxicity: updates on molecular targets. *Trends Mol. Med.* 25, 1123–1132. doi: 10.1016/j.molmed.2019.08.002

He, Z., Fang, Q., Li, H., Shao, B., Zhang, Y., Zhang, Y., et al. (2019). The role of FOXG1 in the postnatal development and survival of mouse cochlear hair cells. *Neuropharmacology* 144, 43–57. doi: 10.1016/j.neuropharm.2018.10.021

He, Z., Guo, L., Shu, Y., Fang, Q., Zhou, H., Liu, Y., et al. (2017). Autophagy protects auditory hair cells against neomycin-induced damage. *Autophagy* 13, 1884–1904. doi: 10.1080/15548627.2017.1359449

He, Z.-H., Li, M., Fang, Q.-J., Liao, F.-L., Zou, S.-Y., Wu, X., et al. (2021). FOXG1 promotes aging inner ear hair cell survival through activation of the autophagy pathway. *Autophagy*. doi: 10.1080/15548627.2021.191 6194

He, Z.-H., Zou, S.-Y., Li, M., Liao, F.-L., Wu, X., Sun, H.-Y., et al. (2020). The nuclear transcription factor FoxG1 affects the sensitivity of mimetic aging hair cells to inflammation by regulating autophagy pathways. *Redox Biol.* 28:101364. doi: 10.1016/j.redox.2019.101364

Hoppins, S., Lackner, L., and Nunnari, J. (2007). The machines that divide and fuse mitochondria. *Annu. Rev. Biochem.* 76, 751–780. doi: 10.1146/annurev.biochem.76.071905.090048

Hudson, G., Amati-Bonneau, P., Blakely, E. L., Stewart, J. D., He, L., Schaefer, A. M., et al. (2008). Mutation of OPA1 causes dominant optic atrophy with external ophthalmoplegia, ataxia, deafness and multiple mitochondrial DNA deletions: a novel disorder of mtDNA maintenance. *Brain* 131(Pt 2), 329–337. doi: 10.1093/brain/awm272

Hutchin, T. P., and Cortopassi, G. A. (2000). Mitochondrial defects and hearing loss. *Cell. Mol. Life Sci.* 57, 1927–1937. doi: 10.1007/PL00000673

Ishihara, N., Fujita, Y., Oka, T., and Mihara, K. (2006). Regulation of mitochondrial morphology through proteolytic cleavage of OPA1. *EMBO J.* 25, 2966–2977. doi: 10.1038/sj.emboj.7601184

Itoh, K., Nakamura, K., Iijima, M., and Sesaki, H. (2013). Mitochondrial dynamics in neurodegeneration. *Trends Cell Biol.* 23, 64–71. doi: 10.1016/j.tcb.2012.10.006

Kjer, P. (1959). Infantile optic atrophy with dominant mode of inheritance: a clinical and genetic study of 19 Danish families. *Acta Ophthalmol. Suppl.* 164(Suppl. 54), 1–147.

Leruez, S., Milea, D., Defoort-Dhellemmes, S., Colin, E., Crochet, M., Procaccio, V., et al. (2013). Sensorineural hearing loss in OPA1-linked disorders. *Brain* 136(Pt 7):e236. doi: 10.1093/brain/aws340

Li, A., You, D., Li, W., Cui, Y., He, Y., Li, W., et al. (2018). Novel compounds protect auditory hair cells against gentamycin-induced apoptosis by maintaining the expression level of H3K4me2. *Drug Deliv.* 25, 1033–1043. doi: 10.1080/10717544.2018.1461277

Li, H., Song, Y., He, Z., Chen, X., Wu, X., Li, X., et al. (2018). Meclofenamic acid reduces reactive oxygen species accumulation and apoptosis, inhibits excessive autophagy, and protects hair cell-Like HEI-OC1 cells from cisplatin-induced damage. *Front. Cell. Neurosci.* 12:139. doi: 10.3389/fncel.2018.00139

Li, Y., Li, A., Wu, J., He, Y., Yu, H., Chai, R., et al. (2016). MiR-182-5p protects inner ear hair cells from cisplatin-induced apoptosis by inhibiting FOXO3a. *Cell Death Dis.* 7:e2362. doi: 10.1038/cddis.2016.246

Liu, L., Chen, Y., Qi, J., Zhang, Y., He, Y., Ni, W., et al. (2016). Wnt activation protects against neomycin-induced hair cell damage in the mouse cochlea. *Cell Death Dis.* 7:e2136. doi: 10.1038/cddis.2016.35

Liu, W., Xu, L., Wang, X., Zhang, D., Sun, G., Wang, M., et al. (2021). PRDX1 activates autophagy via the PTEN-AKT signaling pathway to protect against cisplatin-induced spiral ganglion neuron damage. *Autophagy*. doi: 10.1080/15548627.2021.1905466

Liu, W., Xu, X., Fan, Z., Sun, G., Han, Y., Zhang, D., et al. (2019). Wnt Signaling Activates TP53-induced glycolysis and apoptosis regulator and protects against cisplatin-induced spiral ganglion neuron damage in the mouse cochlea. *Antioxid. Redox Signal.* 30, 1389–1410. doi: 10.1089/ars.2017.7288

Liu, Y., Qi, J., Chen, X., Tang, M., Chu, C., Zhu, W., et al. (2019). Critical role of spectrin in hearing development and deafness. *Sci. Adv.* 5:eaav7803. doi: 10.1126/sciadv.aav7803

Loson, O. C., Song, Z., Chen, H., and Chan, D. C. (2013). Fis1, Mff, MiD49, and MiD51 mediate Drp1 recruitment in mitochondrial fission. *Mol. Biol. Cell* 24, 659–667. doi: 10.1091/mbc.E12-10-0721

Lv, J., Fu, X., Li, Y., Hong, G., Li, P., Lin, J., et al. (2021). Deletion of in mice does not alter auditory function. *Front. Cell Dev. Biol.* 9:630361. doi: 10.3389/fcell.2021.630361

Meire, F., De Laey, J. J., de Bie, S., van Staey, M., and Matton, M. T. (1985). Dominant optic nerve atrophy with progressive hearing loss and chronic progressive external ophthalmoplegia (CPEO). *Ophthalmic Paediatr. Genet.* 5, 91–97. doi: 10.3109/13816818509007861

Mishra, P., and Chan, D. C. (2014). Mitochondrial dynamics and inheritance during cell division, development and disease. *Nat. Rev. Mol. Cell Biol.* 15, 634–646. doi: 10.1038/nrm3877

Mukhopadhyay, P., Horvath, B., Zsengeller, Z., Zielonka, J., Tanchian, G., Holovac, E., et al. (2012). Mitochondrial-targeted antioxidants represent a promising approach for prevention of cisplatin-induced nephropathy. *Free Radic. Biol. Med.* 52, 497–506. doi: 10.1016/j.freeradbiomed.2011.11.001

Olichon, A., Emorine, L. J., Descoins, E., Pelloquin, L., Brichese, L., Gas, N., et al. (2002). The human dynamin-related protein OPA1 is anchored to the mitochondrial inner membrane facing the inter-membrane space. *FEBS Lett.* 523, 171–176. doi: 10.1016/s0014-5793(02)02985-x

Pabla, N., and Dong, Z. (2008). Cisplatin nephrotoxicity: mechanisms and renoprotective strategies. *Kidney Int.* 73, 994–1007. doi: 10.1038/sj.ki.5002786

Palmer, C. S., Elgass, K. D., Parton, R. G., Osellame, L. D., Stojanovski, D., and Ryan, M. T. (2013). Adaptor proteins MiD49 and MiD51 can act independently of Mff and Fis1 in Drp1 recruitment and are specific for mitochondrial fission. *J. Biol. Chem.* 288, 27584–27593. doi: 10.1074/jbc.M113.479873

Patten, D. A., Wong, J., Khacho, M., Soubannier, V., Mailloux, R. J., Pilon-Larose, K., et al. (2014). OPA1-dependent cristae modulation is essential for cellular adaptation to metabolic demand. *EMBO J.* 33, 2676–2691. doi: 10.15252/embj.201488349

Pidoux, G., Witczak, O., Jarnaess, E., Myrvold, L., Urlaub, H., Stokka, A. J., et al. (2011). Optic atrophy 1 is an A-kinase anchoring protein on lipid droplets that mediates adrenergic control of lipolysis. *EMBO J.* 30, 4371–4386. doi: 10.1038/emboj.2011.365

Qi, J., Liu, Y., Chu, C., Chen, X., Zhu, W., Shu, Y., et al. (2019). A cytoskeleton structure revealed by super-resolution fluorescence imaging in inner ear hair cells. *Cell Discov.* 5:12. doi: 10.1038/s41421-018-0076-4

Qiao, P., Zhao, F., Liu, M., Gao, D., Zhang, H., and Yan, Y. (2017). Hydrogen sulfide inhibits mitochondrial fission in neuroblastoma N2a cells through the Drp1/ERK1/2 signaling pathway. *Mol. Med. Rep.* 16, 971–977. doi: 10.3892/mmr.2017.6627

Rogers, C., Fernandes-Alnemri, T., Mayes, L., Alnemri, D., Cingolani, G., and Alnemri, E. S. (2017). Cleavage of DFNA5 by caspase-3 during apoptosis mediates progression to secondary necrotic/pyroptotic cell death. *Nat. Commun.* 8:14128. doi: 10.1038/ncomms14128

Rybak, L. P., Mukherjea, D., Jajoo, S., and Ramkumar, V. (2009). Cisplatin ototoxicity and protection: clinical and experimental studies. *Tohoku J. Exp. Med.* 219, 177–186. doi: 10.1620/tjem.219.177

Santel, A., and Fuller, M. T. (2001). Control of mitochondrial morphology by a human mitofusin. *J. Cell Sci.* 114(Pt 5), 867–874.

Schacht, J., Talaska, A. E., and Rybak, L. P. (2012). Cisplatin and aminoglycoside antibiotics: hearing loss and its prevention. *Anat. Rec.* 295, 1837–1850. doi: 10.1002/ar.22578

Siddik, Z. H. (2003). Cisplatin: mode of cytotoxic action and molecular basis of resistance. *Oncogene* 22, 7265–7279. doi: 10.1038/sj.onc.1206933

Suen, D. F., Norris, K. L., and Youle, R. J. (2008). Mitochondrial dynamics and apoptosis. *Genes Dev.* 22, 1577–1590. doi: 10.1101/gad.1658508

Tezze, C., Romanello, V., Desbats, M. A., Fadini, G. P., Albiero, M., Favaro, G., et al. (2017). Age-Associated Loss of OPA1 in muscle impacts muscle mass, metabolic homeostasis, systemic inflammation, and epithelial senescence. *Cell Metab.* 25, 1374–1389.e6. doi: 10.1016/j.cmet.2017.04.021

Treft, R. L., Sanborn, G. E., Carey, J., Swartz, M., Crisp, D., Wester, D. C., et al. (1984). Dominant optic atrophy, deafness, ptosis, ophthalmoplegia, dystaxia, and myopathy. A new syndrome. *Ophthalmology* 91, 908–915. doi: 10.1016/s0161-6420(84)34214-2

van Gisbergen, M. W., Voets, A. M., Starmans, M. H., de Coo, I. F., Yadak, R., Hoffmann, R. F., et al. (2015). How do changes in the mtDNA and mitochondrial dysfunction influence cancer and cancer therapy? Challenges, opportunities and models. *Mutat. Res. Rev. Mutat. Res.* 764, 16–30. doi: 10.1016/j.mrrev.2015.01.001

Varanita, T., Soriano, M. E., Romanello, V., Zaglia, T., Quintana-Cabrera, R., Semenzato, M., et al. (2015). The OPA1-dependent mitochondrial cristae remodeling pathway controls atrophic, apoptotic, and ischemic tissue damage. *Cell Metab.* 21, 834–844. doi: 10.1016/j.cmet.2015.05.007

Wai, T., García-Prieto, J., Baker, M. J., Merkwirth, C., Benit, P., Rustin, P., et al. (2015). Imbalanced OPA1 processing and mitochondrial fragmentation cause heart failure in mice. *Science* 350:aad0116. doi: 10.1126/science.aad0116

Wang, D., and Lippard, S. J. (2005). Cellular processing of platinum anticancer drugs. *Nat. Rev. Drug Discov.* 4, 307–320. doi: 10.1038/nrd1691

Williams, P. A., Morgan, J. E., and Votruba, M. (2010). Opa1 deficiency in a mouse model of dominant optic atrophy leads to retinal ganglion cell dendropathy. *Brain* 133, 2942–2951. doi: 10.1093/brain/awq218

Yarosh, W., Monserrate, J., Tong, J. J., Tse, S., Le, P. K., Nguyen, K., et al. (2008). The molecular mechanisms of OPA1-mediated optic atrophy in *Drosophila* model and prospects for antioxidant treatment. *PLoS Genet.* 4:e6. doi: 10.1371/journal.pgen.0040006

Zhang, S., Zhang, Y., Dong, Y., Guo, L., Zhang, Z., Shao, B., et al. (2020). Knockdown of Foxg1 in supporting cells increases the trans-differentiation of supporting cells into hair cells in the neonatal mouse cochlea. *Cell. Mol. Life Sci.* 77, 1401–1419. doi: 10.1007/s00018-019-03291-2

Zhang, Y., Li, W., He, Z., Wang, Y., Shao, B., Cheng, C., et al. (2019). Pre-treatment With Fasudil prevents neomycin-induced hair cell damage by reducing the accumulation of reactive oxygen Species. *Front. Mol. Neurosci.* 12:264. doi: 10.3389/fnmol.2019.00264

Zhong, Z., Fu, X., Li, H., Chen, J., Wang, M., Gao, S., et al. (2020). Citicoline protects auditory hair cells against neomycin-induced damage. *Front. Cell Dev. Biol.* 8:712. doi: 10.3389/fcell.2020.00712

Zhou, H., Qian, X., Xu, N., Zhang, S., Zhu, G., Zhang, Y., et al. (2020). Disruption of Atg7-dependent autophagy causes electromotility disturbances, outer hair cell loss, and deafness in mice. *Cell Death Dis.* 11:913. doi: 10.1038/s41419-020-03110-8

2

Long-Term Release of Dexamethasone With a Polycaprolactone-Coated Electrode Alleviates Fibrosis in Cochlear Implantation

Dongxiu Chen[1,2], Yanjing Luo[1,2], Jing Pan[1,2], Anning Chen[1,2], Dong Ma[3], Muqing Xu[1,2], Jie Tang[2,4,5] and Hongzheng Zhang[1,2]**

[1] Department of Otolaryngology Head and Neck Surgery, Zhujiang Hospital, Southern Medical University, Guangzhou, China, [2] Hearing Research Center, Southern Medical University, Guangzhou, China, [3] Key Laboratory of Biomaterials of Guangdong Higher Education Institutes, Department of Biomedical Engineering, Jinan University, Guangzhou, China, [4] Department of Physiology, School of Basic Medical Sciences, Southern Medical University, Guangzhou, China, [5] Key Laboratory of Mental Health of the Ministry of Education, Southern Medical University, Guangzhou, China

***Correspondence:**
Jie Tang
jietang@smu.edu.cn
Hongzheng Zhang
redtrue@smu.edu.cn

Cochlear implantation (CI) is the major treatment for severe sensorineural hearing loss. However, the fibrotic tissue forming around the electrodes reduces the treatment effectiveness of CI. Dexamethasone (DEX) is usually applied routinely in perioperative treatment of cochlear implantation (CI), but its diffusion in the inner ear after systemic administration is limited. In the present study, an electrode coated with polycaprolactone (PCL) loaded with dexamethasone was developed with a simple preparation process to maintain the stability of the electrode itself. The DEX-loaded PCL coating has good biocompatibility and does not change the smoothness, flexibility, or compliance of the implant electrode. Stable and effective DEX concentrations were maintained for more than 9 months. Compared with the pristine electrode, decreasing intracochlear fibrosis, protection of hair cells and spiral ganglion cells, and better residual hearing were observed 5 weeks after PCL-DEX electrode implantation. The PCL-DEX electrode has great potential in preventing hearing loss and fibrosis by regulating macrophages and inhibiting the expression of the fibrosis-related factors IL-1β, TNF-α, IL-4, and TGF-β1. In conclusion, the PCL-DEX electrode coating shows promising application in CI surgery.

Keywords: cochlear implantation, fibrosis, PCL, inflammation, TGF-β1

INTRODUCTION

Cochlear implantation (CI) is the main treatment for severe sensorineural hearing loss (Li et al., 2017). This procedure requires the insertion of electrodes into the cochlea, by which electrical signals containing external sound information are delivered to cochlear neurons, enabling hearing restoration in patients with sensorineural deafness. Over 5% of the world's population—or 466 million people have disabling hearing loss (432 million adults and 34 million children). The long-term efficacy of CI is critical for patients.

However, there are still many problems in CI that need to be improved. Among them, fibrotic tissue forming around the electrodes normally decreases the curative effect of CI. Autopsy pathology studies on human temporal bone specimens of CI recipients found that fibrotic tissue existed in most cochleae (Seyyedi and Nadol, 2014; O'Malley et al., 2017) and fibrous sheaths were usually formed around the electrode in the implanted cochleae (Ishai et al., 2017). A dense fibrotic sheath increases the impedance of the electrode array, resulting in unstable electrical signals and increasing power consumption (Clark et al., 1995; Sanderson et al., 2019). A tracking of 85 cases showed that various degrees of hearing loss occurred in 38% of patients 5 years after CI surgery (Rowe et al., 2016; Foggia et al., 2019). The progressive loss of CI restored hearing was not significantly related to electrode type or the insertion method (*via* round window or cochlear fenestration) but was related to the changes in electrical impedance, which was probably induced by fibrosis around the electrode array (Clark et al., 1995).

Moreover, severe fibrosis in the cochlea causes trauma to the fine structure in the cochlea and blocks the sound vibration conducting to the cochlear basilar membrane (Choi and Oghalai, 2005). Fibrosis in the cochlea is one of the main reasons for the loss of residual hearing after CI, affecting the availability of an acoustic-electricity combined stimulation model in the rehabilitation of CI. In addition, fibrosis in the cochlea makes it difficult and risky to reimplant the electrode in the cochlea (Côté et al., 2007). In many second implantation operation cases, fibrosis in the scala tympani impedes the insertion of electrode arrays and even causes surgical failure. Therefore, a strategy reducing the formation of fibrosis is urgently needed to improve the long-term effect of CI (Eshraghi et al., 2020).

Clinically, glucocorticoids, such as DEX, are applied systemically or locally to reduce the inflammation and foreign body response of CI. However, due to the lack of stable and efficient delivery of drugs in the cochlea or significant side effects of long-term systemic treatment, the current clinical treatment effects vary and are not obvious, limiting the usage of glucocorticoid treatment (Cortés Fuentes et al., 2020).

In many previous studies, multiple bioactive materials and coatings have been applied to preserve the neural function and reduce the inflammation and fibrosis (Liu et al., 2018; Shang et al., 2018; Guo J. H. et al., 2020; Guo et al., 2021; Han et al., 2020; Xia et al., 2020; Zhao et al., 2020; Yang et al., 2021). In the present study, we proposed a drug-loaded electrodes for CI. We employed polycaprolactone (PCL), a polymer that has been approved for clinical use, for long-term release of loaded DEX by coating on CI electrodes (Gaharwar et al., 2014; Zhou et al., 2018). Our data showed that the PCL-DEX coating significantly attenuated inflammation and the formation of fibrosis after CI in rats, preventing the progressive loss of residual hearing induced by fibrosis in the cochlea. Our study suggests that polycaprolactone is a promising material for the long-term release of loaded drugs into the cochlea by coating implants in CI.

MATERIALS AND METHODS

Electrode Coating

Silicone dummies (MEDEL, Innsbruck, Austria) 10 mm in length were used for preparing coating electrodes for cochlear implantation, with marker at 3 and 6 mm, measuring 0.2 mm in diameter at the tip and 0.3 mm at a position 6 mm from the tip. The polycaprolactone (PCL) pellets (AiKe, China) and dexamethasone powder (DEX, purity $\geq$ 98%) (Meryer, Shanghai, China) were mixed in different ratios (95:5, 90:10, and 80:20). The mixture was then dissolved in dichloromethane [10% (w/w)] (Aladdin, China) at RT (room temperature, 27°C). Then the PCL-DEX copolymer was coated on the tip of silicone dummy by dipping the dummy ($\sim$10 mm) into the mixture for 10 s for one time (Luo et al., 2021). The coated electrodes were dried at RT for 24-h for further characterization. The coating thickness was measured by an optic microscope. The loading capacity was determined as following:

$$\textbf{The drug loading capacity} = \frac{\textbf{weight of DEX in the coating}}{\textbf{weight of PCL and DEX in the coating}}\ \textbf{100\%}$$

Scanning Electron Microscopy

The coated electrodes were sputter-coated with thin layers of gold, and the surface morphologies of the coated electrodes were examined by SEM (Ultra55, Zeiss, Germany).

Tensile Testing

To determine effects of PCL coating on the flexibility of the coated electrodes, tensile testing was performed by an electronic universal testing machine (BL-GRW005 K, Zwick/Roell, Germany). The electrode/dummy length was set as 70 mm, and the crosshead speed was 1 mm/min. The displacement-pressure curves were recorded and mean values were calculated.

Dexamethasone Release Measurement

Silicone dummy (35 mm long with an 8 mm diameter) coated with PCL-DEX copolymer was soaked in 3.8 mL artificial perilymph (1.3 $CaCl_2$, 1.8 $MgCl_2$, 5.4 KCl, 137 NaCl, 5 glucose, 5 HEPES, in mmol/L) at 37°C, allowing the DEX released from the copolymer. Aliquots (540 μL) of artificial perilymph were taken out to measure the DEX concentration from 1 h to 270 days. After each measurement, the same volume of fresh artificial perilymph was replenished. DEX mass and concentration in artificial perilymph were determined using a high- performance fluid chromatography (HPLC) (Agilent 1260, United States) at 275 nm.

Cell Culture and Viability Assays

L929-T-25mice fibroblasts cells and House Ear Institute-Organ of Corti 1 (HEI-OC1) cells were used to examine the biocompatibility of the PCL-DEX copolymer. The 35 mm petri dishes were pre-coated with PCL. Cells were cultured in 35 mm Petri dishes with/without PCL-DEX coating in a CO_2 incubator. L929 cells were cultured in RPMI-1640 complemented with 10% FBS (Gibco, United States), 5% CO_2 at 37°C. HEI-OC1 cells were cultured in DMEM medium (Gibco, United States) complemented with 10% FBS, 10% CO_2 at 33°C. After 48 h, the cell densities were calculated under an optic microscope.

For cell viability assays, L929 cells or OC1 cells were seeded into 96-well plate at 5×10^3 cells per well for 24 h. For preparation of leached solution, 0.1 wt% DEX and 1 cm long electrodes coated with PCL, PCL- 5%DEX, PCL- 20%DEX were, respectively, immersed in culture media for 24 h. The leached solution were collected and sterile filtered using a filter of 0.22 μm pore. The culture medium was replaced with leached solution or normal fresh culture medium. 24 h later, a CCK-8 kit (Beyotime, Shanghai, China) was used to examine the cell viability by following the standard protocol.

Animal Surgery

CIs were performed monaurallyin normal hearing SD rats aged 5–7 weeks. Rats were anesthetized with an intraperitoneal injection of pentobarbital sodium (45 mg/kg). Additional doses were given as needed. A retroauricular incision was made, and the nearby muscles and skin were separated to expose the bulla. The bulla was opened under a microscope using a delicate drill. The round-window membrane was then incised with a bent forceps. The electrode was gently inserted through the incision into the scala tympani, to a depth of 3 mm. In DEX group, 0.1 mL of DEX (5 mg/mL) was injected into the cochlea in the scala tympani after insertion of pristine electrodes. In sham group, no electrode was implanted and all other surgical operations remained consistent with the implanted groups. The round window was patched with a small piece of muscle in case of sustained leaking of perilymph. Mobility and integrity of the ear drum and ossicular chain was monitored by microscopic examination during all stages of the surgery. After the surgery, wounds were carefully sutured and animals were sent back to their home cages.

Auditory Brainstem Response

Auditory brainstem response was examined to evaluate hearing function as described in our previous study (Hang et al., 2016). In brief, anesthetized rat (pentobarbital sodium, 45 mg/kg, i. p.) was placed on a vibration isolation table in an electromagnetically and acoustically shielded room. Three subcutaneous needle electrodes were placed on the vertex (recording) of skull, the loose skin behind the tested ears (reference) and the opposite ears (ground). 5 ms tone bursts with different frequency (2, 4, 8, 16, 24, and 32 kHz) and intensity were generated by the software SigGenRP and delivered by a speaker placed 15 cm away from the ear at a rate if 10/s. The ABR waveforms were amplified, recorded, averaged, and stored by a software BioSigRZ (Tucker-Davis Technology, Alachua, FL, United States). During recording, the contralateral ear (non-operated) was plugged with a silicon putty earplug (Mack's, United States). The amplified evoked responses with 256 sweeps were averaged in real time. The ABR thresholds were defined as the highest sound level at which no response was detectable. After recovery from the anesthesia, animal was sent back to its home cage.

Histology and Immunostaining

After the last ABR recording, the animal was scarified and the cochlea was dissected. The cochlea was fixed by 4% paraformaldehyde at 4°C overnight and decalcified for 10 days. The organs of Corti (OC) were isolated and cut evenly into three pieces for immunostaining. To quantify the fibrosis size, the cochlea was sectioned serially in the axial plane at a thickness of 20 μm. Usually, 50–100 slides containing fibrosis were collected and photoed under a Nikon optical microscope. The outline of the fibrous tissue and the scala tympani were tracked by the software Image-Pro Plus. The whole volume of fibrous tissue and scala tympani were calculated by these slides, and the percentage of fibrous tissue in scala tympani was determined. Sections from the modiolar plane were stained with an H&E kit (Beyotime, Shanghai, China) using standard protocols.

Representative sections and OCs were used for immunofluorescence staining. Samples were permeabilized by 0.3% Triton X-100 in PBS (Sigma, United States) and blocked with 10% normal goat serum (Sigma, United States) for 1 h at RT. Sections or tissues were incubated with primary antibodies α-SMA (1:1,000, Sigma, United States), type I collagen (1:1,000, Sigma, United States), Map2 (1:1,000, Protein Tech, Chicago, IL, United States), Myosin 7a (1:1,000, Protein Tech, Chicago, IL, United States), and CD68 (1:1,000, Sigma, United States). After the primary antibodies were completely washed out with PBS, samples were incubated with Alexa Fluor 568-conjugated or Alexa Fluor 488-conjugated secondary antibody (BBI Life Science, China) for 2 h at RT. The fluorescence images were acquired using a confocal laser scanning microscopy (Nikon, Japan) at 20× magnification.

Western Blotting and ELISA Measurement

The protein extracted from the whole cochlea was used for western blotting. 30 μg protein sample was separated by SDS–PAGE gels and transferred to polyvinylidene fluoride (PVDF) membrane (Millipore, Bedford, MA, United States). After blocking with 5 % non-fat milk in TBS-T (Beyotime, Shanghai, China) for 2 h at RT, the membrane was incubated with the primary antibodies α-SMA (Sigma, United States), type I collagen (Sigma, United States), TGF-β1 (Abcam, England), or TNF-α (Abcam, England) overnight at 4°C. The PVDF membrane was washed and incubated with secondary antibodies conjugated to the HRP (BBI Life Sciences, Shanghai, China) for 2 h. Protein bands were detected with a chemiluminescence detection system (Image 600, GE Healthcare, Chicago, IL, United States). Protein grayscale was analyzed with software Image Quant TL (GE Healthcare, Chicago, IL, United States).

The levels of IL-1β and IL-4 released in cochleae after electrode implantation were measured using an ELISA kits (Abcam, United States). The perilymph and tissue lysate were collected from the cochlea. For each group, data was calculated as percentage compared to the level in the control groups.

Data Analysis

The data analysis was performed using SPSS 22.0 (IBM, United States). The quantitative analyses were independently performed by two of the authors in a blind manner to ensure the consistency across all data. Student's *t*-test was performed for the comparison of two groups and comparisons among multiple groups were analyzed by analysis of variance (ANOVA) followed by multiple comparison tests for *post hoc* analysis. Significance was defined as $p < 0.05$. GraphPad Prism 7 (GraphPad Software, SanDiego, CA, United States) was used for was used for statistical analyses and graphical display.

RESULTS

To evaluate the postimplantation effects on the hearing of the implanted ear, silicone dummies were implanted into the rat cochlea, and the ABRs were measured from the implanted ear before and after implantation. As shown in **Figure 1A**, compared with the ABRs before implantation (pre., gray dashed line and open circles), no significant ABR threshold shift was observed at any sound frequency in the sham group (sham, black line and open circles) 1 week after the operation ($p > 0.05$, ANOVA). The ABR thresholds remained unchanged in the sham group from week one to week eight ($p > 0.05$, ANOVA). For the silicone electrode implantation group (implant, black lines and filled circles), the ABR thresholds at all sound frequencies were significantly elevated from the first week after implantation (vs. sham group, $p < 0.001$, ANOVA), indicating the impairment in hearing of pristine electrode insertion. However, the time course of ABR threshold changes was diverse for different sound frequencies. For tones of 2 and 4 kHz, the ABR thresholds increased progressively with implantation time and reached the maximal threshold shift at week 3 after implantation (**Figure 1B**). The ABRs for 2 and 4 kHz tones were responded to by the apical portion of the cochlea; therefore, these threshold shifts indicate progressive functional impairment of the apical cochlea by implantation. However, the cochlear implant resulted in severe hearing loss for 16 and 32 kHz tones with a mean ABR threshold shift > 35 dB from the first week after implantation (**Figure 1B**), implying a possible impairment at the high-frequency end of the cochlea by implant. In the following experiments, the ABR threshold at 2 kHz was chosen to evaluate the chronic effects of electrode implantation.

The cochlear implant causes a foreign body response with associated fibrosis. As shown by a representative cochlear cross section in **Figure 1C** significant fibrous tissue was found around the electrode 5 weeks after implantation. By measuring the volume of fibrous tissue and scala tympani of each implantation, we calculated the percentage of scala tympani occupied by the fibrosis to evaluate the extent of fibrosis. Pooled data showed that fibrosis varied greatly in different individuals, and only a weak correlation was found between the size of fibrosis and the implantation time ($r = 0.441$, $p = 0.0352$, **Figure 1D**). Moreover, no correlation was observed between the ABR threshold shifts (at 2 kHz) and the implantation time ($r = 0.398$, $p = 0.0599$, **Figure 1E**). These results suggest that the implantation time may not be the key factor causing fibrosis and hearing loss. Further analysis showed that this ABR threshold shift increased with the size of fibrosis ($r = 0.339$, $p < 0.0001$, **Figure 1F**), and their strong relationship indicates that fibrosis is the major pathogenetic factor in the hearing loss observed after cochlear implantation.

The tissue responses to silicone dummies were assessed by immunostaining of α-SMA, type I collagen, and TGF-β1 in proliferative tissue. α-SMA and type I collagen are markers of myofibroblasts and major components of the extracellular matrix in fibrotic tissue, respectively. As shown in the representative images, robustα-SMA immunoreactivity was observed in the proliferative tissue surrounding the implant, and strong type I collagen expression was distributed throughout the proliferative tissue (**Figure 2A**). Moreover, immunoreactivity of TGF-β1, which regulates the proliferation and differentiation of myofibroblasts and promotes the secretion of extracellular matrix, was also found in proliferative tissue surrounding the implant and in generation of fibrosis (**Figure 2B**). These results confirmed that proliferative tissue is the typical fibrous tissue in our experiments.

Currently, the therapeutic method to treat fibrosis after cochlear implantation in clinical practice is administration of dexamethasone. However, side effects of systemic administration limit long-term application. The synthesized PCL-DEX was designed to achieve sustained drug release and maintain protective DEX concentrations as the coating of the electrode implanted into the cochlea along with the electrode (**Figure 3A**). The thickness of the coating was also determined to be 48.66 ± 0.35 μm by optical microscopy (**Figure 3B**).

In the present study, 5, 10, and 20% DEX were used to prepare the PCL-DEX electrodes. The microstructure of the PCL (MW = 36 k) coating surface was examined by SEM. As shown by the SEM images in **Figure 3C**, a smooth appearance was observed in PCL coating surfaces with and without DEX loaded. High magnification images revealed the fine texture of the surfaces, and pore-like apertures were observed. DEX was contained in these apertures and released when PCL was degraded slowly in the cochlea. Abundant apertures with homogenic and small sizes are instrumental in the steady and sustained release of DEX.

Good mechanical flexibility is required when PCL-coated electrodes are inserted into the cochlear coil. Tensile displacement was applied to determine the flexibility of PCL-coated electrodes with two different PCL molecular weights (MW = 36 and 60 k). At the maximal bending displacement, no cracking in the PCL coating was observed for any electrode tested. The flexibility of all PCL-DEX electrodes was acceptable for cochlear implantation compared to pristine electrodes (**Figure 3D**). These images suggest that the PCL-DEX electrode prepared with 20% DEX may achieve sufficient and steady DEX release. These results indicate that the physical features of PCL-DEX-coated electrodes meet the requirement of cochlear implantation.

The release properties of the PCL-DEX electrodes were further evaluated by soaking PCL-DEX electrodes in artificial perilymph to test the DEX concentration by HPLC. DEX was released very quickly and reached a stable concentration within 1 day. The stable concentration was maintained for 270 days (**Figures 4A,B**). DEX was released in a slow rate. Slow and sustained release of DEX can lead to enhanced potency (**Figure 4C**). To evaluate the DEX loading capacity in PCL-DEX electrodes, the cumulative amount of DEX released and the percentages in total DEX loading were counted. The PCL-20%DEX (MW36k) electrode had the most cumulative amount of DEX (1.05 mg ± 0.02 mg) released in 270 days and the lowest percentage (19.4 ± 0.42%) in total DEX carried by PCL

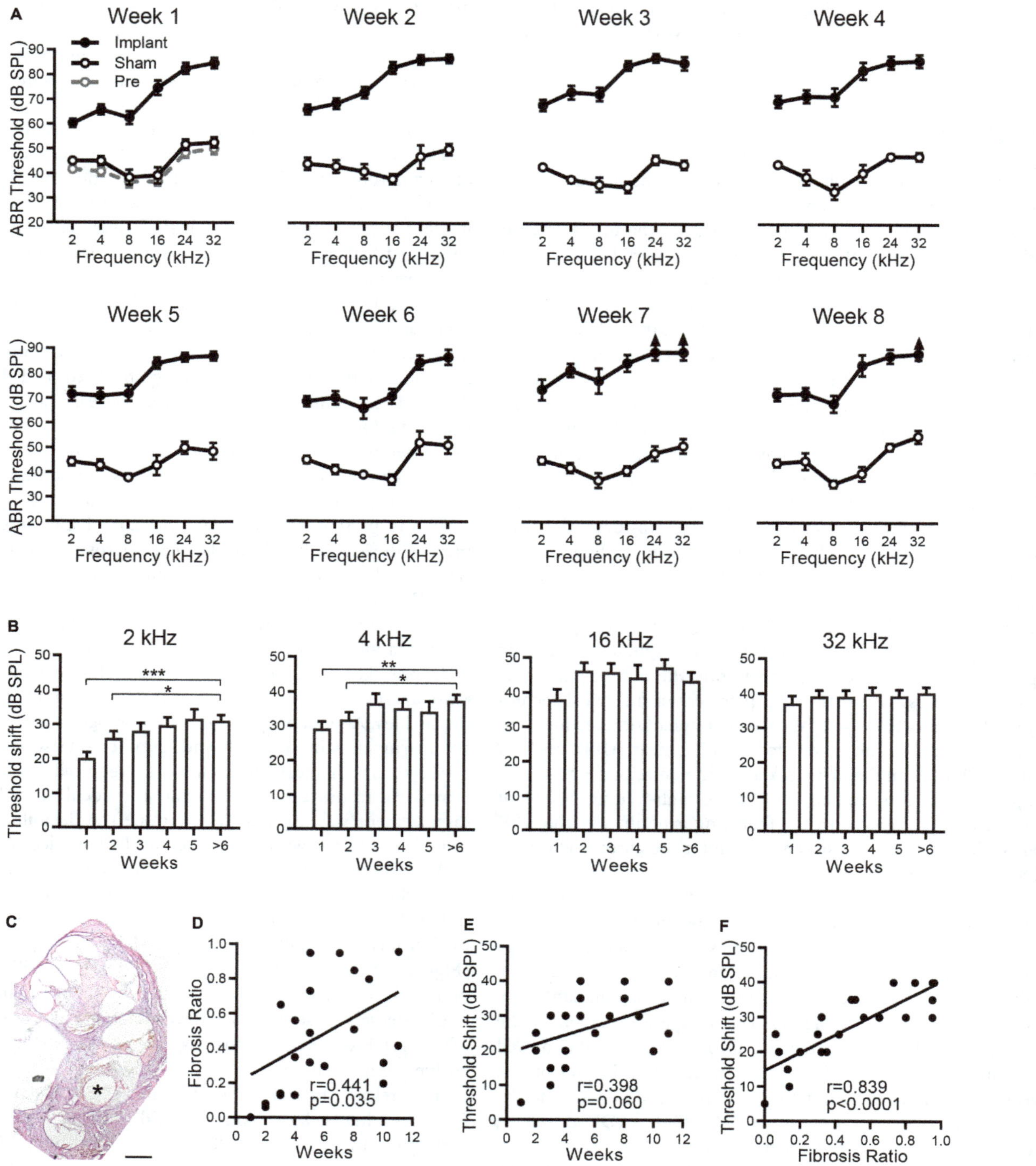

FIGURE 1 | Hearing loss is associated with fibrosis after CI. **(A)** The effects of electrode implantation on the ABR thresholds at different implantation times. The ABR threshold-frequency curves of the implant (filled circles) and sham groups (open circles) were plotted in the same panel from week 1 to week 8. For the implant group, n = 18, 20, 21, 18, 21, 7, 5, and 11 for weeks 1 to 8, respectively. For the sham group, $n = 6$ for each week. The ABR thresholds before implantation (Pre-Op, gray open circles, $n = 6$) are plotted in the panel of week 1. The data are presented as the mean ± SE. For some data points, the arrows indicate the thresholds above the limit of measurement (90 dB SPL). **(B)** ABR threshold shifts at 2, 4, 16, and 32 kHz versus the sham group at different implantation times. Data are presented as the mean and SE. $^{*}p < 0.05$; $^{**}p < 0.01$; $^{***}p < 0.001$. n = 18, 20, 21, 18, 21, and 23 for weeks 1, 2, 3, 4, 5, and > 6, respectively. **(C)** Optical microscope image of a representative H&E-stained cross section of a rat cochlea implanted with electrode for 5 weeks. "*" indicates the trajectory of the electrode insertion. Scale bar = 500 μm. The percentage of fibrous tissue in scala tympani was determined as fibrosis ratio. **(D,E)** The pooled data show the proliferative tissue volume **(D)** and the ABR threshold shifts at 2 kHz **(E)** distributed over the implantation time. **(F)** The relationship between ABR threshold shifts and proliferative tissue volume. The line indicates the linear correlation coefficient.

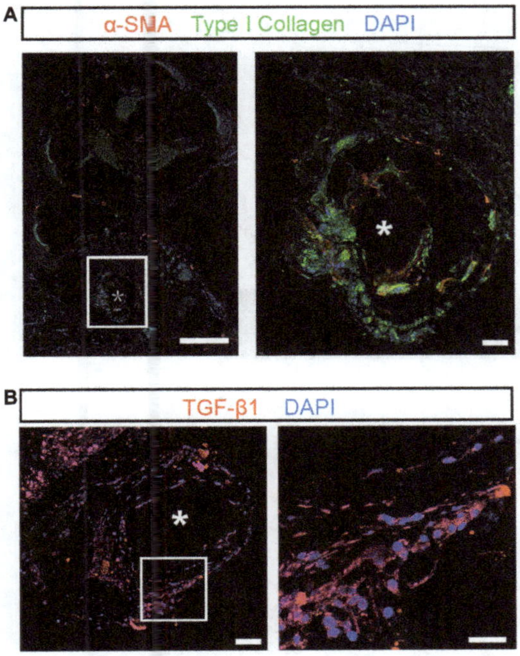

FIGURE 2 | Confocal images of the proliferative tissue after electrode insertion in the cochlea. **(A)** Representative immunostaining images showing the proliferative tissue in the tympanic scala 5 weeks after implantation. α-SMA (red) and type I collagen (green) were evident in the proliferative tissue (magnified view, right panel). Scale bar = 500 and 50 μm for the left and right panels, respectively. **(B)** Left panel: representative immunostaining images showing the expression of TGF-β1 (red) in the proliferative tissue 5 weeks after implantation. Scale bar = 50 μm. Right panel: the enlarged plot of the white box in the left panel. Scale bar = 50 μm. "*" indicates the trajectory of the electrode insertion.

carried by PCL (**Figures 4C,D**). And for PCL-20%DEX electrode, stable and effective DEX concentrations (0.073 ± 0.002 mg/mL) had been maintained for more than 9 months. Combining clinical needs, the PCL-20%DEX electrodes were chosen for implantation (**Figure 4D**). This result indicated that the drug loading content was sufficiently adequate to achieve sustained and effective release. DEX was completely encapsulated in the PCL coating, which slowly released DEX for approximately 270 days at relatively stable concentrations.

HEI-OC1 cell line, which derived from the conditionally immortalized mouse auditory cells, were commonly used cell line in many previous reports (He et al., 2017, 2021; Li et al., 2018; Zhang et al., 2019, 2021). Here HEI-OC1 cells and L929 cells were cultured on the PCL-coated surface to confirm the biocompatibility of our coating. No significant difference in the cell density was observed on the PCL surface compared to that of the normal culture dish for either cell type (**Figure 4E**, $p > 0.05$, Student's *t*-test). The effects of PCL loaded with different DEM concentrations on cell viability were then examined by using the CCK-8 assay. Compared with the cells cultured in normal culture medium, no significant difference in cell viability was found for either cell type cultured in the soaking solution of PCL, PCL-5% DEX, PCL-20% DEX, and culture medium containing 0.1% DEX (**Figure 4F**, $p > 0.05$, one-way ANOVA). Together with the physical feature data, these results indicate that our PCL-DEX coating is safe and suitable for cochlear implantation. The formula of 20% DEX loaded with 36 k MW PCL (denoted as PCL-DEX hereafter) was selected for the following *in vivo* experiments.

Fibrosis was examined in the cochleae at week five after the implantation of a bare silicone electrode (pristine), silicone electrode coated with PCL-DEX, or silicone electrode coated with PCL only. Meanwhile, in a group of bare silicone electrode implantations, one dose of local DEX was applied at insertion to mimic the clinical treatment. As shown by the representative cross sections in **Figure 5A**, in the pristine, PCL, and DEX groups, large fibrotic tissue around the implants compared to the control and sham groups was observed, and little fibrosis was found in the PCL-DEX group. The quantified data showed that the volume of fibrotic tissue was significantly decreased for PCL-DEX-coated implants (**Figure 5B**). This coating presented average reductions of 96, 93, and 95% in fibrosis compared with the uncoated, PCL-coated, and one-dose DEX treatment groups, respectively ($p < 0.001, p = 0.0057, p < 0.001$, respectively, one-way ANOVA). The hearing of the implanted ear was protected by the PCL-DEX coating, as demonstrated by a significantly smaller ABR threshold shift than that of the uncoated, PCL-coated, and one-dose DEX treatment groups (**Figure 5C**, $p < 0.001$, $p = 0.0011$, $p < 0.001$, respectively, one-way ANOVA). The expression of α-SMA and type I collagen, markers of fibrotic tissue, was measured in the cochleae to further confirm the inhibition of fibrosis by PCL-DEX coating. Significantly lowerα-SMA (**Figure 5D**, $p = 0.0013$, one-way ANOVA) and type I collagen (**Figure 5E**, $p < 0.001$, one-way ANOVA) expression was observed in the PCL-DEX-coated implants than in the uncoated implants, while the expression was the same in the local DEX treatment group ($p > 0.05$ for both expression levels, one-way ANOVA).

The protective effects of the PCL-DEX coating may benefit from less progressive impairment-induced cell loss in hair cells (HCs) and spiral ganglion neurons (SGNs) (Zhou et al., 2020). As shown in **Figure 6A**, compared with the controls, significant loss of HCs was observed along the whole cochlea at week 5 after the implantation of pristine electrodes ($p < 0.001$ for all three positions, one-way ANOVA). The cell loss at apical segments of the cochlea, at which the electrode did not directly reach, indicates a progressive impairment of HCs in addition to the possible direct trauma of the basal cochlea by implant insertion. This loss of HCs was significantly reduced by the implantation of the PCL-DEX-coated electrode (**Figure 6A**, $p < 0.001$ for all three positions, one-way ANOVA). The protective effect of the PCL-DEX coating was also observed for SGNs. The densities of SGNs at the middle and basal cochlea were decreased at week 5 after the implantation of pristine electrodes (**Figure 6B**, $p < 0.001$ for both positions, one-way ANOVA). Such loss of SGNs was alleviated by the PCL-DEX-coated electrode (for both positions $p < 0.001$ vs. pristine, one-way ANOVA), and no significant loss of SGNs was found compared with the controls ($p > 0.05$ vs. controls, one-way ANOVA). These results are consistent with our functional measurements of ABR recordings.

It is of great significance to reveal the possible mechanisms of how the PCL-DEX-coated implant protected SGNs and

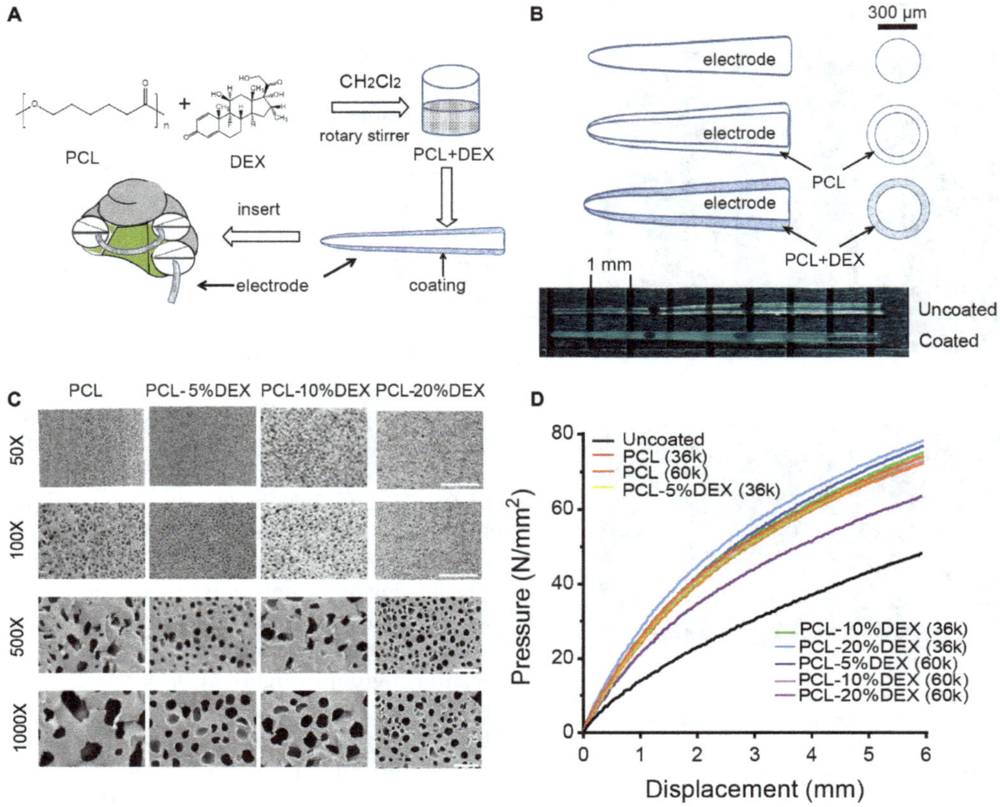

FIGURE 3 | Cochlear implant PCL-coated electrodes and their physical properties. **(A)** Schematic showing the PCL-DEX coating process of the cochlear implant electrode. **(B)** Top panels show diagrams of the electrode and its coating. Bottom photographs show the tips of uncoated (pristine) and PCL-DEX-coated electrodes. **(C)** Scanning electron microscopic images show the surface of electrodes coated with PCL, PCL-5%DEX, PCL-10%DEX, and PCL-20% DEX (MW = 36 k). Scale bar = 100, 20, 10, and 5 μm for 50×, 100×, 500×, and 1,000× magnifications, respectively. **(D)** Color coded lines show the pressure produced by the pristine and coated electrodes at different bend displacements.

HCs, reduced fibrotic tissue, and restored hearing. The role of inflammation in the foreign body response resulting in fibrosis and cell death has been well recognized. In the present study, inflammation-related factors were examined to determine the effects of PCL-DEX-coated implants. The western blotting in **Figure 7A** shows that the expression of TGF-β1 was increased by pristine implants with/without local DEX treatment, indicating an increase in the foreign body response in the cochlea (for both implants, $p < 0.001$ vs. controls, one-way ANOVA). This TGF-β1 increase was significantly reduced by the PCL-DEX coating ($p < 0.001$ vs. pristine and DEX only, one-way ANOVA). TNF-α and IL-1β, two factors in the early inflammation phase, were measured in cochleae by western blotting and ELISA (**Figures 7B,C**). Compared with the controls, the expression of both factors was increased by the implantation of pristine electrodes ($p < 0.001$ and $p < 0.05$, respectively, one-way ANOVA). The PCL-DEX coating reduced the increase in these factors ($p < 0.01$ and $p < 0.05$, respectively, one-way ANOVA), while local DEX treatment exhibited a weak influence only on IL-1β ($p < 0.05$, one-way ANOVA). IL-4, a factor in the later inflammation phase, was examined 3 days after implantation (**Figure 7D**). Similar to the effects on TNF-α and IL-1β, the PCL-DEX coating reduced the expression of IL-4 induced by the implant ($p < 0.05$ vs. pristine, one-way ANOVA), and the reduction was more significant than local DEX treatment ($p < 0.05$, one-way ANOVA).

For the foreign body response, macrophages play a key role in inflammation and the formation of fibrotic tissue. As shown in the cochlear cross section 5 weeks postimplantation of the uncoated electrode, CD68-marked macrophages were found in the fibrotic tissue around the pristine implant (**Figure 8A**). However, in the intact contralateral cochlea, no macrophages were observed in the OC, stria vascularis (SV), and spiral ligament (SL) regions (**Figure 8B**). To investigate how macrophages invade the cochlea after cochlear implantation, we examined the distribution of macrophages in the cochlea. CD68 staining 1 week postimplantation showed that macrophages first appeared in the SL regions in the uncoated electrode-implanted cochlea (**Figures 8C1,C2**), while macrophages were rarely observed in the PCL-DEX-implanted cochlea (**Figures 8C3,C4**). At 5 weeks postimplantation of the uncoated implant, macrophages were observed in fibrotic tissue, while macrophages were also found in the SV, OC, and SL regions (**Figures 8D1,D2**). The PCL-DEX-coated implant showed much

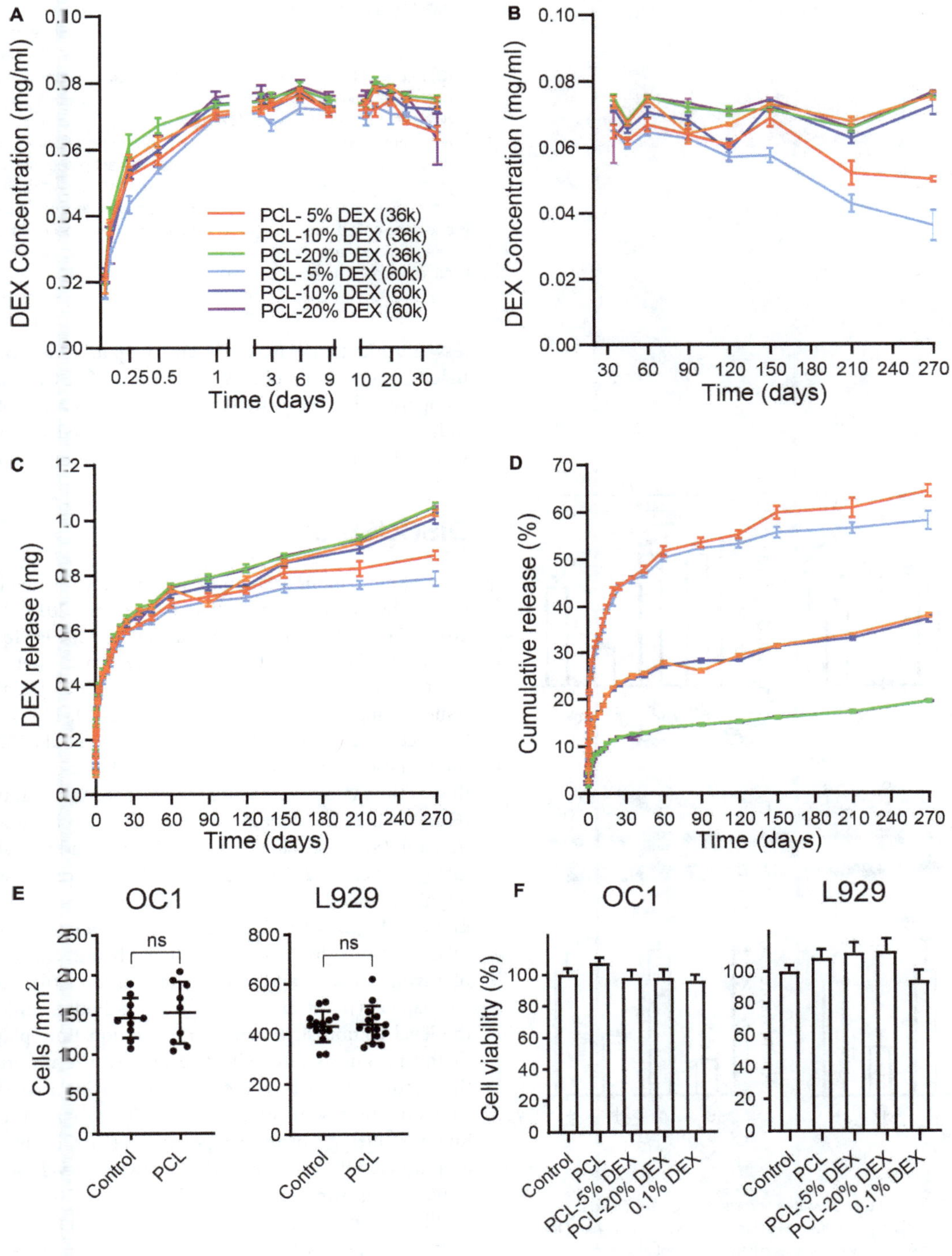

FIGURE 4 | The release of DEX. **(A,B)** The concentration of dexamethasone released by PCL-DEX-coated electrodes in artificial perilymph fluids each day in the short term [**(A)** within 30 days] and long term [**(B)** 30–270 days]. Color-coded lines indicate the electrodes coated with different molecular weights of PCL (MW36k or 60k) containing DEX from 5 to 20%. **(C)** Cumulative mass of DEX released by different PCL-DEX-coated electrodes in 3.6 ml of artificial perilymph fluids. DEX mass was measured from day 0 to 270. **(D)** The percentage of total DEX loaded in PCL released from day 0 to day 270 for different PCL-DEX formulas. The color code fits **(A–D)**. The data are presented as the mean ± SE. $n = 10$ for each group. **(E)** Cell density of HEI-OC1 cells and L929 cells cultured in PCL-coated and noncoated (control) plates. The data are presented as the mean ± SE. ns: no significant difference, $p > 0.05$, $n = 10$ for each group. **(F)** The cell viability of HEI-OC1 and L929 cells cultured in normal medium (control) and leach solution of PCL, PCL-5%DEX, PCL-10%DEX, and PCL-20% DEX and 0.1%DEX. The data are presented as the mean ± SE. $n = 13$ for OC1 cells and $n = 23$ for L929 cells.

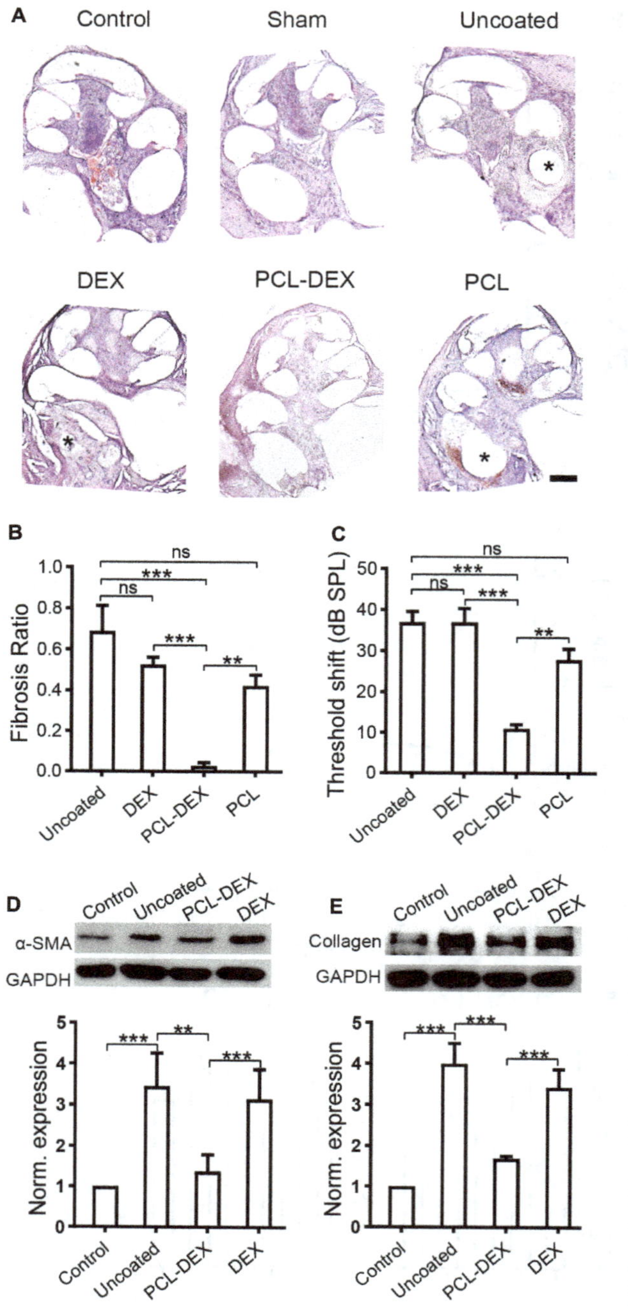

FIGURE 5 | PCL-DEX electrode alleviates fibrosis after CI. **(A)** Optical microscopy images show representative H&E-stained cross sections of the cochlea before (control) and 5 weeks after different implantation procedures. "Sham" for cochlea 5 weeks after sham surgery. "Pristine" for pristine electrode implant. "DEX" for pristine electrode implantation with one dose of DEX applied *via* a round window. "PCL" for implantation with a PCL-coated electrode containing no DEX. "PCL-DEX" for implantation with a PCL-coated electrode containing 20% DEX. Scale bar = 500 μm for all panels. **(B)** The fibrosis ratio 5 weeks after different implant procedures. **(C)** The ABR threshold shift at 2 kHz 5 weeks after different implantation procedures. The data in panels **(B,C)** are presented as the mean ± SE. ns: no significant difference, $p > 0.05$; $^{*}p < 0.05$; $^{**}p < 0.01$; $^{***}p < 0.001$, Student's *t*-test. *(Continued)*

FIGURE 5 | (Continued)
$n = 5$ for each group. **(D)** The effects of different implant treatments on the expression of fibroblastic proliferation-related proteins in the cochlea. **(D)** Representative immune bands (upper panel) and normalized expression level (lower panel) of α-SMA in the cochlea before (control) and 5 weeks after different implant procedures. **(E)** Representative immune bands (upper panel) and normalized expression level (lower panel) of type I collagen in the cochlea before (control) and 5 weeks after different implant procedures. "Pristine" for pristine electrode implant. "PCL-DEX" for implantation with a PCL-coated electrode containing 20% DEX. "DEX" for pristine electrode implantation with one dose of DEX applied *via* a round window. The experiment was repeated three times in each group. All datapoints are presented as the mean ± SD. ns: no significant difference, $p > 0.05$; $^{*}p < 0.05$; $^{**}p < 0.01$; $^{***}p < 0.001$.

less fibrotic tissue in the scala tympani. Moreover, very few macrophages were observed in the SV, OC, and SL regions compared to the uncoated implant (**Figures 8D3,D4**). These data indicate that the PCL-DEX coating resulted in fewer activated macrophages recruited to the cochlea after implantation.

DISCUSSION

In mammal's inner ear, sound wave is transformed into electrical signals by cochlear hair cells (Guo et al., 2019; Liu W. et al., 2019; Qi et al., 2019, 2020; Tan et al., 2019; He et al., 2020; Zhang et al., 2020; Chen et al., 2021) and then these signals are transduced to auditory cortex by spiral ganglion neurons (Guo et al., 2016, 2021; Fang et al., 2019; Liu Y. et al., 2019; Zhao et al., 2019; Guo R. et al., 2020; Liu et al., 2021). Cochlear implantation can perfectly replace the function of hair cells, and thus is the major treatment for severe sensorineural hearing loss (Guo J. H. et al., 2020). However, fibrotic tissue after cochlear implantation (O'Malley et al., 2017) may lead to residual hearing loss (Reiss et al., 2015) in patients. In the present study, hearing impairment and fibrosis after CI were also observed in our animal models (**Figures 1A–C**). Our results (**Figure 2**) together with related studies have indicated that fibrotic tissue is composed of myofibroblasts and extracellular matrix (for example, type I collagen) (Jia et al., 2016). Since individual differences exist, the level of fibrosis but not implantation time plays a key role in the prognosis after CI. The greater the fibrotic volume in the cochlea, the worse the residual hearing loss (**Figures 1D–F**). Consistent with the present study, individual differences in humans during fibrotic progression after CI have been found, and no significant correlation between level of fibrosis and implantation time was found (Ishai et al., 2017). These clinical problems are expected to be solved with long-term release of dexamethasone with a PCL-coated electrode. Corresponding to the location of the implant that is vulnerable to direct mechanical damage from the electrodes, hearing thresholds at high frequencies did not vary significantly with changes in the level of fibrosis. However, hearing thresholds at low frequency (2 kHz) vary as a function of the level of fibrosis, where the apical turn of the cochlea far away from the implant. Two reasons may involve in the hearing loss. First, fibrosis after CI may attenuate the vibration of perilymph. Secondly, the release of profibrotic factors and inflammation producers during the progression of

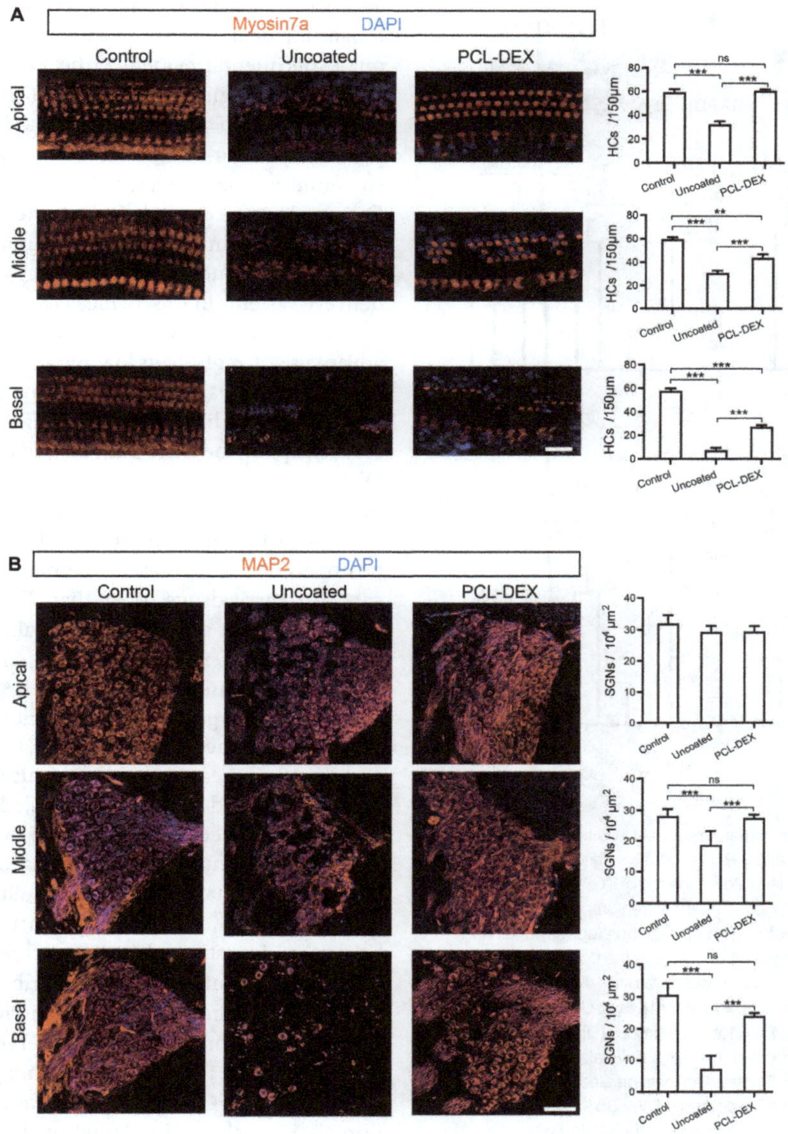

FIGURE 6 | The effects of different implant treatments on HCs and SGNs. **(A)** Representative immunofluorescence staining for myosin 7a (red) as a marker for HC (left panel) and HC density (right panel) at the basal, middle, and apical turns from cross sections of the cochlea before (control) and 5 weeks after implantation with pristine and PCL-DEX electrodes. Scale bar = 20 μm. **(B)** Representative immunofluorescence staining for MAP2 (red) as a marker for SGN (left panel) and SGN density (right panel) at the basal, middle, and apical turns from cross sections of the cochlea before (control) and 5 weeks after implantation with pristine and PCL-DEX electrodes. Scale bar = 30 μm. The data are presented as the mean ± SE. ns: no significant difference, $p > 0.05$, $n = 3$ for each group. $^{**}p < 0.01$; $^{***}p < 0.001$.

fibrosis causes damage to hair cells and SGNs (**Figure 6**). In the present study, dexamethasone was selected to alleviate fibrosis in cochlear implantation. Long-term release of dexamethasone with a PCL-coated electrode alleviated fibrosis and improved hearing function after CI compared with the uncoated electrode (**Figure 5**). Hair cells and spiral ganglion cells were well preserved by the PCL-DEX electrode (**Figure 6**).

Polycaprolactone is an attractive biomedical polymer with slow biodegradability, good biocompatibility, good drug permeability, and relatively low production cost (Wei et al., 2009). PCL has been used in basic research and approved for some clinical use, including wound healing, tissue regeneration, and drug control delivery systems (Liang et al., 2020). Although it has not been applied to intracochlear administration, PCL did not affect the survival of cells and or the microenvironment in the cochlea (**Figures 4E,F**). Moreover, abundant apertures that were homogenic and small in size were instrumental in the steady and sustained release of DEX (**Figure 3C**), that was supported by our *in vitro* data (**Figure 4**). Clinically, glucocorticoids are administered systemically or locally to treat fibrosis following implantation (Stathopoulos et al., 2014). Due to individual differences and other reasons, the current clinical efficacy

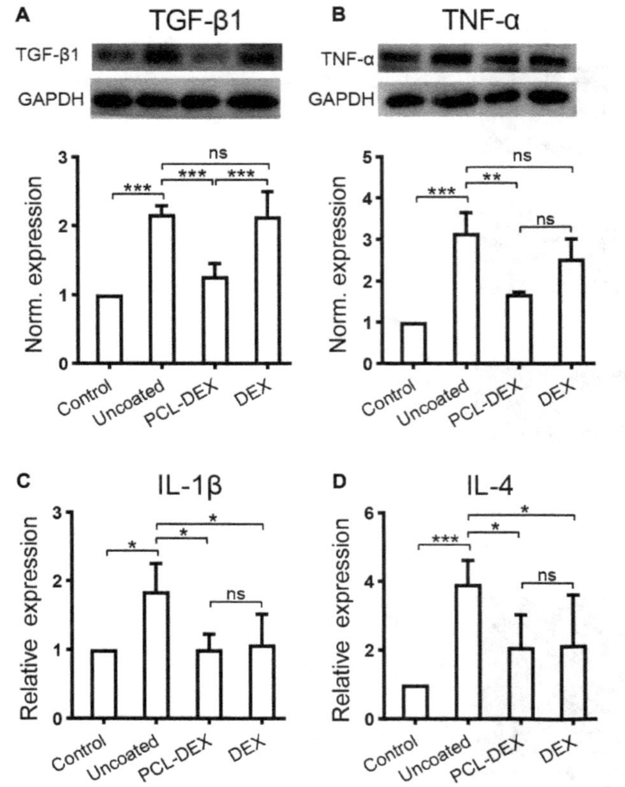

FIGURE 7 | The effects of different implant treatments on the expression of inflammatory factors in the cochlea. **(A)** Representative immune bands (upper panel) and normalized expression level (lower panel) of TGF-β1 in the contralateral cochlea (control) and 7 days after different implant procedures. $n = 4$ for each group. **(B)** Representative immune bands (upper panel) and normalized expression level (lower panel) of TNF-α in the contralateral cochlea (control) and 1 day after different implant procedures. $n = 4$ for each group. **(C)** ELISA shows the normalized expression of IL-1β in cochlear lysates 1 day after different implant procedures. $n = 4$ for each group. **(D)** ELISA shows the normalized expression of IL-4 in cochlear lysates 7 days after different implant procedures. $n = 5$ for each group. "Pristine" for pristine electrode implant. "PCL-DEX" for implantation with a PCL-coated (MW = 36 k) electrode containing 20% DEX. "DEX" for pristine electrode implantation with one dose of DEX applied *via* a round window. The experiment was repeated at least three times in each group. All data points are presented as the mean ± SD. ns: no significant difference, $p > 0.05$; $^{*}p < 0.05$; $^{**}p < 0.01$; $^{***}p < 0.001$, Student's *t*-test.

varies and is not significant. Systemic and local dexamethasone delivery cannot be continued for a long time because of side effects and technical difficulties. After discontinuation of DEX administration, fibrosis progresses and the effectiveness of cochlear implantation decreases, suggesting that sustained interventions should be carried out (Mamelle et al., 2017). Since fibrotic reactions continuously develop, fibrosis will further develop after discontinuation of DEX (Liu et al., 2015). PCL was reported to achieve controlled release with a relatively low release rate (Song et al., 2014). Our PCL-DEX electrodes controlled drug delivery system managed to release DEX at a stable and effective concentration for a much longer time. The effectiveness of our PCL-DEX electrode lies in the fact that it can reach all cochlear locations that electrodes reach, and it can persist longer for dexamethasone to work (**Figures 4A–D**). Implied by our experimental evidence, the PCL-DEX electrode had better efficacy than a single dose of DEX (**Figure 5**).

Drug elution from the cochlear implant has been explored previously using a mini-osmotic pump or drug loaded in a gel surrounding the implant (Mamelle et al., 2017; Xu et al., 2018). Other reported drug delivery systems are not able to achieve long-term continuous administration or maintain a therapeutic level of drug concentration for a long time. Some reported drug delivery systems in the cochlea lasted only approximately 3 weeks after surgery. In our study, the PCL-DEX-coated electrode has the advantage of high drug loading efficiency compared with other methods, such as capsuling drugs or drug pumping (Richardson et al., 2009). Additionally, when DEX was carried by PCL into the scala tympani, the DEX was released directly into the cochlea, and DEX release lasted longer, resulting in a decrease in fibrosis. Our findings support the hypothesis that coated implant in the cochlea enables sustained release of the drug reduces fibrosis caused by postoperative implantation trauma. In addition, the PCL coating can also carry drugs other than DEX to target fibrosis in the cochlea (Puga et al., 2012; Zhao et al., 2012).

This treatment also allows us to further explore the mechanism of inhibiting fibrosis better and find more precise therapeutic targets, enabling more specific and accurate treatment. In the early stage after CI, the expression of TNF-α and IL-1β increased in the cochlea (Yamahara et al., 2018). In the advanced stage of fibrosis, the expression of IL-4 and TGF-β1 increased and the TGF-β1was observed in the fibrous tissue around the electrode implanted (**Figures 2**, **7**). Fibrosis-associated mechanisms have been elucidated in various organs, such as the liver, kidney, lung, heart, and skin, but they need to be further investigated in the cochlea. IL-1β, TNF-α, and IL-4 are critical proinflammatory contributors to the pathogenesis of inflammation and fibrosis (Weiskirchen et al., 2019). Significant increases in expression were observed for inflammatory genes after cochlear implantation (Zhang et al., 2015; Eshraghi et al., 2019). TGF-β1 plays a leading role in the process of fibrosis in cochlear implantation by stimulating myofibroblast differentiation and collagen synthesis and deposition (Bas et al., 2020). The PCL-DEX electrode reduced the expression of TNF-α, IL-1β, IL-4, and TGF-β1 (**Figure 7**) and thus reduced myofibroblast infiltration and decreased collagen deposition (**Figure 5**). The PCL-DEX electrode achieved a therapeutic effect by blocking the TGF-β1 signaling pathway.

Local macrophage is a main source of TGF-β1 during fibrosis (Chung et al., 2018; Tang et al., 2019). Macrophages and foreign body giant cells (FBGCs) were found in a previous pathologic study of the temporal bone after cochlear implantation (Bas et al., 2020). Previous studies have shown that the activation of myofibroblasts and the production of extracellular matrix induced by the production of TGF-β1 by macrophages are key links in the process of fibrosis in other organs (Wynn and Ramalingam, 2012). After uncoated electrode implantation, macrophages migrate to the surface of the electrode (Bellamri et al., 2019). Foreign body reactions can lead to the degradation of CI biomaterials. It is presumed that these biomaterials are

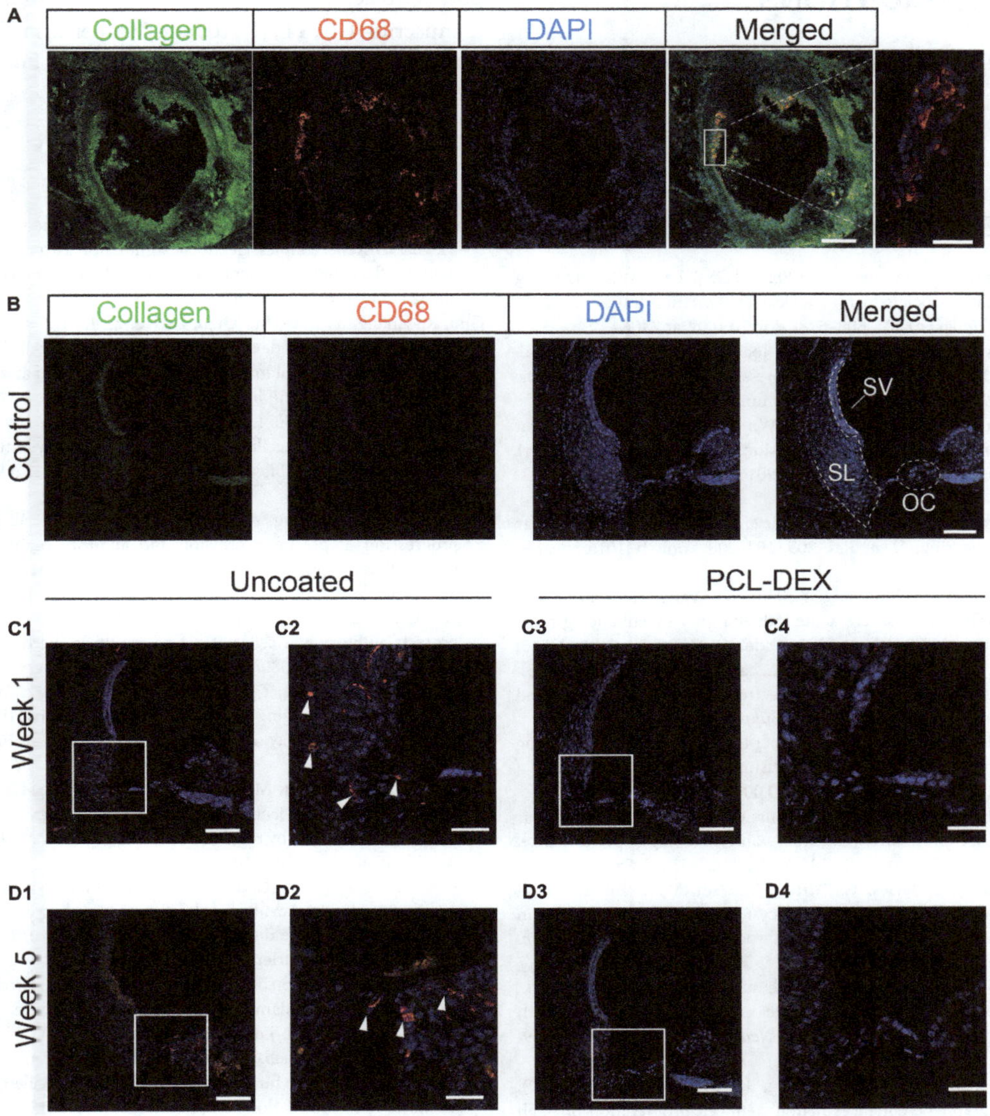

FIGURE 8 | Confocal images of macrophages expressed in the cochlea. **(A)** Representative immunostaining images showing the proliferative tissue in the tympanic scala 5 weeks after implantation. CD68 (red) and type I collagen (green) were evident in the proliferative tissue, especially on the surface of the electrode (magnified view, right panel). Scale bar = 100 and 20 μm for the left and right panels, respectively. **(B)** Representative immunostaining images showing the spiral ligament in the control cochlea. SL, spiral ligament; SV, stria vascularis; OC, organ of Corti. **(C)** Representative immunostaining images showing the spiral ligament of the basal turn in the cochlea implanted with pristine or PCL-DEX electrodes for 1 week **(C1,C3)** and 5 weeks **(D1,D3)**. **(C2,C4,D2,D4)** are magnified views of panels **(C1,C3,D1,D3)**, respectively, and solid white arrows indicate macrophages positive for CD68 (red). Scale bar = 100 μm.

subject to mediators of degradation released by macrophages and FBGCs and undergo phagocytosis in an attempt to clear the debris (Liu et al., 2018; Yan et al., 2018; Wu et al., 2020). FBGCs were seen at the interface between the electrode and the fibrous capsule (**Figure 8A**). Correspondingly, the number of macrophages increased after uncoated electrode implantation. PCL-DEX electrodes carried more DEX and had a longer DEX release time than other approaches (Lehner et al., 2019), and the number of macrophages decreased after PCL-DEX electrode implantation (**Figure 8**). Together, these data suggest that PCL-DEX electrodes reduce fibrosis by inhibiting the proliferation of macrophage cells, the secretion of fibrosis-related factors, and inhibiting the proliferation of myofibroblasts into the scala tympani. Therefore, the coating of PCL-DEX is beneficial to improve the long-term effect after cochlear implantation.

ETHICS STATEMENT

The animal study was reviewed and approved by Institutional Animal Care and Use Committee (IACUC) of Southern Medical University.

AUTHOR CONTRIBUTIONS

HZ and JT designed the experiments. DM provided technical assistance with preparation and performance detection on the polycaprolactone coated electrode. DC, JT, and HZ wrote the manuscript. DC, YL, JP, AC, and MX performed experiments. All authors reviewed, edited, and approved the final manuscript.

REFERENCES

Bas, E., Anwar, M. R., and Van De Water, T. R. (2020). TGF β-1 and WNT signaling pathways collaboration associated with cochlear implantation trauma-induced fibrosis. *Anat. Rec. (Hoboken)* 303, 608–618. doi: 10.1002/ar.24064

Bellamri, N., Viel, R., Morzadec, C., Lecureur, V., Joannes, A., de Latour, B., et al. (2019). TNF-α and IL-10 control CXCL13 expression in human macrophages. *J. Immunol.* 204, 2492–2502. doi: 10.4049/jimmunol.1900790

Chen, Y., Gu, Y., Li, Y., Li, G. L., Chai, R., Li, W., et al. (2021). Generation of mature and functional hair cells by co-expression of Gfi1, Pou4f3, and Atoh1 in the postnatal mouse cochlea. *Cell Rep.* 35:109016. doi: 10.1016/j.celrep.2021.109016

Choi, C. H., and Oghalai, J. S. (2005). Predicting the effect of post-implant cochlear fibrosis on residual hearing. *Hear. Res.* 205, 193–200. doi: 10.1016/j.heares.2005.03.018

Chung, S., Overstreet, J. M., Li, Y., Wang, Y., Niu, A., Wang, S., et al. (2018). TGF-β promotes fibrosis after severe acute kidney injury by enhancing renal macrophage infiltration. *JCI Insight* 3:e123563. doi: 10.1172/jci.insight.123563

Clark, G. M., Shute, S. A., Shepherd, R. K., and Carter, T. D. (1995). Cochlear implantation: osteoneogenesis, electrode-tissue impedance, and residual hearing. *Ann. Otol. Rhinol. Laryngol. Suppl.* 166, 40–42.

Cortés Fuentes, I. A., Videhult Pierre, P., and Engmér Berglin, C. (2020). Improving clinical outcomes in cochlear implantation using glucocorticoid therapy: a review. *Ear Hear.* 41, 17–24. doi: 10.1097/AUD.0000000000000740

Côté, M., Ferron, P., Bergeron, F., and Bussières, R. (2007). Cochlear reimplantation: causes of failure, outcomes, and audiologic performance. *Laryngoscope* 117, 1225–1235. doi: 10.1097/MLG.0b013e31805c9a06

Eshraghi, A. A., Shahal, D., Davies, C., Mittal, J., Shah, V., Bulut, E., et al. (2020). Evaluating the efficacy of L-N-acetylcysteine and dexamethasone in combination to provide otoprotection for electrode insertion trauma. *J. Clin. Med.* 9:716. doi: 10.3390/jcm9030716

Eshraghi, A. A., Wolfovitz, A., Yilmazer, R., Garnham, C., Yilmazer, A. B., Bas, E., et al. (2019). Otoprotection to implanted cochlea exposed to noise trauma with dexamethasone eluting electrode. *Front. Cell. Neurosci.* 13:492. doi: 10.3389/fncel.2019.00492

Fang, Q., Zhang, Y., Chen, X., Li, H., Cheng, L., Zhu, W., et al. (2019). Three-dimensional graphene enhances neural stem cell proliferation through metabolic regulation. *Front. Bioeng. Biotechnol.* 7:436. doi: 10.3389/fbioe.2019.00436

Foggia, M. J., Quevedo, R. V., and Hansen, M. R. (2019). Intracochlear fibrosis and the foreign body response to cochlear implant biomaterials. *Laryngoscope Investig. Otolaryngol.* 4, 678–683. doi: 10.1002/lio2.329

Gaharwar, A. K., Nikkhah, M., Sant, S., and Khademhosseini, A. (2014). Anisotropic poly (glycerol sebacate)-poly (ϵ-caprolactone) electrospun fibers promote endothelial cell guidance. *Biofabrication* 7:15001. doi: 10.1088/1758-5090/7/1/015001

Guo, J. H., Yu, Y., Sun, L., Zhang, Z., Zhao, Y., and Chai, R. (2020). Bio-inspired multicomponent carbon nanotube microfibers from microfluidics for supercapacitor. *Chem. Eng. J.* 397:125517. doi: 10.1016/j.cej.2020.125517

Guo, R., Li, J., Chen, C., Xiao, M., Liao, M., Hu, Y., et al. (2021). Biomimetic 3D bacterial cellulose-graphene foam hybrid scaffold regulates neural stem cell proliferation and differentiation. *Colloids Surf. B Biointerfaces* 200:111590. doi: 10.1016/j.colsurfb.2021.111590

Guo, R., Ma, X., Liao, M., Liu, Y., Hu, Y., Qian, X., et al. (2019). Development and application of cochlear implant-based electric-acoustic stimulation of spiral ganglion neurons. *ACS Biomater. Sci. Eng.* 5, 6735–6741. doi: 10.1021/acsbiomaterials.9b01265

Guo, R., Xiao, M., Zhao, W., Zhou, S., Hu, Y., Liao, M., et al. (2020). 2D Ti3C2TxMXene couples electrical stimulation to promote proliferation and neural differentiation of neural stem cells. *Acta Biomater.* S1742–7061, 30749–30752. doi: 10.1016/j.actbio.2020.12.035

Guo, R., Zhang, S., Xiao, M., Qian, F., He, Z., Li, D., et al. (2016). Accelerating bioelectric functional development of neural stem cells by graphene coupling: implications for neural interfacing with conductive materials. *Biomaterials* 106, 193–204. doi: 10.1016/j.biomaterials.2016.08.019

Han, S., Xu, Y., Sun, J., Liu, Y., Zhao, Y., Tao, W., et al. (2020). Isolation and analysis of extracellular vesicles in a Morpho butterfly wing-integrated microvortex biochip. *Biosens. Bioelectron.* 154:112073. doi: 10.1016/j.bios.2020.112073

Hang, J., Pan, W., Chang, A., Li, S., Li, C., Fu, M., et al. (2016). Synchronized progression of prestin expression and auditory brainstem response during postnatal development in rats. *Neural Plast.* 2016:4545826. doi: 10.1155/2016/4545826

He, Z., Guo, L., Shu, Y., Fang, Q., Zhou, H., Liu, Y., et al. (2017). Autophagy protects auditory hair cells against neomycin-induced damage. *Autophagy* 13, 1884–1904. doi: 10.1080/15548627.2017.1359449

He, Z. H., Li, M., Fang, Q. J., Liao, F. L., Zou, S. Y., Wu, X., et al. (2021). FOXG1 promotes aging inner ear hair cell survival through activation of the autophagy pathway. *Autophagy* 19, 1–22. doi: 10.1080/15548627.2021.1916194

He, Z. H., Zou, S. Y., Li, M., Liao, F. L., Wu, X., Sun, H. Y., et al. (2020). The nuclear transcription factor FoxG1 affects the sensitivity of mimetic aging hair cells to inflammation by regulating autophagy pathways. *Redox Biol.* 28:101364. doi: 10.1016/j.redox.2019.101364

Ishai, R., Herrmann, B. S., Nadol, J. B. Jr., and Quesnel, A. M. (2017). The pattern and degree of capsular fibrous sheaths surrounding cochlear electrode arrays. *Hear. Res.* 348, 44–53. doi: 10.1016/j.heares.2017.02.012

Jia, H., François, F., Bourien, J., Eybalin, M., Lloyd, R. V., Van De Water, T. R., et al. (2016). Prevention of trauma-induced cochlear fibrosis using intracochlear application of anti-inflammatory and antiproliferative drugs. *Neuroscience* 316, 261–278. doi: 10.1016/j.neuroscience.2015.12.031

Lehner, E., Gündel, D., Liebau, A., Plontke, S., and Mäder, K. (2019). Intracochlear PLGA based implants for dexamethasone release: challenges and solutions. *Int. J. Pharm. X* 1:100015. doi: 10.1016/j.ijpx.2019.100015

Li, H., Song, Y., He, Z., Chen, X., Wu, X., Li, X., et al. (2018). Meclofenamic acid reduces reactive oxygen species accumulation and apoptosis, inhibits excessive autophagy, and protects hair cell-like HEI-OC1 cells from cisplatin-induced damage. *Front. Cell. Neurosci.* 23:139. doi: 10.3389/fncel.2018.00139

Li, J. N., Chen, S., Zhai, L., Han, D. Y., Eshraghi, A. A., Feng, Y., et al. (2017). The advances in hearing rehabilitation and cochlear implants in China. *Ear Hear.* 38, 647–652. doi: 10.1097/AUD.0000000000000441

Liang, R., Zhao, J., Li, B., Cai, P., Loh, X. J., Xu, C., et al. (2020). Implantable and degradable antioxidant poly(ε-caprolactone)-lignin nanofiber membrane for effective osteoarthritis treatment. *Biomaterials* 230:119601. doi: 10.1016/j.biomaterials.2019.119601

Liu, W., Xu, L., Wang, X., Zhang, D., Sun, G., Wang, M., et al. (2021). PRDX1 activates autophagy via the PTEN-AKT signaling pathway to protect against cisplatin-induced spiral ganglion neuron damage. *Autophagy* 12, 1–23. doi: 10.1080/15548627.2021.1905466

Liu, W., Xu, X., Fan, Z., Sun, G., Han, Y., Zhang, D., et al. (2019). Wnt signaling activates TP53-induced glycolysis and apoptosis regulator and protects against cisplatin-induced spiral ganglion neuron damage in the mouse cochlea. *Antioxid. Redox Signal.* 30, 1389–1410. doi: 10.1089/ars.2017.7288

Liu, Y., Jolly, C., Braun, S., Janssen, T., Scherer, E., Steinhoff, J., et al. (2015). Effects of a dexamethasone-releasing implant on cochleae: a functional, morphological and pharmacokinetic study. *Hear. Res.* 327, 89–101. doi: 10.1016/j.heares.2015.04.019

Liu, Y., Qi, J., Chen, X., Tang, M., Chu, C., Zhu, W., et al. (2019). Critical role of spectrin in hearing development and deafness. *Sci. Adv.* 5:eaav7803. doi: 10.1126/sciadv.aav7803

Liu, Z., Tang, M., Zhao, J., Chai, R., and Kang, J. (2018). Looking into the future: toward advanced 3D biomaterials for stem-cell-based regenerative medicine. *Adv. Mater.* 30:e1705388. doi: 10.1002/adma.201705388

Luo, Y., Chen, A., Xu, M., Chen, D., Tang, J., Ma, D., et al. (2021). Preparation, characterization, and in vitro/vivo evaluation of dexamethasone/poly(ε-caprolactone)-based electrode coatings for cochlear implants. *Drug Deliv.* 28, 1673–1684. doi: 10.1080/10717544.2021.1960927

Mamelle, E., Kechai, N. E., Granger, B., Sterkers, O., Bochot, A., Agnely, F., et al. (2017). Effect of a liposomal hyaluronic acid gel loaded with dexamethasone in a guinea pig model after manual or motorized cochlear implantation. *Eur. Arch. Otorhinolaryngol.* 274, 729–736. doi: 10.1007/s00405-016-4331-8

O'Malley, J. T., Burgess, B. J., Galler, D., and Nadol, J. B. (2017). Foreign body response to silicone in cochlear implant electrodes in the human. *Otol. Neurotol.* 38, 970–977. doi: 10.1097/MAO.0000000000001454

Puga, A. M., Rey-Rico, A., Magariños, B., Alvarez-Lorenzo, C., and Concheiro, A. (2012). Hot melt poly-ε-caprolactone/poloxamine implantable matrices for sustained delivery of ciprofloxacin. *Acta Biomater.* 8, 1507–1518. doi: 10.1016/j.actbio.2011.12.020

Qi, J., Liu, Y., Chu, C., Chen, X., Zhu, W., Shu, Y., et al. (2019). A cytoskeleton structure revealed by super-resolution fluorescence imaging in inner ear hair cells. *Cell Discov.* 5:12. doi: 10.1038/s41421-018-0076-4

Qi, J., Zhang, L., Tan, F., Liu, Y., Chu, C., Zhu, W., et al. (2020). Espin distribution as revealed by super-resolution microscopy of stereocilia. *Am. J. Transl. Res.* 12, 130–141.

Reiss, L. A., Reiss, L. A., Stark, G., Nguyen-Huynh, A. T., Spear, K. A., Zhang, H., et al. (2015). Morphological correlates of hearing loss after cochlear implantation and electro-acoustic stimulation in a hearing-impaired Guinea pig model. *Hear. Res.* 327, 163–174. doi: 10.1016/j.heares.2015.06.007

Richardson, R. T., Wise, A. K., Thompson, B. C., Flynn, B. O., Atkinson, P. J., and Fretwell, N. J. (2009). Polypyrrole-coated electrodes for the delivery of charge and neurotrophins to cochlear neurons. *Biomaterials* 30, 2614–2624. doi: 10.1016/j.biomaterials.2009.01.015

Rowe, D., Chambers, S., Hampson, A., Eastwood, H., Campbell, L., and O'Leary, S. (2016). Delayed low frequency hearing loss caused by cochlear implantation interventions via the round window but not cochleostomy. *Hear. Res.* 333, 49–57. doi: 10.1016/j.heares.2015.12.012

Sanderson, A. P., Rogers, E. T. F., Verschuur, C. A., and Newman, T. A. (2019). Exploiting routine clinical measures to inform strategies for better hearing performance in cochlear implant users. *Front. Neurosci.* 12:1048. doi: 10.3389/fnins.2018.01048

Seyyedi, M., and Nadol, J. B. Jr. (2014). Intracochlear inflammatory response to cochlear implant electrodes in humans. *Otol. Neurotol.* 35, 1545–1551. doi: 10.1097/MAO.0000000000000540

Shang, L. R., Yu, Y. R., Gao, W., Wang, Y. T., Qu, L. L., Zhao, Z., et al. (2018). Bio-inspired anisotropic wettability surface from dynamic ferrofluid assembled templates. *Adv. Funct. Mater.* 28:1705802. doi: 10.1002/adfm.201705802

Song, Z., Zhu, W., Liu, N., Yang, F., and Feng, R. (2014). Linolenic acid-modified PEG-PCL micelles for curcumin delivery. *Int. J. Pharm.* 471, 312–321. doi: 10.1016/j.ijpharm.2014.05.059

Stathopoulos, D., Chambers, S., Enke, Y. L., Timbol, G., Risi, F., Miller, C., et al. (2014). Development of a safe dexamethasone-eluting electrode array for cochlear implantation. *Cochlear Implants Int.* 15, 254–263. doi: 10.1179/1754762813Y.0000000054

Tan, F., Chu, C., Qi, J., Li, W., You, D., Li, K., et al. (2019). AAV-ie enables safe and efficient gene transfer to inner ear cells. *Nat. Commun.* 10:3733. doi: 10.1038/s41467-019-11687-8

Tang, P. M., Nikolic-Paterson, D. J., and Lan, H. Y. (2019). Macrophages: versatile players in renal inflammation and fibrosis. *Nat. Rev. Nephrol.* 15, 144–158. doi: 10.1038/s41581-019-0110-2

Wei, X., Gong, C., Gou, M., Fu, S., Guo, Q., Shi, S., et al. (2009). Biodegradable poly(epsilon-caprolactone)-poly (ethylene glycol) copolymers as drug delivery system. *Int. J. Pharm.* 381, 1–18. doi: 10.1016/j.ijpharm.2009.07.033

Weiskirchen, R., Weiskirchen, S., and Tacke, F. (2019). Organ and tissue fibrosis: molecular signals, cellular mechanisms and translational implications. *Mol. Aspects Med.* 65, 2–15. doi: 10.1016/j.mam.2018.06.003

Wu, P., Luo, X., Wu, H., Zhang, Q., Dai, Y., and Sun, M. (2020). Efficient and targeted chemo-gene delivery with self-assembled fluoro-nanoparticles for liver fibrosis therapy and recurrence. *Biomaterials* 261:120311. doi: 10.1016/j.biomaterials.2020.120311

Wynn, T. A., and Ramalingam, T. R. (2012). Mechanisms of fibrosis: therapeutic translation for fibrotic disease. *Nat. Med.* 18, 1028–1040. doi: 10.1038/nm.2807

Xia, S., Shang, Y., Chen, X., Li, H., Xu, X., Liu, W., et al. (2020). Oriented neural spheroid formation and differentiation of neural stem cells guided by anisotropic inverse opals. *Front. Bioeng. Biotechnol.* 8:848. doi: 10.3389/fbioe.2020.00848

Xu, M., Ma, D., Chen, D., Cai, J., He, Q., Shu, F., et al. (2018). Preparation, characterization and application research of a sustained dexamethasone releasing electrode coating for cochlear implantation. *Mater. Sci. Eng. C Mater. Biol. Appl.* 90, 16–26. doi: 10.1016/j.msec.2018.04.033

Yamahara, K., Nishimura, K., Ogita, H., Ito, J., Nakagawa, T., Furuta, I., et al. (2018). Hearing preservation at low frequencies by insulin-like growth factor 1 in a guinea pig model of cochlear implantation. *Hear. Res.* 368, 92–108. doi: 10.1016/j.heares.2018.07.004

Yan, W., Liu, W., Qi, J., Fang, Q., Fan, Z., Sun, G., et al. (2018). A three-dimensional culture system with matrigel promotes purified spiral ganglion neuron survival and function in vitro. *Mol. Neurobiol.* 55, 2070–2084. doi: 10.1007/s12035-017-0471-0

Yang, Y., Gao, B., Hu, Y., Wei, H., Zhang, C., Chai, R., et al. (2021). Ordered inverse-opal scaffold based on bionic transpiration to create a biomimetic spine. *Nanoscale* 13, 8614–8622. doi: 10.1039/D1NR00731A

Zhang, H., Stark, G., and Reiss, L. (2015). Changes in gene expression and hearing thresholds after cochlear implantation. *Otol. Neurotol.* 36, 1157–1165. doi: 10.1097/MAO.0000000000000787

Zhang, S., Dong, Y., Qiang, R., Zhang, Y., Zhang, X., Chen, Y., et al. (2021). Characterization of Strip1 expression in mouse cochlear hair cells. *Front. Genet.* 12:625867. doi: 10.3389/fgene.2021.625867

Zhang, S., Zhang, Y., Dong, Y., Guo, L., Zhang, Z., Shao, B., et al. (2020). Knockdown of Foxg1 in supporting cells increases the trans-differentiation of supporting cells into hair cells in the neonatal mouse cochlea. *Cell. Mol. Life Sci.* 77, 1401–1419. doi: 10.1007/s00018-019-03291-2

Zhang, Y., Li, W., He, Z., Wang, Y., Shao, B., Cheng, C., et al. (2019). Pre-treatment with fasudil prevents neomycin-induced hair cell damage by reducing the accumulation of reactive oxygen species. *Front. Mol. Neurosci.* 12:264. doi: 10.3389/fnmol.2019.00264

Zhao, C., Chen, G., Wang, H., Zhao, Y., and Chai, R. (2020). Bio-inspired intestinal scavenger from microfluidic electrospray for detoxifying lipopolysaccharide. *Bioact. Mater.* 6, 1653–1662. doi: 10.1016/j.bioactmat.2020.11.017

Zhao, J., Tang, M., Cao, J., Ye, D., Guo, X., Xi, J., et al. (2019). Structurally tunable reduced graphene oxide substrate maintains mouse embryonic stem cell pluripotency. *Adv. Sci.* 6:1802136. doi: 10.1002/advs.201802136

Zhao, P., Liu, L., Feng, X., Wang, C., Shuai, X., and Chen, Y. (2012). Molecular nanoworm with PCL core and PEO shell as a non-spherical carrier for drug delivery. *Macromol. Rapid Commun.* 33, 1351–1355. doi: 10.1002/marc.201200172

Zhou, H., Qian, X., Xu, N., Zhang, S., Zhu, G., Zhang, Y., et al. (2020). Disruption of Atg7-dependent autophagy causes electromotility disturbances, outer hair cell loss, and deafness in mice. *Cell Death Dis.* 11:913. doi: 10.1038/s41419-020-03110-8

Zhou, Z., Yan, H., Liu, Y., Xiao, D., Li, W., Wang, Q., et al. (2018). Adipose-derived stem-cell-implanted poly(ϵ-caprolactone)/chitosan scaffold improves bladder regeneration in a rat model. *Regen. Med.* 13, 331–342. doi: 10.2217/rme-2017-0120

3

A Porcine Congenital Single-Sided Deafness Model, Its Population Statistics and Degenerative Changes

Wei Ren[1,2,3,4†], Cong Xu[1,2,3,4†], Fan-jun Zheng[1,2,3,4†], Ting-ting Lin[5†], Peng Jin[6], Yue Zhang[1,2,3,4], Wei-wei Guo[1,2,3,4], Chuan-hong Liu[5], Xiao-yang Zhou[5], Lu-lu Wang[5], Yong Wang[5‡], Hui Zhao[1,2,3,4‡] and Shi-ming Yang[1,2,34‡]*

[1] College of Otolaryngology Head and Neck Surgery, Chinese PLA General Hospital, Beijing, China, [2] National Clinical Research Center for Otolaryngologic Diseases, Beijing, China, [3] Key Lab of Hearing Science, Ministry of Education, Beijing, China, [4] Beijing Key Lab of Hearing Impairment for Prevention and Treatment, Beijing, China, [5] Department of Laboratory Animal Science, College of Basic Medical Science, Army Medical University, Chongqing, China, [6] Department of Human Genetics, Emory University School of Medicine, Atlanta, GA, United States

***Correspondence:**
Shi-ming Yang
shm_yang@163.com

[†] These authors have contributed equally to this work and share first authorship

[‡] These authors have contributed equally to this work and shared co-corresponding authorship

Objective: To describe and study the population statistics, hearing phenotype, and pathological changes of a porcine congenital single-sided deafness (CSSD) pedigree.

Methods: Click auditory brainstem response (ABR), full-frequency ABR, and distortion product otoacoustic emission (DPOAE) were used to assess the hearing phenotype of the strain. Tympanogram was used to assess the middle ear function since birth. Celloidin embedding–hematoxylin–eosin (CE-HE) stain and scanning electron microscopy (SEM) were used to study the pathological changes of cochlear microstructures. Chi-square analysis was used to analyze the relation between hearing loss and other phenotypes.

Results: The mating mood of CSSD with CSSD was most efficient in breeding-targeted CSSD phenotype (47.62%), and the prevalence of CSSD reached 46.67% till the fifth generation, where 42.22% were bilateral hearing loss (BHL) and 9.00% were normal hearing (NH) individuals. Hearing loss was proved to have no relation with coat color ($P = 0.0841 > 0.05$) and gender ($P = 0.4621 > 0.05$) by chi-square analysis. The deaf side of CSSD offspring in the fifth generation had no relation with that of their maternal parent ($P = 0.2387 > 0.05$). All individuals in this strain exhibited congenital severe to profound sensorineural hearing loss with no malformation and dysfunction of the middle ear. The good hearing ear of CSSD stayed stable over age. The deaf side of CSSD and BHL presented cochlear and saccular degeneration, and the hair cell exhibited malformation since birth and degenerated from the apex to base turn through time. The pathology in BHL cochlea progressed more rapidly than CSSD and till P30, the hair cell had been totally gone. The stria vascularis (SV) was normal since birth and degenerated through time and finally exhibited disorganization of three layers of cells.

Conclusion: This inbred porcine strain exhibited high and stable prevalence of CSSD, which highly resembled human non-syndromic CSSD disease. This porcine model could be used to further explore the etiology of CSSD and serve as an ideal tool for the studies of the effects of single-sided hearing deprivation on neural, cognitive, and behavioral developments and the benefits brought by CI in CSSD individuals.

Keywords: porcine (pig) model, deafness (hearing loss), ABR, DPOAE, pathology

INTRODUCTION

Single-sided deafness (SSD) is defined as profound sensorineural hearing loss in one ear with normal hearing on the opposite side. Congenital SSD (CSSD) often refers to those who did not pass the newborn hearing screening and then was diagnosed with unilateral hearing loss at birth. The incidence of sensorineural hearing loss is estimated to be 1.86 per 1,000 newborns; among them, 30–40% are unilateral (Fitzpatrick et al., 2017; van Wieringen et al., 2019), but the CSSD incidence varies among researches because populations of different ages were involved, for children from 6 to 19 years old. The estimated CSSD incidence was 0.7–0.8% (Ross et al., 2010). In South Korea, the prevalence of unilateral hearing loss (UHL) was 9.31%, among which SSD accounts for 5.98% in the population over 12 years old; however, the prevalence of CSSD was unknown (Jun et al., 2015). Because of the lack of international or regional epidemiology study, the incidence of CSSD needs further study.

Many researches had tried to find etiologies of CSSD; some identified risk factors including cochlear nerve deficiency (Clemmens et al., 2013; Lipschitz et al., 2020), congenital cytomegalovirus, congenital inner ear malformation, and bacterial and viral meningitis, but more than 60% of the CSSD was of unknown etiology (van Wieringen et al., 2019). Unilateral and asymmetric hearing loss in a Waardenburg Syndrome Type 2 (WS2) pedigree was reported to be caused by mutation in *KIT* or *KITLG*. KIT-KITLG signaling pathway and MITF were suggested to mutually interact in the migration process of melanocyte from the neural crest to stria vascularis (SV). The imbalanced migration and distribution of melanocytes in stria vascularis might be cause by laterality of hearing (Zazo Seco et al., 2015; Hamadah et al., 2019). However, most cases of CSSD in the clinic were non-syndromic and reported to be not correlated with other systematic symptoms.

Besides the high prevalence, CSSD gradually catches clinical physicians' attention because there is a growing consensus that children with CSSD have difficulties in hearing, sound localization, and speech discrimination in a noisy environment. Moreover, CSSD also negatively influences the neural, cognitive, language, and behavioral development and neural network working mode (Kral and O'Donoghue, 2010; Maslin et al., 2013). A large body of researches had verified that the duration and onset of UHL were two key factors impacting the auditory restoration, cochlear implantation (CI) outcome, and cortical speech processing (Kral and Sharma, 2012; Vanderauwera et al., 2020). Clinically, CI might be the only way to restore hearing, but its outcome was controversial. A longitudinal study on six CSSD infants with early CI intervention demonstrated that children showed beneficial outcome in language, cognitive development, and hearing compared to non-implanted samples (Sangen et al., 2019). Additionally, early CI also helped avoid neurofunctional dominance of the hearing ear and would be beneficial to the neural development in deaf cats (Kral et al., 2013), indicating early CI in the case of CSSD.

Few clinical studies separate CSSD and acquired SSD (ASSD) in neuroscientific studies. The mechanism and the onset of neural reorganization might differ for CSSD and ASSD, which should be considered (Vanderauwera et al., 2020). Since clinical research cannot reveal the pathological changes and the observation period for brain and auditory system function changes is usually very long, researchers referred to animal models. Different species of animals have been used in the hearing research, including chinchilla, white deaf cats, mouse, rat, and dogs with pigmentation. Various methods have been tried to establish the SSD animal model, among which cochlear ablation is the most often used method. Other ways include local injection of high dose of gentamicin or neomycin at early postnatal days to cochleae to mimic the congenital SSD to study the impact of monaural hearing deprivation on cortical development or deafening adult animals by injecting drugs to the middle ear, posterior canal, and round window at different ages to study the impact of sudden SSD on the trajectory changes of cortical, visual, and language processing (Jakob et al., 2016; Liu et al., 2016; Banakis Hartl et al., 2019; Cheng et al., 2019; Ding et al., 2020; Zhong et al., 2020).

The postnatal artificial SSD could not fully mimic congenital SSD, and the influence of CSSD on cortical development started long before birth. How imbalanced sound signal input affect the neural development since embryo stage remains unknown because of lack of CSSD animal models. Congenitally unilateral deaf animal was reported in feline, canine, and horse breeds. Various reports indicated that deaf white cats (DWCs) were feline homolog of the human Waardenburg syndrome (Schwartz and Higa, 2009) because the coat and iris pigmentation were correlated with hearing loss and several relating genes had been reported, like *PAX3* and *KIT* (David et al., 2014). Andrej Kral explored how unilateral hearing affected cortex plastic reorganizations by using two CSSD white cats (Kral et al., 2013), which were reported and inbred by Heid et al. (1998). However, the CSSD phenotype in cats were very rare and appeared occasionally instead of in a stable inheritable mood. Congenital canine deafness had been observed since 1896 in over 80 breeds (Strain, 2004) with prevalence from 7.0 to 32.3%, among which CSSD accounted for 1.3–18.0% (Rak and Distl, 2005). Most studies focused on the Dalmatian because of its highest hearing loss prevalence with approximately 5.3–8% bilateral deafness and 9.4–21.9% CSSD, or total of up to 30% affected (Strain et al., 1992; Rak and Distl, 2005). Hearing loss in most not all canine breeds also positively corelated with blue iris and coat color pigmentation (Famula et al., 1996). However, the inheritance mechanism and responsible genes remained unknown; the most possible candidate genes include merle (M locus) and *piebald* allele (S locus), which would influence the differentiation and migration of melanocytes in cochlea during embryogenesis (Rak and Distl, 2005). People also failed to inbreed a canine pedigree with stable prevalence of deafness.

Although the above animal breeds exhibited high prevalence of deafness, however, few hereditary components were verified, and nearly all breeds mentioned above mimicked the phenotypes of human Waardenburg syndrome, and the prevalence of CSSD was casual. In our study, we describe a naturally occurring inbred CSSD porcine pedigree with high and stable prevalence of CSSD. Auditory physiology and pathological presentations of different hearing phenotypes in the pedigree were uniform and detailly described.

MATERIALS AND METHODS

Animals

All animals of this inbred Bama Miniature pig pedigree in this paper were provided by the Laboratory Animal Science Center of College of Basic Medicine in the Army Military Medical University (Chongqing, China). All animals were raised in a standard pathogen-free (SPF) condition. Animals younger than P30 were raised in the Lab Animal Science Center in Chongqing; animals older than P30 were delivered to the Lab Animal Center of PLA General Hospital and being raised in the same condition.

Anesthesia

In all experiments, animals were anesthetized with 1.5–5% Isoflurane in 3:3 mixture of oxygen and air by inhalation machine for animal use (Medical Supplies and Services Int. Ltd., United Kingdom). Animals were put on a heating pad to maintain body temperature.

Click-ABR Tests

Since the full-frequency auditory brainstem response (ABR) measurement would take about 2 h, pigs under P30 could not stand long-time anesthesia. Therefore, for the pigs younger than P30, only stimulus click (Intelligent Smart EP, United States) was used to diagnose if they are deaf or not, and hearing tests were taken in a small sound-proof booth for animals. Insert ear plug was put into the ear and sealed the external ear canal. Ground electrode was put at the apex nasi; reference electrodes were put in the ipsilateral earlobes of the tested ear, and recording electrode was inserted into the skin of the calvaria along the centerline. The click ABR tests only took about 10 min each pig.

Full-Frequency ABR Tests

Tucker Davis Technology RZ6 (TDT RZ6) was used to apply the full-frequency—from 1 to 32 kHz—ABR tests in pigs over P30. Electrodes were put in the same position as described above. This part of hearing tests was conducted in a standard soundproof booth. A loudspeaker (MF1 2356) was put in the external ear canal meatus, and the untested ear was masked by a calibrated 60 dB SPL white noise by an inserted earphone.

Tympanogram and DPOAE

Titan (Interacoustics, Denmark) was used to do the tympanometry, which reflected the function of the middle ear, and parameters like middle ear compliance and volume were obtained. Distortion product otoacoustic emission (DPOAE) from 500 to 10 kHz was measured by Titan, which reflected the function of outer hair cells (OHCs). Tympanogram and DPOAE were tested at P1 and P30.

Celloidin Embedding–Hematoxylin–Eosin Stain and Scanning Electron Microscopy

Celloidin embedding–hematoxylin–eosin (CE-HE) stained cochlear section and scanning electron microscopy (SEM) samples were made following the methods described in our previous studies. Animals were sacrificed in accordance with the Care and Use of the of Laboratory Animals. Cochleae were extracted from the temporal bone within 10 min and being postfixed in 4% paraformaldehyde (CE-HE) or 2.5% glutaraldehyde (SEM) at 4°C overnight. After being washed in 1% phosphate-buffered saline (PBS) three times, each time 10 min, the cochleae were shifted into 10% ethylenediaminetetraacetic acid (EDTA) solution for decalcification at room temperature (RT) on a shaker for 2 weeks.

For the HE staining, the cochleae were dehydrated using graded ethanol (50, 75, 80, 90, 95, and 100%), and each grade would take 2 days. Then, the cochleae were transferred into graded celloidin (2.5, 5.0, 8, 10, 12.5, and 15%), and each grade would take 7 days at RT. The cochleae were embedded in 15% celloidin in a glass dish for 1–2 months until solidification. Then, the samples were put into 75% ethanol for 2–5 days. The samples were sectioned (15 μm each slice) using a freezing microtome (Leica CM1900) and stained with hematoxylin and eosin. The images were visualized and captured using a Leica DMI3000 microscope. For the SEM, decalcified cochleae were postfixed for 2 h in 1% osmium at RT, dehydrated in graded ethanol (50, 75, 80, 90, 95, and 100%), treated with 2% tannin acid for 2 h at RT, rinsed in 0.24 M phosphate buffer (pH 7.4) for 2 h at RT, and dried in a critical point dryer (HCP-2, Hitachi) using liquid CO_2. Fixed sections were then coated using a sputter coater and examined under a scanning electron microscope (Helios Nanolab 600i).

Spiral Ganglion Cell Counting of the CE-HE Specimen

Spiral ganglion cells were counted, using the CE-HE specimen under a Leica DMI3000 light microscope. Two cochleae of each hearing phenotype were counted; 12 serial sections, 15 μm each specimen, containing modiolus were counted, and for each specimen, apical, middle, and basal turn ganglion cells were counted, respectively. The mean values of the above 12 serial sections at each turn were used as the ganglion cell counting number for each turn. Only the cells with clear nucleus were counted (**Supplementary Figure 4**).

Statistical Methods

Prism GraphPad 8.4.0 was used to do statistical analysis and draw graphs. Chi-squared test was used to analyze the possible hereditary mode. Unpaired *t*-test was used to analyze the statistical difference of tympanogram parameters and ganglion cell counting number of each group compared to the normal group, and $P < 0.05$ was considered as statistical different.

Ethical Approval

All experiments and procedures in this paper were conducted under the guidelines of the Care and Use of the Laboratory Animals and approved by both the Animal Ethics Committee of Army Military Medical University and PLA General Hospital.

RESULTS

The Mating Strategy of CSSDs Female With Male Individuals Was the Most Efficient Way to Stabilize the Pedigree

Figure 1A showed the family tree of this porcine pedigree. In order to explore the most efficient mating strategy to build up the pedigree and rise the occurrence rate of targeted hearing phenotypes, we tried different mating strategies to explore the phenotype distribution. Under the strategy of CSSD mating with CSSD individuals, the number of targeted CSSD phenotype reached the highest with 20 CSSDs accounting for 47.62% of all offspring, 19 bilateral hearing losses (BHLs) for 45.24%, and only 3 NHs for 7.14%. When CSSD was mating with BHL, the BHLs (10/71.42%) exceeded CSSDs (2/14.28%) by four times. In the mode of BHL mating with BHL, BHL equaled NHs by six (37.5%), and four CSSDs accounted for about 25% of the offspring. When BHL mated with NH, 31 (88.57%) were NHs with only 3 (8.57%) CSSDs and 1 (2.86%) BHL (**Figure 1E** and **Table 1**). Thereafter, we mated CSSDs in the fourth generation to get the fifth generation for further studies.

Coat Color Had No Relation With Hearing Loss

The wild type Bama Miniature pig exhibited "liang-tou-wu" coat color with black head; the hip and tail and other parts of the body exhibited white color. However, in this pedigree, we observed pigmentation. The association between hearing loss and coat color in the fifth generation is listed in **Table 2**. In NHs, normal and abnormal coat color accounted for 50 and 50%, respectively, while in hearing loss populations, the proportions were 7.5 and 92.5%, respectively. As shown by chi-square with Yates correction (chi-square = 2.984, df = 1), no correlation between hearing loss and coat color changes was observed ($P = 0.0841 > 0.05$). Since we also observed the pigmentation of iris color in some pigs within the pedigree, we listed the iris color change in different phenotypes (**Table 3**). As shown by chi-square with Yates correction (chi-square = 0.003, df = 1), $p = 0.9568 > 0.05$, hearing loss had no correlation with iris pigmentation.

The Deaf Side of CSSDs Had No Relation With Gender

In the whole pedigree, female individuals amounted to 16 (55.17%) and male individuals 13 (44.83%). The ratio of female CSSD to male CSSD was 1.23:1, close to 1. In the whole pedigree, L-CSSDs amounted to 14 (48.28%), and R-CSSD totaled 15 (51.72%) with a ratio of 1:1.07. Among female CSSDs, the proportion of L-CSSD (9/56.25%) to R-CSSD (7/43.75%) was

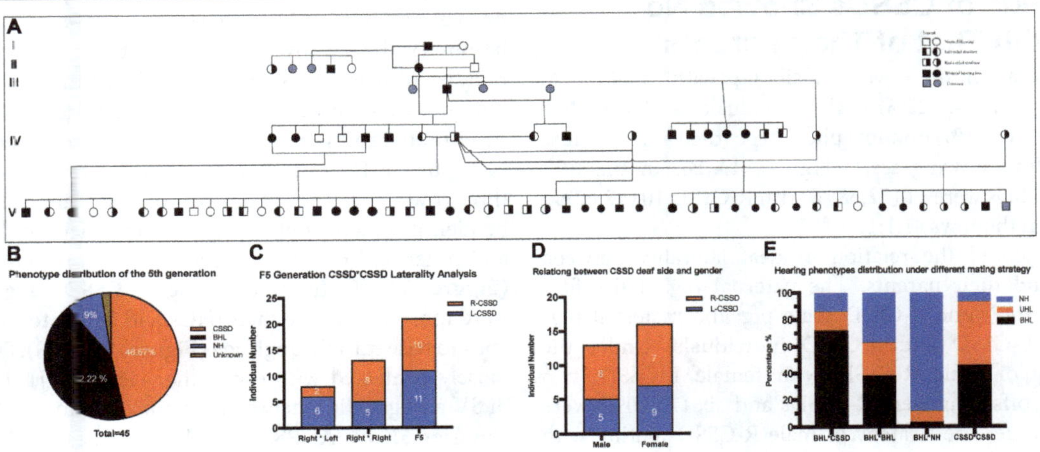

FIGURE 1 | Congenital single-sided deafness (CSSD) pedigree information. **(A)** CSSD pedigree information that consists five generations. **(B)** Hearing phenotype distribution of the fifth generation with different mating strategies. **(C)** Relation of the deaf side between CSSD siblings and their parents. **(D)** Relation between CSSD deaf side and gender. **(E)** Hearing phenotypes distribution under a different mating strategy. L-CSSD, left-sided CSSD; R-CSSD, right-sided CSSD. The individuals with red star in Panel **(A)** were selected to do whole genome resequencing.

TABLE 1 | The Iris color and the hearing loss in 5th Generation.

Hearing Phenotype	BHL	L-CSSD	R-CSSD	NH	Total
Bilateral Normal	2	0	1	3	6
Light color (left)	2	1	1	0	4
Light color (right)	2	2	2	1	7
Bilateral pigmentation	13	7	5	0	25
Total	19	10	9	4	42

The pig with unknown hearing phenotype was excluded from counting. The iris color of one L-CSSD and one R-CSSD individuals were not recorded and excluded from analyzing.

TABLE 2 | The phenotype distribution under different mating strategies in 4th generation.

Father	Mother	BHL(%)	CSSD(%)	NH(%)	Individuals
BHL	NH (6)	1(2.86)	3(8.57)	31(88.57)	35
BHL	BHL (3)	6(37.5)	4(25)	6(37.5)	16
CSSD	CSSD (6)	19(45.24)	20(47.62)	3(7.14)	42
BHL	CSSD (2)	10(71.42)	2(14.28)	2(14.28)	14

TABLE 3 | The Coat color and the hearing loss of 5th Generation.

Hearing Phenotype	BHL	L-CSSD	R-CSSD	NH	Total
Normal	2	1	0	2	5
Abnormal	17	10	10	2	39
Total	19	11	10	4	44

The individual of unknown hearing phenotype was excluded from analysis.

1.28:1. Among the male CSSDs, the proportion of L-CSSD (5/38.46%) to R-CSSD (8/71.54%) was 1:1.6 (**Figure 1D**). As shown by the Fisher's exact test, no correlation between gender and the deaf side of CSSD was observed ($P = 0.4621 > 0.05$).

The Deaf Side of CSSDs Showed No Relation With That of Their Parents

In the fifth generation, there were 45 siblings with 21 (46.67%) CSSD individuals, 19 (42.22%) BHL individuals, 4 (9.00%) NH individuals, and 1 (2.11%) unknow phenotype (died at P1 because of diarrhea before hearing test) (**Figures 1A,B**). In the fifth generation, L-CSSDs were 11 (52.38%) with R-CSSD 10 (47.62%); the ratio between them was 1.1:1.

Next, we explored the relation of deaf laterality between the offspring and their parents. The paternal pig of the fifth generation was the same R-CSSD male pig; the maternal pigs included both L-CSSD and R-CSSD individuals. Under the mating strategy of Male R-CSSD with female L-CSSD, two (25.00%) of the offspring were R-CSSDs and six (75.00%) were L-CSSDs, and under the strategy of male R-CSSD mating with female R-CSSD, eight (61.64%) of the offspring were R-CSSDs and five (48.36%) were L-CSSDs (**Figure 1C**). As shown by the Yates corrected chi-square test, no correlation between the maternal deaf side and that of the offspring was observed ($P = 0.2387 > 0.05$).

CSSD and BHL Presented Congenital Profound Sensorineural Hearing Loss

bilateral hearing losses and the deaf ear of CSSD individuals presented congenital profound sensorineural hearing loss since P1 through all frequencies. NHs and the normal side of CSSD showed normal hearing thresholds since P1 through all frequencies (**Figure 2A**). The hearing function of both normal and deaf side of CSSD remained stable through age, the normal side would not be influenced by the loss of hearing of the contralateral side (**Figure 2B**). In NHs and the normal side of CSSD ABR waveforms, seven waves could be evoked by each stimulus from click to 32 kHz (**Figure 2C** and **Supplementary Figure 1**). In BHLs and the deaf side of CSSD, no waveform of clear response could be identified at all frequencies (**Figure 2D** and **Supplementary Figure 1**).

The volume and the compliance of middle ear showed that there were no statistical differences among each group of the CSSD pedigree (**Figures 3A,C,E,G,J**). This result excluded the possibility of middle ear malfunction. The OHCs of NHs and normal sides of CSSDs responded well to the DPOAE stimuli from 500 to 10kHz (**Figures 3B,D**), while the OHCs of BHLs and the deaf sides of CSSDs showed no responses to the DPOAE stimuli (**Figures 3F,H**) with signal-to-noise ratio (SNR) largely below six (**Figure 3I**). The above result demonstrated the loss of function of OHCs since birth.

Deaf Sides of CSSD HCs Degenerated From Apex to Base Turn and Through Age

Figure 4A shows the three-dimensional (3D) reconstruction images of the cochleae in the pedigree. All cochleae exhibited normal structures: the coiling of the cochlear capsule reached three and a half turns, three semicanals were mutually vertical to each other. The cross-section showed the microstructure of the cochlear (**Supplementary Figure 4**). **Figure 4B** showed the overall pathologic changes of HCs in the pedigree. In NH and normal side of CSSD cochleae, four rows of hair cells could be observed (one row of IHCs and three rows of OHCs). The bundles of hair cells shaped like "V". In the deaf side of CSSD, bundles were fused and HCs disorganized. For BHLs, HCs deteriorated and were replaced by non-hearing sensory cells.

In the CE-HE images of NHs and the normal sides of CSSDs, three rows of OHCs and one row of inner hair cells (IHCs) could be identified, and supporting cells like Dieter cells, Hansen cell, and inner and outer pillar cells closely and regularly arranged (**Figures 5A–H**). In the deaf sides of CSSDs (**Figure 5I**), OHCs were more vulnerable than IHCs and began to degenerate from apex to base turn through age (**Figures 6A,D,G**). Supporting cells loosely contacted with each other (**Figure 5J**) the morphology of SV and ganglion neurons remained normal in CE-HE images (**Figures 5K,L**). At P8, few cells were observed on the BM at apex turn, loss of OHCs could be observed on the mid turn and nearly normal BM on the base turn (**Supplementary Figures 2B, F, and J**). Till P80, no HCs could be observed on the BM; sporadic IHCs and OHCs with fused bundles scattered along middle and basal BM (**Figures 6A–I**). At P154, no HCs were

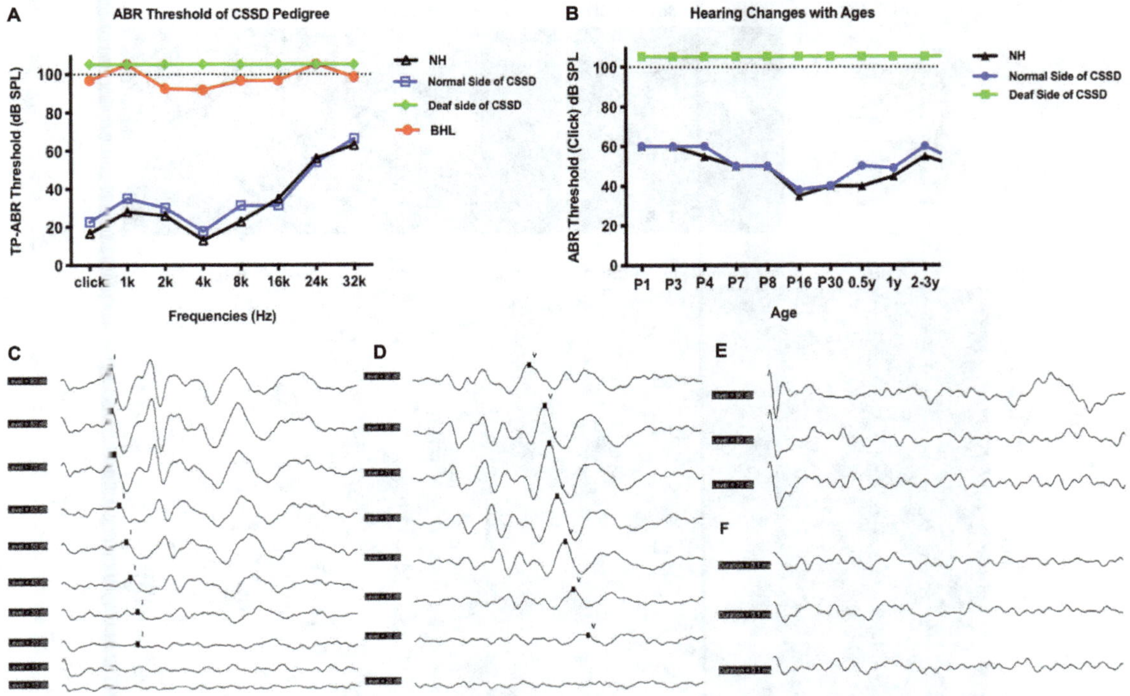

FIGURE 2 | Auditory brainstem response (ABR) hearing thresholds of congenital single-sided deafness (CSSD) pedigree. **(A)** ABR thresholds from 1 to 32 kHz of different hearing phenotypes in CSSD pedigree. **(B)** ABR thresholds changes in the CSSD individuals with age compared to NHs. In Panels **(A,B)**, the threshold of 105 dB SPL means that no response was evoked at 100 dB SPL. **(C,D)** ABR waves triggered by click of NH and normal side of CSSD, respectively. **(E,F)** ABR waves triggered by click of deaf side of CSSD and bilateral hearing loss (BHL), respectively.

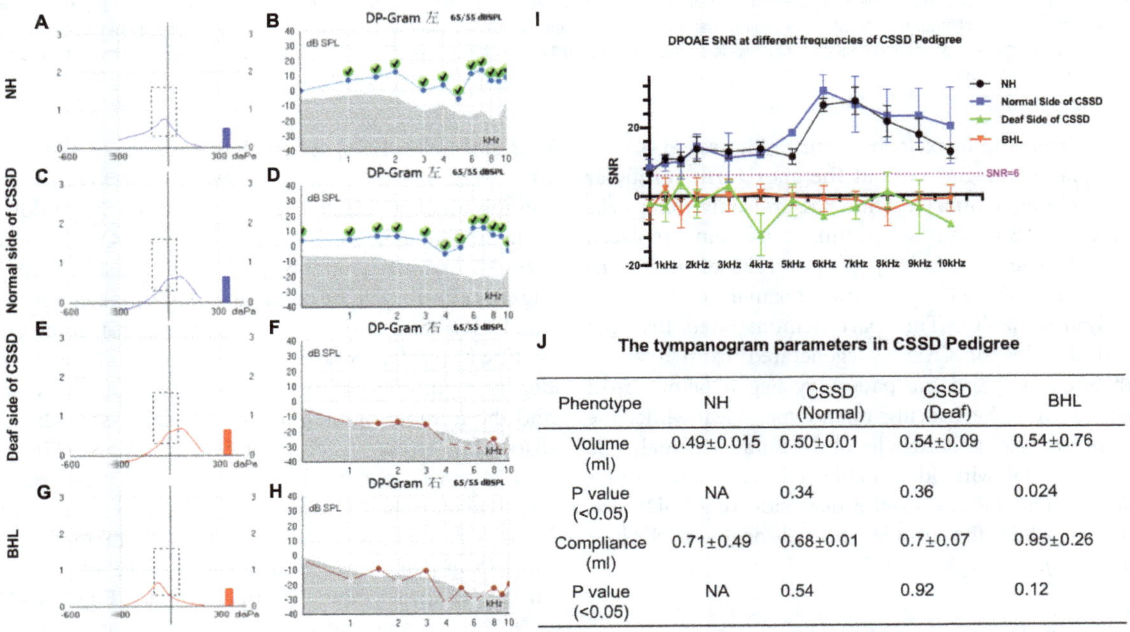

J The tympanogram parameters in CSSD Pedigree

Phenotype	NH	CSSD (Normal)	CSSD (Deaf)	BHL
Volume (ml)	0.49±0.015	0.50±0.01	0.54±0.09	0.54±0.76
P value (<0.05)	NA	0.34	0.36	0.024
Compliance (ml)	0.71±0.49	0.68±0.01	0.7±0.07	0.95±0.26
P value (<0.05)	NA	0.54	0.92	0.12

FIGURE 3 | Distortion product otoacoustic emission (DPOAE) and tympanogram results of congenital single-sided deafness (CSSD) pedigree. **(A,C,E,G)** Tympanograms of each phenotype in the CSSD pedigree. **(B,D,F,H)** DPOAE results from 500 Hz to 10 kHz of each phenotype in the CSSD pedigree at P1. **(I)** Signal-to-noise ratio (SNR) of DPOAE at each frequency of different phenotypes in the pedigree. **(J)** Volume and compliance of the middle ear of each phenotype in the pedigree ($P < 0.05$ was considered statistical different).

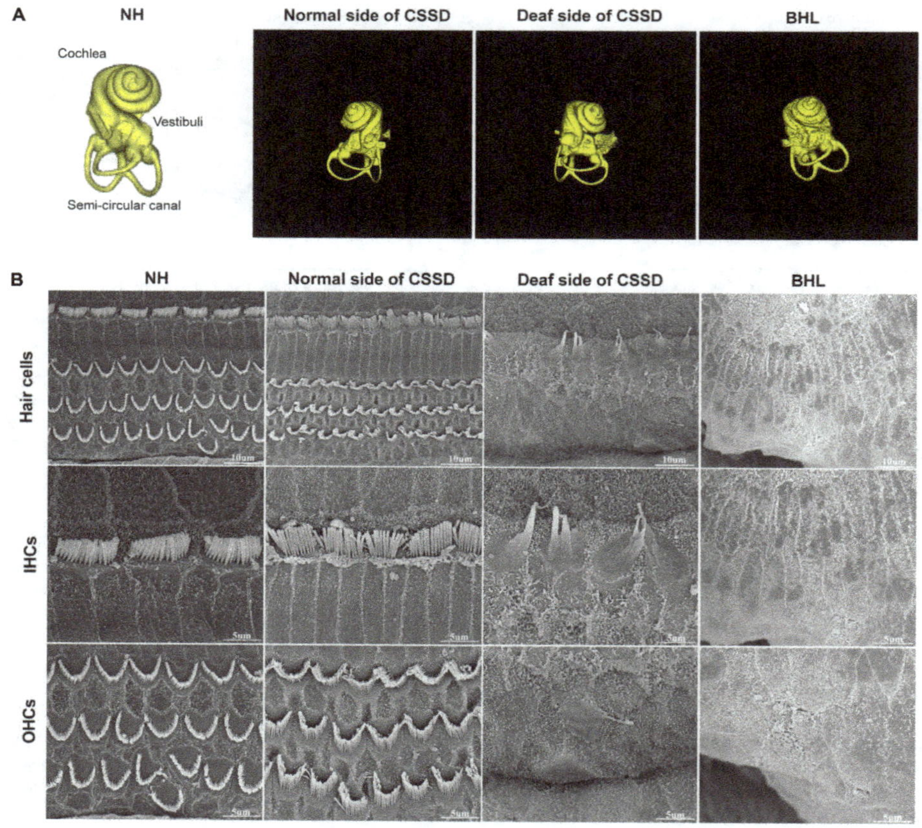

FIGURE 4 | The micro-CT images of different phenotypes and SEM images of inner ear basal membrane in congenital single-sided deafness (CSSD) pedigree. **(A)** Micro-CT 3D reconstructions of the cochlear of different phenotypes in the pedigree. **(B)** SEM images of the inner ear basal membrane. The normal side of a CSSD individual exhibited normal inner ear structure as the normal hearing (NH) ones. Sporadic inner hair cells (IHCs) with fused hair bundles were left in the deaf side of CSSD individuals. In bilateral hearing loss (BHL) individuals, nearly no hair cells were left on the basal membrane. The BHL showed more severe deterioration compared to the deaf side of CSSD.

left on the BM from the apex to base turn (**Figures 6J–L**). At P180, fibers replaced the BM cells at the apex turn; vestibular membrane was closely contacted with BM and only pillar cells were left under the BM with supporting cells being replaced (**Figures 6M–O**). The morphology of hair cells of each turn in good hearing ear of CSSDs remained normal at P80, P154 and P180 (**Figures 6P–T**). This part demonstrated that the BM of the deaf sides of CSSDs degenerated from apex to base turn through age, and the pathology began before birth which coincided with the hearing phenotype. Meanwhile, the morphology of saccule and utricle of NH and normal side of CSSD were normal with identifiable hair cells and otolith (**Figures 7A–H**). The saccule of the deaf side of CSSDs was identical to NH while the utricle showed degenerated hair cells (**Figures 7I–L**).

BHL Showed the Same, but More Severe and Rapid Pathological Progress as CSSD

In the BHLs, HC damage progressed the same trajectory as the CSSD but was more severe and rapid compared to the deaf sides of CSSDs. At P1, hair bundles of IHCs at the apex turn were fused; OHCs were disorganized with fused bundles (**Supplementary Figures 4A–C**). IHCs of the middle and basal turn exhibited nearly normal structure. OHCs at the middle were disorganized and began to degenerate (**Supplementary Figures 4D–F**). Till the basal turn, IHCs were in normal structure and OHCs were in three lines, but bundles in some OHCs began to fuse (**Supplementary Figures 4G–I**). At P8, hair cells had degenerated, only the nucleus of inner hair cell could be seen and the number of supporting cells decreased which led to the disruption of the structure of organ of Corti (**Figures 5M–P**). At P14, no HCs could be observed at the apex turn; few HCs could be identified at the middle turn, and nearly all HCs could be seen at the basal turn; bundles of remained HCs were all fused (**Supplementary Figures 4J–L**). Till P30, no HCs were left on the basal membrane (**Supplementary Figures 4M–O**). The SEM results coincided with the CE-HE results (**Supplementary Figure 3**). The above results demonstrated that BHL follow the same pathological trajectory as CSSD, but the progress was more rapid and severe. As for the vestibular organ, the structure of saccule remained normal and the hair cells in utricle had degenerated since P1 (**Figures 7M,O–Q**).

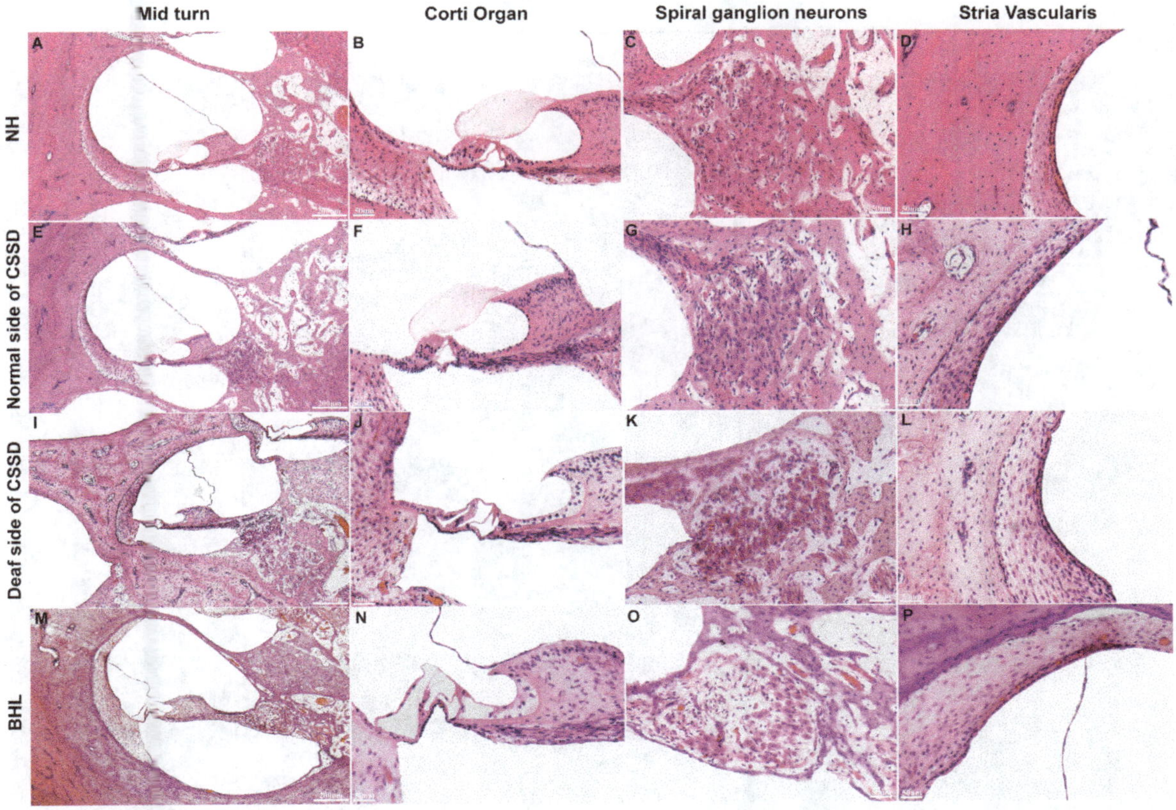

FIGURE 5 | Celloidin embedding–hematoxylin–eosin (CE-HE) results of each phenotype at P8 in congenital single-sided deafness (CSSD) pedigree. Panels **(A,E,I,M)** were at low magnification (10×). The other images are all high magnification (40×). Panels **(B,F,J,N)** showed fine structure of the organ of Corti; panels **(J,N)** showed loss of hair cells in the deaf side of CSSD and bilateral hearing loss (BHL) individuals. Panels **(C,G,K,O)** showed the changes in spiral ganglion cells. Panels **(D,H,L,P)** showed the fine structure of stria vascularis of each phenotype in CSSD pedigree.

The Ganglion Cells of NS of CSSD Declined Compared to the NH

The ganglion cells counting number of BHL, deaf side (DS) of CSSD, and normal side (NS) of CSSD showed significant decrease compared to the NH and that of the DS of CSSD showed significant reduction compared to the NS of CSSD; about 76, 77.4, and 66.7% cells survived for BHL, DS of CSSD, and NS of CSSD, respectively (**Figure 8A** and **Table 4**). For the apex turn, both DS and NS of CSSD showed sever cell loss and significantly less than the BHL individuals (**Figure 8B**). For the mid and base turn, ganglion cells of BHL and DS of CSSD both showed clear reduction compared to the NS of CSSD and NH individuals (**Figures 8C,D**). The loss of ganglion cells was most severe in the apex turn for the CSSD individuals and was equal for each turn for BHL individuals.

The Stria Vascularis Degenerated Over Time After Birth

In NHs, the stria vascularis was composed of three layers of cells: marginal cells, intermediate cells, and basal cells. Marginal cells (star) were tightly attached with each other by gap junction. Basal cells (triangle) were interconnected to separate stria vascularis (SV) from spiral ligament. Intermediate cells (circle) were in the middle layer in which melanin spots could be identified. At P30, the SV of NHs and both sides of CSSDs were of normal structure, while in BHL, SV was disorganized with only two layers of cells survived (**Figure 9**).

The structure of SV degenerated through age. In DS of CSSD cochleae, the structure of SV remained normal till P154. At P180, the SV was dominated by marginal and basal cells; the intermediate cells declined (**Supplementary Figure 6**). In BHL cochleae, the structure of the SV remained normal. However, at P30, the cells in SV were disorganized, the same as that in DS of CSSD. The SV was composed of two layers of cells, mainly marginal and basal cells; intermediate cells were hardly identified (**Supplementary Figure 7**).

DISCUSSION

Sensorineural hearing loss is often induced by loss of HCs and SGNs in the inner ear cochlea (Liu et al., 2016, 2019; Zhong et al., 2020). HC transduces the sound waves into electric signals (Qi et al., 2019), while SGNs transfer these signals into the auditory cortex to have the hearing ability (Guo et al., 2016,

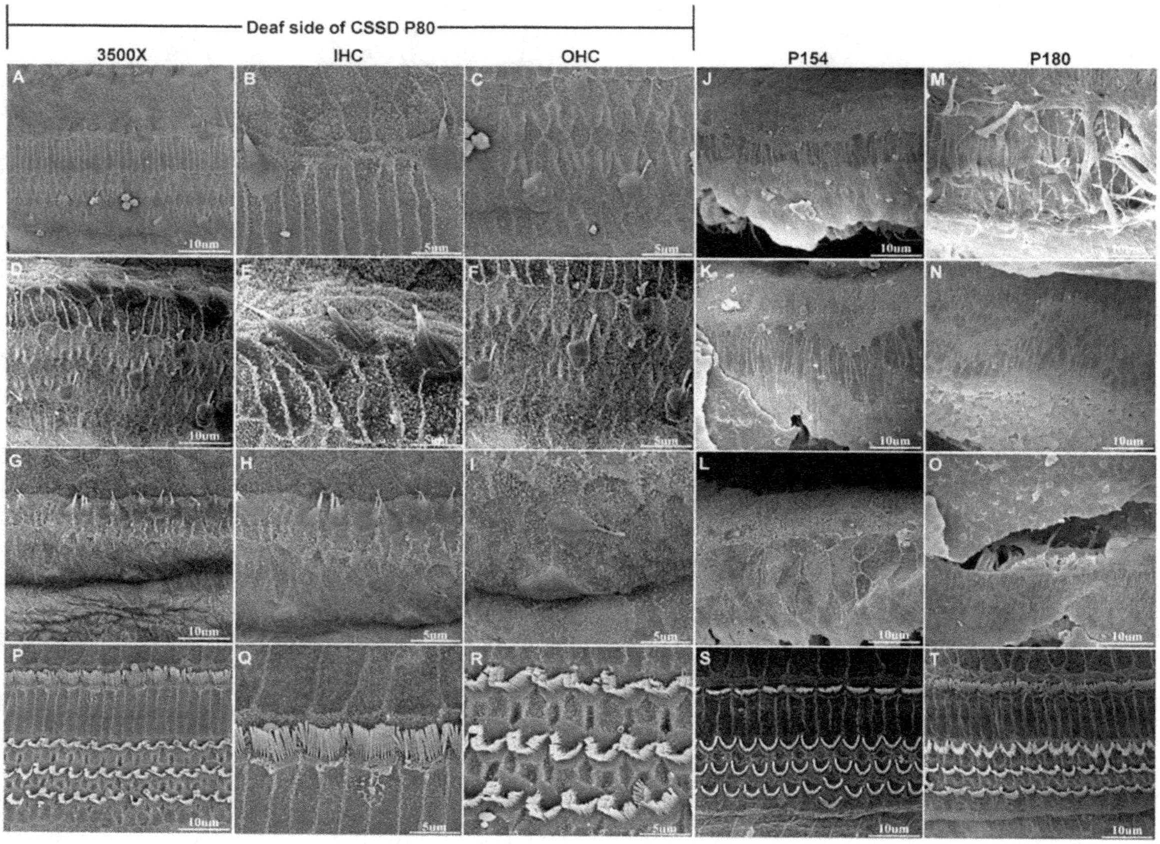

FIGURE 6 | SEM results of the basal membrane of congenital single-sided deafness (CSSD) individual at different ages. **(A–I)** Images of the basal membrane of the deaf side of CSSD at P80. **(A,D,G)** Images from the apex to base turn of the cochlear at low magnification of 3,500×. **(B–I)** Inner (IHCs) and outer hair cells (OHCs) from the apex to base turn at high magnification of 8,000×. **(J–L)** Images of the basal membrane from the apex to base turn of the deaf side of the CSSD at P154; nearly no HCs were left on P154. **(M–O)** Images of the basal membrane from the apex to base turn of the deaf side of the CSSD at P180. **(P–T)** Images of the contralateral normal side of the CSSD individuals at P80, P154, and P180, respectively.

2019, 2020). WHO reported that 466 million people are suffering with hearing loss worldwide, caused by genetic factors, infectious diseases, chronic cochlear infections, aging, exposure to noise, and ototoxic drugs (He et al., 2017, 2020; Tan et al., 2019; Zhang et al., 2020; Zhou et al., 2020; Lv et al., 2021); for children from 6 to 19 years old, the estimated CSSD incidence was 0.7–0.8%. In this study, we reported a Bama miniature pedigree with high and stable incidence of CSSD, which reached 46.67% under the mating mode of paternal CSSD with maternal CSSD pigs. In this pedigree, the hearing phenotypes varies with different mating modes. Under the mode of CSSD with CSSD, BHLs accounted for 42.22% and CSSDs 46.67%, NHs only accounted for 9%. All hearing loss individuals exhibited congenital severe sensorineural hearing loss with no ABR, DPOAE response being evoked since birth. Normal tympanogram had excluded the possibility of middle ear diseases. Phenotype of hearing loss was not correlated with coat color and gender. The deaf side of the offspring had no relation with the deaf side of their parents. This porcine model highly mimicked the human non-syndromic CSSD in the clinics and might be the first porcine model with high and stable presence rate of CSSD being reported in the world.

In this paper, we studied the auditory physiology and pathology of BHL, NH, and CSSD individuals. All the deaf cochlear showed cochlear-saccular degeneration, also known as Scheibe dysplasia. For DS of CSSD and BHL, bundles of hair cells were fused since birth, and hair cells degenerated from the apex to the base. In the CSSDs, sporadic hair cells could be identified at P80–P154; basal membrane was replaced by the epithelial cells. BHL showed the same but more severe and rapid pathological process; till P30, hair cells and supporting cells could not be identified, and the Reissner's membrane tensely attached to the basal membrane. Only sporadic pillar cells survived. The ipsilateral saccule exhibited degenerated hair cells since P1. Scheibe dysplasia had been proven to occur in many animals, like deaf white cats, Dalmatian dogs, waltzing guinea pigs, and mice (Schuknecht et al., 2009). It was reported that the Scheibe dysplasia occurred in 70% of the cases with hereditary hearing loss (Lalwani et al., 1997), which is similar to our porcine deafness model. The structure of SV in the deaf ear degenerated through age; in CSSDs, the disorganization could be observed from P180, while in BHL, the malformation presented no later than P30. This time course corresponds to that of the hair cells, which might

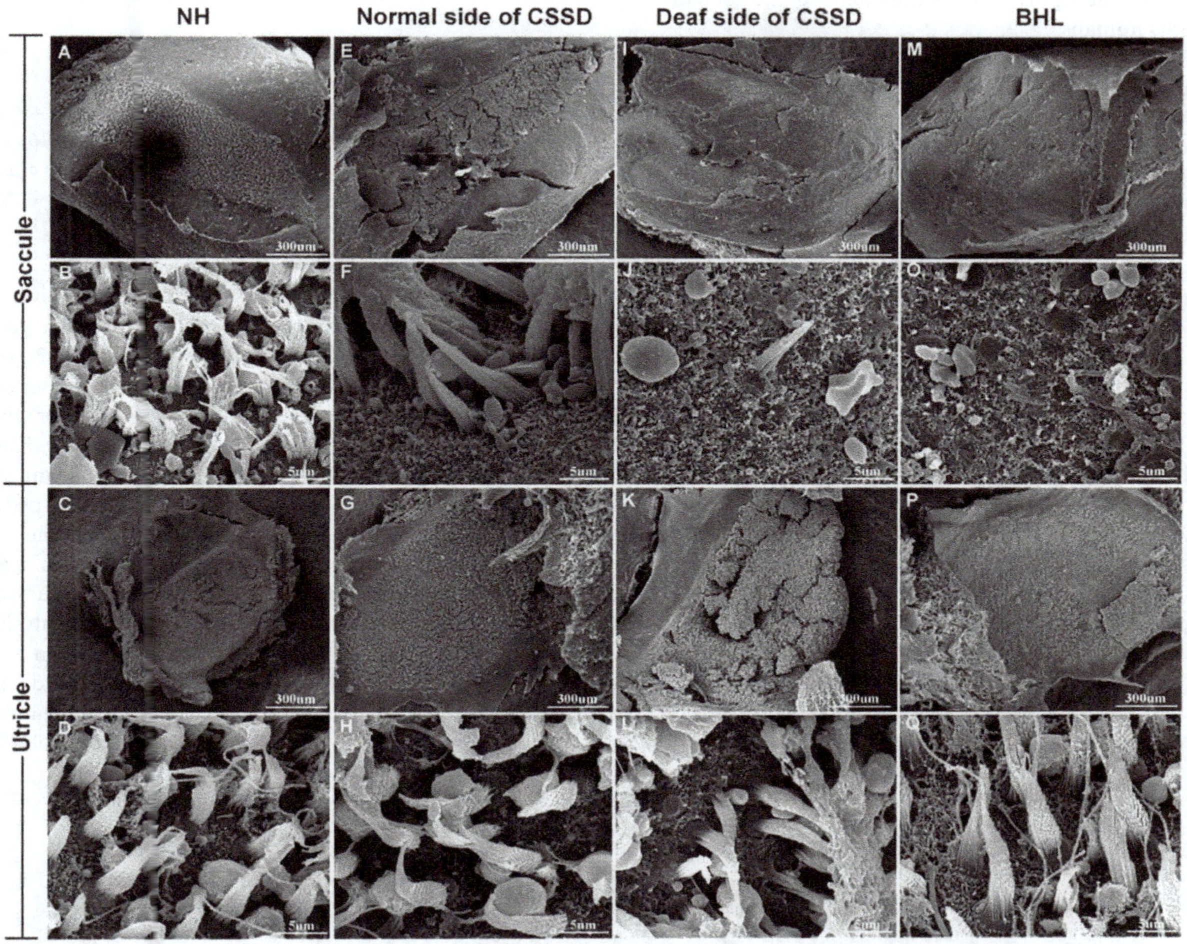

FIGURE 7 | The SEM of saccule and utricle in congenital single-sided deafness (CSSD) pedigree. The deaf side of the CSSD individuals exhibited congenital hair cell malformation with sporadic hair cells left and infused hair bundles. The bilateral hearing loss (BHL) individuals showed the same pathology changes as the deaf side of the CSSD. The microstructure of the utricles in different phenotypes of CSSD pedigree were normal with normal hair cells and otolith.

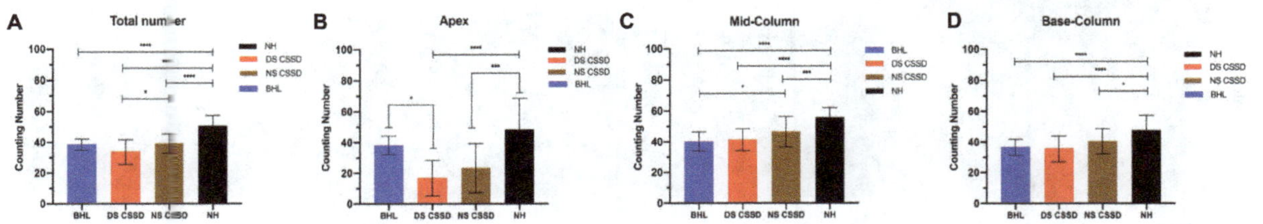

FIGURE 8 | Spiral ganglion cell counting at P30. **(A)** Averaged total ganglion cell counting number from the apex to base turns. **(B)** Ganglion cell counting number in the apex turn in different hearing phenotypes. **(C)** Ganglion cell counting number in the mid turn in different hearing phenotypes. **(D)** Ganglion cell counting number in the base turn in different hearing phenotypes. $^{*}p < 0.05$, $^{**}p < 0.01$, $^{***}p < 0.001$, $^{****}p < 0.0001$.

indicate that the SV degeneration was not responsible for hearing loss but an outcome of hearing loss.

For the degeneration of the ganglion, we did not have enough animals at different ages, so we chose pigs of P30 to analyze the pathology of ganglion cells. The pathology changes in each hearing phenotype were uniform in this pedigree. Significant reduction in ganglion cells of BHL, DS of CSSD, and NS of CSSD could be observed. For BHL, the ganglion cell counting number at each turn decreased proportionately. For CSSDs, the most severe cell loss occurred in the apex turn; we should also pay attention to the NS of CSSD; the total ganglion cell number and that of each turn showed a significant reduction compared to NHs. This might indicate that the NS of CSSD might be vulnerable to factors that harm hearing like noise exposure and ototoxic drugs. This coincided with the reports of the vulnerability of the good hearing ear of CSSD humans.

We also calculated the ganglion cell number of BHL at P1; the mean value for apex, mid, and base turns were 38.20 ± 6.14 (P = 0.19 > 0.05), 40.77 ± 7.70 (P < 0.0001), 36.00 ± 6.06 (P < 0.0001), respectively, and the counting number at apex turn showed no significant differences with the NH. Meanwhile, the organ of Corti was flattened, and supporting cells vanished at the apex and mid turn at P1 (**Supplementary Figure 3**). For the deaf side of the CSSD individuals, the counting number of ganglion cells for the apex, mid, and base turns were 11.7 ± 8.47 (P < 0.001), 37.10 ± 7.16 (P < 0.001), and 31.30 ± 7.14 (P < 0.001), while the organ of Corti showed the same but much milder pathological changes. These results indicated that the pathological process started from embryogenesis period because the degeneration of supporting cells occurring after the acquired hearing loss would trigger the neural degeneration at least 2 weeks away (Schuknecht et al., 2009).

Congenital single deafness of white cat, dog, and horse were also reported. In canine deafness model, the unilateral deafness reached 21.9% in a Dalmatian breed; however, no underlying inheritance mechanism and contributing genes had been revealed. Hayward et al. (2020) did genome-wide association study (GWAS) in 3 canine breeds; 14 suggestive genes were found, but none was located in the areas causing WS as their symptoms indicated, and the genes had no overlap between species. Numerous labs had tried to find the causative gene for the natural deafness canine breeds; only few identified genes, like SOX10 (Hansen et al., 2010) and OTOF (Cargill, 2004), were verified genes responsible for human deafness. One possibility of why no suggestive genes overlap among breeds was that they were caused by different underlying genetic mechanisms. Therefore, GWAS could not be done by using samples from different pedigree; the best would be samples from one inbred pedigree.

TABLE 4 | The ganglion cell counting number of each hearing phenotype at P30.

Hearing Phenotype	BHL	NS-CSSD	DS-CSSD	NH
Apex	38.2 ± 6.14	23.40 ± 15.99	16.83 ± 11.56	48.53 ± 19.99
Mid	40.18 ± 6.31	46.58 ± 9.76	41.31 ± 7.09	55.71 ± 6.43
Base	36.59 ± 6.35	40.46 ± 8.25	35.54 ± 8.38	47.67 ± 9.60
Total	38.50 ± 3.71	39.21 ± 6.27	33.76 ± 8.06	50.65 ± 6.75

In our study, we also could not locate the possible responsible genes and identify the possible inheritance mode. Neither a dominant nor a recessive simple Mendelian mode of transmission could be proven by chi-square analysis in the pedigree. Gender differences and correlation between coat color and hearing loss were also not observed; the deaf side of CSSD had no relation with their parent deaf side. Unlike the DWC, deaf dog, and horse breeds with pigmentation and iris color change,

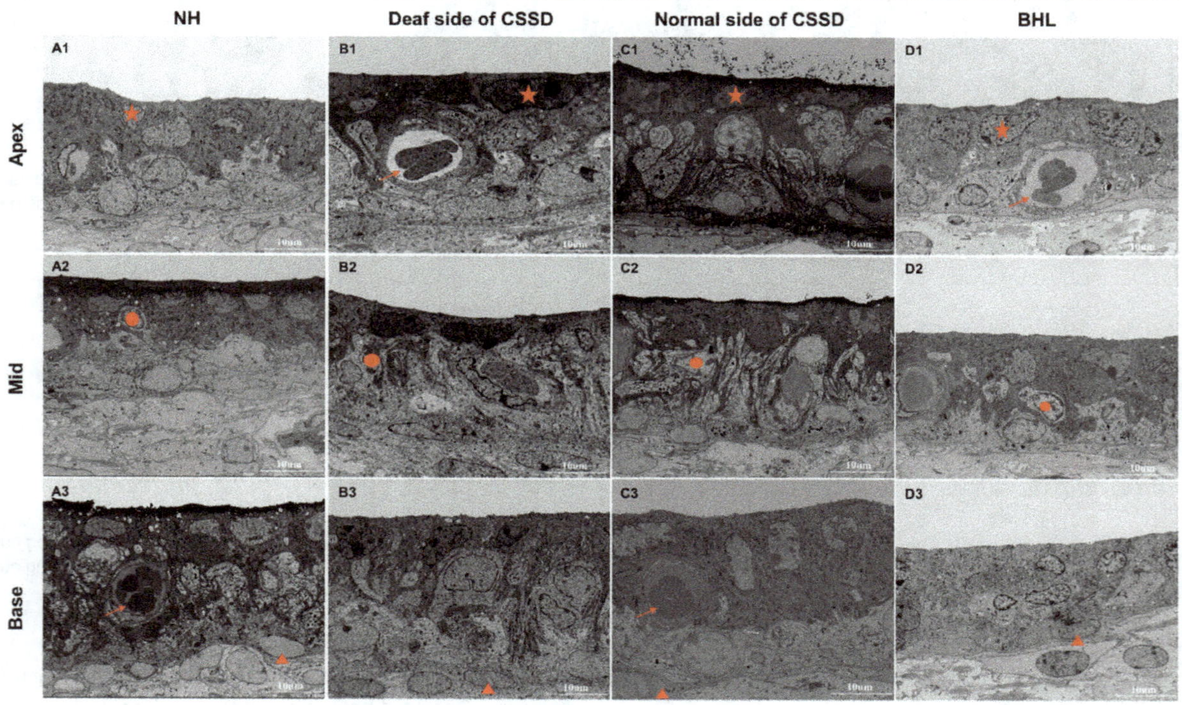

FIGURE 9 | The SEM images of stria vascularis of different phenotypes in the congenital single-sided deafness (CSSD) pedigree at P30. **(A1-D3)** SEM images of the stria vascularis at different turns of normal hearing (NH), deaf side (DS) of CSSD, normal side (NS) of CSSD, and bilateral hearing loss (BHL). For NH, three layers of cell could be clearly identified: star, marginal cell; circle, intermediate cell; and triangle, basal cell. Vascularis (arrow) could be seen in some parts of the stria vascularis. No obvious malformation was observed in the DS of CSSD and NS of CSSD; in the BHL, the three layers of cells were disorganized, and the stria vascularis was thinner than normal.

the pigs in our pedigree presented non-syndromic hearing loss and cochlear–saccular degeneration, much more like the CSSD patients in the clinics. However, the interaction between genes associated with coat and iris color and that with hearing loss was unclear. The genetics underlying the disease is very complex. One reason is that the matching rate of human and animal deafness causative genes is very low; the other is that other elements also affect the expression, like epigenetic and transcriptomic factors.

Pigs have become an important biomedical model due to their genetic, anatomical, and physiological similarities with human, as well as the short generation interval (~114 days), broad availability, large litter size, and lower ethical concern because they are of a kind of food source instead of companion animals like cats and dogs (Schook et al., 2015). Pigs are also widely used in the studies of human disease, like cancer model, cardiovascular model, metabolic and gastrointestinal disease model, and hearing loss model. The porcine cochlear anatomy and auditory physiology highly resembles that of human. Unlike rodent lab animals, the porcine cochlear size was much larger and may provide us a chance to study the hearing and behavioral changes and the cortex reorganization brought by CI in CSSD animals, which might give an indication on the time window of CI in CSSD children clinically. Additionally, the pig's brain resembles that of the human in size, anatomy, development, and importantly the cognitive development (Lind et al., 2007; Elmore et al., 2012). This would allow us to gain a deep insight into the impact of CSSD on cognitive development and the benefits of CI. In the future study, pedigree genome and RNA sequencing will be combined to find the possible responsible genes that might reveal the mechanism underlying CSSD.

ETHICS STATEMENT

The animal study was reviewed and approved by The Ethics Committee of Chinese PLA General Hospital. Written informed consent was obtained from the owners for the participation of their animals in this study.

AUTHOR CONTRIBUTIONS

WR, CX, and F-JZ mainly conducted the experiment. YW, T-TL, C-HL, X-YZ and L-LW were mainly in charge of breeding and maintaining the pedigree. YZ mainly conducted the SEM and TEM studies and illustrated the relative results. HZ, W-WG, PJ, and S-MY designed the study, analyzed the data, and illustrated the pathology results of the pedigree. WR finally contributed to the writing of the article, figures, and tables. All authors contributed to the article and approved the submitted version.

ACKNOWLEDGMENTS

We would like to thank the Center for Biological Imaging (CBI), Institute of Biophysics, Chinese Academy of Sciences for the scanning electric microscope (SEM, Helios Nanolab 600i), and we are grateful to Professor Xi-Xia Li for her help in making SEM samples and analyzing images.

SUPPLEMENTARY MATERIAL

Supplementary Figure 1 | The ABR waveform at different frequencies of the CSSD individual. Panels **(A–H)** showed that on the deaf side of CSSD, no ABR response was triggered from 1kHz to 32kHz. Panels **(I–P)** showed that on the normal side of CSSD, identifiable ABR responses were evoked and the thresholds of each frequency showed no statistical difference from the NHs.

Supplementary Figure 2 | The CH-HE images of CSSD cochlear at P8. Panels **(A–D)** showed the images of the apex turn, no sensory cells were left on the BM. Panels **(E–H)** showed the images of the mid turn, supporting cells and OHCs were left on the BM. Panels **(I–L)** showed the images of the base turn, IHC, OHC and supporting cells all could be seen. Panels **(M–P)** showed the contralateral normal side of CSSD individual.

Supplementary Figure 3 | The CH-HE images of BHL cochlear at P30. Panels **(A–D)** showed the images of the apex turn, no sensory cells were left on the BM. Panels **(E–H)** showed the images of the mid turn, only supporting cells were left on the BM. Panels **(I–L)** showed the images of the base turn, sporadic hair cells could be seen at P30.

Supplementary Figure 4 | CH-HE image of 4X magnification. This specimen was the normal side of CSSD with mid-modiolus, the coiling of the cochlear adequate reached three turns. In the above image, 1 and 2 were apex turn, 3 and 4 were mid turn, 5 and 6 were base turn and 7 was the very end of the basal membrane named hook region. Ganglion cells inside the black dotted line were counted.

Supplementary Figure 5 | SEM results of Basal membrane of BHL individual at different ages. Panels **(A,D,G)** were images of P1 BHL cochlear from apex to base turn at low magnification of 3500X. Panels **(B–I)** showed the inner and outer hair cells at higher magnification of 8000X. Panels **(J–L)** were images of P14 BHL cochlear from apex to base turn. Panels **(M–O)** showed images of P30 BHL cochlear from apex to base turn.

Supplementary Figure 6 | TEM results of Stria Vascularis of the deaf side of CSSD individuals at different ages. Panels **(A1-3,B1-3,C1-3)** were stria vascularis images of DS of CSSD from apex to base turn at magnification of 3500X at P80, P154, and P180. The structure of stria vascularis at P80 was nearly normal, three layers of cells (marginal, intermediate and basal cells) were identified. Till P180, the stria vascularis remained nearly normal.

Supplementary Figure 7 | TEM results of Stria Vascularis of BHL individual at different ages. Panels **(A1–3,B1–3,C1–3)** were stria vascularis images of P1 BHL cochlear from apex to base turn at magnification of 3500X at P1, P14, and P30. The structure of stria vascularis at P1 was normal, three layers of cells (marginal, intermediate and basal cells) were identified. Till P30, the stria vascularis was disorganized, only the marginal cells could be clearly identified.

REFERENCES

Banakis Hartl, R. M., Greene, N. T., Benichoux, V., Dondzillo, A., Brown, A. D., and Tollin, D. J. (2019). Establishing an Animal Model of Single-Sided Deafness in Chinchilla lanigera. *Otolaryngol. Head Neck. Surg.* 161, 1004–1011. doi: 10.1177/0194599819877649

Cargill, E. J. (2004). *Development of a Multiplexing Strategy for Whole Genome Scans of the Domestic Dog and Analysis of Hereditary Deafness in the Dalmatian.* Nebraska: University of Nebraska-Lincoln.

Cheng, C., Wang, Y., Guo, L., Lu, X., Zhu, W., Muhammad, W., et al. (2019). Age-related transcriptome changes in Sox2+ supporting cells in the mouse cochlea. *Stem. Cell. Res. Ther.* 10:365.

Clemmens, C. S., Guidi, J., Caroff, A., Cohn, S. J., Brant, J. A., Laury, A. M., et al. (2013). Unilateral Cochlear Nerve Deficiency in Children. *Otolaryngol. Head Neck. Surg.* 149, 318–325.

David, V. A., Menotti-Raymond, M., Wallace, A. C., Roelke, M., Kehler, J., Leighty, R., et al. (2014). Endogenous Retrovirus Insertion in theKITOncogene DeterminesWhiteandWhite spottingin Domestic Cats. *G3* 4, 1881–1891. doi: 10.1534/g3.114.013425

Ding, Y., Meng, W., Kong, W., He, Z., and Chai, R. (2020). The Role of FoxG1 in the Inner Ear. *Front. Cell. Dev. Biol.* 8:614954. doi: 10.3389/fcell.2020.614954

Elmore, M. R., Dilger, R. N., and Johnson, R. W. (2012). Place and direction learning in a spatial T-maze task by neonatal piglets. *Anim. Cogn.* 15, 667–676. doi: 10.1007/s10071-012-0495-9

Famula, T. R., Oberbauer, A. M., and Sousa, C. A. (1996). A threshold model analysis of deafness in Dalmatians. *Mamm. Genome* 7, 650–653. doi: 10.1007/s003359900199

Fitzpatrick, E. M., Al-Essa, R. S., Whittingham, J., and Fitzpatrick, J. (2017). Characteristics of children with unilateral hearing loss. *Int. J. Audiol.* 56, 819–828.

Guo, R., Ma, X., Liao, M., Liu, Y., Hu, Y., Qian, X., et al. (2019). Development and Application of Cochlear Implant-Based Electric-Acoustic Stimulation of Spiral Ganglion Neurons. *ACS Biomater. Sci. Eng.* 5, 6735–6741. doi: 10.1021/acsbiomaterials.9b01265

Guo, R., Xiao, M., Zhao, W., Zhou, S., Hu, Y., Liao, M., et al. (2020). *2D Ti 3C 2T x Mxene Couples Electrical Stimulation to Promote Proliferation and Neural Differentiation of Neural Stem Cells.* Available online at: https://ssrn.com/abstract=3677369 (accessed September 23, 2020).

Guo, R., Zhang, S., Xiao, M., Qian, F., He, Z., Li, D., et al. (2016). Accelerating bioelectric functional development of neural stem cells by graphene coupling: implications for neural interfacing with conductive materials. *Biomaterials* 106, 193–204. doi: 10.1016/j.biomaterials.2016.08.019

Hamadah, I., Chisti, M., Haider, M., Al Dosssari, H., Alhumaidan, R., Meyer, B. F., et al. (2019). A novel KIT mutation in a family with expanded syndrome of piebaldism. *JAAD Case. Rep.* 5, 627–631. doi: 10.1016/j.jdcr.2019.01.021

Hansen, I. A., Sommerlad, S., McRae, A. F., McDonald, B., Johnstone, I., Cuttell, L., et al. (2010). Congenital Sensorineural Deafness in Australian Stumpy-Tail Cattle Dogs Is an Autosomal Recessive Trait That Maps to CFA10. *PLoS One* 5:e13364. doi: 10.1371/journal.pone.0013364

Hayward, J. J., Kelly-Smith, M., Boyko, A. R., Burmeister, L., De Risio, L., Mellersh, C., et al. (2020). A genome-wide association study of deafness in three canine breeds. *PLoS One* 15:e0232900. doi: 10.1371/journal.pone.0232900

He, Z., Guo, L., Shu, Y., Fang, Q., Zhou, H., Liu, Y., et al. (2017). Autophagy protects auditory hair cells against neomycin-induced damage. *Autophagy* 13, 1884–1904. doi: 10.1080/15548627.2017.1359449

He, Z. H., Zou, S. Y., Li, M., Liao, F. L., Wu, X., Sun, H. Y., et al. (2020). The nuclear transcription factor FoxG1 affects the sensitivity of mimetic aging hair cells to inflammation by regulating autophagy pathways. *Redox. Biol.* 28:101364. doi: 10.1016/j.redox.2019.101364

Heid, S., Hartmann, R., and Klinke, R. (1998). A model for prelingual deafness, the congenitally deaf white cat - Population statistics and degenerative changes. *Hear. Res.* 115, 101–112. doi: 10.1016/s0378-5955(97)00182-2

Jakob, T. F., Rosskothen-Kuhl, N., and Illing, R. B. (2016). Induction of single-sided deafness in the newborn rat and its consequence for cochlear nucleus volume development. *Hear. Res.* 333, 210–215. doi: 10.1016/j.heares.2015.09.002

Jun, H. J., Hwang, S. Y., Lee, S. H., Lee, J. E., Song, J. J., and Chae, S. (2015). The prevalence of hearing loss in South Korea: data from a population-based study. *Laryngoscope* 125, 690–694. doi: 10.1002/lary.24913

Kral, A., Heid, S., Hubka, P., and Tillein, J. (2013). Unilateral hearing during development: hemispheric specificity in plastic reorganizations. *Front. Syst. Neurosci.* 7:93. doi: 10.3389/fnsys.2013.00093 eCollection 2013.

Kral, A., and O'Donoghue, G. M. (2010). Medical Progress: profound Deafness in Childhood. *N. Engl. J. Med.* 363, 1438–1450. doi: 10.1056/nejmra0911225

Kral, A., and Sharma, A. (2012). Developmental neuroplasticity after cochlear implantation. *Trends Neurosci.* 35, 111–122. doi: 10.1016/j.tins.2011.09.004

Lalwani, A. K., Linthicum, F. H., Wilcox, E. R., and Moore, J. K. A. (1997). five-generation family with late-onset progressive hereditary hearing impairment due to cochleo-saccular degeneration. *Audiol. nd Neuro. Otol.* 2, 139–154. doi: 10.1159/000259237

Lind, N. M., Moustgaard, A., Jelsing, J., Vajta, G., Cumming, P., and Hansen, A. K. (2007). The use of pigs in neuroscience: modeling brain disorders. *Neurosci. Biobehav. Rev.* 31, 728–751. doi: 10.1016/j.neubiorev.2007.02.003

Lipschitz, N., Kohlberg, G. D., Scott, M., and Greinwald, J. H. (2020). Imaging findings in pediatric single-sided deafness and asymmetric hearing loss. *Laryngoscope* 130, 1007–1010. doi: 10.1002/lary.28095

Liu, L., Chen, Y., Qi, J., Zhang, Y., He, Y., Ni, W., et al. (2016). Wnt activation protects against neomycin-induced hair cell damage in the mouse cochlea. *Cell. Death Dis.* 7:e2136. doi: 10.1038/cddis.2016.35

Liu, Y., Qi, J., Chen, X., Tang, M., Chu, C., Zhu, W., et al. (2019). Critical role of spectrin in hearing development and deafness. *Sci. Adv.* 5:eaav7803. doi: 10.1126/sciadv.aav7803

Lv, J., Fu, X., Li, Y., Hong, G., Li, P., Lin, J., et al. (2021). Deletion of Kcnj16 in Mice Does Not Alter Auditory Function. *Front. Cell. Dev. Biol.* 9:630361. doi: 10.3389/fcell.2021.630361

Maslin, M. R. D., Munro, K. J., and El-Deredy, W. (2013). Evidence for multiple mechanisms of cortical plasticity: a study of humans with late-onset profound unilateral deafness. *Clin. Neurophysiol.* 124, 1414–1421. doi: 10.1016/j.clinph.2012.12.052

Qi, J., Liu, Y., Chu, C., Chen, X., Zhu, W., Shu, Y., et al. (2019). A cytoskeleton structure revealed by super-resolution fluorescence imaging in inner ear hair cells. *Cell. Discov.* 5:12.

Rak, S. G., and Distl, O. (2005). Congenital sensorineural deafness in dogs: a molecular genetic approach toward unravelling the responsible genes. *Vet. J.* 169, 188–196. doi: 10.1016/j.tvjl.2004.01.015

Ross, D. S., Visser, S. N., Holstrum, W. J., Qin, T. L., and Kenneson, A. (2010). Highly Variable Population-Based Prevalence Rates of Unilateral Hearing Loss After the Application of Common Case Definitions. *Ear Hear.* 31, 126–133. doi: 10.1097/aud.0b013e3181bb69db

Sangen, A., Dierckx, A., Boudewyns, A., Dhooge, I., Offeciers, E., Wouters, J., et al. (2019). Longitudinal linguistic outcomes of toddlers with congenital single-sided deafness-Six with and twelve without cochlear implant and nineteen normal hearing peers. *Clin. Otolaryngol.* 44, 671–676. doi: 10.1111/coa.13347

Schook, L. B., Collares, T. V., Darfour-Oduro, K. A., De, A. K., Rund, L. A., Schachtschneider, K. M., et al. (2015). Unraveling the swine genome: implications for human health. *Annu. Rev. Anim. Biosci.* 3, 219–244. doi: 10.1146/annurev-animal-022114-110815

Schuknecht, H. F., Icarashi, M., and Gacek, R. R. (2009). The Pathological Types of Cochleo-Saccular Degeneration. *Acta Oto. Laryngol.* 59, 154–170. doi: 10.3109/00016486509124549

Schwartz, I. R., and Higa, J. F. (2009). Correlated Studies of the Ear and Brainstem in the Deaf White Cat: changes in the Spiral Ganglion and the Medial Superior Olivary Nucleus. *Acta Oto. Laryngol.* 93, 9–18. doi: 10.3109/00016488209130847

Strain, G. M. (2004). Deafness prevalence and pigmentation and gender associations in dog breeds at risk. *Vet. J.* 167, 23–32. doi: 10.1016/s1090-0233(03)00104-7

Strain, G. M., Kearney, M. T., Gignac, I. J., Levesque, D. C., Nelson, H. J., Tedford, B. L., et al. (1992). Brainstem auditory-evoked potential assessment of congenital deafness in Dalmatians: associations with phenotypic markers. *J. Vet. Intern. Med.* 6, 175–182. doi: 10.1111/j.1939-1676.1992.tb00333.x

Tan, F., Chu, C., Qi, J., Li, W., You, D., Li, K., et al. (2019). AAV-ie enables safe and efficient gene transfer to inner ear cells. *Nat. Commun.* 10: 3733.

van Wieringen, A., Boudewyns, A., Sangen, A., Wouters, J., and Desloovere, C. (2019). Unilateral congenital hearing loss in children: challenges and potentials. *Hear. Res.* 372, 29–41. doi: 10.1016/j.heares.2018.01.010

Vanderauwera, J., Hellemans, E., and Verhaert, N. (2020). Research Insights on Neural Effects of Auditory Deprivation and Restoration in Unilateral Hearing Loss: a Systematic Review. *J Clin Med* 9:812. doi: 10.3390/jcm9030812

Zazo Seco, C., Serrão de Castro, L., van, N. J. W., Morín, M., Jhangiani, S., and Verver, E. J. J. (2015). *Am. J. Hum. Genet.* 97, 647–660.

Zhang, S., Zhang, Y., Dong, Y., Guo, L., Zhang, Z., Shao, B., et al. (2020). Knockdown of Foxg1 in supporting cells increases the trans-differentiation of supporting cells into hair cells in the neonatal mouse cochlea. *Cell. Mol. Life Sci.* 77, 1401–1419. doi: 10.1007/s00018-019-03291-2

Zhong, Z., Fu, X., Li, H., Chen, J., Wang, M., Gao, S., et al. (2020). Citicoline Protects Auditory Hair Cells Against Neomycin-Induced Damage. *Front. Cell. Dev. Biol.* 8:712. doi: 10.3389/fcell.2020.00712

Zhou, H., Qian, X., Xu, N., Zhang, S., Zhu, G., Zhang, Y., et al. (2020). Disruption of Atg7-dependent autophagy causes electromotility disturbances, outer hair cell loss, and deafness in mice. *Cell. Death Dis.* 11:913.

4

SMPX Deficiency Causes Stereocilia Degeneration and Progressive Hearing Loss in CBA/CaJ Mice

Hailong Tu[1], Aizhen Zhang[1], Xiaolong Fu[1], Shiqi Xu[2], Xiaohui Bai[3], Haibo Wang[1,3]* and Jiangang Gao[1]**

[1] School of Life Sciences, Shandong Provincial ENT Hospital, Shandong University, Jinan, China, [2] University of Edinburgh Institute, Zhejiang University School of Medicine, Zhejiang University, Haining, China, [3] Otolaryngology-Head and Neck Surgery, Shandong Provincial ENT Hospital, Jinan, China

***Correspondence:**
Haibo Wang
whboto11@163.com
Xiaolong Fu
fuxiaolongshifan@163.com
Jiangang Gao
jggao@sdu.edu.cn

The small muscle protein, x-linked (*SMPX*) encodes a small protein containing 88 amino acids. Malfunction of this protein can cause a sex-linked non-syndromic hearing loss, named X-linked deafness 4 (DFNX4). Herein, we reported a point mutation and a frameshift mutation in two Chinese families who developed gradual hearing loss with age. To explore the impaired sites in the hearing system and the mechanism of DFNX4, we established and validated an *Smpx* null mouse model using CRISPR-Cas9. By analyzing auditory brainstem response (ABR), male *Smpx* null mice showed a progressive hearing loss starting from high frequency at the 3rd month. Hearing loss in female mice was milder and occurred later compared to male mice, which was very similar to human beings. Through morphological analyses of mice cochleas, we found the hair cell bundles progressively degenerated from the shortest row. Cellular edema occurred at the end phase of stereocilia degeneration, followed by cell death. By transfecting exogenous fluorescent Smpx into living hair cells, Smpx was observed to be expressed in stereocilia. Through noise exposure, it was shown that Smpx might participate in maintaining hair cell bundles. This *Smpx* knock-out mouse might be used as a suitable model to explore the pathology of DFNX4.

Keywords: *Smpx*, hair cell, stereocilia degeneration, hearing loss, CRISPR-Cas9

INTRODUCTION

X-linked hearing loss accounts for 1-2% of all non-syndromic hearing loss (NSHL) cases. Five genes have been associated with x-linked hearing loss, including *PRPS1* for DFNX1, *POU3F4* for DFNX2, *SMPX* for DFNX4, *AIFM1* for DFNX5, and *COL4A6* for DFNX6[1].

Mechanosensory hair cells are primary cells that enable mammals to sense and distinguish sounds with different frequencies and intensities. These cells, located in the inner ear, can convert sound-induced vibrations into electrical signals. The inner ear can responds to sound-induced vibrations of less than a nanometer and amplify signals by more than 100-fold, and has a wide dynamic range of hearing enabling humans to perceive frequencies from 20 Hz to 20 kHz (Schwander et al., 2010).

[1] https://hereditaryhearingloss.org/xlinked-genes

Outer hair cell (OHC) bundles are composed of 3 height-ranked rows of stereocilia-modified microvilli packed with highly cross-linked actin filaments (Corvino et al., 2018; Qi et al., 2019, 2020; Liu Y. et al., 2019). Stereocilia, the mechanosensory actin protrusions on the roof of hair cells, play a key role in the transduction of vibration into electrical signals (Wang et al., 2017; Zhu et al., 2018; Cheng et al., 2021). The vertebrate auditory epithelium displays a gradient of stereocilia bundles, the lengths of which is inversely proportional to the frequency of the sound detected by cell tuning (Crawford and Fettiplace, 1985; Howard and Hudspeth, 1987; Ricci et al., 2000; Petit and Richardson, 2009). Although stereocilia are extremely sensitive to mechanical vibration, they are easily damaged by over-stimulation, such as sharp, high-decibel sound. Stereocilia share many construction principles with the formations of actin in microvilli and filopodia. Yet, the length of different stereocilia in a single cell can vary from 1 up to 120 μm and persist for a lifetime. The length of stereocilia may be influenced by actin treadmills, cross-links within the actin core, plasma membrane tension, interstereociliary links, and the overlying extracellular structures (Manor and Kachar, 2008). The turnover of actin filaments has long been considered to reflect the treadmilling behavior. However, recently studies have identified that filament barbed ends can be used for both elongation and disassembly (Romet-Lemonne and Jégou, 2021). In these aspects, actin binding proteins (ABP) are the main parts regulating the length of stereocilia.

The small muscle protein, x-linked (*SMPX*), originally identified and mapped in Patzak et al. (1999) is abundantly expressed in heart and skeletal muscles. In muscle cells (Kemp et al., 2001; Palmer et al., 2001) SMPX has an important function in protecting the sarcolemmal plasma membrane from mechanical stress. In Huebner et al. (2011); Schraders et al. (2011) proposed *SMPX* as the causative gene to DFNX4 in two Dutch families, one German family, and one Spanish family. Palmer et al. (2001) found that *Smpx*-null mice had no obvious developmental defects in the heart or skeletal muscle, which indicated functional redundancy. However, after the identification of hearing loss-associated gene *SMPX*, there are no detailed reports on how this gene causes hearing loss *in vivo*. In this study, we established a progressive hearing loss mouse model *via* CRISPR-Cas9 (Jinek et al., 2012; Cong et al., 2013), which is highly consistent with the DFNX4 displayed in humans.

MATERIALS AND METHODS

Information Collection on Hearing Loss in Two Chinese Families

Data on individual patients were gathered and provided by the Institute of Otolaryngology, West Hospital of Shandong Provincial Hospital. NGS sequencing and data analyses identified three heterozygous mutations that were potentially pathogenic. After that, all exons and intron/exon boundaries containing or surrounding *SMPX* mutations were PCR-amplified using specific primers. The protocols for PCR reaction and amplification were described in a previous study (Zhang et al., 2016, 2018). Sanger sequencing of *SMPX* mutations was performed using the following primers: forward 5′-GCTTATGGCCCAAAG AGATC-3′ and reverse 5′-GGCCCAAAAACTTGGCTTAAC-3′. *SMPX* mRNA (RefSeq NM_014332) was used as a reference to align the sequences using Lasergene-SeqMan software.

Phylogenetic analysis of *SMPX* was performed with multiple sequence alignment using Clustal Omega software. The sequences included NP_055147.1 (Homo sapiens), XP_003317426.1 (Pan troglodytes), XP_001086790.2 (Macaca mulatta), NP_445847.1 (Rattus norvegicus), NP_001032715.1 (Bos taurus), XP_854567.1 (Canis lupus), and NP_001239520.1 (Mus musculus).

Generation of *Smpx* Knockout Mice

Smpx knockout mice were generated in the animal facility of School of Life Sciences, Shandong University. Animal management was performed in strict accordance with the standards of the Animal Ethics Committee of Shandong University. All animals were housed in a quiet environment with a temperature of 22 ± 1°C, relative humidity of 50 ± 1%, and a light/dark cycle of 12/12 h.

Gene knockout mice were generated using the CRISPR-Cas9 gene-editing system. To avoid aging-related hearing loss resulting from Cdh23 single nucleotide substitutions carried by C57BL/6 mice, CBA/CaJ mice were used instead. CRISPR/Cas9 genome editing in mice was performed as previously described (Shen et al., 2013). PUC57-sgRNA expression vector containing single guide RNA scaffold (Addgene ID: #51132) and pST1374-NLS-flag-linker-Cas9 containing humanized Cas9 (hCas9) (Addgene ID: #44758) were obtained from Addgene. Two pairs of primers (**Table 1**) were used to amplify sgRNA transcription templates. Target sequence (20 bps) was directly cloned in the forward primer to avoid the enzyme digestion process. The vector of pST1374-NLS-flag-linker-Cas9 was linearized by SpaI. Cas9 mRNA and SgRNA were synthesized *in vitro* using AM1345 (Ambion) and AM1354 (Ambion).

CBA/CaJ female mice were superovulated and mated with CBA/CaJ male mice. Fertilized eggs were isolated from the oviducts of the female mice. Mixed RNAs were then microinjected into the pronucleus and cytoplasm of the fertilized eggs under an inverted microscope. The injected fertilized eggs were incubated in KSOM-AA medium (Millipore) for ten minutes and then transferred into the oviducts of pseudopregnant CD1 female mice.

To identify the mutant mice, genomic DNA was extracted from the toes of pups, and a DNA fragment surrounding the target site was PCR amplified. PCR products were subjected to sequencing or cloned using the T/A cloning kit and then sequenced.

Analysis of Off-Target Mutations

Predictable off-targeting sites were found by using Off-Spotter[2]. Five potential sequences and corresponding amplification primers were shown in **Table 2**. To reduce the impact of off-targeting, *Smpx* null mice were consecutively outcrossed with wild-type CBA/CaJ mice for five generations.

[2]https://cm.jefferson.edu/Off-Spotter/

TABLE 1 | The primers used in KO mouse generation.

sgRNA transcription template construction:	
Target 1 forward primer: 5′-CCTAATACGACTCACTATAGGCTGCTTCGACATATTCACAGTTTAGAGCTAGAAATAG	
Target 2 forward primer: 5′-CTAATACGACTCACTATAGGCGAATATCAATATTCCAAGTTTAGAGCTAGAAATAG	
Reverse primer: 5′-AAAAAAAGCACCGACTCGGTGCCAC	
Genotyping sequence:	
Smpx Target1 seq F: 5′-GGGGTGCTCTAGTGTTCC	**Smpx target1 seq R:** 5′-TCTGCCTCCTTAGCCTTAT
Smpx target2 seq F: 5′-TTACAGGAAGGAGGTGGC	**Smpx target2 seq R:** 5′-GGGACTCTGGAGGAAACA
Clone primers:	
Smpx clone forward: 5′-CGGAATTCATGTCGAAGCAGCCAATTTCC	
Smpx clone reverse: 5′-CGGGATCCCTACTGTTCACCTTTGGGGAC	

Red: T7 promoter Blue: A part of sgRNA scaffold Green:Target sequence

Auditory Brainstem Response and Distortion Product Otoacoustic Emission

Auditory brainstem responses (ABRs) of wild type, heterozygous, and homozygous -null mice were recorded from 1 to 5 months after birth. Mice were anesthetized with 0.007 g/ml sodium pentobarbital and placed in a soundproof box. All ABR recordings were captured by three subdermal needle electrodes. The positive electrode was inserted subcutaneously into the midline of vertex, the negative electrode was into the mastoid of the right ear and the ground electrode was into the rear region above the tail. ABR tone pips at frequencies of 4, 8, 16, and 32 kHz were generated using a Tucker Davis Technologies (TDT) workstation running the SigGen32 software and ABR data were recorded using the BioSig32 software. The stimuli were created and equalized with the audio editing software Audacity Portable. The ABR threshold was defined by a visual detection of the third peak in the waveform for click stimulus and at least one of the waves in response to the tone stimulus. The sound intensity was decreased from 90 to 20 dB until the lowest response waveform could not be identified.

Statistical analyses were performed using the GraphPad Prism 9 software. Different threshold groups collected in ABR were compared using the two-way ANOVA, followed by Fisher's LSD test. A total of 90 mice were used in these experiments (n = 12 in 1 month WT and KO male mice groups; n = 11 in 3 months male WT and KO male mice groups; n = 8 in 5 months WT and KO male mice groups; n = 7 in all female mice groups). Mean values and standard deviation(SD) were used to describe the variability. A p-Value of <0.05 indicated statistical significance. Cohen's d with Hedges' g correction was used to calculate the effect sizes of ABRs, which reflected the influence of variables such as knock-out processing.

At 24 h following ABR recordings, DPOAEs at 2f1-f2 from mice that were anesthetized in the way above were obtained using the Real-time Signal Processing System III from Tucker-Davis Technologies. The primary tone produced by two separate speakers was placed as a combination microphone/speaker system in the animal's sealed ear canal near the tympanic membrane. The DPOAE recordings were made with a low-noise microphone. All stimuli were digitally synthesized using TDT SigGen32 software. Primary tone frequencies (f1 and f2) differed by a factor of 1.25. The test frequencies were at 4, 8, 12, 16, 24, and 32 kHz and the levels were reduced in 10-dB steps from 80 to 20 dB. A fast Fourier Transform (FFT) was applied to obtain the magnitude of the 2f1-f2 distortion product. A peak at 2f1-f2 in the spectrum was accepted as DPOAE. Four WT mice and five KO mice of 3 months were used in this experiment.

Immunostaining of Cochlea Basilar Membrane Stretching Preparation

Cochleae of wild-type and *Smpx* KO mice were isolated from mice aged 1, 3, and 5 months (3 mice each group). In each cochlea, a part of the cupula cochlea was removed. Paraformaldehyde (4% in PBS) was gently perfused into the cochlea through the opening. Then, the entire cochlea was immersed in a fixative solution for 2 hours at room temperature, followed by washing with 10 mM PBS. After that, the cochleae were decalcified in 10% EDTA overnight at 4°C. Softened cochleae were dissected into three or four parts of the basilar membrane, including the apical, middle, and basal turns. After 3 washes by PBS, samples were blocked with goat serum at 37°C for an hour and then stained with anti-myosin VIIa polyclonal antibody (rabbit, Proteus-Bioscience) overnight at 4°C. After that, the samples were incubated with secondary antibodies for 1 h at 37°C, followed by washing in PBS. Finally, samples were stained with rhodamine-phalloidin (Sigma) and DAPI (Sigma), followed by a final wash in PBS. Sections were visualized under an LSM 700 confocal microscope.

FM1-43 Uptake Assay

The electromechanical conversion function of OHCs mainly depend on MET Channel on OHC bundles. To examine if there were any changes of MET channel on degenerated OHC bundles, FM1-43 uptake was carried out. FM1-43, a fluorescent dye that permeated the transduction channels, was used as a preliminary exploration of MET channel. The FM1-43 uptake assay was performed as previously described (Lelli et al., 2009). Cochleae were dissected from wild-type and *Smpx*-null mice, and basilar membranes were acquired following the same protocol explained in the immunostaining assay. Samples were treated with 2 μmol FM1-43 dye (Invitrogen) in PBS for 20 s and then fixed with 4% PFA overnight at 4°C. After three times washing in 10 mM PBS, the sections were visualized under an LSM 700 confocal microscope. Seven middle turn areas were captured in each

TABLE 2 | The potential off-target site and their amplification primers.

	Potential off-target site:			
	Potential mismatch sequence	**Amplification primer**	**Chromosome**	**NCBI reference ID**
Target 1	GCTGCTgaCAaATATTCACA-tgg	F:TTGGGGTGGCATGAAATAGGG R:TGTTCACCACAGCCCAGAAA	17	NC_000083.7
	tgTGtTTaGACATATTCACA-agg	F:ATGGGAAATGGGGCTTTGGT R:GAGCTGTCGCTAATCCCCAA	1	AC113043.7
Target 2	tGgGAAaATaAATATTCCAA-agg	F:AGAGGCACGTACAGTGGGAT R:AAGCACACAGATCTGGGAAAAT	5	AC164419.3
	cagGAATATCAgTATTCCAA-ggg	F:CAGTTACCTGAACACCAACAGA R:TGTGAGATACCTGTTTCCTTGTC	X	AL732291.11
	caCaAATATCAATgTTCCAA-tgg	F:TGTGAGATACCTGTTTCCTTGTC R:AACCCCTGCAAGTGGCTAAG	4	LO018688.1

Red color means the mismatched sites.

group. The fluorescence intensity was calculated by ImageJ software and the relative fluorescence units were used to represent the results.

Scanning Electron Microscopy

Under sodium pentobarbital anesthesia, wild-type (5 male and 2 female) and *Smpx* KO mice (7 male and 4 female) were transcardially perfused with 4% PFA. The cochleae were isolated and immersed in 2.5% glutaraldehyde for 10 hours at 4°C. In order to soften the tissue, the cochleae were decalcified in 10% EDTA overnight at 4°C. The basilar membranes were dissected from softened cochleae and post-fixed in 1% osmium tetroxide (diluted by ddH_2O) for 1 hour and washed in ddH_2O. Then, the samples were dehydrated using a gradient ethanol series, dried and mounted. Finally, the samples were sputter-coated with nanogold. The stereocilia bundles of the cochleae were examined using a Hitachi S-4800 Field-Emission scanning electron microscope.

Transmission Electron Microscopy

The basilar membranes were dissected, fixed and dehydrated. To be embedded in resin, ethyl alcohol in tissue was successively replaced with acetone and resin. After this step, tissues were placed into grooves of a mold filled with resin. The mold was transferred into an oven at 50°C overnight. The samples were cut to slices with a thickness of 50nm using a cryo diamond knife and stretched on the water. The collected ultrathin sections were attached to a copper grid and stained with uranyl acetate and lead citrate. Images were acquired using a JEOL-1200 electron microscope. Three KO male mice and two WT male mice were used in this experiment.

Noise Exposure

In this study, 1- to 2-month-old male mice were divided into two groups (5 mice per group): a control group (wild-type mice) and an experimental group (*Smpx* knock-out mice). All mice were anesthetized according to the ABR method. Then they were placed in the sound-proof box and exposed to noise limited to the 8-16 kHz octave band at 105 db SPL for 2 h. The auditory brainstem responses of these mice were recorded at four time points: 3 h, 7 days, 14 days, and 30 days after noise exposure. The sound was generated by the noise generator (SF-06, Random Noise Generator, RION, United States), amplified by the power amplifier (CDi 1000 Power Amplifier, Crown, United States), and transmitted to a microphone. The noise files were created and equalized with audio editing software (Audacity Portable). Sound levels were calibrated at multiple locations within the sound chamber to ensure uniformity of the stimulus.

In vivo Transfection by Injectoporation

Plasmid pEGFP-N2 (Clontech) was used as a backbone to express Smpx in living outer hair cells. The whole open reading frame (ORF) was cloned using primers shown in **Table 1**. pEGFP-N2 and PCR products were digested by *Eco*RI and *Bam*HI (NEB). Mixed products were incubated 10 min at 22°C with T4 DNA ligase (Thermo). Heat inactivation was conducted at 65°C for 10 min. Then, the plasmids were transferred into Trans 5α competent cells. The positive bacteria strains were screened by kanamycin.

Injectoporation was performed as previously described (Xiong et al., 2014). In brief, the otic vesicles from mice between postnatal day 0 (P0) and P8 were dissected from the skull, and the bony capsules were removed and the Corti organ was exposed. The remaining cochlear ducts were transferred to the lid of a 35-mm Petri dish. During the entire procedure, the tissue was covered with a solution to prevent mechanical damage. The tissue was placed on the bottom of the dish attaching to its surface. A microinjection pipette was controlled by a micromanipulator. Smpx-EGFP expression plasmid was injected into the space surrounding the hair cell bodies by a microinjection pipette and the electroporation electrodes were activated. These procedures were controlled by micromanipulators. After overnight culturing, the tissues were examined by an LSM 800 confocal microscope after overnight culture.

RESULTS

Clinical Presentation

In the screened subjects, Two mutations were found to be associated with DFNX4 (SMPX:c.140delC and SMPX:c.262C > G). The patients from family F42* and F177* showed an X-linked non-syndromic sensorineural hearing loss (**Figures 1A,B**). Due to the limitation of the tested families, only the adult patient information was obtained. A 26-year-old male subject (F177* III-3) suffered a significant high-frequency hearing loss, but had a nearly normal low-frequency hearing. Elderly subjects (F177* II-7, F42* II-1, F42* II-3) exhibited a severer hearing loss at all frequencies. Four female subjects(F42* I-2, F42* II-6, F42* II-8, F177* II-4) exhibited various degrees of hearing loss apparently more mild than males.

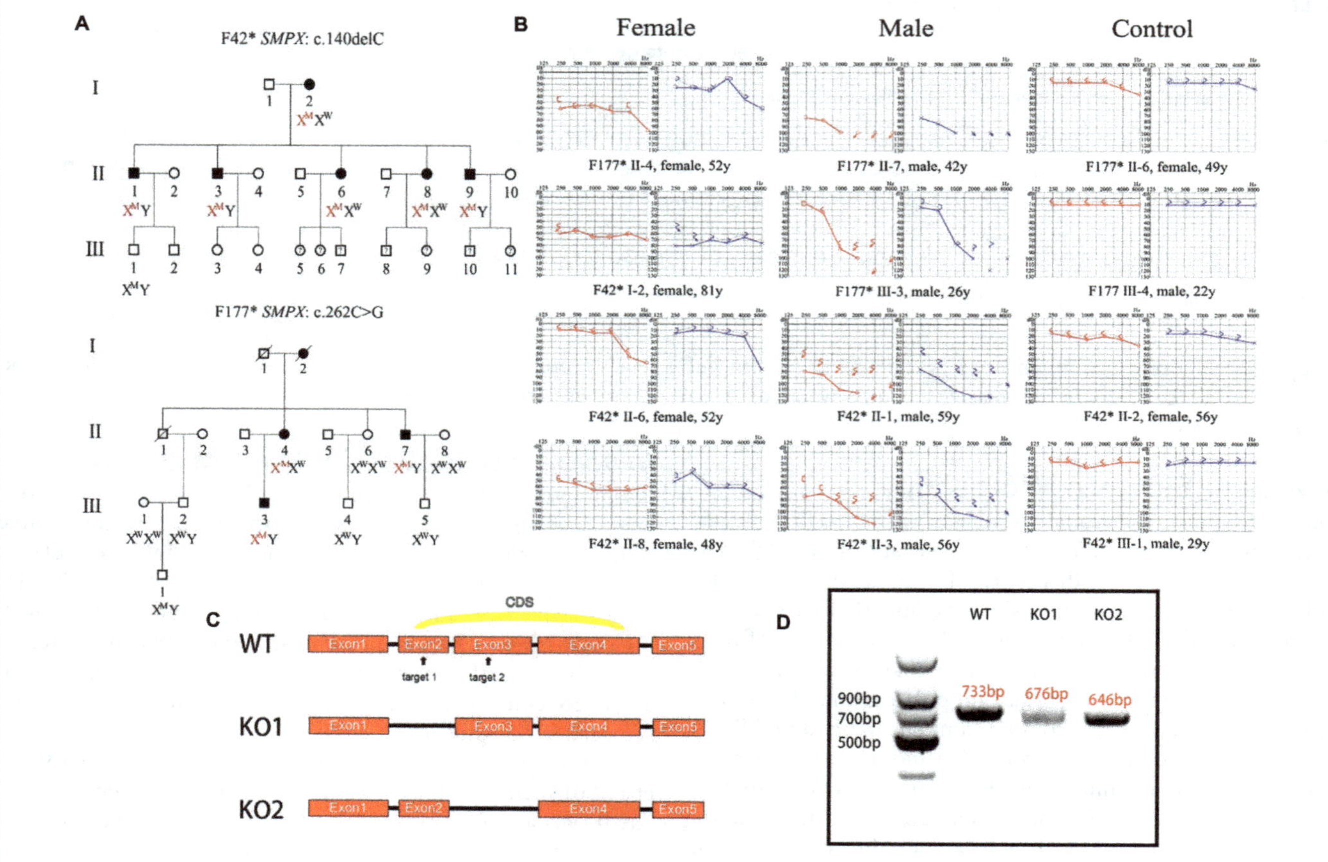

FIGURE 1 | Clinical phenotype and mouse model construction. **(A)** Pedigree of two Chinese families affected by DFNX4. Solid objects mean gene defect; hollow objects mean unaffected members; squares represent males; circles represent females. This pedigree indicated an X-linked dominant inheritance. **(B)** Audiograms of affected family members. Red indicates right ear and blue indicates left ear. We discovered that the hearing threshold of two ears was almost the same except F177* II-4's; hearing loss was more serious in male than female mice; Hearing loss was significantly worse in high frequency than that in low and medium frequencies and varied among individuals. **(C)** Schematic diagram of Smpx KO mouse construction. Two target sites were chosen in exon 2 and 3 (arrowed); two KO models were obtained. **(D)** Agarose gel electrophoresis of cDNAs acquired from knock-out mice. We cloned the whole Smpx CDS of these two knock-out pattern and discovered 57 and 87 bps deletions, which were exactly the whole length of exons 2 and 3.

Generation of *Smpx* Knock-Out Mouse

Mouse full length Smpx protein has only 85 aa. The coding sequence (CDS) contains 3 exons (**Figure 1C**). We chose two target sites in exon 2 and 3, respectively. The mixed mRNA was injected into 100 zygotes of CBA/CaJ background by cytoplasm microinjection. After 2 h of culturing, 50 plump zygotes were transferred into the oviduct ampullary of two pseudopregnancy mothers. Twenty-three fetuses were born (F0) after 19 days of pregnancy, and 11 of them were found with different indels (insertion and deletions) by genotyping. Nine indels were theoretically effective. We then selected 86 base pairs (bps) deletion mutations in the second exon and a 620 bps insertion mutation in the third exon as our experimental subjects (**Figure 1C**).

To test these knock-out effects, the entire RNA was extracted from the cochlear of knock-out mouse and reversibly transcribed to cDNA (primers were shown in **Table 1**). cDNAs were cloned into pMD18-T and sequenced. Interestingly, the whole exon 2 in mutation 1 disappeared, and exon 3 vanished in mutation 2. We believed this occurred due to the following reasons. In mutation 1, the deletion led to the loss of the GT-AG splice site, which in turn caused the spicing to skip through the 2nd exon. In mutation 2, the 620bps recombination sequence disrupted the 87bps exon3, which potentially led to the failure to identify the splice site by snRNP. All potential off-target sequences were amplified using primers (**Table 2**) and sequenced. Fortunately, no mutations on these sites were identified (data not shown).

Progressive Hearing Loss in *Smpx* Knock-Out Mice

Pedigree of X-linked dominant inheritance hearing loss DFNX4 was displayed in **Figure 1A**. Considering that *Smpx* was an X chromosome-linked gene, *Smpx* KO mice were separated into male and female two groups. We detected auditory brainstem response (ABR) of mice aged 1, 3, and 5 months in both groups (**Figure 2**). The responses to broadband click stimuli included varying degrees of hearing loss in both male and female mice. The threshold shifts first appeared at a younger age in male mice (3 months) compared to female mice (5 months) (**Figures 2A,B**).

In addition, the male mice showed a greater elevation of mean threshold compared to the mild increase in female mice. These results were consistent with human audiograms which suggested that hearing loss in males was more severe than that in females (**Figure 1B**). Moreover, threshold shift appeared earlier in high frequency, which was observed from pure tone stimuli ABR (F177* III-3 in **Figures 1B**, **2C-G**). Hearing loss gradually spread from high to low frequency until the whole spectrum was affected by the 5th month. Due to individual difference, all KO curves (dotted line in **Figure 2E** and the thresholds in detail were shown in **Supplementary Table 1A**) at 5th month were plotted to show more details of hearing loss in KO mice. We found that both normal hearing and completely deafness accounted for 11% of mice. This conformed to the normal distribution. Mixed effect ANOVAs were performed to evaluate the effect of KO on overall hearing (male click, p = 0.0049; female click, p = 0.0108) and the difference was significant. We also analyzed the effect sizes of the ABRs with Hedges' g (**Supplementary Table 1B**). In brief, the KO caused a medium to large effect on mice hearing from the 3rd month both in male and female mice. In male mice, the KO was effective at all frequencies, whereas it was shown to have a negligible effect at low frequencies in female mice. By comparing effect sizes with audiograms, we found that the KO had already slightly affected the hearing before there was a significant difference (see 3-month female click and 3-month male pure tone).

We also tested DPOAE (**Figure 2H**) and compared it with ABR. As shown in ABR, hearing loss varied in *Smpx*$^{-/-}$ mice. Some mice normally displayed WT phenotype. However, in DPOAE, the mice concurrently exhibited threshold shifts, which revealed problems in outer hair cells. At the age of 3 months, the tested KO mice showed significant threshold shifts at frequency of 12, 16, 20, and 32 kHz, which represented the middle to high frequency. This result led us to pay more attention to outer hair cells.

Progressive Degeneration of Stereocilia

To determine the changes caused by *Smpx* deficiency, the cochlear hair cell stereocilia bundles were stained with FITC-phalloidin. The cell body was marked by Myo7a (**Figure 3**). At p30, the OHCs were neatly arranged and no significant cell loss was detected. Nevertheless, abnormal bundles were found on the top of the cuticular plate (**Figures 3d-f**). At p150, OHC numbers began to gradually decrease (**Figures 3g-i**). All the above results were confirmed by quantitative analysis (**Figures 3j,k**). On the basis of this phenotype, a scanning electron microscope was utilized to examine the morphology of the stereocilia in detail (**Figure 4**).

In male mice, OHC stereocilia degeneration began from p30 and existed only at the end of basal turn near the oval window. The shortest-row of OHC bundles showed a shorter or normal length (data not shown). At p60, most stereocilia in the shortest row of OHC bundles at the basal turn were degenerated. Stereocilia degeneration spread from the base to the apex and some stereocilia in the middle row started to shorten in the basal turn (**Figures 4d-f**). At p150, OHC stereocilia in the basal turn were usually completely degenerated, or if still present, they were very short and showed signs of fusion (**Figure 4i**). The shortest row of OHC bundle in the middle and apical turn were mostly degenerated (**Figures 4g,h**). In female mice, stereocilia degeneration started at p150, and the degeneration process was milder. The shortest row of OHC stereocilia began to degenerate in the basal turn, while those were normal at middle and apical turns (**Figures 4j-l**). We analyzed this process in a quantitative way by computing the stereocilia loss rate (**Figures 4m-o**). These results might explain why DFNX4 in females was milder, and the high-frequency hearing deteriorated earlier in both male and female mice.

Although OHC stereocilia showed progressive degeneration, no changes were observed in IHC stereocilia compared to WT mice. To confirm whether OHC stereocilia degeneration was consistent with hearing loss and whether the remaining stereocilia were still sensitive to the vibration, a pair of sister mice's data (#43,#44) were individually shown (**Figure 5**). ABR was tested 1 day before the basilar membrane was dissected and observed under SEM. We chose two locations as the targets (**Figure 5b**). Site A was on the middle turn of the basilar membrane, responding to the medium frequency hearing. Site B was on the basal turn, responding to the high-frequency hearing. Broadband click stimuli ABR suggested that these subjects had a varing degree of hearing loss (**Figure 5a**). For #44 (**Figures 5c,d,g,h**), stereocilia in site A were intact and straight. In site B, some OHCs were lost, and a whole row of stereocilia disappeared in the remaining cells. These changes were reflected in the ABR thresholds. Low and medium frequencies hearing were normal, while there was a 25 dB threshold shifted in 32 kHz. For #43 (**Figures 5e,f,i,j**), some stereocilia degenerated in site A. In site B, large numbers OHCs were lost, and only some longest-row stereocilia remained. These changes were reflected in the ABR thresholds. 8-16 kHz hearing had a 10-20 dB threshold shift and hearing in 32 kHz was nearly lost. These evidence supported the observations from DPOAEs and the affected OHCs were likely to be largely responsible for the hearing impairment.

FM1-43 Uptake

Previous studies have reported that the mechanically gated ion channel is on the top of stereocilia and located at the lower tip-link end (Beurg et al., 2009). To explore whether the MET channel was still present, an simple assay for FM1-43 uptake was performed in the hair cells of 2-month-old mice (**Figures 6a,b**). A clear fluorescence dye uptake was observed in WT and KO living hair cells. The relative fluorescence unit was computed by the ImageJ software. The results indicated that ion channel decreased to some extent with statistical difference (**Figure 6c**). We describe earlier that middle turn OHCs of 2-month-old mice were still present, although their shortest row of stereocilia had degenerated (**Figures 4d-f**). Combined with the results of the FM1-43 assay, it was likely that the remaining stereocilia still maintained a mechanical-electrical transduction function.

Cell Death in *Smpx*-Null Mice

At the 5th month, a large number of OHC deaths, especially at the basal turn of the basilar membrane, were observed in *Smpx*-null mice. With aging, cell death spread from the base to the

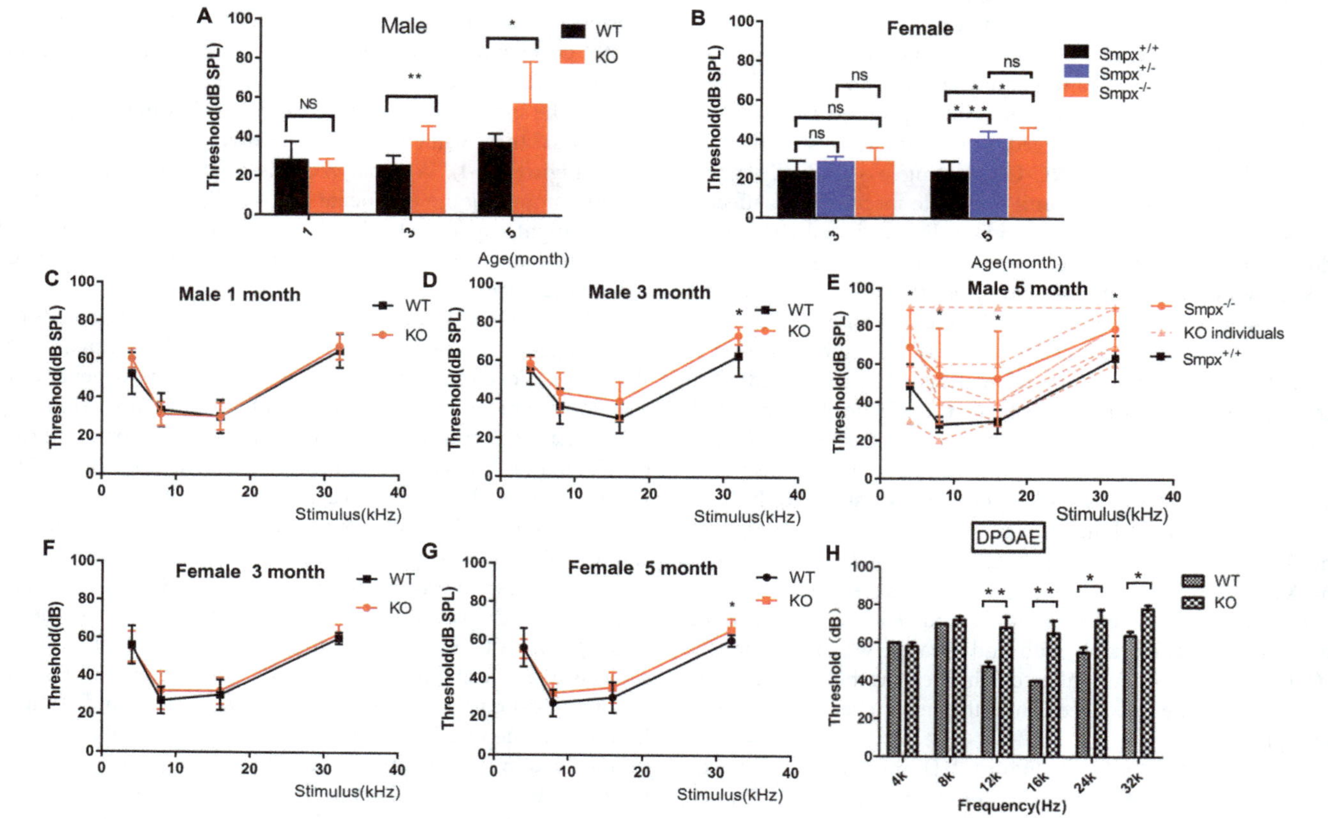

FIGURE 2 | Progressive hearing loss was displayed in ABR and DPOAE. **(A)** Broadband click stimuli induced ABR in male mice. Hearing loss started from the 3rd month and the hearing gradually decreased with aging. **(B)** Broadband click stimuli induced ABR of female mice. Hearing loss started from the fifth month, and homozygous and heterozygous mutation mice displayed similarities with aging. The hearing loss in female mice had a later onset and more mild than that in the males **(C-E)**. Frequency-specific pure tone induced ABR of male mice aged 1, 3, and 5 months. These ABRs indicated that hearing loss started at the 3rd month. The situation deteriorated from high to low frequency. In the 5th month, there was a 20 db threshold shift in 4 kHz pure tone. However, the individual difference was significant shown in panel **(D)**. Two-way ANOVA was used to compare the difference between two groups. $^{*}p < 0.05$; $^{**}p < 0.01$; and $^{***}p < 0.001$. **(F,G)** Frequency-specific pure tone induced ABR in female mice at the 3rd and 5th month. Compared to male mice, the threshold shift occurred later and was milder. **(H)** DPOAE test on wild type and Smpx KO 3-month-old male mice. Threshold shift appeared from 12 to 32 kHz, which did not appear in low frequency at this time. This result was consistent with that in ABR **(D)**.

apex, and outer hair cell survival at the basal turn was decreased. Based on the fact that OHC death came later than stereocilia degeneration, we assumed that OHC death might be secondary to stereocilia degeneration.

We used TEM to examine the condition of the outer hair cell body after stereocilia degeneration (**Figures 6d,e**). At 5000X, we discovered an obvious transformation corresponding to the characteristics of cellular edema (Xu et al., 2017). There were some substantial edematous changes in the organelles and vacuolation of the mitochondria. The cellular contents were disturbed by water, and swelling appeared on the surface of the membrane. Remarkably, this phenomenon in the cell body had already taken place before stereocilia completely degenerated (**Figures 6f,g**). The cell body was filled with water, while the stereocilia were still present (**Figure 6g**). These data suggested that stereocilia degeneration might be linked to cellular swelling and final cell death.

Localization of *Smpx* in Hair Cells

To verify the localization of Smpx in outer hair cells, we tried nearly all the commercial antibodies against Smpx, but none of them worked well. Instead, we used injectoporation to deliver pEGFP and pEGFP-Smpx plasmids to mechanosensory hair cells (**Figure 7**). Smpx was made of 85 amino acids. In order to test if the EGFP would interrupt the localization of Smpx, the plasmids were first transfected into Hela cells (**Figures 7k,l**). GFP-Smpx were concentrated in the nuclear skeleton and lamellipodia (arrowed) where actin was found, while GFP was diffusely located throughout the cytoplasm. After being delivered into outer hair cells by injectoporation, an obvious expression along the whole cell body was detected in the GFP and Smpx + GFP groups. Although GFP was abundantly expressed in the cell body, no signal was detected on bundles (**Figure 7b**). On the contrary, an obvious "V" shape on the cuticular plate was observed, indicating that Smpx-GFP was located in stereocilia (**Figure 7e**).Three-dimensional images displayed a clearer expression of GFP and

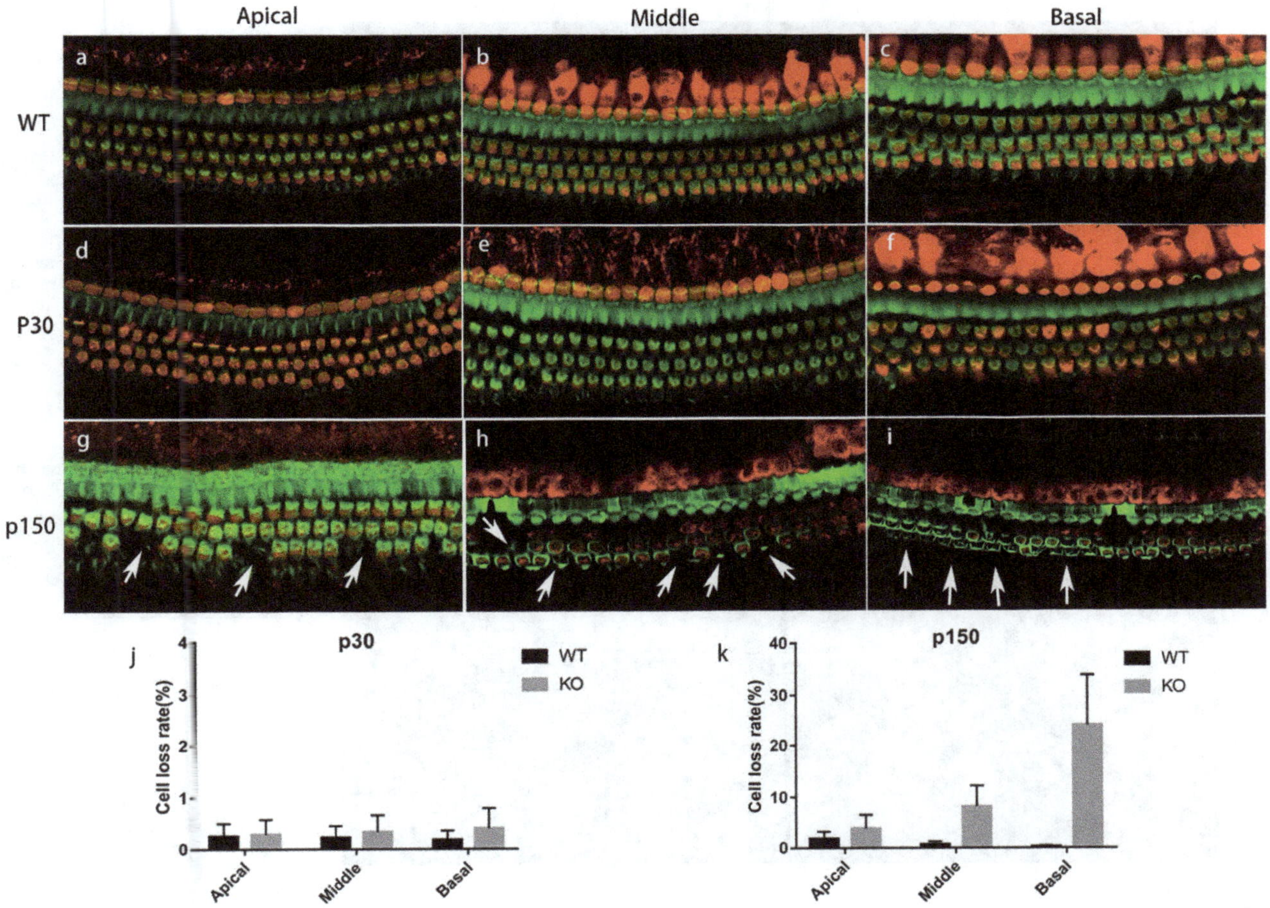

FIGURE 3 | Immunostaining of cochlea basilar membrane. Red: Myo7a, marking the cell bodies; Green: phalloidin, marking the stereocilia. **(a-c)** Basilar membranes from a p150 WT mouse. **(c-f)** Basilar membranes from a P30 Smpx KO mouse. No cell loss was detected, but some OHC bundles were out of shape. **(g-i)** Basilar membrane from p150 Smpx KO mice. Cells loss was sporadically detected at the apical and middle turn, and a large number of cells loss were detected at the basal turn. Scale bar: 20 μm. **(j,k)** OHC loss rate of mice at p30 and p150. This data indicated a progressive OHC loss consisting with the images above.

Smpx + GFP throughout the cell (**Figures 7g-j**). Localization of Smpx to the OHC stereocilia provided good evidence that Smpx-deficiency was closely linked with stereocilia degeneration. In addition, this experiment confirmed the expression of Smpx in stereocilia, but could not exclude its existence in the cytoplasm.

Noise Exposure

We found that mice within 3 months of age had a normal hearing, but the stereocilia had already degenerated at p60. To examine whether hearing of KO mice was more vulnerable to loud sound under 3 months. we exposed two groups of 1- to 2-month-old mice (WT and KO mice) to loud noise (**Supplementary Figure 1**). Both groups showed 20-30 dB threshold shift in ABR after 2 h of noise exposure. Thresholds of WT mice recovered after one week and thresholds of KO mice did not recover, which suggested that noise-exposure had induced a permanent injury to the outer hair cells of the KO mice. The unrecoverable hearing loss in KO mice indicated that the absence of Smpx had already affected the mice hearing within 3 months of age. It took some intense stimulation for the influence to show up. These results suggested that the DFNX4 patients should avoid excessively loud sound exposure as much as possible.

DISCUSSION

Sensorineural hearing loss affects nearly 300 million individuals. It mainly arises from damage or death of auditory hair cells (Liu et al., 2016; Liu W. et al., 2019; Gao et al., 2020; Chen et al., 2021; He et al., 2021) and spiral ganglion neurons (SGN) (Liu Y. et al., 2019; Ding et al., 2020; Guo et al., 2020; Liu et al., 2021; Yuan et al., 2021), which can be caused by environmental insults (such as overexposure to loud sounds or exposure to aminoglycoside antibiotics or chemotherapeutics) (He Z. et al., 2017; He et al., 2020; Gao et al., 2020; Jiang et al., 2020; Zhang et al., 2020; Zhong et al., 2020; Zhou et al., 2020), or genetic alteration (He Y. et al., 2017; Fang et al., 2019; He et al., 2019; Qian et al., 2020;

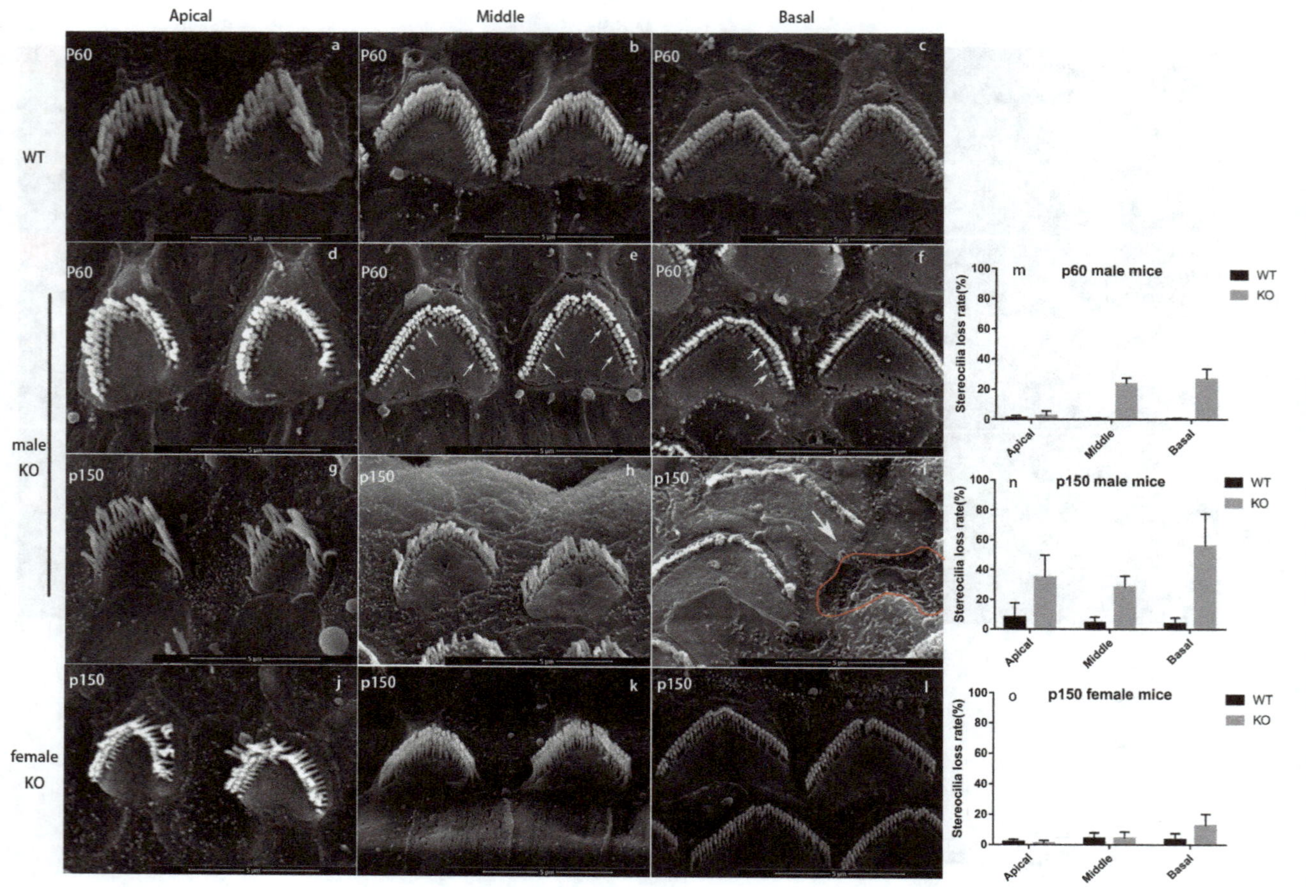

FIGURE 4 | Scanning electron microscope of WT and KO mice. **(a-c)** OHC bundles of wild-type male mouse at p60. There are three rows of stereocilia ("M" shape) on the cuticular plate (heart shape). Scale bar = 5 nm. **(d-f)** OHC bundles of Smpx KO male mouse at p60. The loss of shortest row stereocilia from apex to base showed a trend from less to more (arrowed). However, the middle and longest rows were normal, and the "M" shape was still sharp and clear. **(g-i)** OHC bundles of Smpx KO male mouse at p150. The stereocilia degeneration appeared at the apical turn and the conditions were more severe at the middle and basal turns. The middle and longest rows of OHC stereocilia started to degenerate and the "M" shape was indistinct at the middle turn. The whole bundle degenerated at the basal turn. Some OHCs were dead and left a pit on the basilar membrane (red line). **(j-l)** OHC bundles of Smpx KO female mouse at p150. The bundles were normal in apical and middle turn. A number of the shortest row stereocilia was degenerated at the basal turn. **(m-o)** OHC stereocilia loss rate of p60 male mice, p150 male mice, and p150 female mice. This data indicated a progressive OHC stereocilia degeneration and this process was more mild and had a later onset in female mice.

Fu et al., 2021; Lv et al., 2021; Zhang et al., 2021). Sound is collected and conducted by the external and middle ear, and transformed into electrical signals by cochlear inner and outer hair cells, Then the electrical signals are transduced to the auditory cortex through spiral ganglion neurons (Martin et al., 2003; Sun et al., 2016; Guo et al., 2019, 2021; Zhao et al., 2019; Hu et al., 2021). *SMPX* is closely linked to sex-linked non-syndromic hearing loss DFNX4. It was first identified and mapped in 1999. Within the 88 amino acids of SMPX protein, the predicted peptide showed no significant homologies to known structural elements (Patzak et al., 1999). Previous studies have reported that mutations in *Smpx* cause progressive autosomal recessive non-syndromic deafness DFNX4. The *Smpx* deficient mice made on C57BL/6 background showed no obvious phenotype (Huebner et al., 2011; Schraders et al., 2011; Abdelfatah et al., 2013). Therefore, this mice strain was not further preserved.

In this study, we established and validated Smpx KO mice using CRISPR/Cas9-mediated genomic editing technology in CBA/CaJ mice to explore the function of Smpx and the underlying mechanism its action in the hearing system. With the cooperation of the Institute of Otolaryngology, West Hospital of Shandong Provincial Hospital, we also obtained some patients data and new mutation sites of DFNX4, which had never been reported. The male subjects displayed a more severe hearing loss than the female subjects and high frequency hearing seemed worse in both males and females. To confirm whether our mouse model was suitable, we tested the ABR of *Smpx* KO mice. In male mice, definite hearing loss started from the 3rd month for high frequencies and gradually increased with time. Female mice had a milder hearing impairment and developed hearing loss later than male mice. This progressive hearing loss process was highly consistent with that in DFNX4 patients, which

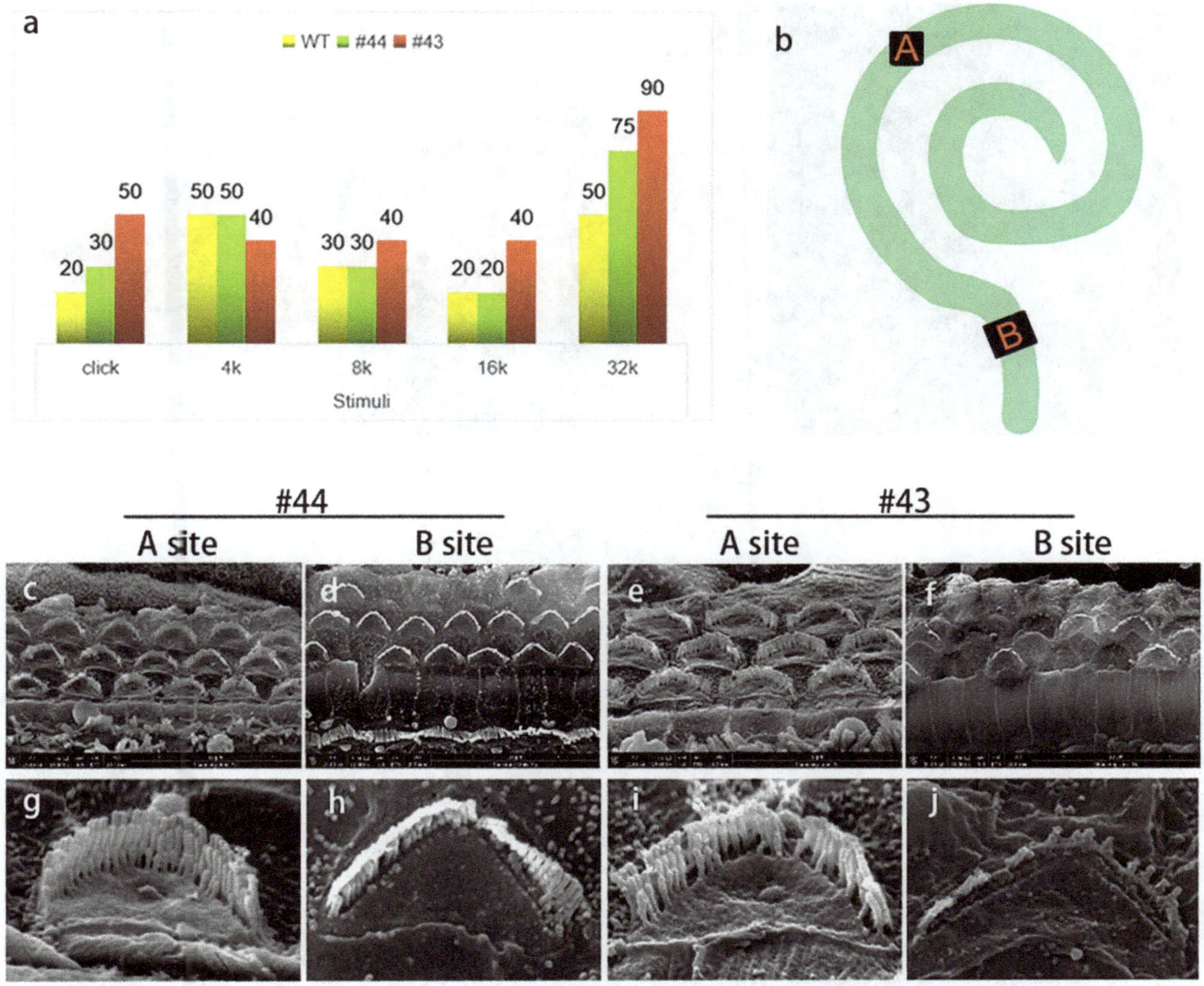

FIGURE 5 | The condition of outer hair cells was closely related to the hearing of the Smpx KO mouse. **(a)** Auditory brainstem response to a pair of sister mice (#43, #44) with different levels of hearing loss. Two mice were both 1-year-old. **(b)** Schematic diagram of the whole basilar membrane. Site A represents the middle turn and responses to medium frequency sound waves; site B represents the basal turn and responses to high-frequency sound waves. **(c-j)** SEM of basilar membranes from the cochlea of #43 and #44 and the amplified image. Comparing **(c,g)** with panels **(e,i)**, middle turn hair bundles in panel **(g)** is normal. The Shortest-row of stereocilia in panel **(i)** starts to degenerate. Reflected in the ABR, there are 10 and 20 dB threshold shifts in #43 at 8 and 16 kHz (medium-frequency), but it is normal in #44. Comparing **(d,h)** with panels **(f,j)**, stereocilia degeneration in #43 is badly worse than that in #44. Large numbers of hair cells' death in panel **(f)** resulted in the loss of hearing in a high frequency of #43. The remaining hair cells and stereocilia ensured that #43 maintained a low-level hearing in high frequency.

suggested that Smpx KO mouse could be used as an mouse model for DFNX4 research.

The deficiency of some actin binding proteins expressed in stereocilia can lead to the shortening or even degeneration of stereocilia. As an actin binding protein, Smpx expression site is essential in determining whether Smpx is functional in stereocilia. The most common way to prove the localization of Smpx in hair cells is the positive staining using a corresponding antibody. Unfortunately we didn't find a suitable commercial antibody that worked. Instead, we used injectoporation to deliver a plasmid containing an ORF of Smpx binding with EGFP into living hair cells. After 24 hours of culture and expression, we detected the fluorescence signal of Smpx-EGFP in stereocilia and cell body, while EGFP was only expressed in the cell body. The null mutation of Smpx led to stereocilia degeneration after p60. Since Smpx was localized on stereocilia, we speculated that Smpx might play a role in maintaining OHC bundles.

At the age of 2 months, stereocilia of KO male mice started to degenerate from the shortest row of OHC bundles. Also at the age of 2 months, FM1-43 uptake in OHCs of KO mice was a little lower than that of WT mice, but the hair cells were still positively stained. This result implied that degeneration of the shortest row stereocilia in OHC bundle didn't greatly affect ion channel. As a simple way, FM1-43 uptake was an imperfect method to test

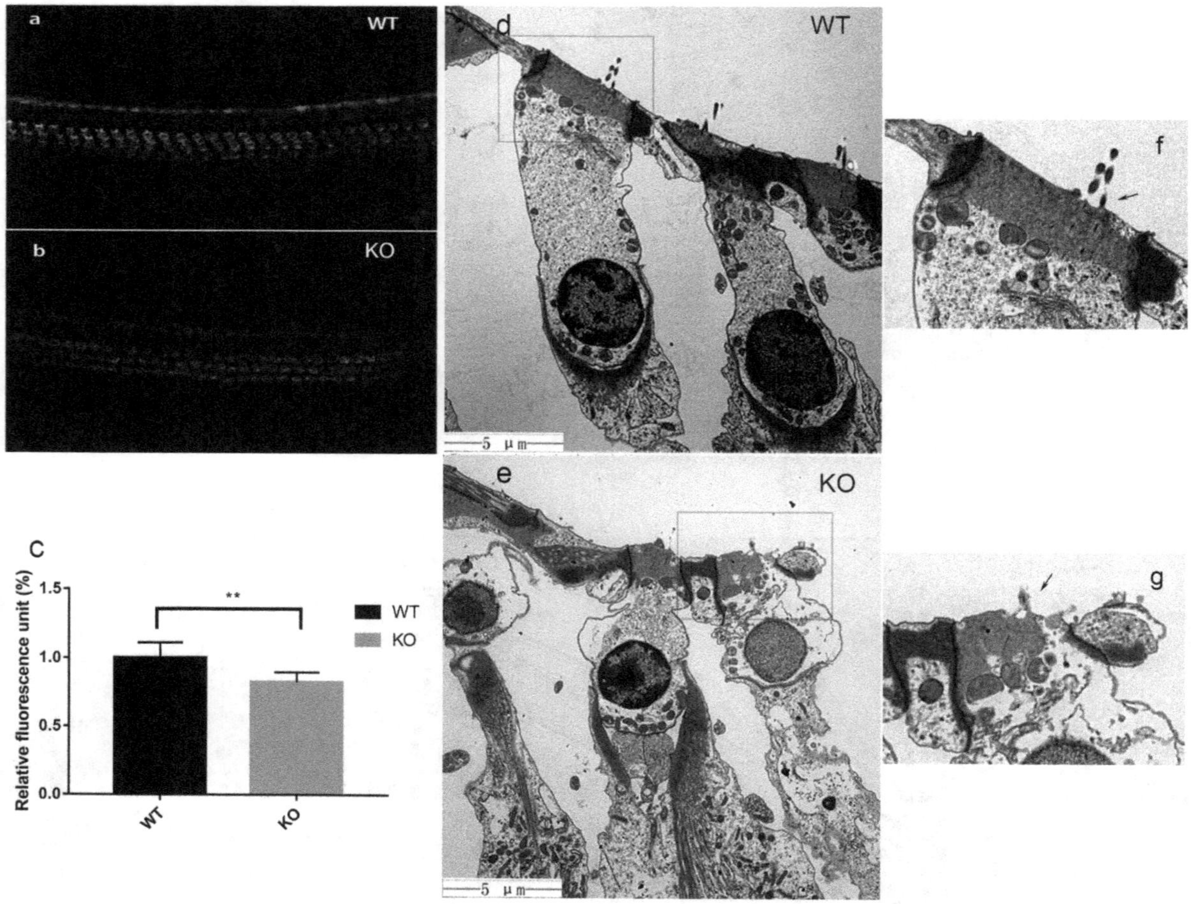

FIGURE 6 | In KO mice, the FM1-43 uptake decreased and cell edema began to appear at the end phase of stereocilia degeneration. **(a,b)** FM1-43 uptake in hair cells of WT and Smpx KO mouse at p60. This image indicated that the shortest row stereocilia degeneration did not greatly affect the uptake of FM1-43. **(c)** relative fluorescence unit of FM1-43 uptake. The uptake in KO mice at p60 was reduced by 17%. **(d,e)** Transmission electron microscope of hair cells in WT and Smpx KO mouse at p150. In panel **(e)**, the cellular contents were disturbed by water, and swelling appeared on the surface of cell membrane. Undoubtedly, these were characteristics of cell edema. This state of hair cells was more sensitive. **(f,g)** Magnified image of panels **(d,e)**. In panel **(g)**, the longest row was still remaining (arrowed), which indicated that cellular edema occurred during the stereociliary degenerating process but not after the process. ** means $0.01 > p$ value > 0.001.

the MET channel. Yet, these findings still gave us a preliminary indication whether MET channel function was affected.

Smpx Knock-Out Mouse Is an Ideal Model for Examining DFNX4 and Stereocilia Degeneration

Animal models are extremely important for investigation of the roles played by genes in the hearing process. The genetic background of mice sometimes affects the phenotype of mutant mice. Thus, it is crucial to use an appropriate animal strain with regard to a specific research field such as hearing. For example, C57BL/6 mice carry the Ahl allele of Cdh23 which predisposes them to early onset presbycusis and is therefore not always an ideal choice for auditory research. In a previous study (Palmer et al., 2001), *Smpx* KO mouse models with age-related hearing loss (ARHL) were generated by gene-targeting based on C57/BL6 background. We could not tell if the ARHL was caused by genetic mutation or mouse background. In this study, no obvious abnormities were found in mice and the inbreeding of mice strain was discontinued (confirmed by e-mail). CBA/CaJ mouse without ARHL is a better choice in hearing research especially when studying progressive hearing loss.

Comparing the audiograms, we showed that our mouse model could mimic the progressive hearing loss observed in humans. To date, no mice cochleae with *Smpx* mutation have been histologically studied. Using the *Smpx*-null mouse model, we investigated the degeneration of OHC stereocilia bundles and the resulting effect on Smpx function in the outer hair cells. With the OHC stereocilia degeneration mouse model, we can further study OHC bundle structures, such as MET channel and tip-link. Moreover, using SEM, we found the degeneration of OHC stereocilia at the shortest row in the 2nd month. In the test of FM1-43 uptake, there was a 17% signal reduction in KO OHCs which indicated the weakened function of MET channel. Interestingly, the hearing loss started from the 3rd month. For a

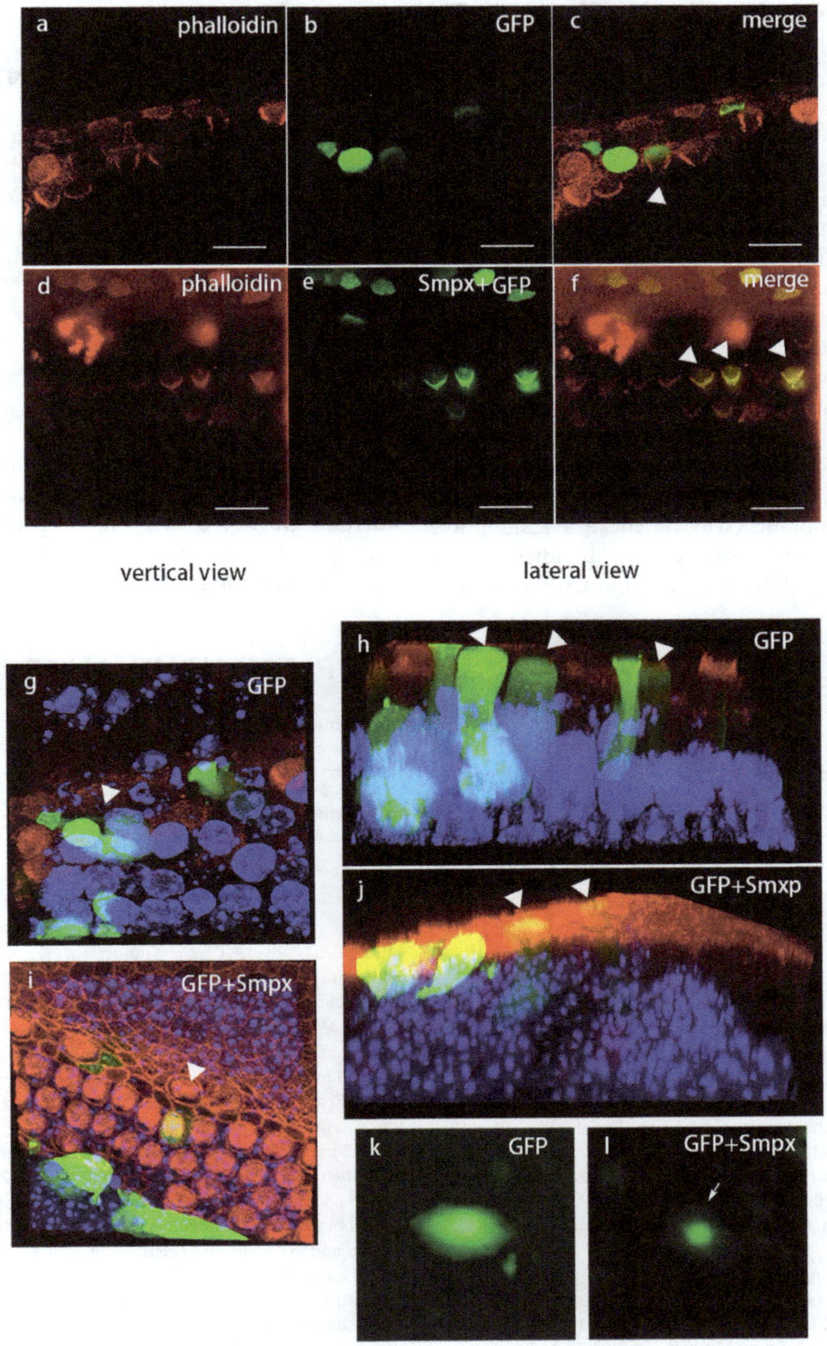

FIGURE 7 | Localization of *Smpx* in hair cells *via in vivo* electrotransfection (injectoporation). Red, phalloidin; Green, GFP. **(a-c)** Hair cells transfected with pEGFP. These images showed GFP was expressed in the cell body but not in the stereocilia. **(d-f)** Hair cells transfected with pEGFP-Smpx. The obvious "V" shape indicated that GFP-Smpx was located in stereocilia. **(g-j)** Three-dimensional image of transfected hair cells. Red, phalloidin; Green, GFP; blue, DAPI. 3D images displayed a clearer expression of GFP and GFP-Smpx. **(k,l)** Hela cells transfected with pEGFP and pEGFP-Smpx. The fusion protein GFP-Smpx should be tested before injectoporation to confirm if GFP would affect the localization of Smpx.

further research, we put the WT and KO mice (under 2 months of age) exposed to a certain intensity noise. The WT mice recovered after a week as expected while the KO mice suffered a permanent injury to their hearing. In a conclusion, though young mice under 2 months of age had a normal hearing, they were more sensitive to loud noise. This gave us a hint that, DFNX4 patients were more susceptible to noise and they should stay away from excessively loud noise to avoid serious hearing loss.

Smpx May Play a Role in Maintaining Hair Cell Bundles

In OHCs, the stereocilia contain a core of actin filaments associated with actin binding proteins. As an ABP, Smpx was also expressed in OHC stereocilium. Degeneration of the OHC stereocilia and the unrecovered hearing after noise exposure gave us a hint that Smpx might play a role in maintaining the hair cell bundles. In the previous study (Palmer et al., 2001; Eftestøl et al., 2014), Smpx was shown to be expressed in pleural segment muscle where its functions included binding the sarcomere to cytomembrane. The localization where Smpx expressed in muscle cells could be described as the bridge rib, which not only connected but also supported the sarcomere (actin filament) to the cytomembrane. We will make a assumption that Smpx may have a similar role in hair bundles, i.e., it may provide a supporting link between the actin core and surrounding structures.

ETHICS STATEMENT

The studies involving human participants were reviewed and approved by Ethics Committee of the Shandong University. The patients/participants provided their written informed consent to participate in this study. The animal study was reviewed and approved by Ethics Committee of the Shandong University.

AUTHOR CONTRIBUTIONS

JG and HW supervised the project. HW and XB provided the information of human DFNX4 patients. AZ, HT, and XF generated the *Smpx* KO mouse model. HT and SX performed the statistical analysis and acquired the data. HT performed the experiment and analyzed and interpreted the results. HT and JG wrote the manuscript. All authors approved the submitted version.

ACKNOWLEDGMENTS

We thank Linzhi Zou and Wei Xiong's lab from the School of Life Sciences, Tsinghua University, for injectoporation and microimaging. We also thank plasmid sharing of Xingxu Huang's lab from the Model Animal Research Center of Nanjing University.

SUPPLEMENTARY MATERIAL

Supplementary Figure 1 | Noise exposure of mice less than 2 months old. The KO mice suffered permanent hearing impairment, while the WT mice recovered in a week.

Supplementary Table 1 | Thresholds of KO male mice at 5 months of age and the effect size of ABRs.

REFERENCES

Abdelfatah, N., Merner, N., Houston, J., Benteau, T., Griffin, A., Doucette, L., et al. (2013). A novel deletion in SMPX causes a rare form of X-linked progressive hearing loss in two families due to a founder effect. *Hum. Mutat.* 34, 66–69. doi: 10.1002/humu.22205

Beurg, M., Fettiplace, R., Nam, J. H., and Ricci, A. J. (2009). Localization of inner hair cell mechanotransducer channels using high-speed calcium imaging. *Nat. Neurosci.* 12, 553–558. doi: 10.1038/nn.2295

Chen, Y., Gu, Y., Li, Y., Li, G. L., Chai, R., Li, W., et al. (2021). Generation of mature and functional hair cells by co-expression of Gfi1, Pou4f3, and Atoh1 in the postnatal mouse cochlea. *Cell Rep.* 35:109016. doi: 10.1016/j.celrep.2021.109016

Cheng, C., Hou, Y., Zhang, Z., Wang, Y., Lu, L., Zhang, L., et al. (2021). Disruption of the autism-related gene Pak1 causes stereocilia disorganization, hair cell loss, and deafness in mice. *J. Genet. Genomics* 48, 324–332. doi: 10.1016/j.jgg.2021.03.010

Cong, L., Ran, F. A., Cox, D., Lin, S., Barretto, R., Habib, N., et al. (2013). Multiplex genome engineering using CRISPR/Cas systems. *Science* 339, 819–823. doi: 10.1126/science.1231143

Corvino, V., Apisa, P., Malesci, R., Laria, C., Auletta, G., and Franzé, A. X. - (2018). Linked sensorineural hearing loss: a literature review. *Curr. Genomics* 19, 327–338. doi: 10.2174/1389202919666171218163046

Crawford, A. C., and Fettiplace, R. (1985). The mechanical properties of ciliary bundles of turtle cochlear hair cells. *J. Physiol.* 364, 359–379. doi: 10.1113/jphysiol.1985.sp015750

Ding, Y., Meng, W., Kong, W., He, Z., and Chai, R. (2020). The role of FoxG1 in the inner ear. *Front. Cell Dev. Biol.* 8:614954. doi: 10.3389/fcell.2020.614954

Eftestøl, E., Alver, T. N., Gundersen, K., and Bruusgaard, J. C. (2014). Overexpression of SMPX in adult skeletal muscle does not change skeletal muscle fiber type or size. *PLoS One* 9:e99232. doi: 10.1371/journal.pone.0099232

Fang, Q., Zhang, Y., Da, P., Shao, B., Pan, H., He, Z., et al. (2019). Deletion of Limk1 and Limk2 in mice does not alter cochlear development or auditory function. *Sci. Rep.* 9:3357. doi: 10.1038/s41598-019-39769-z

Fu, X., An, Y., Wang, H., Li, P., Lin, J., Yuan, J., et al. (2021). Deficiency of Klc2 induces low-frequency sensorineural hearing loss in C57BL/6 J mice and human. *Mol. Neurobiol.* doi: 10.21203/rs.3.rs-277106/v1

Gao, S., Cheng, C., Wang, M., Jiang, P., Zhang, L., Wang, Y., et al. (2020). Blebbistatin inhibits neomycin-induced apoptosis in hair cell-like HEI-OC-1 cells and in cochlear hair cells. *Front. Cell. Neurosci.* 13:590. doi: 10.3389/fncel.2019.00590

Guo, R., Li, J., Chen, C., Xiao, M., Liao, M., Hu, Y., et al. (2021). Biomimetic 3D bacterial cellulose-graphene foam hybrid scaffold regulates neural stem cell proliferation and differentiation. *Colloids Surf. B Biointerfaces* 200:111590. doi: 10.1016/j.colsurfb.2021.111590

Guo, R., Ma, X., Liao, M., Liu, Y., Hu, Y., Qian, X., et al. (2019). Development and application of cochlear implant-based electric-acoustic stimulation of spiral ganglion neurons. *ACS Biomater. Sci. Eng.* 5, 6735–6741. doi: 10.1021/acsbiomaterials.9b01265

Guo, R., Xiao, M., Zhao, W., Zhou, S., Hu, Y., Liao, M., et al. (2020). 2D Ti3C2TxMXene couples electrical stimulation to promote proliferation and neural differentiation of neural stem cells. *Acta Biomater.* doi: 10.1016/j.actbio.2020.12.035

He, Y., Lu, X., Qian, F., Liu, D., Chai, R., and Li, H. (2017). Insm1a is required for zebrafish posterior lateral line development. *Front. Mol. Neurosci.* 10:241. doi: 10.3389/fnmol.2017.00241

He, Z. H., Li, M., Fang, Q. J., Liao, F. L., Zou, S. Y., Wu, X., et al. (2021). FOXG1 promotes aging inner ear hair cell survival through activation of the autophagy pathway. *Autophagy* doi: 10.1080/15548627.2021.1916194

He, Z. H., Zou, S. Y., Li, M., Liao, F. L., Wu, X., Sun, H. Y., et al. (2020). The nuclear transcription factor FoxG1 affects the sensitivity of mimetic aging hair cells to inflammation by regulating autophagy pathways. *Redox Biol.* 28:101364. doi: 10.1016/j.redox.2019.101364

He, Z., Fang, Q., Li, H., Shao, B., Zhang, Y., Zhang, Y., et al. (2019). The role of FOXG1 in the postnatal development and survival of mouse cochlear hair cells. *Neuropharmacology* 144, 43–57. doi: 10.1016/j.neuropharm.2018.10.021

He, Z., Guo, L., Shu, Y., Fang, Q., Zhou, H., Liu, Y., et al. (2017). Autophagy protects auditory hair cells against neomycin-induced damage. *Autophagy* 13, 1884–1904. doi: 10.1080/15548627.2017.1359449

Howard, J., and Hudspeth, A. J. (1987). Mechanical relaxation of the hair bundle mediates adaptation in mechanoelectrical transduction by the bullfrog's saccular hair cell. *Proc. Natl. Acad. Sci. U.S.A.* 84, 3064–3068. doi: 10.1073/pnas.84.9.3064

Hu, Y., Li, D., Wei, H., Zhou, S., Chen, W., Yan, X., et al. (2021). Neurite extension and orientation of spiral ganglion neurons can be directed by superparamagnetic iron oxide nanoparticles in a magnetic field. *Int. J. Nanomed.* 16, 4515–4526. doi: 10.2147/IJN.S313673

Huebner, A. K., Gandia, M., Frommolt, P., Maak, A., Wicklein, E. M., Thiele, H., et al. (2011). Nonsense mutations in SMPX, encoding a protein responsive to physical force, result in X-chromosomal hearing loss. *Am. J. Hum. Genet.* 88, 621–627. doi: 10.1016/j.ajhg.2011.04.007

Jiang, P., Zhang, S., Cheng, C., Gao, S., Tang, M., Lu, L., et al. (2020). The roles of exosomes in visual and auditory systems. *Front. Bioeng. Biotechnol.* 8:525. doi: 10.3389/fbioe.2020.00525

Jinek, M., Chylinski, K., Fonfara, I., Hauer, M., Doudna, J. A., and Charpentier, E. (2012). A programmable dual-RNA-guided DNA endonuclease in adaptive bacterial immunity. *Science* 337, 816–821. doi: 10.1126/science.1225829

Kemp, T. J., Sadusky, T. J., Simon, M., Brown, R., Eastwood, M., Sassoon, D. A., et al. (2001). Identification of a novel stretch-responsive skeletal muscle gene (Smpx). *Genomics* 72, 260–271. doi: 10.1006/geno.2000.6461

Lelli, A., Asai, Y., Forge, A., Holt, J. R., and Géléoc, G. S. (2009). Tonotopic gradient in the developmental acquisition of sensory transduction in outer hair cells of the mouse cochlea. *J. Neurophysiol.* 101, 2961–2973. doi: 10.1152/jn.00136.2009

Liu, L., Chen, Y., Qi, J., Zhang, Y., He, Y., Ni, W., et al. (2016). Wnt activation protects against neomycin-induced hair cell damage in the mouse cochlea. *Cell Death Dis.* 7:e2136. doi: 10.1038/cddis.2016.35

Liu, W., Xu, L., Wang, X., Zhang, D., Sun, G., Wang, M., et al. (2021). PRDX1 activates autophagy *via* the PTEN-AKT signaling pathway to protect against cisplatin-induced spiral ganglion neuron damage. *Autophagy* 12, 1–23. doi: 10.1080/15548627.2021.1905466

Liu, W., Xu, X., Fan, Z., Sun, G., Han, Y., Zhang, D., et al. (2019). Wnt signaling activates TP53-induced glycolysis and apoptosis regulator and protects against cisplatin-induced spiral ganglion neuron damage in the mouse cochlea. *Antioxid. Redox Signal.* 30, 1389–1410. doi: 10.1089/ars.2017.7288

Liu, Y., Qi, J., Chen, X., Tang, M., Chu, C., Zhu, W., et al. (2019). Critical role of spectrin in hearing development and deafness. *Sci. Adv.* 5:eaav7803. doi: 10.1126/sciadv.aav7803

Lv, J., Fu, X., Li, Y., Hong, G., Li, P., Lin, J., et al. (2021). Deletion of Kcnj16 in mice does not alter auditory function. *Front. Cell Dev. Biol.* 9:630361. doi: 10.3389/fcell.2021.630361

Manor, U., and Kachar, B. (2008). Dynamic length regulation of sensory stereocilia. *Semin. Cell Dev. Biol.* 19, 502–510. doi: 10.1016/j.semcdb.2008.07.006

Martin, P., Bozovic, D., Choe, Y., and Hudspeth, A. J. (2003). Spontaneous oscillation by hair bundles of the bullfrog's sacculus. *J. Neurosci.* 23, 4533–4548. doi: 10.1523/JNEUROSCI.23-11-04533.2003

Palmer, S., Groves, N., Schindeler, A., Yeoh, T., Biben, C., Wang, C. C., et al. (2001). The small muscle specific protein Csl modifies cell shape and promotes myocyte fusion in an insulin-like growth factor 1-dependent manner. *J. Cell Biol.* 153, 985–998. doi: 10.1083/jcb.153.5.985

Patzak, D., Zhuchenko, O., Lee, C. C., and Wehnert, M. (1999). Identification, mapping, and genomic structure of a novel X-chromosomal human gene (SMPX) encoding a small muscular protein. *Hum. Genet.* 105, 506–512. doi: 10.1007/s004399900171

Petit, C., and Richardson, G. P. (2009). Linking genes underlying deafness to hair-bundle development and function. *Nat. Neurosci.* 12, 703–710. doi: 10.1038/nn.2330

Qi, J., Liu, Y., Chu, C., Chen, X., Zhu, W., Shu, Y., et al. (2019). A cytoskeleton structure revealed by super-resolution fluorescence imaging in inner ear hair cells. *Cell Discov.* 5:12. doi: 10.1038/s41421-018-0076-4

Qi, J., Zhang, L., Tan, F., Liu, Y., Chu, C., Zhu, W., et al. (2020). Espin distribution as revealed by super-resolution microscopy of stereocilia. *Am. J. Transl. Res.* 12, 130–141.

Qian, F., Wang, X., Yin, Z., Xie, G., Yuan, H., Liu, D., et al. (2020). The slc4a2b gene is required for hair cell development in zebrafish. *Aging* 12, 18804–18821. doi: 10.18632/aging.103840

Ricci, A. J., Crawford, A. C., and Fettiplace, R. (2000). Active hair bundle motion linked to fast transducer adaptation in auditory hair cells. *J. Neurosci.* 20, 7131–7142. doi: 10.1523/JNEUROSCI.20-19-07131.2000

Romet-Lemonne, G., and Jégou, A. (2021). The dynamic instability of actin filament barbed ends. *J. Cell Biol.* 220:e202102020. doi: 10.1083/jcb.202102020

Schraders, M., Haas, S. A., Weegerink, N. J., Oostrik, J., Hu, H., Hoefsloot, L. H., et al. (2011). Next-generation sequencing identifies mutations of SMPX, which encodes the small muscle protein,X-linked, as a cause of progressive hearing impairment. *Am. J. Hum. Genet.* 88, 628–634. doi: 10.1016/j.ajhg.2011.04.012

Schwander, M., Kachar, B., and Müller, U. (2010). Review series: the cell biology of hearing. *J. Cell Biol.* 190, 9–20. doi: 10.1083/jcb.201001138

Shen, B., Zhang, J., Wu, H., Wang, J., Ma, K., Li, Z., et al. (2013). Generation of gene-modified mice *via* Cas9/RNA-mediated gene targeting. *Cell Res.* 23, 720–723. doi: 10.1038/cr.2013.46

Sun, G., Liu, W., Fan, Z., Zhang, D., Han, Y., Xu, L., et al. (2016). The three-dimensional culture system with matrigel and neurotrophic factors preserves the structure and function of spiral ganglion neuron *in vitro*. *Neural Plast.* 2016:4280407. doi: 10.1155/2016/4280407

Wang, Y., Li, J., Yao, X., Li, W., Du, H., Tang, M., et al. (2017). Loss of CIB2 causes profound hearing loss and abolishes mechanoelectrical transduction in mice. *Front. Mol. Neurosci.* 10:401. doi: 10.3389/fnmol.2017.00401

Xiong, W., Wagner, T., Yan, L., Grillet, N., and Müller, U. (2014). Using injectoporation to deliver genes to mechanosensory hair cells. *Nat. Protoc.* 9, 2438–2449. doi: 10.1038/nprot.2014.168

Xu, L. X., Lv, Y., Li, Y. H., Ding, X., Wang, Y., Han, X., et al. (2017). Melatonin alleviates brain and peripheral tissue edema in a neonatal rat model of hypoxic-ischemic brain damage: the involvement of edema related proteins. *BMC Pediatr.* 17:90. doi: 10.1186/s12887-017-0824-x

Yuan, T. F., Dong, Y., Zhang, L., Qi, J., Yao, C., Wang, Y., et al. (2021). Neuromodulation-based stem cell therapy in brain repair: recent advances and future perspectives. *Neurosci. Bull.* 37, 735–745. doi: 10.1007/s12264-021-00667-y

Zhang, C., Wang, M., Xiao, Y., Zhang, F., Zhou, Y., Li, J., et al. (2016). Novel nonsense mutation of POU4F3 gene causes autosomal dominant hearing loss. *Neural Plast.* 2016:1512831. doi: 10.1155/2016/1512831

Zhang, F., Xu, L., Xiao, Y., Li, J., Bai, X., and Wang, H. (2018). Three MYO15A mutations identified in one chinese family with autosomal recessive nonsyndromic hearing loss. *Neural Plast.* 2018:5898025. doi: 10.1155/2018/5898025

Zhang, S., Dong, Y., Qiang, R., Zhang, Y., Zhang, X., Chen, Y., et al. (2021). Characterization of strip1 expression in mouse cochlear hair cells. *Front. Genet.* 12:625867. doi: 10.3389/fgene.2021.625867

Zhang, S., Zhang, Y., Dong, Y., Guo, L., Zhang, Z., Shao, B., et al. (2020). Knockdown of Foxg1 in supporting cells increases the trans-differentiation of supporting cells into hair cells in the neonatal mouse cochlea. *Cell. Mol. Life Sci.* 77, 1401–1419. doi: 10.1007/s00018-019-03291-2

Zhao, J., Tang, M., Cao, J., Ye, D., Guo, X., Xi, J., et al. (2019). Structurally tunable reduced graphene oxide substrate maintains mouse embryonic stem cell pluripotency. *Adv. Sci.* 6:1802136. doi: 10.1002/advs.201802136

Zhong, Z., Fu, X., Li, H., Chen, J., Wang, M., Gao, S., et al. (2020). Citicoline protects auditory hair cells against neomycin-induced damage. *Front. Cell Dev. Biol.* 8:712. doi: 10.3389/fcell.2020.00712

Zhou, H., Qian, X., Xu, N., Zhang, S., Zhu, G., Zhang, Y., et al. (2020). Disruption of Atg7-dependent autophagy causes electromotility disturbances, outer hair cell loss, and deafness in mice. *Cell Death Dis.* 11:913. doi: 10.1038/s41419-020-03110-8

Zhu, C., Cheng, C., Wang, Y., Muhammad, W., Liu, S., Zhu, W., et al. (2018). Loss of ARHGEF6 causes hair cell stereocilia deficits and hearing loss in mice. *Front. Mol. Neurosci.* 11:362. doi: 10.3389/fnmol.2018.00362

5

Disruption of Glutamate Release and Uptake-Related Protein Expression After Noise-Induced Synaptopathy in the Cochlea

Kefeng Ma[1†], Anran Zhang[1,2†], Xiaojun She[1], Honglian Yang[1], Kun Wang[1], Yingwen Zhu[1], Xiujie Gao[1] and Bo Cui[1,2*]*

[1] Tianjin Institute of Environmental and Operational Medicine, Tianjin, China, [2] Shandong Academy of Occupational Health and Occupational Medicine, Shandong First Medical University & Shandong Academy of Medical Sciences, Jinan, China

***Correspondence:**
Xiujie Gao
xjgao@ustc.edu
Bo Cui
iamcuibo@sina.com

† These authors have contributed equally to this work and share first authorship

High-intensity noise can cause permanent hearing loss; however, short-duration medium-intensity noise only induces a temporary threshold shift (TTS) and damages synapses formed by inner hair cells (IHCs) and spiral ganglion nerves. Synaptopathy is generally thought to be caused by glutamate excitotoxicity. In this study, we investigated the expression levels of vesicle transporter protein 3 (Vglut3), responsible for the release of glutamate; glutamate/aspartate transporter protein (GLAST), responsible for the uptake of glutamate; and Na^+/K^+-ATPase α1 coupled with GLAST, in the process of synaptopathy in the cochlea. The results of the auditory brainstem response (ABR) and CtBP2 immunofluorescence revealed that synaptopathy was induced on day 30 after 100 dB SPL noise exposure in C57BL/6J mice. We found that GLAST and Na^+/K^+-ATPase α1 were co-localized in the cochlea, mainly in the stria vascularis, spiral ligament, and spiral ganglion cells. Furthermore, Vglut3, GLAST, and Na^+/K^+-ATPase α1 expression were disrupted after noise exposure. These results indicate that disruption of glutamate release and uptake-related protein expression may exacerbate the occurrence of synaptopathy.

Keywords: noise, synaptopathy, Vglut3, GLAST, Na^+/K^+-ATPase α1, glutamate excitotoxicity

INTRODUCTION

High-level noise, which can cause sensorineural hearing loss accompanied by permanent threshold shift, has become a major threat to human health. Short-duration medium-intensity noise (e.g., 98, 100, 106 dB SPL, 2 h), which only causes a temporary threshold shift (TTS), is distinguished from high-level noise exposure (Furman et al., 2013; Liberman et al., 2015; Bakay et al., 2018; Fernandez et al., 2020; Wei et al., 2020). In the inner ear, the mechanical vibration of sound wave was transformed into the electric signals by cochlear hair cells (Wang et al., 2017; Liu Y. et al., 2019; Qi et al., 2019, 2020; Zhang Y. et al., 2020); while spiral ganglion neurons mainly function as the neural auditory transduction cells (Sun et al., 2016; Guo et al., 2019, 2021; Liu W. et al., 2019b; Zhao et al., 2019). Noise induced hearing loss includes damage of cochlear hair cells (Liu et al., 2016; He et al., 2017, 2021; Zhou et al., 2020; Cheng et al., 2021; Fu et al., 2021), cochlear supporting cells (Lu et al., 2017; Cheng et al., 2019; Tan et al., 2019; Zhang S. et al., 2019, 2020; Zhang Y. et al., 2020;

Chen et al., 2021), spiral ganglion neurons (Guo et al., 2016, 2020, 2021; Sun et al., 2016; Liu et al., 2021) and ribbon synaptopathy (Furman et al., 2013; Shi et al., 2013; Kujawa and Liberman, 2015; Liberman et al., 2015; Bakay et al., 2018; Fernandez et al., 2020; Kohrman et al., 2020; Tserga et al., 2020a; Wei et al., 2020; Song et al., 2021). It has been reported that the wave I amplitude of the auditory brainstem response (ABR) is permanently reduced and ribbon synapses between inner hair cells (IHCs) and spiral ganglion nerves are damaged after exposure to short-duration medium intensity noise (Liberman et al., 2015; Fernandez et al., 2020; Wei et al., 2020). Glutamate excitotoxicity is known to be a major factor in the damage to ribbon synapses (Kurabi et al., 2017; Sebe et al., 2017; Hu et al., 2020), but it is unknown how glutamate-associated proteins are altered after noise exposure.

Vesicle transporter protein 3 (Vglut3), encoded by the SLC17A8 gene, is important for the development and maturation of the inner ear (Obholzer et al., 2008; Ruel et al., 2008; Kim et al., 2019). Within IHCs, Vglut3 facilitates the packaging of glutamate into vesicles which is subsequently secreted into the postsynaptic membrane during exocytosis, to transduce acoustic signals into neural signals. Disrupted expression or deletion of Vglut3 can lead to tinnitus (Zhang W. et al., 2020) and deafness (Ruel et al., 2008; Seal et al., 2008; Akil et al., 2012); previous studies have suggested that knocking out the Vglut3 allele results in decreased ribbon synapse density and the number of spiral ganglion nerves (Kim et al., 2019). Moreover, ototoxic drugs (Zhang Y. et al., 2020) and aging (Peng et al., 2013) can also affect the expression of Vglut3.

Glutamate/aspartate transporter protein (GLAST) is widely expressed in the central and peripheral nervous systems (CNS and PNS, respectively), and is mainly expressed in the pillar cells (PCs) surrounding IHCs, the main site of glutamate uptake in the inner ear (Glowatzki et al., 2006). Hakuba et al. (2000) found that cochlear glutamate levels were much higher in $GLAST^{-/-}$ animals compared to wild-type animals, which may result from glutamate uptake dysfunction. Glutamate uptake through the GLAST is dependent on the Na^+ concentration gradient, which is primarily maintained by Na^+/K^+-ATPase (Zhang et al., 2016). Na^+/K^+-ATPase consists of α, β, and γ subunits, which are further divided into $\alpha 1$, $\alpha 2$, and $\alpha 3$ subunits. CNS studies have shown that GLAST interacts with Na^+/K^+-ATPase, especially through the $\alpha 1$ subunit to co-uptake extracellular glutamate to protect neurons from excitotoxic injury (Bauer et al., 2012; Zhang et al., 2016). It is unclear whether GLAST interacts with Na^+/K^+-ATPase $\alpha 1$ in the cochlea.

A cycle consisting of Vglut3 and GLAST maintains low concentrations of glutamate in the cochlea. Excitotoxicity may occur when this cycle is disrupted. Therefore, we wanted to study how Vglut3, GLAST, and Na^+/K^+-ATPase $\alpha 1$ changed after ribbon synaptopathy. First, we investigated whether GLAST interacts with Na^+/K^+-ATPase $\alpha 1$ in the inner ear. Second, we constructed a ribbon synaptopathy model using 100 dB SPL white noise, and then measured the expression of Vglut3, GLAST, and Na^+/K^+-ATPase $\alpha 1$ at four different time points (2 h, 1 day, 7 days, and 30 days), after exposure to noise.

MATERIALS AND METHODS

Animals and Groups

Six-week-old male C57BL/6J mice ($N = 55$) were purchased from Vital River (Beijing, China). The animals were housed in a 12 h light/dark cycle for 1 week in an animal laboratory room, where the ambient noise was maintained below 50 dB SPL, and food and water were provided *ad libitum*. Fifteen mice were used for immunoprecipitation experiments before noise exposure, and the remaining 40 mice were divided into two groups. Ten mice were included in the control group (Ctr) without noise exposure; one mouse died due to an overdose of anesthetic injection during the ABR measurement. Thirty mice were included in the noise exposure group. ABR and immunofluorescence were detected on day 1 (1 d), day 7 (7 d), and day 30 (30 d) after noise exposure. All experiments were approved by the ethics committee of the Tianjin Institute of Environmental and Operational Medicine.

Noise Exposure

Mice were placed in a small cage woven with wire and placed under an amplifier (IBO, BA-215, China) at a distance of 10 cm from the mouse's ears. Mice were exposed to a 100 dB SPL white noise stimulus for 2 h produced by a sound generator (SKC, GZ009, China). The sound intensity was calibrated with a sound level meter (BSWA, 308, China) at the mouse's ear position, from different directions. The average noise level was 100 ± 1.9 dB SPL.

ABR Detection

Auditory brainstem response was measured in an electroacoustic shielded room before noise exposure and on days 1, 7, and 30 after noise exposure. Mice were anesthetized using ketamine (100 mg/kg) and thiazide (3 mg/kg), and the recording needle was inserted into the Fz point of the head, the reference needle was placed in the mastoid of both ears, and the grounding needle was inserted into the skin of the forepaw. ABR waveforms were recorded at 4, 8, 12, and 16 kHz pure-tone (3,000 μs) stimulations. Sound intensity was decreased in 10 dB steps at high levels of stimulation and in 5 dB steps near the hearing threshold. Because wave II was easily recognized, the lowest stimulus intensity of wave II was used as the hearing threshold, and was repeated it three times to confirm the threshold intensity. A wave I amplitude of 90 dB was detected at each frequency.

Immunofluorescence

Mice were anesthetized with ketamine (100 mg/kg) and thiazide (3 mg/kg) and the cochleae were carefully removed and fixed with 4% paraformaldehyde (PFA). Briefly, the muscle tissue was carefully removed under a body microscope (Olympus, SZX7, Japan), and a hole was drilled at the top of the cochlea. PFA was slowly injected into the cochlea from the round window, with a syringe until the top of cochlea flowed clear liquid; the cochleae were then fixed overnight at 4°C in 4% PFA. The fixed cochlea was placed in 10% ethylene diamine tetra-acetic acid at room temperature overnight. For whole-mount staining, cochlear basilar membranes were carefully isolated and rinsed three times with Phosphate Buffered Saline (PBS). For frozen sections, cochleae were rinsed three times with PBS and dehydrated overnight in 30% sucrose. Then, cochleae were cut into 20 μm sections after incubation in embedding agent for 3 days. Tissues were incubated in PBS containing 1% Triton-X 100 for 30 min at room temperature, followed by incubation with PBS containing 0.5% Triton-X 100 and 5% BSA for 1 h at room temperature. Rabbit anti-CtBP2 (1:100; Bioworld, BS2287), rabbit anti-GLAST (1:1,000, Abcam, Ab416), and mouse anti-Na^+/K^+-ATPase α1 (1:500, Millipore, #05-369) were applied overnight or for 2 h at room temperature. Tissues were rinsed three times for 10 min each with PBS containing 1% Triton-X 100. Tissue sections were incubated in secondary antibodies conjugated with dylight 488 (1:500, Bioworld, BS10015) or dylight 549 (1:500, Bioworld, BS10023), for 1 h at room temperature. Tissues were rinsed three times for 10 min each with PBS containing 1% Triton-X 100. The tissues were mounted on glass slides after nuclei staining.

Confocal and Fluorescence Microscopy

For whole-mount staining, tissues were photographed with a 63× oil objective using 546 nm wave with a laser confocal microscope (Leica, SP8, Germany). Meanwhile, the field of view was 1.8 digital zoom. All photographs were taken in 0.5 μm steps with equal laser intensity and exposure time. For frozen sections, photographs were taken under a normal fluorescence microscope (Olympus BX51, Japan). Panoramic and local photographs were taken under 20× and 100× objectives, respectively, with equal fluorescence intensity and exposure time.

Immunoprecipitation

The basilar membrane, spiral ligament, and osseous spiral lamina, which were removed from the ear unexposed to noise, were placed in IP lysate (60 μL, containing 1% inhibitor cocktail) on ice. Tissues were homogenized with a pestle and lysed on ice for 30 min. The supernatant (approximately 50 μL) was collected after centrifugation at 10,000 rpm for 15 min at 4°C. GLAST or IgG antibody (1 μL; CST, #5684, Santa Cruz, sc-2025, respectively) and supernatant were co-incubated overnight at 4°C in a shaker. An equal volume of beads (Santa Cruz, sc-2003) were added. The mixture was incubated at room temperature for 4 h, followed by centrifugation at 3,000 rpm for 5 min at 4°C. The beads were rinsed three times with IP lysis solution, and finally resuspended in 30 μl of IP lysis solution. Western Blotting was performed after adding 30 μl of loading buffer to boil.

Western Blot

To extract total protein, cochleae were homogenized in radioimmunoprecipitation assay buffer (containing 1% enzyme inhibitor), and the bones were removed. Samples were loaded according to total protein amount, which was calculated by measuring the gray level of β-actin (1:200, Santa Cruz, sc-47778). Proteins were separated using sodium dodecyl sulfate-polyacrylamide gel electrophoresis. After electrophoresis, the proteins were transferred onto a nitrocellulose membrane and blocked with 5% degreased milk powder in PBS plus 0.1% Tween 20 (PBST). The membrane was incubated with primary antibodies at 4°C overnight and washed three times (10 min per wash) with PBST. The membranes were then incubated with the secondary antibodies for 2 h. After the membrane was washed, the protein bands were visualized by electrochemiluminescence.

Statistical Analysis

All data are expressed as the mean ± standard error of the mean. All statistical analyses were performed using GraphPad Prism version 8. ABR threshold and amplitude data were analyzed by two-way analysis of variance (ANOVA). CtBP2 count and protein expression levels were analyzed by one-way ANOVA.

RESULTS

ABR Threshold and Wave I Amplitude Detection

To examine the effects of noise on the peripheral auditory system, we first compared hearing thresholds between the control and noise groups on days 1, 7, and 30-post exposure. There was no change in the 4 kHz hearing threshold (**Figure 1B**). Hearing thresholds at 8 kHz were only significantly elevated on day 1 after exposure (**Figure 1C**), and significantly higher than that of the control on days 1 and 7 after noise exposure, at both 12 kHz and 16 kHz (**Figures 1A,D,E**). The thresholds of all pure tones were not significantly different from controls on day 30 post-exposure (**Figures 1A–E**). These ABR threshold results indicate that the TTS is caused by noise. Furthermore, hair cell damage was not detected on days 1, 7, or 30 after noise exposure, compared to the Ctr (**Figure 1F**).

We then measured the change in wave I amplitude and found that the wave I amplitude of all pure tones was significantly lower than that of the Ctr (**Figures 2A–E**). On day 1 after noise exposure, the amplitude of wave I was the lowest at all frequencies (**Figures 2B–E**). On day 7, the amplitude recovered compared to day 1 (**Figures 2B–E**). On day 30, there was a significant decrease in amplitude compared with the Ctr, as well as a decrease compared to day 7 (**Figures 2B–E**). These amplitude results indicate that nerve transmission was damaged by noise exposure. It seems that the latency of wave I was delayed after noise exposure (**Figure 2A**). Through statistical analysis, no significant difference was found in latency of wave I on day 30 (data not show), which is consistent with previous studies (Kujawa and Liberman, 2015; Liberman et al., 2015; Fernandez et al., 2020; Kohrman et al., 2020; Wei et al., 2020; Song et al., 2021).

Ribbon Synaptopathy Caused by Noise Exposure

Since the amplitude of ABR wave I indicates the total activity of the SGN (Plack et al., 2016), we stained for CtBP2 on day 1, 7, and 30 after noise exposure, to determine whether the decrease in wave I amplitude was caused by ribbon synaptopathy. Punctate CtBP2 was distributed around IHCs as well as within the nuclei, and in supporting cells (**Figure 3A**). In the apical region, CtBP2 numbers decreased significantly on day 1 after noise exposure; however, CtBP2 numbers recovered significantly on days 7 and 30, but this difference was not significant compared to that of day 1 (**Figures 3A,B**). In the middle region, the number

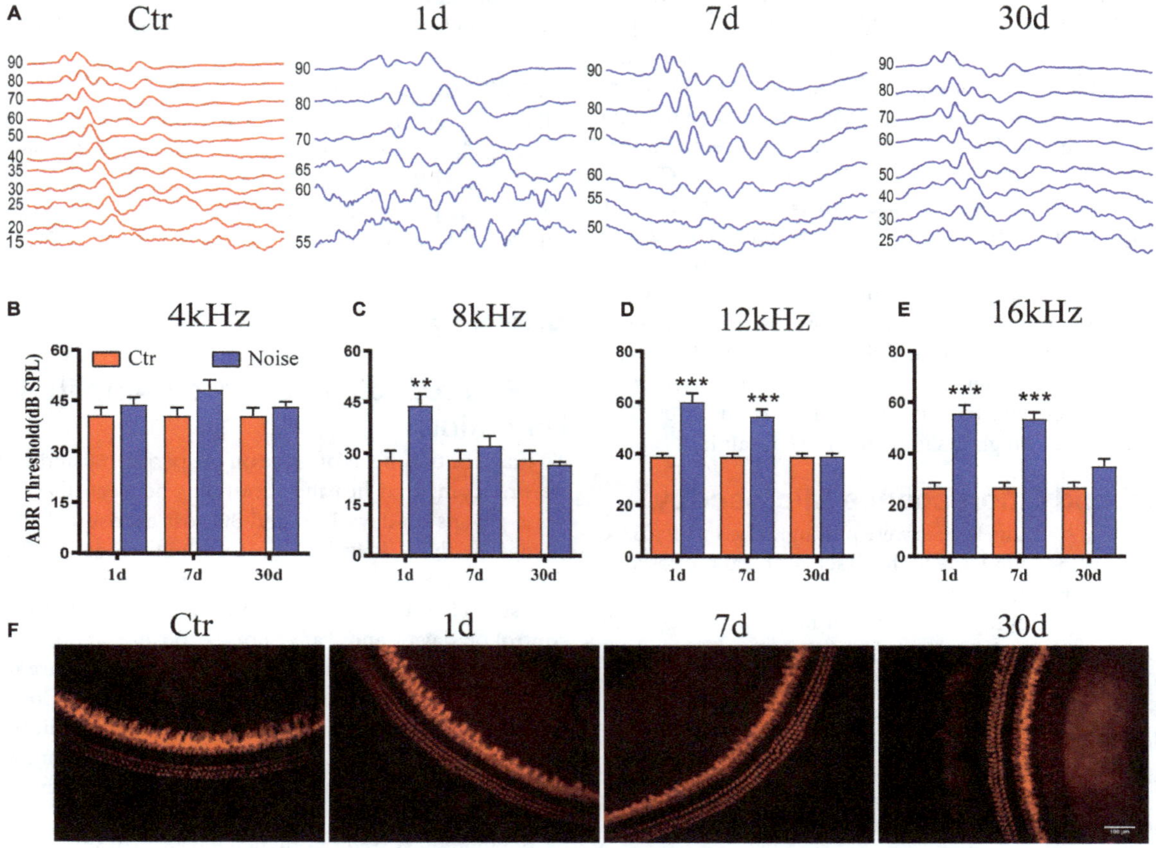

FIGURE 1 | Auditory brainstem response (ABR) threshold following noise exposure. **(A)** The waveform of control and day 1, 7, and 30 after noise exposure with 90 dB SPL pure tone stimulation at 16 kHz. **(B–E)** Statistical analysis of ABR threshold showed temporary threshold shift at 4 kHz **(B)**, 8 kHz **(C)**, 12 kHz **(D)**, and 16 kHz **(E)** (n = 9–10). **(F)** Immunofluorescence image of hair cells at middle turn in the basilar membrane with anti-myosin VIIa antibody at 20x objective, scale bar = 100 μm. **vs. Ctr, $p < 0.01$; ***vs. Ctr, $p < 0.001$.

of CtBP2 decreased on day 1 after noise exposure, but there was no significant difference compared with the Ctr. On day 7 after exposure, the numbers were equivalent to controls and recovered compared with day 1 after noise exposure. The CtBP2 numbers were significantly lower than those in the Ctr on day 30, after noise exposure (**Figures 3A,C**). In the apical and middle regions, the recovery of CtBP2 may suggest the presence of synaptic remodeling. In the base region, the number of CtBP2 decreased significantly on days 1, 7, and 30 after noise exposure (**Figures 3A,D**). The change in CtBP2 numbers is consistent with the change in wave I amplitude.

The Interaction of GLAST and Na^+/K^+-ATPase α1 in Cochlea

Studies of the CNS have shown a clear interaction between GLAST and Na^+/K^+-ATPase α1 (Bauer et al., 2012; Zhang et al., 2016). To investigate the relationship between GLAST and Na^+/K^+-ATPase α1 in the cochlea, we performed immunoprecipitation and immuno co-localization within the cochlea. After purification of the protein with GLAST antibody, immunoblotting of GLAST and Na^+/K^+-ATPase α1 on the same membrane was performed sequentially, and clear bands were observed in the input lane and the GLAST lane, but not in the IgG lane (**Figure 4A**). Following, we detected immunoreactivity of GLAST and Na^+/K^+-ATPase α1 in the cochlear basilar membrane; only GLAST immuno-positivity was identified (**Figure 4B**). To determine immunoreactivity in other structures, we performed immunofluorescence using frozen sections. We found co-localization of GLAST and Na^+/K^+-ATPase α1 in the stria vascularis (**Figure 4C**, white dovetailed arrowhead, D), the spiral ligament (**Figure 4C**, white flat-tailed arrowhead, D), and spiral ganglion cells (**Figures 4C,D**). Na^+/K^+-ATPase α1 was only expressed in hair cells in the Organ of Cotti. There is no evidence that GLAST and Na^+/K^+-ATPase α1 are co-expressed in PCs which are major cells to take in glutamate (**Figures 4B–D**).

Noise Exposure Disorders Vglut3, GLAST and Na^+/K^+-ATPase α1 Expression

To determine the changes in Vglut3, GLAST or Na^+/K^+-ATPase α1, we examined the expression levels of these proteins at 2 h, 1 day, 7 days, and 30 days after noise exposure (**Figure 5A**). Vglut3

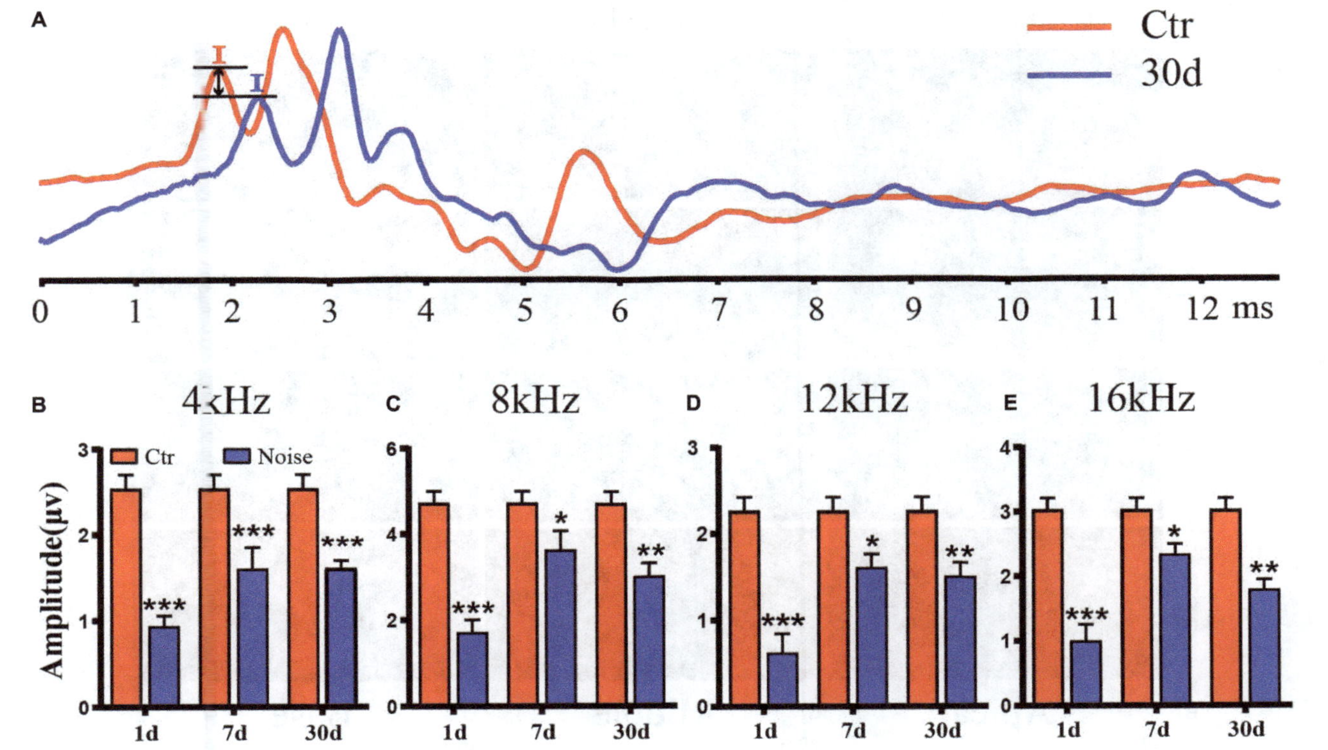

FIGURE 2 | Auditory brainstem response (ABR) wave I amplitude after noise exposure. **(A)** The comparison of wave I amplitude of the control group and day 30 after noise exposure with 90 dB SPL pure tone stimulation at 16 kHz. **(B–E)** Statistical analysis of wave I amplitude at 4 kHz **(B)**, 8 kHz **(C)**, 12 kHz **(D)**, and 16 kHz **(E)** (n = 9–10). *vs. Ctr, $p < 0.05$; **vs. Ctr, $p < 0.01$; ***vs. Ctr, $p < 0.001$.

expression level was lowest at 2 h after noise exposure. Vglut3 expression level recovered on day 1, but it was still lower than that of the Ctr. On day 7, the Vglut3 expression level increased significantly compared to that of the control at hour 2 or day 1 (**Figure 5B**). Vglut3 expression level decreased on day 30 but was still significantly higher than that in the control at hour 2, or day 1 (**Figure 5B**). The expression levels of GLAST and Na^+/K^+-ATPase α1 were completely opposite to those of Vglut3. The expression level of GLAST gradually increased between hour 2 and day 7, it recovered until on day 30 after noise exposure (**Figure 5C**). The change in Na^+/K^+-ATPase α1 was consistent with GLAST at 2 h and 1 day after noise exposure, but returned to normal levels on day 7 after noise exposure, and significantly decreased on day 30 compared to day 1 (**Figure 5D**). These results indicate an enhanced ability to release glutamate and a decreased ability to uptake glutamate on day 30 after noise exposure, which may be the main mediator of synaptopathy.

DISCUSSION

The cochlear hair cells are sensitive to aging, acoustic trauma, ototoxic drugs, and environmental or genetic influences (Zhu et al., 2018; Fang et al., 2019; He et al., 2020; Jiang et al., 2020; Qian et al., 2020; Lv et al., 2021; Zhang et al., 2021). Previous reports have shown that oxidative stress and cell apoptosis play important roles in noise induced hair cell loss and ribbon synaptopathy (Sun et al., 2014; Yu et al., 2017; Li et al., 2018; Gao et al., 2019; He et al., 2019; Zhang Y. et al., 2019; Zhong et al., 2020). In this study, we confirmed the interaction between GLAST and Na^+/K^+-ATPase α1 in the cochlea of C57BL/6J mice; protein expression was mainly co-localized in the stria vascularis, spiral ligament, and spiral ganglion cells, but not in the PCs, the major site of glutamate uptake. On day 30 after noise exposure, C57BL/6J mice experienced a TTS, a decrease in wave I amplitude at the 4, 8, 12, and 16 kHz cochlear regions, and a decrease in the amount of the presynaptic protein CtBP2. Meanwhile, the expression level of Vglut3 was upregulated on day 30 after exposure, and the expression level of GLAST remained almost unchanged, however, the expression level of Na^+/K^+-ATPase α1, which is directly coupled to GLAST, was downregulated. These findings may reveal an intrinsic link between noise-induced glutamate excitotoxicity and ribbon synaptopathy.

Vglut3 dysfunction or deficiency disrupts nerve conduction in the peripheral auditory system. LSP5-2157, an inhibitor of Vglut3, inhibited the compound action potential of the peripheral auditory system in guinea pigs (Poirel et al., 2020). Animals lose hearing after knockout of the Vglut3 allele; however, it can be restored using an adenoviral vector delivery system to re-establish Vglut3 expression (Akil et al., 2015; Akil and Lustig, 2019; Kim et al., 2019). In our study, the expression of Vglut3 was lowest at 2 h, slightly recovered on day 1, was highest on day 7, and

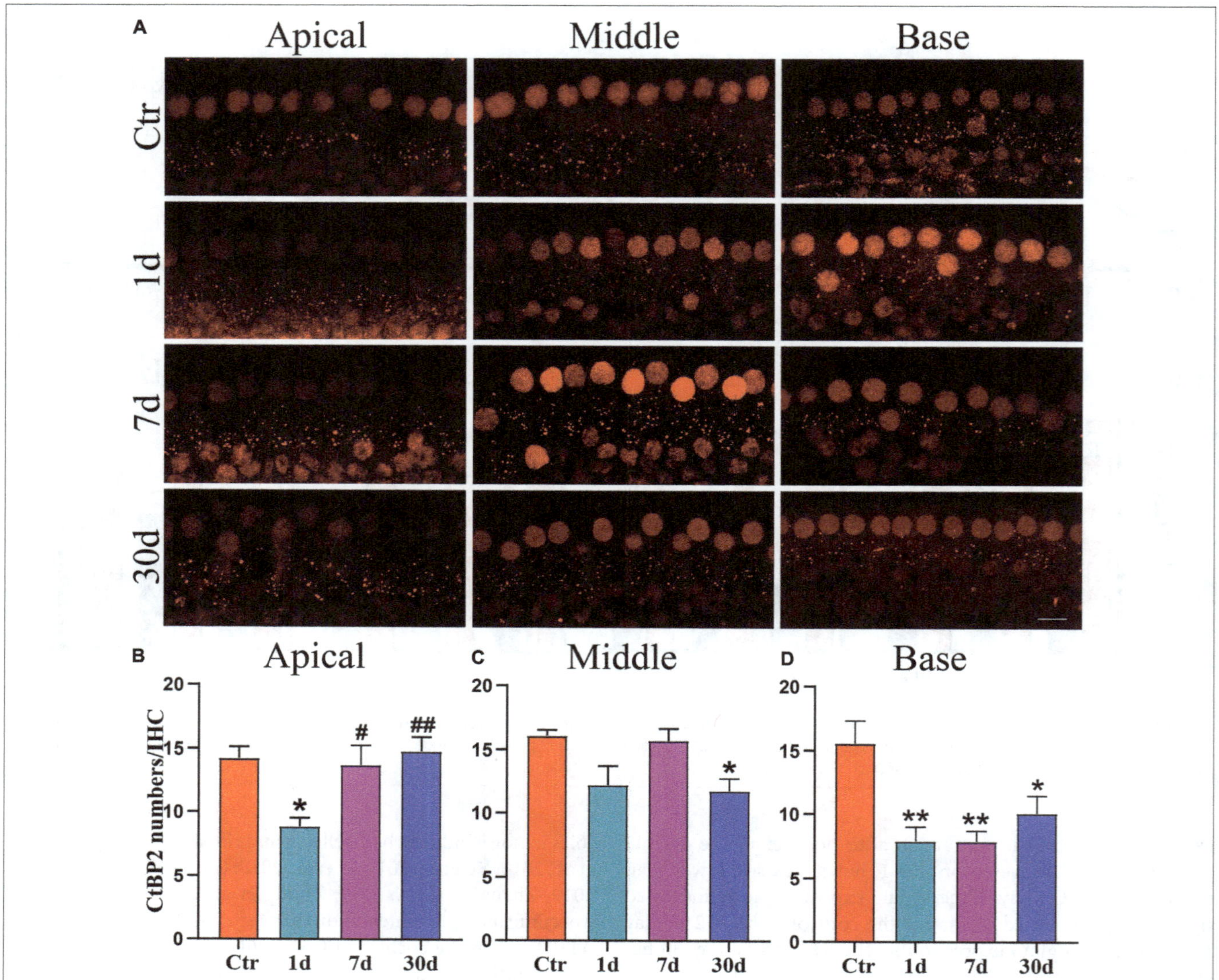

FIGURE 3 | Changes of CtBP2 numbers after noise exposure. **(A)** Immunofluorescence images was taken by confocal microscope with a 63x oil objective. Punctate CtBP2 was labeled with a CtBP2 antibody in IHCs; IHCs and supporting cells' nuclei were also stained, scale bars = 10 μm. **(B–D)** Statistical analysis of CtBP2 in each group (n = 4–5 ears) on day 1, day 7, and day 30 after noise exposure. *vs. Ctr, $p < 0.05$; **vs. Ctr, $p < 0.01$; #vs. 1 day, $p < 0.05$; ##vs. 1 day, $p < 0.01$.

slightly lowered on day 30 which was almost consistent with the observed change in wave I amplitude. Hu et al. (2020) and Sebe et al. (2017) considered that noise-induced ribbon synaptopathy is caused by over-activation of Ca^{2+}-permeable AMPA receptors (CP-AMPARs), which lack GluR2, and mediate excessive inward Ca^{2+} which can damage presynaptic ribbons and postsynaptic receptors. Kim et al. (2019) revealed the role of the Vglut3 in CP-AMPAR-mediated glutamatergic excitotoxicity. They found that a single copy of the Vglut3 gene was sufficient to cause ribbon synaptopathy after noise exposure, and deletion of the Vglut3 allele reduced excitotoxicity induced by noise. Our study found that the intensity of CtBP2 significantly reduced in the apical and base regions on day 1 after noise exposure, compared to that of the Ctr, and that the expression of CtBP2 in the middle region was reduced compared to the Ctr (not statistically significant). Although Vglut3 expression levels decreased on day 1 after noise exposure, the ribbon synapse structure was also damaged, which means that low levels of glutamate can also cause ribbon synaptopathy under the influence of noise. Synapses recovered on day 7 (apical and middle region) or day 30 (apical region) after exposure, suggesting the presence of synaptic reconstruction. ABR thresholds and wave I amplitudes of $Vglut3^{WT}$ animals recovered better than $Vglut3^{+/-}$ mice exposed to 94 dB SPL noise, indicating that Vglut3 or glutamate release contributed to hearing recovery (Kim et al., 2019). Glutamate release may also help to construct synapses (Akil et al., 2012; Shi et al., 2013; Song et al., 2021). Synaptic remodeling was not observed on day 7 in the base region, and it is possible that the base region is more susceptible to noise and the development of ribbon synaptopathy. Our results are consistent with those of the previous studies.

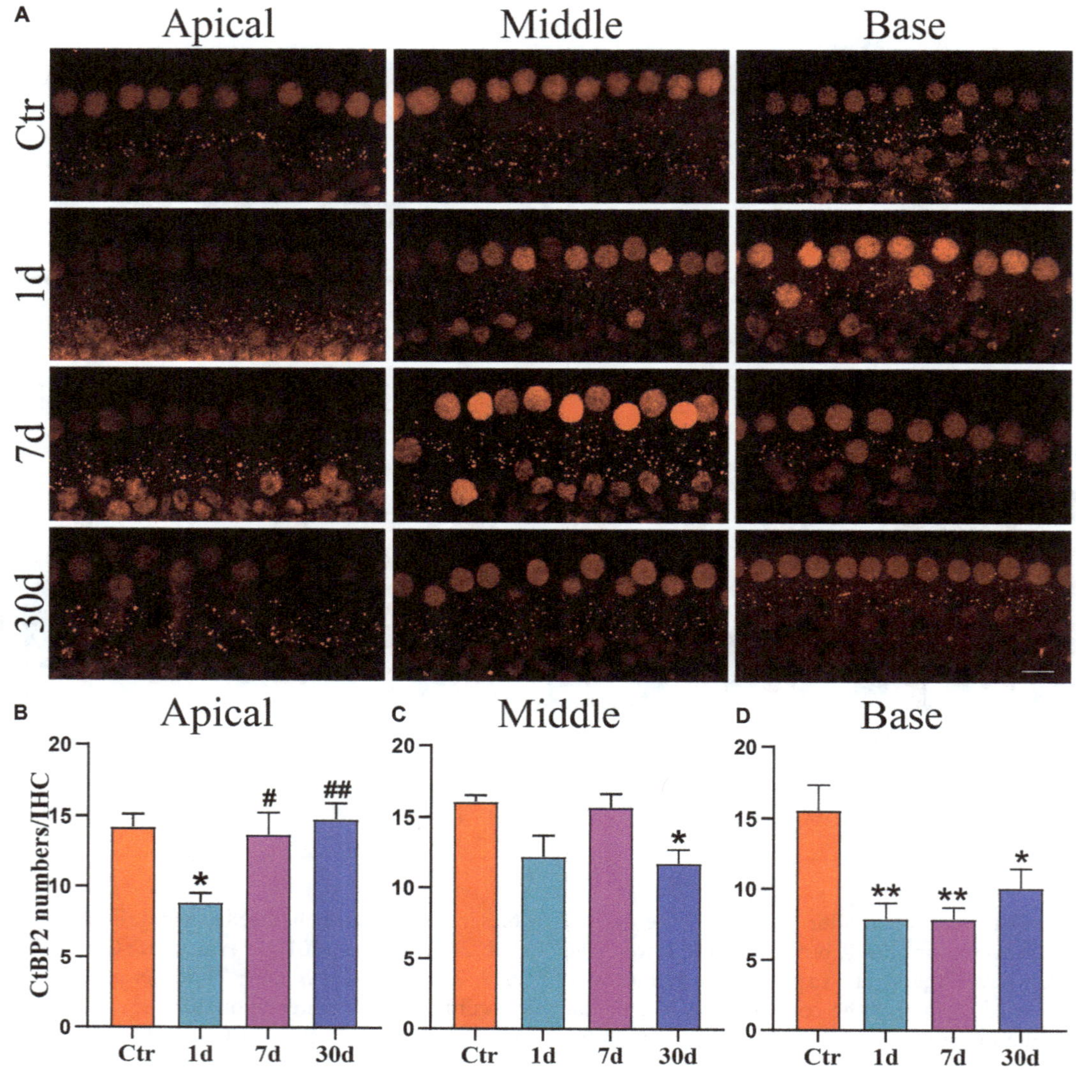

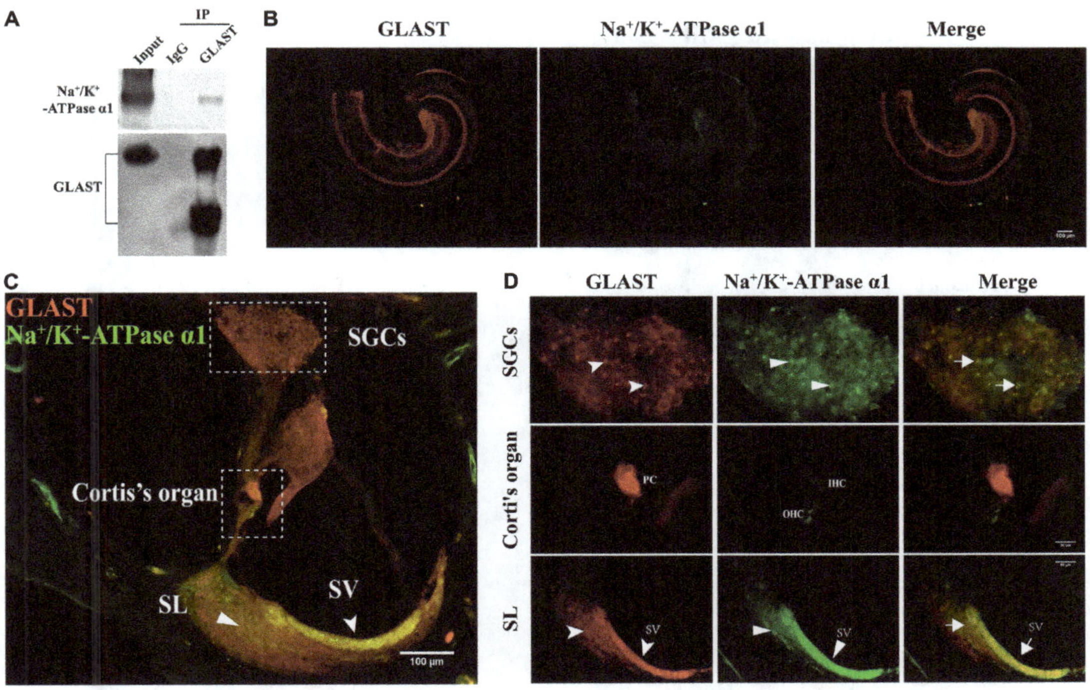

FIGURE 4 | Interaction of GLAST and Na^+/K^+-ATPase α1. **(A)** Immunoprecipitation of GLAST from cochlear tissue. Anti-GLAST antibody or IgG was used for Immunoprecipitation from cochlea lysates (*n* = 10 ears). Except for the IgG lane, endogenous Na^+/K^+-ATPase α1 and GLAST were all detected on the same membrane. **(B)** Immunofluorescence image of apical turn in the basilar membrane, scale bar = 100 μm. **(C)** Frozen sections of noise-unexposed C57BL/6J cochlea were stained with anti-GLAST antibody (red) and anti- Na^+/K^+-ATPase α1 (green) antibody, scale bar = 100 μm; the dovetailed arrowhead represents SV; the flat-tailed arrowhead represents SL. **(D)** Corti's organ and spiral ganglion cells (SGCs) were magnified under 100x oil objective, scale bars = 20 μm; spiral ligament is magnified under 40x objective, scale bars = 50 μm; GLAST (the dovetailed arrowhead), Na^+/K^+-ATPase α1 (the flat-tailed arrowhead) and merged immunopositive fluorescence (the arrow) were point out in particular. SGCs, spiral ganglion cells; SV, stria vascularis; SL, spiral ligament; PCs, pillar cells; OHCs, out hair cells; IHCs, inner hair cells.

Reduced ribbon synapses may promote the expression of Vglut3 protein to maintain physiological signal transduction.

The main function of GLAST transport extracellular glutamate, while the uptake drive depends on the Na^+ concentration gradient inside and outside of cells; Na^+/K^+-ATPase maintains the Na^+ gradient concentration difference by hydrolyzing ATP (Robinson and Jackson, 2016). Studies on astrocytes and the CNS have shown that Na^+/K^+-ATPase is directly coupled to GLAST *via* the α subunit (Rose et al., 2009; Bauer et al., 2012; Robinson and Jackson, 2016; Zhang et al., 2016). In the peripheral auditory system, GLAST and Na^+/K^+-ATPase α1 are both expressed in PCs surrounding IHCs (Glowatzki et al., 2006; McLean et al., 2009; Sundaresan et al., 2016; Liu W. et al., 2019a; Stephenson et al., 2021). In our study, we found an interaction between GLAST and Na^+/K^+-ATPase α1; however, immuno co-localization revealed that the sites of interaction were in the stria vascularis, spiral ligament, and SGCs. There was no α1 subunit immunoreactivity in the PCs. Immunoreactivity of Na^+/K^+-ATPase α1 have been demonstrated in stria vascularis, spiral ligament and support cells in the human cochlea (Stephenson et al., 2021). Our findings on Na^+/K^+-ATPase α1 were consistent with published researches on stria vascularis, spiral ligament, SGCs and hair cells (Clemens Grisham et al., 2013; Yamaguchi et al., 2014; Ding et al., 2018; Liu W. et al., 2019a; Stephenson et al., 2021). Our findings in PCs differ from studies done in rats (McLean et al., 2009). PCs and IHCs are adjacent in spatial structure, which maybe an account for no immunoreactivity of Na^+/K^+-ATPase α1 in PCs. Na^+/K^+-ATPase α1 not expressing simultaneously in PCs or IHCs can reduce structural and functional redundancy.

The functional deficiency of GLAST affects hearing sensitivity and synaptic integrity (Yu et al., 2016; Tserga et al., 2020b). Glutamate levels in the endolymph fluid were twice as high in GLAST knockout animals compared to wild-type mice, after noise exposure, revealing that noise-induced hearing loss and ribbon synaptopathy may be caused by glutamate excitotoxicity (Hakuba et al., 2000). The combined exogenous inhibitor and glutamate perfusion further demonstrated the importance of GLAST in the hearing system (Chen et al., 2010). In our study, GLAST expression levels gradually increased after noise exposure and recovered on day 30, possibly indicating that the inner ear prevented glutamate toxicity by increasing GLAST expression levels. However, Vglut3 expression level increased on day 7, thereby increasing the release of glutamate. The extent of GLAST increase may not be sufficient to fully take in glutamate due to increased Vglut3 expression level, resulting in excitotoxicity. Aminoglycosides,

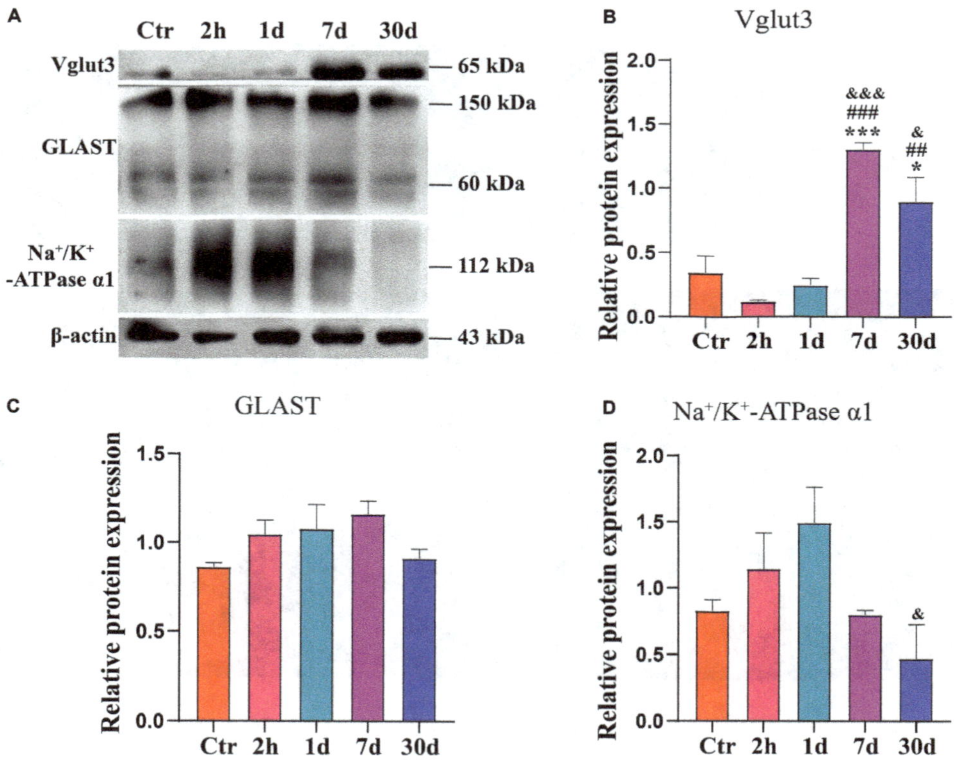

FIGURE 5 | Expression levels of GLAST, Na^+/K^+-ATPase α1 and Vglut3 were disrupted after noise exposure. **(A)** Western blot of Vglut3, GLAST and Na^+/K^+-ATPase α1 from normal cochlea and noise-exposure cochlea on hour 2, day 1, day 7, day 30 after noise (n = 6–8 ears). **(B–D)** Quantification of expression levels of Vglut3, GLAST and Na^+/K^+-ATPase α1. The statistics were repeated three times. *vs. Ctr, $p < 0.05$; ***vs. Ctr, $p < 0.001$. ##vs. 2 h, $p < 0.01$; ###vs. 2 h, $p < 0.001$; &vs. 1 day, $p < 0.05$; &&&vs. 1 day, $p < 0.001$.

like noise, are excitotoxic to the peripheral auditory system (Kohrman et al., 2020). Kanamycin, an aminoglycoside, induced high expression of cochlear GLAST mRNA, which returned to normal until the 12th day after treatment (Matsuda et al., 1999). Although there is no significantly difference in expression of GLAST in our study, we found that there is the tendency for decreasing of excitotoxicity through increasing of GLAST. In our study, the expression pattern of GLAST induced by noise was consistent with that of kanamycin (Matsuda et al., 1999).

The interaction of Na^+/K^+-ATPase α1 with GLAST determines its important role in glutamate uptake. Ouabain, a selective inhibitor of Na^+/K^+-ATPase, can cause pathological changes in the rodent cochlea, mainly type I SGN damage (Lang et al., 2005; Fu et al., 2012; Yuan et al., 2014; Zhang et al., 2017; Schomann et al., 2018). Low spontaneous rate fiber damage in type I fibers is an important feature of synaptopathy (Furman et al., 2013; Kujawa and Liberman, 2015). Inhibition of Na^+/K^+-ATPase activity may significantly reduce the ability of GLAST to take-up glutamate (Rose et al., 2009). In our study, we found that the expression of GLAST and Na^+/K^+-ATPase α1 were almost identical within a week after noise exposure, which is reasonable for reducing excitotoxicity. The expression level of Na^+/K^+-ATPase α1 was reduced on day 30 after noise exposure, which may limit the function of GLAST, and the expression of Vglut3 increased, resulting in a pathological concentration of glutamate in the synaptic cleft, causing ribbon synaptopathy.

SUMMARY

In this study, we found an interaction between GLAST and Na^+/K^+-ATPase α1 in the cochlea of C57BL/6J mice. Based on the present results, we conclude that noise exposure influences ribbon synapses in two ways: (1) Noise briefly downregulated the expression of Vglut3 and upregulated the expression of GLAST and Na^+/K^+-ATPase α1, which trend to help to reduce glutamate toxicity in the synaptic cleft; (2) Noise damages ribbon synapses, and Vglut3 expression is upregulated for the normal transmission of auditory signals, but further downregulation of Na^+/K^+-ATPase α1 limits the uptake function of GLAST on day 30, which may further increase glutamate toxicity. Our study may provide a new approach for the prevention and treatment of ribbon synaptopathy.

ETHICS STATEMENT

The animal study was reviewed and approved by Laboratory Animal Welfare Ethics Committee of Tianjin Institute of Environmental and Operational Medicine.

AUTHOR CONTRIBUTIONS

KM and AZ performed whole experimental work. KM wrote the manuscript. XS contributed to ABR experiment. XS, HY, KW, and YZ contributed to data analysis. HY, XG, and BC contributed to the experimental design. XG and BC revised the manuscript. KM and BC secured funding for the study. All authors discussed the results and approved the final manuscript.

REFERENCES

Akil, O., and Lustig, L. (2019). AAV-Mediated Gene Delivery to the Inner Ear. *Methods Mol. Biol.* 1950, 271–282. doi: 10.1007/978-1-4939-9139-6_16

Akil, O., Rouse, S. L., Chan, D. K., and Lustig, L. R. (2015). Surgical method for virally mediated gene delivery to the mouse inner ear through the round window membrane. *J. Vis. Exp.* 97:e52187. doi: 10.3791/52187

Akil, O., Seal, R. P., Burke, K., Wang, C., Alemi, A., During, M., et al. (2012). Restoration of hearing in the VGLUT3 knockout mouse using virally mediated gene therapy. *Neuron* 75, 283–293. doi: 10.1016/j.neuron.2012.05.019

Bakay, W. M. H., Anderson, L. A., Garcia-Lazaro, J. A., McAlpine, D., and Schaette, R. (2018). Hidden hearing loss selectively impairs neural adaptation to loud sound environments. *Nat. Commun.* 9:4298. doi: 10.1038/s41467-018-06777-y

Bauer, D. E., Jackson, J. G., Genda, E. N., Montoya, M. M., Yudkoff, M., and Robinson, M. B. (2012). The glutamate transporter, GLAST, participates in a macromolecular complex that supports glutamate metabolism. *Neurochem. Int.* 61, 566–574. doi: 10.1016/j.neuint.2012.01.013

Chen, Y., Gu, Y., Li, Y., Li, G. L., Chai, R., Li, W., et al. (2021). Generation of mature and functional hair cells by co-expression of Gfi1, Pou4f3, and Atoh1 in the postnatal mouse cochlea. *Cell Rep.* 35:109016. doi: 10.1016/j.celrep.2021.109016

Chen, Z., Kujawa, S. G., and Sewell, W. F. (2010). Functional roles of high-affinity glutamate transporters in cochlear afferent synaptic transmission in the mouse. *J. Neurophysiol.* 103, 2581–2586. doi: 10.1152/jn.00018.2010

Cheng, C., Hou, Y., Zhang, Z., Wang, Y., Lu, L., Zhang, L., et al. (2021). Disruption of the autism-related gene Pak1 causes stereocilia disorganization, hair cell loss, and deafness in mice. *J. Genet. Genomics* [Epub Online ahead of print]. doi: 10.1016/j.jgg.2021.03.010

Cheng, C., Wang, Y., Guo, L., Lu, X., Zhu, W., Muhammad, W., et al. (2019). Age-related transcriptome changes in Sox2+ supporting cells in the mouse cochlea. *Stem Cell Res. Ther.* 10:365. doi: 10.1186/s13287-019-1437-0

Clemens Grisham, R., Kindt, K., Finger-Baier, K., Schmid, B., and Nicolson, T. (2013). Mutations in *ap1b1* cause mistargeting of the Na^+/K^+-ATPase pump in sensory hair cells. *PloS One*, 8:e60866. doi: 10.1371/journal.pone.0060866

Ding, B., Walton, J. P., Zhu, X., and Frisina, R. D. (2018). Age-related changes in Na, K-ATPase expression, subunit isoform selection and assembly in the stria vascularis lateral wall of mouse cochlea. *Hear. Res.* 367, 59–73. doi: 10.1016/j.heares.2018.07.006

Fang, Q., Zhang, Y., Da, P., Shao, B., Pan, H., He, Z., et al. (2019). Deletion of Limk1 and Limk2 in mice does not alter cochlear development or auditory function. *Sci. Rep.* 9:3357. doi: 10.1038/s41598-019-39769-z

Fernandez, K. A., Guo, D., Micucci, S., De Gruttola, V., Liberman, M. C., and Kujawa, S. G. (2020). Noise-induced Cochlear Synaptopathy with and Without Sensory Cell Loss. *Neuroscience* 427, 43–57. doi: 10.1016/j.neuroscience.2019.11.051

Fu, X., An, Y., Wang, H., Li, P., Lin, J., Yuan, J., et al. (2021). Deficiency of Klc2 Induces Low-Frequency Sensorineural Hearing Loss in C57BL/6 J Mice and Human. *Mol. Neurobiol.* [Epub Online ahead of print]. doi: 10.1007/s12035-021-02422-w

Fu, Y., Ding, D., Jiang, H., and Salvi, R. (2012). Ouabain-induced cochlear degeneration in rat. *Neurotox. Res.* 22, 158–169. doi: 10.1007/s12640-012-9320-0

Furman, A. C., Kujawa, S. G., and Liberman, M. C. (2013). Noise-induced cochlear neuropathy is selective for fibers with low spontaneous rates. *J. Neurophysiol.* 110, 577–586. doi: 10.1152/jn.00164.2013

Gao, S., Cheng, C., Wang, M., Jiang, P., Zhang, L., Wang, Y., et al. (2019). Blebbistatin Inhibits Neomycin-Induced Apoptosis in Hair Cell-Like HEI-OC-1 Cells and in Cochlear Hair Cells. *Front. Cell Neurosci.* 13:590. doi: 10.3389/fncel.2019.00590

Glowatzki, E., Cheng, N., Hiel, H., Yi, E., Tanaka, K., and Ellis-Davies, G. C. (2006). The glutamate-aspartate transporter GLAST mediates glutamate uptake at inner hair cell afferent synapses in the mammalian cochlea. *J. Neurosci.* 26, 7659–7664. doi: 10.1523/jneurosci.1545-06.2006

Guo, R., Li, J., Chen, C., Xiao, M., Liao, M., Hu, Y., et al. (2021). Biomimetic 3D bacterial cellulose-graphene foam hybrid scaffold regulates neural stem cell proliferation and differentiation. *Colloids Surf. B Biointerfaces* 200:111590. doi: 10.1016/j.colsurfb.2021.111590

Guo, R., Ma, X., Liao, M., Liu, Y., Hu, Y., Qian, X., et al. (2019). Development and Application of Cochlear Implant-Based Electric-Acoustic Stimulation of Spiral Ganglion Neurons. *ACS Biomater. Sci. Eng.* 5, 6735–6741. doi: 10.1021/acsbiomaterials.9b01265

Guo, R., Xiao, M., Zhao, W., Zhou, S., Hu, Y., Liao, M., et al. (2020). 2D $Ti_3C_2T_x$MXene couples electrical stimulation to promote proliferation and neural differentiation of neural stem cells. *Acta Biomater.* [Epub Online ahead of print]. doi: 10.1016/j.actbio.2020.12.035

Guo, R., Zhang, S., Xiao, M., Qian, F., He, Z., Li, D., et al. (2016). Accelerating bioelectric functional development of neural stem cells by graphene coupling: implications for neural interfacing with conductive materials. *Biomaterials* 106, 193–204. doi: 10.1016/j.biomaterials.2016.08.019

Hakuba, N., Koga, K., Gyo, K., Usami, S. I., and Tanaka, K. (2000). Exacerbation of noise-induced hearing loss in mice lacking the glutamate transporter GLAST. *J. Neurosci.* 20, 8750–8753. doi: 10.1523/jneurosci.20-23-08750.2000

He, Z., Fang, Q., Li, H., Shao, B., Zhang, Y., Zhang, Y., et al. (2019). The role of FOXG1 in the postnatal development and survival of mouse cochlear hair cells. *Neuropharmacology* 144, 43–57. doi: 10.1016/j.neuropharm.2018.10.021

He, Z., Guo, L., Shu, Y., Fang, Q., Zhou, H., Liu, Y., et al. (2017). Autophagy protects auditory hair cells against neomycin-induced damage. *Autophagy* 13, 1884–1904. doi: 10.1080/15548627.2017.1359449

He, Z. H., Li, M., Fang, Q. J., Liao, F. L., Zou, S. Y., Wu, X., et al. (2021). FOXG1 promotes aging inner ear hair cell survival through activation of the autophagy pathway. *Autophagy* [Epub Online ahead of print]. doi: 10.1080/15548627.2021.1916194

He, Z. H., Zou, S. Y., Li, M., Liao, F. L., Wu, X., Sun, H. Y., et al. (2020). The nuclear transcription factor FoxG1 affects the sensitivity of mimetic aging hair cells to inflammation by regulating autophagy pathways. *Redox Biol.* 28:101364. doi: 10.1016/j.redox.2019.101364

Hu, N., Rutherford, M. A., and Green, S. H. (2020). Protection of cochlear synapses from noise-induced excitotoxic trauma by blockade of Ca^{2+}-permeable AMPA receptors. *Proc. Natl. Acad. Sci. U. S. A.* 117, 3828–3838. doi: 10.1073/pnas.1914247117

Jiang, P., Zhang, S., Cheng, C., Gao, S., Tang, M., Lu, L., et al. (2020). The Roles of Exosomes in Visual and Auditory Systems. *Front. Bioeng. Biotechnol.* 8:525. doi: 10.3389/fbioe.2020.00525

Kim, K. X., Payne, S., Yang-Hood, A., Li, S. Z., Davis, B., Carlquist, J., et al. (2019). Vesicular Glutamatergic Transmission in Noise-Induced Loss and Repair of Cochlear Ribbon Synapses. *J. Neurosci.* 39, 4434–4447. doi: 10.1523/jneurosci.2228-18.2019

Kohrman, D. C., Wan, G., Cassinotti, L., and Corfas, G. (2020). Hidden Hearing Loss: a Disorder with Multiple Etiologies and Mechanisms. *Cold Spring Harb. Perspect. Med.* 10:a035493. doi: 10.1101/cshperspect.a035493

Kujawa, S. G., and Liberman, M. C. (2015). Synaptopathy in the noise-exposed and aging cochlea: primary neural degeneration in acquired sensorineural hearing loss. *Hear. Res.* 330, 191–199. doi: 10.1016/j.heares.2015.02.009

Kurabi, A., Keithley, E. M., Housley, G. D., Ryan, A. F., and Wong, A. C. (2017). Cellular mechanisms of noise-induced hearing loss. *Hear. Res.* 349, 129–137. doi: 10.1016/j.heares.2016.11.013

Lang, H., Schulte, B. A., and Schmiedt, R. A. (2005). Ouabain induces apoptotic cell death in type I spiral ganglion neurons, but not type II neurons. *J. Assoc. Res. Otolaryngol.* 6, 63–74. doi: 10.1007/s10162-004-5021-6

Li, A., You, D., Li, W., Cui, Y., He, Y., Li, W., et al. (2018). Novel compounds protect auditory hair cells against gentamycin-induced apoptosis by maintaining the expression level of H3K4me2. *Drug Deliv.* 25, 1033–1043. doi: 10.1080/10717544.2018.1461277

Liberman, L. D., Suzuki, J., and Liberman, M. C. (2015). Dynamics of cochlear synaptopathy after acoustic overexposure. *J. Assoc. Res. Otolaryngol.* 16, 205–219. doi: 10.1007/s10162-015-0510-3

Liu, L., Chen, Y., Qi, J., Zhang, Y., He, Y., Ni, W., et al. (2016). Wnt activation protects against neomycin-induced hair cell damage in the mouse cochlea. *Cell Death Dis.* 7:e2136. doi: 10.1038/cddis.2016.35

Liu, W., Luque, M., Glueckert, R., Danckwardt-Lillieström, N., Nordström, C. K., Schrott-Fischer, A., et al. (2019a). Expression of Na/K-ATPase subunits in the human cochlea: a confocal and super-resolution microscopy study with special reference to auditory nerve excitation and cochlear implantation. *Ups. J. Med. Sci.* 124, 168–179. doi: 10.1080/03009734.2019.1653408

Liu, W., Xu, L., Wang, X., Zhang, D., Sun, G., Wang, M., et al. (2021). PRDX1 activates autophagy via the PTEN-AKT signaling pathway to protect against cisplatin-induced spiral ganglion neuron damage. *Autophagy* [Epub Online ahead of print]. doi: 10.1080/15548627.2021.1905466

Liu, W., Xu, X., Fan, Z., Sun, G., Han, Y., Zhang, D., et al. (2019b). Wnt Signaling Activates TP53-Induced Glycolysis and Apoptosis Regulator and Protects Against Cisplatin-Induced Spiral Ganglion Neuron Damage in the Mouse Cochlea. *Antioxid. Redox Signal.* 30, 1389–1410. doi: 10.1089/ars.2017.7288

Liu, Y., Qi, J., Chen, X., Tang, M., Chu, C., Zhu, W., et al. (2019). Critical role of spectrin in hearing development and deafness. *Sci. Adv.* 5:eaav7803. doi: 10.1126/sciadv.aav7803

Lu, X., Sun, S., Qi, J., Li, W., Liu, L., Zhang, Y., et al. (2017). Bmi1 Regulates the Proliferation of Cochlear Supporting Cells Via the Canonical Wnt Signaling Pathway. *Mol. Neurobiol.* 54, 1326–1339. doi: 10.1007/s12035-016-9686-8

Lv, J., Fu, X., Li, Y., Hong, G., Li, P., Lin, J., et al. (2021). Deletion of Kcnj16 in Mice Does Not Alter Auditory Function. *Front. Cell Dev. Biol.* 9:630361. doi: 10.3389/fcell.2021.630361

Matsuda, K., Ueda, Y., Doi, T., Tono, T., Haruta, A., Toyama, K., et al. (1999). Increase in glutamate-aspartate transporter (GLAST) mRNA during kanamycin-induced cochlear insult in rats. *Hear. Res.* 133, 10–16. doi: 10.1016/s0378-5955(99)00050-7

McLean, W. J., Smith, K. A., Glowatzki, E., and Pyott, S. J. (2009). Distribution of the Na,K-ATPase alpha subunit in the rat spiral ganglion and organ of corti. *J. Assoc. Res. Otolaryngol.* 10, 37–49. doi: 10.1007/s10162-008-0152-9

Obholzer, N., Wolfson, S., Trapani, J. G., Mo, W., Nechiporuk, A., Busch-Nentwich, E., et al. (2008). Vesicular glutamate transporter 3 is required for synaptic transmission in zebrafish hair cells. *J. Neurosci.* 28, 2110–2118. doi: 10.1523/jneurosci.5230-07.2008

Peng, Z., Wang, G. P., Zeng, R., Guo, J. Y., Chen, C. F., and Gong, S. S. (2013). Temporospatial expression and cellular localization of VGLUT3 in the rat cochlea. *Brain Res.* 1537, 100–110. doi: 10.1016/j.brainres.2013.09.019

Plack, C. J., Léger, A., Prendergast, G., Kluk, K., Guest, H., and Munro, K. J. (2016). Toward a Diagnostic Test for Hidden Hearing Loss. *Trends Hear.* 20, 1–9. doi: 10.1177/2331216516657466

Poirel, O., Mamer, L. E., Herman, M. A., Arnulf-Kempcke, M., Kervern, M., Potier, B., et al. (2020). LSP5-2157 a new inhibitor of vesicular glutamate transporters. *Neuropharmacology* 164:107902. doi: 10.1016/j.neuropharm.2019.107902

Qi, J., Liu, Y., Chu, C., Chen, X., Zhu, W., Shu, Y., et al. (2019). A cytoskeleton structure revealed by super-resolution fluorescence imaging in inner ear hair cells. *Cell Discov.* 5:12. doi: 10.1038/s41421-018-0076-4

Qi, J., Zhang, L., Tan, F., Liu, Y., and Chai, R. (2020). Espin distribution as revealed by super-resolution microscopy of stereocilia. *Am. J. Transl. Res.* 12, 130–141.

Qian, F., Wang, X., Yin, Z., Xie, G., Yuan, H., Liu, D., et al. (2020). The slc4a2b gene is required for hair cell development in zebrafish. *Aging* 12, 18804–18821. doi: 10.18632/aging.103840

Robinson, M. B., and Jackson, J. G. (2016). Astroglial glutamate transporters coordinate excitatory signaling and brain energetics. *Neurochem. Int.* 98, 56–71. doi: 10.1016/j.neuint.2016.03.014

Rose, E. M., Koo, J. C., Antflick, J. E., Ahmed, S. M., Angers, S., and Hampson, D. R. (2009). Glutamate transporter coupling to Na,K-ATPase. *J. Neurosci.* 29, 8143–8155. doi: 10.1523/jneurosci.1081-09.2009

Ruel, J., Emery, S., Nouvian, R., Bersot, T., Amilhon, B., Van Rybroek, J. M., et al. (2008). Impairment of SLC17A8 encoding vesicular glutamate transporter-3, VGLUT3, underlies nonsyndromic deafness DFNA25 and inner hair cell dysfunction in null mice. *Am. J. Hum. Genet.* 83, 278–292. doi: 10.1016/j.ajhg.2008.07.008

Schomann, T., Ramekers, D., de Groot, J., van der Ploeg, C. H., Hendriksen, F. G. J., Böhringer, S., et al. (2018). Ouabain Does Not Induce Selective Spiral Ganglion Cell Degeneration in Guinea Pigs. *Biomed. Res. Int.* 2018:1568414. doi: 10.1155/2018/1568414

Seal, R. P., Akil, O., Yi, E., Weber, C. M., Grant, L., Yoo, J., et al. (2008). Sensorineural deafness and seizures in mice lacking vesicular glutamate transporter 3. *Neuron* 57, 263–275. doi: 10.1016/j.neuron.2007.11.032

Sebe, J. Y., Cho, S., Sheets, L., Rutherford, M. A., von Gersdorff, H., and Raible, D. W. (2017). Ca^{2+}-Permeable AMPARs Mediate Glutamatergic Transmission and Excitotoxic Damage at the Hair Cell Ribbon Synapse. *J. Neurosci.* 37, 6162–6175. doi: 10.1523/jneurosci.3644-16.2017

Shi, L., Liu, L., He, T., Guo, X., Yu, Z., Yin, S., et al. (2013). Ribbon synapse plasticity in the cochleae of Guinea pigs after noise-induced silent damage. *PloS One,* 8:e81566. doi: 10.1371/journal.pone.0081566

Song, F., Gan, B., Wang, N., Wang, Z., and Xu, A. T. (2021). Hidden hearing loss is associated with loss of ribbon synapses of cochlea inner hair cells. *Biosci. Rep.* 41:BSR20201637. doi: 10.1042/BSR20201637

Stephenson, R., Mangasarian, A., Ishiyama, G., Hosokawa, K., Hosokawa, S., Ishiyama, A., et al. (2021). Immunohistochemical location of Na^+, K^+-ATPase $\alpha 1$ subunit in the human inner ear. *Hear. Res.* 400:108113. doi: 10.1016/j.heares.2020.108113

Sun, G., Liu, W., Fan, Z., Zhang, D., Han, Y., Xu, L., et al. (2016). The Three-Dimensional Culture System with Matrigel and Neurotrophic Factors Preserves the Structure and Function of Spiral Ganglion Neuron In Vitro. *Neural Plast.* 2016:4280407. doi: 10.1155/2016/4280407

Sun, S., Sun, M., Zhang, Y., Cheng, C., Waqas, M., Yu, H., et al. (2014). In vivo overexpression of X-linked inhibitor of apoptosis protein protects against neomycin-induced hair cell loss in the apical turn of the cochlea during the ototoxic-sensitive period. *Front. Cell Neurosci.* 8:248. doi: 10.3389/fncel.2014.00248

Sundaresan, S., Kong, J. H., Fang, Q., Salles, F. T., Wangsawihardja, F., Ricci, A. J., et al. (2016). Thyroid hormone is required for pruning, functioning and long-term maintenance of afferent inner hair cell synapses. *Eur. J. Neurosci.* 43, 148–161. doi: 10.1111/ejn.13081

Tan, F., Chu, C., Qi, J., Li, W., You, D., Li, K., et al. (2019). AAV-ie enables safe and efficient gene transfer to inner ear cells. *Nat. Commun.* 10:3733. doi: 10.1038/s41467-019-11687-8

Tserga, E., Damberg, P., Canlon, B., and Cederroth, C. R. (2020a). Auditory synaptopathy in mice lacking the glutamate transporter GLAST and its impact on brain activity. *Prog. Brain Res.* 262, 245–261. doi: 10.1016/bs.pbr.2020.04.004

Tserga, E., Moreno-Paublete, R., Sarlus, H., Björn, E., Guimaraes, E., Göritz, C., et al. (2020b). Circadian vulnerability of cisplatin-induced ototoxicity in the cochlea. *FASEB J.* 34, 13978–13992. doi: 10.1096/fj.202001236R

Wang, Y., Li, J., Yao, X., Li, W., Du, H., Tang, M., et al. (2017). Loss of CIB2 Causes Profound Hearing Loss and Abolishes Mechanoelectrical Transduction in Mice. *Front. Mol. Neurosci.* 10:401. doi: 10.3389/fnmol.2017.00401

Wei, W., Shi, X., Xiong, W., He, L., Du, Z. D., and Qu, T. (2020). RNA-seq Profiling and Co-expression Network Analysis of Long Noncoding RNAs and mRNAs Reveal Novel Pathogenesis of Noise-induced Hidden Hearing Loss. *Neuroscience* 434, 120–135. doi: 10.1016/j.neuroscience.2020.03.023

Yamaguchi, T., Nagashima, R., Yoneyama, M., Shiba, T., and Ogita, K. (2014). Disruption of ion-trafficking system in the cochlear spiral ligament prior to permanent hearing loss induced by exposure to intense noise: possible involvement of 4-hydroxy-2-nonenal as a mediator of oxidative stress. *PLoS One* 9:e102133. doi: 10.1371/journal.pone.0102133

Yu, H., Vikhe Patil, K., Han, C., Fabella, B., Canlon, B., Someya, S., et al. (2016). GLAST Deficiency in Mice Exacerbates Gap Detection Deficits in a Model of Salicylate-Induced Tinnitus. *Front. Behav. Neurosci.* 10:158. doi: 10.3389/fnbeh.2016.00158

Yu, X., Liu, W., Fan, Z., Qian, F., Zhang, D., Han, Y., et al. (2017). c-Myb knockdown increases the neomycin-induced damage to hair-cell-like HEI-OC1 cells in vitro. *Sci. Rep.* 7:41094. doi: 10.1038/srep41094

Yuan, Y., Shi, F., Yin, Y., Tong, M., Lang, H., Polley, D. B., et al. (2014). Ouabain-induced cochlear nerve degeneration: synaptic loss and plasticity in a mouse model of auditory neuropathy. *J. Assoc. Res. Otolaryngol.* 15, 31–43. doi: 10.1007/s10162-013-0419-7

Zhang, L. N., Sun, Y. J., Wang, L. X., and Gao, Z. B. (2016). Glutamate Transporters/Na(+), K(+)-ATPase Involving in the Neuroprotective Effect as a Potential Regulatory Target of Glutamate Uptake. *Mol. Neurobiol.* 53, 1124–1131. doi: 10.1007/s12035-014-9071-4

Zhang, S., Dong, Y., Qiang, R., Zhang, Y., Zhang, X., Chen, Y., et al. (2021). Characterization of Strip1 Expression in Mouse Cochlear Hair Cells. *Front. Genet.* 12:625867. doi: 10.3389/fgene.2021.625867

Zhang, S., Liu, D., Dong, Y., Zhang, Z., Zhang, Y., Zhou, H., et al. (2019). Frizzled-9+ Supporting Cells Are Progenitors for the Generation of Hair Cells in the Postnatal Mouse Cochlea. *Front. Mol. Neurosci.* 12:184. doi: 10.3389/fnmol.2019.00184

Zhang, S., Qiang, R., Dong, Y., Zhang, Y., Chen, Y., Zhou, H., et al. (2020). Hair cell regeneration from inner ear progenitors in the mammalian cochlea. *Am. J. Stem Cells* 9, 25–35.

Zhang, W., Peng, Z., Yu, S., Song, Q. L., Qu, T. F., Liu, K., et al. (2020). Exposure to sodium salicylate disrupts VGLUT3 expression in cochlear inner hair cells and contributes to tinnitus. *Physiol. Res.* 69, 181–190. doi: 10.33549/physiolres.934180

Zhang, Y., Li, W., He, Z., Wang, Y., Shao, B., Cheng, C., et al. (2019). Pre-treatment With Fasudil Prevents Neomycin-Induced Hair Cell Damage by Reducing the Accumulation of Reactive Oxygen Species. *Front. Mol. Neurosci.* 12:264. doi: 10.3389/fnmol.2019.00264

Zhang, Y., Zhang, S., Zhang, Z., Dong, Y., and Chai, R. (2020). Knockdown of Foxg1 in Sox9+ supporting cells increases the trans-differentiation of supporting cells into hair cells in the neonatal mouse utricle. *Aging* 12, 19834–19851. doi: 10.18632/aging.104009

Zhang, Z. J., Guan, H. X., Yang, K., Xiao, B. K., Liao, H., Jiang, Y., et al. (2017). Dose-dependent effects of ouabain on spiral ganglion neurons and Schwann cells in mouse cochlea. *Acta Otolaryngol.* 137, 1017–1023. doi: 10.1080/00016489.2017.1324217

Zhao, J., Tang, M., Cao, J., Ye, D., Guo, X., Xi, J., et al. (2019). Structurally Tunable Reduced Graphene Oxide Substrate Maintains Mouse Embryonic Stem Cell Pluripotency. *Adv. Sci.* 6:1802136. doi: 10.1002/advs.201802136

Zhong, Z., Fu, X., Li, H., Chen, J., Wang, M., Gao, S., et al. (2020). Citicoline Protects Auditory Hair Cells Against Neomycin-Induced Damage. *Front. Cell Dev. Biol.* 8:712. doi: 10.3389/fcell.2020.00712

Zhou, H., Qian, X., Xu, N., Zhang, S., Zhu, G., Zhang, Y., et al. (2020). Disruption of Atg7-dependent autophagy causes electromotility disturbances, outer hair cell loss, and deafness in mice. *Cell Death Dis.* 11:913. doi: 10.1038/s41419-020-03110-8

Zhu, C., Cheng, C., Wang, Y., Muhammad, W., Liu, S., Zhu, W., et al. (2018). Loss of ARHGEF6 Causes Hair Cell Stereocilia Deficits and Hearing Loss in Mice. *Front. Mol. Neurosci.* 11:362. doi: 10.3389/fnmol.2018.00362

6

The Rho GTPase Cell Division Cycle 42 Regulates Stereocilia Development in Cochlear Hair Cells

Haibo Du[1], Hao Zhou[1], Yixiao Sun[1], Xiaoyan Zhai[1], Zhengjun Chen[2,3], Yanfei Wang[1] and Zhigang Xu[1,4]**

[1] Shandong Provincial Key Laboratory of Animal Cell and Developmental Biology, School of Life Sciences, Shandong University, Qingdao, China, [2] State Key Laboratory of Cell Biology, Center for Excellence in Molecular Cell Science, Shanghai Institute of Biochemistry and Cell Biology, Chinese Academy of Sciences, Shanghai, China, [3] School of Life Sciences and Technology, ShanghaiTech University, Shanghai, China, [4] Shandong Provincial Collaborative Innovation Center of Cell Biology, Shandong Normal University, Jinan, China

***Correspondence:**
Yanfei Wang
wang_yf@sdu.edu.cn
Zhigang Xu
xuzg@sdu.edu.cn

Stereocilia are actin-based cell protrusions on the apical surface of inner ear hair cells, playing a pivotal role in hearing and balancing sensation. The development and maintenance of stereocilia is tightly regulated and deficits in this process usually lead to hearing or balancing disorders. The Rho GTPase cell division cycle 42 (CDC42) is a key regulator of the actin cytoskeleton. It has been reported to localize in the hair cell stereocilia and play important roles in stereocilia maintenance. In the present work, we utilized hair cell-specific *Cdc42* knockout mice and CDC42 inhibitor ML141 to explore the role of CDC42 in stereocilia development. Our data show that stereocilia height and width as well as stereocilia resorption are affected in *Cdc42*-deficient cochlear hair cells when examined at postnatal day 8 (P8). Moreover, ML141 treatment leads to planar cell polarity (PCP) deficits in neonatal hair cells. We also show that overexpression of a constitutively active mutant CDC42 in cochlear hair cells leads to enhanced stereocilia developmental deficits. In conclusion, the present data suggest that CDC42 plays a pivotal role in regulating hair cell stereocilia development.

Keywords: inner ear, hair cells, stereocilia, CDC42, knockout mice

INTRODUCTION

As the mechanosensitive receptor cells in the inner ear, hair cells are characterized by their hairy-looking hair bundles, which consist of hundreds of actin-based stereocilia and one microtubule-based kinocilium on the apical surface of each cell (Flock and Cheung, 1977). The kinocilium is important for hair bundle development as well as planar cell polarity (PCP) establishment, while the stereocilia are essential for mechano-electrical transduction (MET), the process that converts mechanical signals into electrical signals (Lindeman et al., 1971; Hudspeth and Jacobs, 1979; Jones et al., 2008). In each hair cell, the stereocilia are organized into several rows of increasing heights, forming a staircase-like pattern (Tilney et al., 1980). Deflection of stereocilia toward the taller row direction opens the MET channels at the tips of shorter row stereocilia, eventually leading to the influx of cations into hair cells (Hudspeth and Jacobs, 1979; Beurg et al., 2009).

The actin core of stereocilia consists of a bundle of cross-linked actin filaments (F-actin), with their barbed (plus) ends pointing toward the distal tips (Flock and Cheung, 1977; Tilney et al., 1980). During development, the stereocilia start as short apical microvilli and develop into the final mature morphology by increasing the length and numbers of F-actin core (Tilney et al., 1992;

Krey et al., 2020). In adults, the stereocilia are quite stable and actin polymerization/depolymerization is only detected at the distal tips (Zhang et al., 2012; Drummond et al., 2015; Narayanan et al., 2015). The development and maintenance of stereocilia is tightly regulated, and deficits in this process usually lead to hearing loss or balancing deficits (Ciuman, 2011; Barr-Gillespie, 2015). With the rapid progress of genetic, transcriptomic, and proteomic techniques, many proteins have been identified to participate in the development and/or maintenance of stereocilia (Barr-Gillespie, 2015; McGrath et al., 2017; Ellwanger et al., 2018; Krey and Barr-Gillespie, 2019; Velez-Ortega and Frolenkov, 2019).

The Rho GTPase cell division cycle 42 (CDC42) is a key regulator of the actin cytoskeleton (Sit and Manser, 2011). It has been long known that CDC42 stimulates Arp2/3-dependent actin polymerization and plays an important role in the formation of filopodia, another finger-like actin-based cell protrusion that is similar to stereocilia and microvilli (Rohatgi et al., 1999; Chen et al., 2000; Yang et al., 2006). Recently, Ueyama et al. (2014) reported that CDC42 localizes in the stereocilia of cochlear hair cells, and that *Cdc42* gene disruption causes deficits in stereocilia maintenance. In the present work, we further explore the role of CDC42 in stereocilia development using *Cdc42* conditional knockout mice and CDC42 inhibitor. Our present data suggest that CDC42 regulates hair cell stereocilia development both in a cell autonomous and non-autonomous manner.

MATERIALS AND METHODS

Plasmids and Antibodies

Mouse cDNAs encoding wild-type or mutant CDC42 were subcloned into pEGFP-C2. Rabbit anti-CAPZB2 antibody (Cat. No. AB6017) was purchased from Merck, and its specificity has been validated previously (Avenarius et al., 2017). Rabbit anti-MYO15A antibody was described and validated previously (Zou et al., 2014). Mouse anti-EPS8 antibody (Cat. No. 610143) was purchased from BD Biosciences, and its specificity has been validated previously (Zampini et al., 2011). Other antibodies and additional reagents were as follows: mouse anti-GFP antibody (Abmart, Cat. No. M20004); Alexa Fluor 488-conjugated donkey anti-rabbit IgG (Thermo Fisher Scientific, Cat. No. A21206); Alexa Fluor 488-conjugated donkey anti-mouse IgG (Thermo Fisher Scientific, Cat. No. A21202); Alex Fluor 546-conjugated donkey anti-mouse IgG (Thermo Fisher Scientific, Cat. No. A10036); TRITC-conjugated phalloidin (Sigma-Aldrich, Cat. No. P1951); iFluor 405-conjugated phalloidin (Abcam, Cat. No. ab176752).

Mice

All animal experiments were approved by the Animal Ethics Committee of Shandong University School of Life Sciences (Permit Number: SYDWLL-2020-31) and performed accordingly. $Cdc42^{loxP/+}$ mice were developed as previously reported (van Hengel et al., 2008). $Atoh1^{Cre/+}$ knock-in mice that express Cre recombinase under the control of *Atoh1* promoter were developed as previously reported (Yang et al., 2010).

Scanning Electron Microscopy and Stereocilia Length/Width Quantification

SEM was performed as previously described (Wang et al., 2017). Dissected mouse temporal bone was fixed with 2.5% glutaraldehyde in 0.1 M phosphate buffer overnight at 4°C. The cochleae were then taken out and post-fixed with 1% osmium tetroxide in 0.1 M phosphate buffer at 4°C for 2 h. After dehydration in ethanol and critically point drying using a Leica EM CPD300 (Leica, Germany), samples were mounted and sputter coated with platinum (15 nm) using a Cressington 108 sputter coater (Cressington, United Kingdom). Images were taken using a Quanta250 field-emission scanning electron microscope (FEI, Netherlands) with a beam strength of 5 kV.

Stereocilia length quantification were performed as previously described (Li et al., 2020). Briefly, SEM images were taken in two different imaging planes with a known angle between them, and the relative stereocilia projection length and its angles in the reconstructed three-dimensional coordinates were measured using Photoshop. The stereocilia length was then calculated using the equations mentioned in the above report. Stereocilia width quantification were performed as previously described (McGrath et al., 2021). Briefly, stereocilia with approximately perpendicular orientation in SEM images were used for calculations. A line was drawn perpendicularly across the stereocilium at approximately the same distance above the taper region of each measured stereocilium. The length of this line was then measured using Image J to give rise to the width of the stereocilium.

Whole-Mount Immunostaining

All steps were performed at room temperature unless otherwise indicated. The auditory sensory epithelia were dissected out of the temporal bone and fixed with 4% paraformaldehyde (PFA) in PBS for 20 min, followed by permeabilization and blocking with PBT1 (0.1% Triton X-100, 1% BSA, and 5% heat-inactivated goat serum in PBS, pH 7.3) for 40 min. After that, the samples were incubated with primary antibody in PBT1 at 4°C overnight, followed by sequential incubation with secondary antibody in PBT2 (0.1% Triton X-100 and 0.1% BSA in PBS) for 2 h and phalloidin in PBS for 30 min. The samples were mounted in PBS/glycerol (1:1), and images were taken using a confocal microscope with a 1.4 NA/100 × Kort M27 objective lens (LSM 700, Zeiss, Germany).

Injectoporation

Injectoporation was performed as previously described (Du et al., 2020). Briefly, the cochlear sensory epithelia were isolated from P2 mice and cultured in DMEM/F12 with 1.5 μg/ml ampicillin. Expression plasmids (0.2 μg/μl in Hanks' balanced salt solution) were delivered to hair cells using a glass pipette of 2 μm tip diameter. A series of three pulses at 60 V lasting 15 ms at 1-s intervals were applied by an electroporator (ECM Gemini X2, BTX, CA). The tissues were cultured for 24 h *in vitro* and then incubated with phalloidin in PBS for 30 min. The samples were mounted in PBS/glycerol (1:1), and images were taken using a confocal microscope with a 1.4 NA/63 × Kort M27 objective lens (LSM 900, Zeiss, Germany).

Protein Purification and Localization in Permeabilized Hair Cells

Protein expression and purification was performed as previously described (Cao et al., 2013). Briefly, the coding sequence encoding wild-type or mutant CDC42 fused to EGFP was inserted into expression vector pET-28a, which was then transformed into *Escherichia coli* BL21(DE3) cells. His-tagged EGFP-CDC42 protein was induced in the presence of 0.4 mM isopropyl-β-d-thiogalactopyranoside (IPTG) at 16°C, then purified using Ni-NTA agarose (TransGen) according to manufacturer's instructions.

The subcellular localization of purified protein in permeabilized hair cells was examined as described before (McGrath et al., 2021). All steps were performed at room temperature unless otherwise indicated. Briefly, the cochlear epithelia were dissected out of temporal bone in Hank's balanced salt solution, followed by incubation with 40 μg purified EGFP-CDC42 protein in cytoskeletal buffer (20 mM HEPES, pH 7.5, 138 mM KCl, 4 mM $MgCl_2$, 3 mM EGTA, 1% bovine serum albumin, 0.05% saponin, and 2 mM fresh ATP) for 5 min.

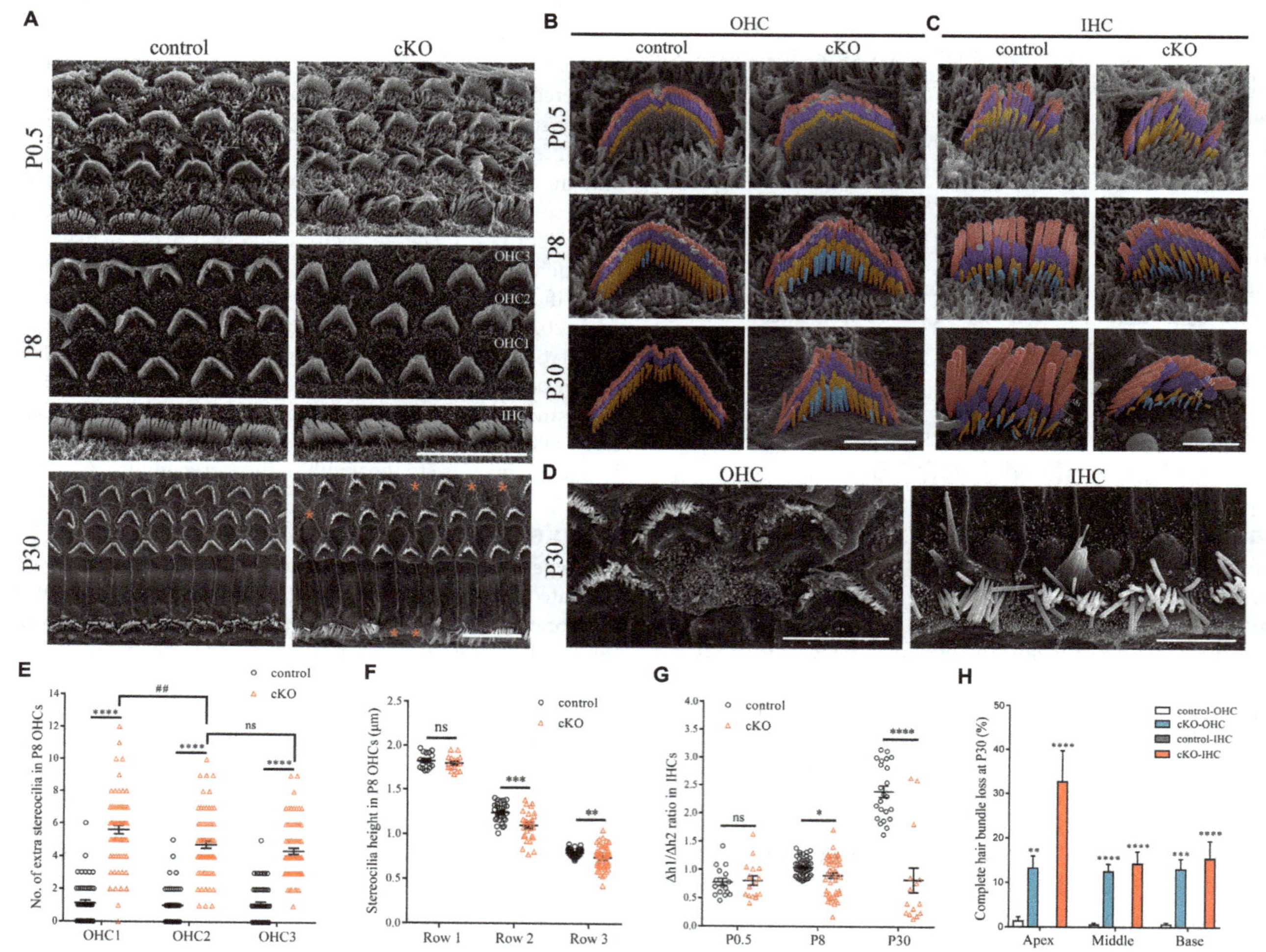

FIGURE 1 | Hair cell-specific *Cdc42* inactivation leads to stereocilia development deficits. **(A)** Low magnification SEM images of the hair bundles from control or cKO mice at different ages as indicated. Shown are images taken from the middle turns. Asterisks indicate complete loss of hair bundles. Scale bar: 10 μm. **(B,C)** High magnification pseudo-colored SEM images of hair bundles from control or cKO OHCs **(B)** and IHCs **(C)** at different ages as indicated. The first, second, and third row stereocilia are indicated by pink, purple, and yellow, respectively. The extra fourth-row stereocilia are indicated by cyan. Δh1 and Δh2 represent the relative distance from 1st row stereocilium tip to its parallel connecting 2nd row stereocilium tip and the 2nd row stereocilium tip to its parallel connecting 3rd row stereocilium tip, respectively. Shown are images taken from the middle turns. Scale bars: 2 μm. **(D)** High magnification SEM images of severely disorganized hair bundles from control or cKO mice at P30. Shown are images taken from the middle turns. Scale bar: 5 μm. **(E)** Number of the extra fourth-row stereocilia per P8 OHC was analyzed according to the results from **(B)**. **(F)** Average stereocilia height in different rows of P8 OHCs were analyzed according to the results from **(B)**. **(G)** The Δh1/Δh2 ratio in IHCs at different ages was analyzed according to the results from **(C)**. **(H)** Percentage of P30 OHCs and IHCs with complete hair bundle loss was calculated according to the results from **(A)**. For statistical analyses in **(E–H)**, images were randomly taken from at least three animals for each group. The bars indicate mean ± SEM values. $^{*}P < 0.05$; $^{**}P < 0.01$; $^{***}P < 0.001$; $^{****}P < 0.0001$; $^{\#\#}P < 0.01$; ns, no significant difference.

Samples were then fixed with 4% PFA for 30 min, followed by blocking with 0.1 M PBS containing 5% (v/v) donkey serum for an hour. Afterward, samples were incubated with mouse anti-GFP antibody in 0.1 M PBS containing 5% (v/v) donkey serum for an hour, then Alex Fluor 546-conjugated donkey anti-mouse IgG in PBST buffer (0.01% Triton X-100 and 0.1% BSA in PBS) for an hour, followed by incubation with iFluor 405-conjugaetd phalloidin in PBS for 30 min. After mounting in PBS/glycerol (1:1), samples were imaged with a confocal microscope with a 1.4 NA/63× Kort M27 objective lens (LSM 900, Zeiss, Germany).

Statistical Analysis

All experiments were performed at least three times independently. The numbers of analyzed animals or cells are indicated in the figures or figure legends. Data were shown as means ± standard error of mean (SEM). Student's two-tailed unpaired t-test was used to determine statistical significance, and $P < 0.05$ was considered statistically significant.

RESULTS

Hair Cell-Specific *Cdc42* Inactivation Leads to Stereocilia Development Deficits

To investigate the potential role of CDC42 in stereocilia development, we first crossed $Cdc42^{loxp/loxp}$ mice with $Atoh1^{Cre/+}$ knock-in mice that express Cre recombinase in developing cochlear hair cells from embryonic day 14.5 (E14.5) (Yang et al., 2010). The resultant $Atoh1^{Cre/+};Cdc42^{loxp/loxp}$ mice are referred to as *Cdc42* cKO mice thereafter in this work. $Atoh1^{Cre/+};Cdc42^{loxp/-}$ and $Cdc42^{loxp/loxp}$ mice were used as controls. Scanning electron microscopy (SEM) was then performed to examine the morphology of hair bundles in *Cdc42* cKO mice and control mice. At postnatal day 0.5 (P0.5), the morphology of hair bundle is largely indistinguishable between *Cdc42* cKO and control cochlear hair cells, with multiple rows of immature stereocilia protruding from the apical surface of hair cells (**Figures 1A–C**). By P8, most of the short-row immature stereocilia are resorbed and only 3 or 4 rows are remained in the control OHCs and IHCs, respectively (**Figures 1B,C**). However, in P8 *Cdc42* cKO OHCs, there are more fourth-row stereocilia remained, suggesting that immature stereocilia resorption is affected by *Cdc42* inactivation (**Figures 1B,E**). The extra fourth-row stereocilia in the *Cdc42* cKO OHCs persist when examined at P30, suggesting that it is a result of reduced stereocilia resorption instead of delayed stereocilia resorption (**Figure 1B**). Meanwhile, the stereocilia number in the regular rows is slightly decreased in the *Cdc42* cKO OHCs (**Supplementary Figures 1A–C**). By P30, stereocilia fusion, fragmentation, or even complete stereocilia loss could be observed in the *Cdc42* cKO OHCs and IHCs (**Figures 1A,D,H**).

The stereocilia height is also affected by *Cdc42* inactivation. By P8, there is significant variability of stereocilia height in the second and third rows in *Cdc42* cKO OHCs and IHCs, which becomes more apparent at P30 (**Figures 1B,C,F**). Moreover, in the *Cdc42* cKO OHCs, the average height of second- and third-row stereocilia is slightly decreased compared with control OHCs (**Figures 1B,F**). The height of IHC stereocilia is difficult to measure because of the imaging angle in most SEM images (**Figure 1C**). Nevertheless, the ratio of height difference between row 1 and row 2 stereocilia to that between row 2 and row 3 stereocilia is significantly decreased in the *Cdc42* cKO IHCs especially at P30 (**Figures 1C,G**).

Albeit the height of the tallest row stereocilia is largely unaffected in the *Cdc42* cKO hair cells, it seems that their width is decreased compared to control mice (**Figures 1B,C**). To examine the width of the tallest stereocilia more precisely, we took SEM images from the side of the tallest row stereocilia and quantified the stereocilia width. The results show that the width of the tallest-row stereocilia of *Cdc42* cKO OHCs is significantly decreased from P8 (**Figures 2A,C**). Similarly, the width of the tallest-row stereocilia of *Cdc42* cKO IHCs is significantly decreased from P0.5 (**Figures 2B,D**). Taken together, our present data suggest that CDC42 plays an important role in stereocilia development.

Stereociliary Tip Localization of Row 1 and 2 Complex Components Is Not Affected in the *Cdc42* cKO Hair Cells

It has been known that stereocilia height is tightly regulated by the so-called row 1 and row 2 complex, which are localized at the tips of the highest-row stereocilia or shorter-row stereocilia, respectively (Krey et al., 2020; McGrath and Perrin, 2020). We then performed whole-mount immunostaining to examine whether *Cdc42* inactivation affects the stereociliary tip localization of known row 1 components MYO15A and EPS8 as well as row 2 component CAPZB2 (Belyantseva et al., 2003; Manor et al., 2011; Zampini et al., 2011; Avenarius et al., 2017). The results show that stereociliary tip localization of these proteins is not affected in the *Cdc42* cKO IHCs (**Figure 2E**) and OHCs (**Supplementary Figure 2**). Therefore, it seems that although *Cdc42* inactivation leads to stereocilia development deficits, it does not affect the general stereocilia row identity.

CDC42 Inhibitor ML141 Treatment Leads to Stereocilia Development Deficits

We next examined the role of CDC42 in stereocilia development using a known CDC42 inhibitor ML141 (Surviladze et al., 2010). The cochlear sensory epithelia from P0.5 wild-type mice were cultured in presence of ML141 at 0, 1, 2.5, or 5 μM for 96 h, followed by fixation and SEM imaging (**Figure 3A**). The results show that 1 μM ML141 treatment leads to significant stereocilia disorganization, which is exaggerated at higher concentration of ML141 (**Figures 3B–E**). Noticeably, the staircase-like pattern of hair bundle is compromised, and more rows of stereocilia are observed in the ML141-treated hair cells (**Figures 3B–E**). Moreover, the PCP of hair cells is also significantly altered. We classified hair cells into three groups according to their PCP phenotypes, namely type I (roughly normal PCP), type

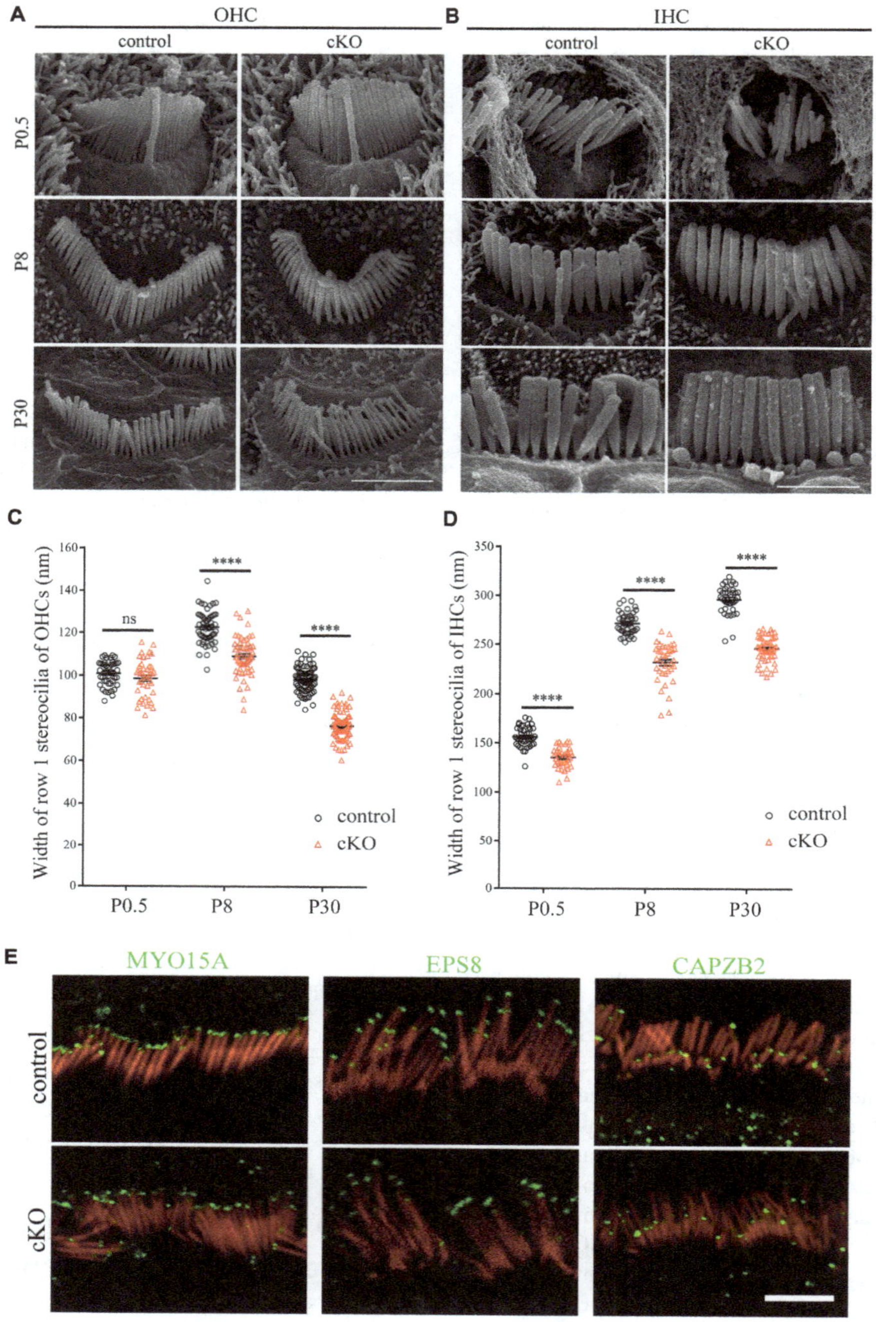

FIGURE 2 | Hair cell-specific *Cdc42* inactivation leads to decreased stereocilia width. **(A,B)** High magnification SEM images of hair bundles (dorsal view) from OHCs **(A)** and IHCs **(B)** at different ages as indicated. Shown are images taken from the middle turns. Scale bars: 2 μm. **(C,D)** Width of the tallest-row stereocilia in OHCs **(C)** and IHCs **(D)** at different ages as indicated were analyzed according to the results from **(A,B)**, respectively. For statistical analyses in **(C,D)**, images were randomly taken from at least 3 animals for each group. The bars indicate mean ± SEM values. ****$P < 0.0001$; ns, no significant difference. **(E)** Whole-mount immunostaining showing localization of MYO15A, EPS8 and CAPZB2 in IHCs of P9 control or cKO mice. TRITC-phalloidin (red) was used to visualize the stereociliary F-actin core. All images were taken from the apical turns of cochlea using a confocal microscope. Scale bar: 5 μm.

II (circle-shaped stereocilia), and type III (reversed PCP) (**Figure 3F**). In the untreated controls, almost all hair cells are type I and only a small fraction of hair cells are type II (**Figure 3G**). However, in the presence of ML141, most hair cells show altered PCP in a dosage-dependent manner (**Figure 3G**). Taken together, our data show that stereocilia development is significantly affected by CDC42 inactivation either genetically or chemically.

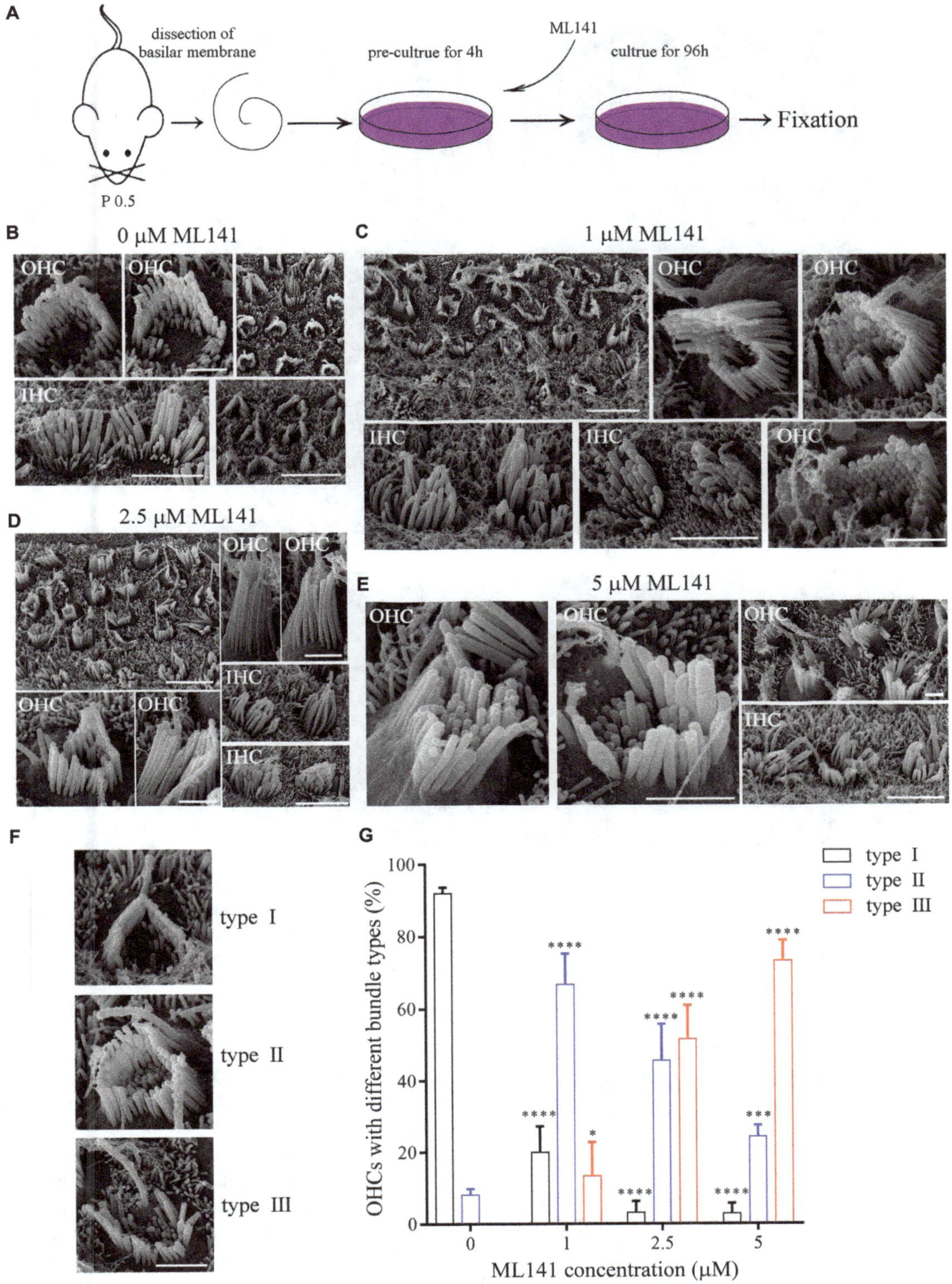

FIGURE 3 | CDC42 inhibitor ML141 treatment leads to stereocilia development deficits. **(A)** Schematic drawing of the strategy of ML141 treatment and SEM imaging. **(B–E)** SEM images of hair bundles after treatment of ML141 at different concentrations as indicated. Scale bars: 5 μm in low magnification images; 1 μm in high magnification OHC images; 3 μm in high magnification IHC images. **(F)** Representative images showing three types of hair bundles with different PCP phenotypes. Scale bar: 1 μm. **(G)** Percentages of hair cells of different types were analyzed from three independent experiments. The bars indicate the mean ± SEM values. *$P < 0.05$; ***$P < 0.001$; ****$P < 0.0001$.

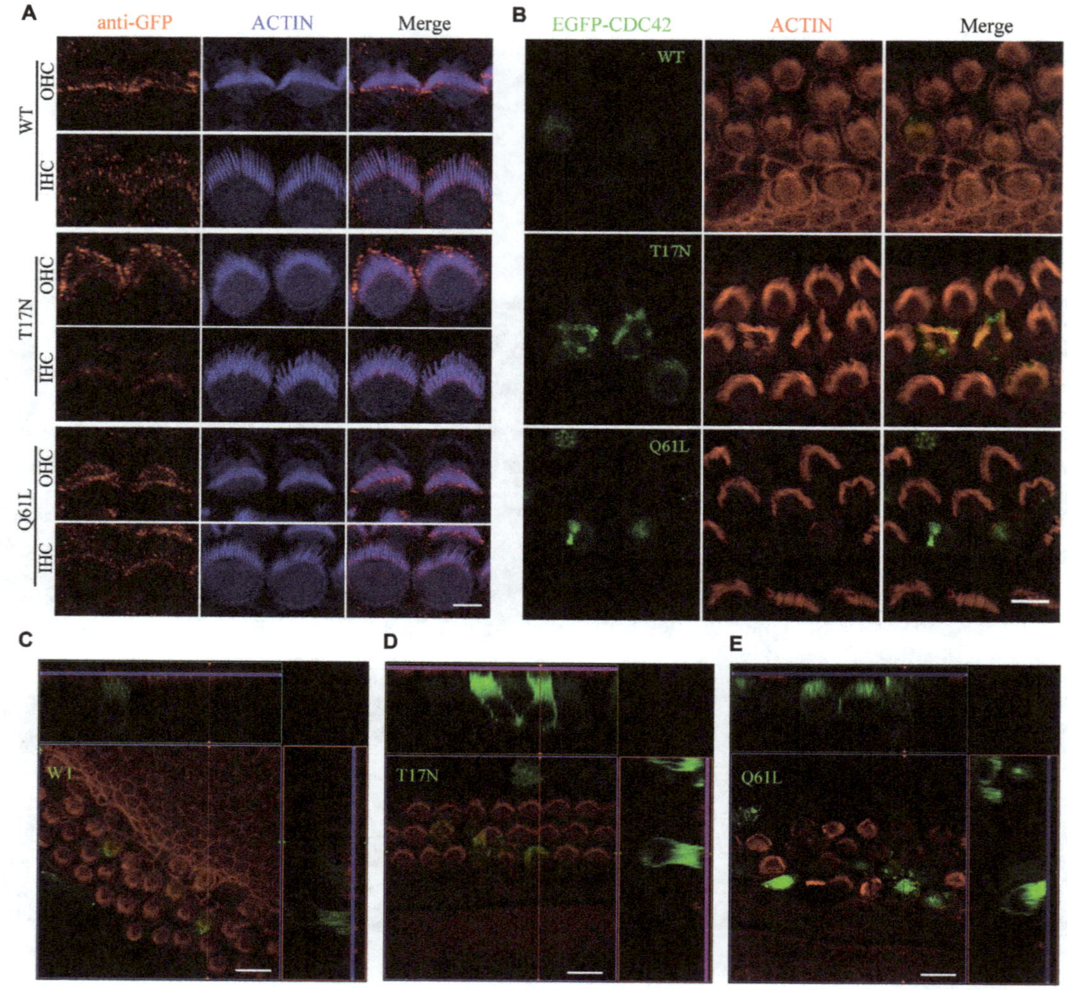

FIGURE 4 | Constitutively active CDC42 mutant leads to enhanced stereocilia deficits. **(A)** Whole-mount staining showing localization of purified exogenous wild-type or mutant CDC42 proteins in saponin-permeabilized P0.5 OHCs and IHCs. iFluor 405-conjugated phalloidin was used to visualize stereociliary F-actin core. GFP antibody was used to amplify the signals of EGFP fused with CDC42 proteins. Scale bar: 2 μm. **(B)** Cochlear explants from P2 wild-type mice were injectoporated with expression vectors to express EGFP-tagged wild-type or mutant CDC42 in hair cells. TRITC-conjugated phalloidin was used to visualize stereociliary F-actin core. Scale bar: 5 μm. **(C–E)** 3D reconstruction showing the side view of hair cells injectoporated with different CDC42 constructs as indicated. Scale bar: 10 μm.

Constitutively Active Mutant CDC42 Leads to Enhanced Stereocilia Deficits

As a small Rho GTPase, CDC42 is reversibly cycling between an active (GTP-bound) and inactive (GDP-bound) state (Hart et al., 1991). We next wanted to examine the effect of CDC42 in different state on stereocilia. We made use of two point mutations that mimic CDC42 in different state, namely inactive CDC42 mutant (T17N) and constitutively active CDC42 mutant (Q61L) (Kozma et al., 1995). We first examined whether exogenous CDC42 mutants could target to the stereocilia following permeabilization of unfixed cochlear sensory epithelia with 0.05% saponin (McGrath et al., 2021). The results show that wild-type CDC42 and two CDC42 mutants all localize in the stereocilia of P0.5 mice, with enrichment at the stereociliary tips (**Figure 4A**). However, all three forms of CDC42 are mainly detected in the cell body of saponin-permeabilized P6 cochlear hair cells, suggesting that CDC42 may show dynamic subcellular localization in the hair cells during development (**Supplementary Figures 3A–C**).

We then examined the effect of different CDC42 mutants on stereocilia development by employing the injectoporation assay and confocal microscopy. CDC42-expression vectors were injectoporated into P2 wild-type cochlear sensory epithelia, followed by *in vitro* culture for 24 h and confocal imaging. Stereociliary F-actin core was visualized using phalloidin. The results show that wild-type and CDC42 T17N mutant localize in the stereocilia as well as cell body of injectoporated hair cells, with largely normal stereocilia morphology (**Figures 4B–D**). In contrast, CDC42 Q61L mutant injectoporation results in complete stereocilia loss in most hair cells (21 out of 24 analyzed cells), suggesting that this constitutively active mutant CDC42 leads to enhanced stereocilia deficits (**Figures 4B,E**).

DISCUSSION

It was recently reported that the Rho GTPase CDC42 is localized in the stereocilia of cochlear hair cells, and that cochlear hair cell stereocilia of *Atoh1-Cre*; *Cdc42*$^{flox/flox}$ mice develop normally but progressively degenerate after maturation, suggesting that CDC42 plays an important role in stereocilia maintenance but not development (Ueyama et al., 2014). In the present work, however, we show that CDC42 is indispensable for normal stereocilia development in cochlear hair cells. One possible reason for this discrepancy might be the different *Atoh1-Cre* mouse lines used in these two works. Ueyama and colleagues used transgenic *Atoh1-Cre* mice (Matei et al., 2005), whereas we used *Atoh1-Cre* knock-in mice (Yang et al., 2010). Therefore, different Cre recombinase activity in these two mouse lines might account for the slightly different stereocilia phenotypes. Another possibility is that the subtle stereocilia development deficits revealed in the present work might have simply been overlooked in the earlier study.

Our SEM results reveal that the morphology of cochlear hair cell stereocilia is largely indistinguishable between P0.5 *Cdc42* cKO mice and control mice. Stereocilia deficits are apparent in P8 *Cdc42* cKO cochlear hair cells, which include increased stereocilia height variation and decreased stereocilia width. Moreover, the height difference between rows is significantly altered in IHCs, and extra shortest row stereocilia exist in OHCs of *Cdc42* cKO mice. Despite of the stereocilia deficits, the stereocilia row identity largely remains normal, given that the stereociliary tip localization of row 1 complex components MYO15A and EPS8 as well as row 2 complex component CAPZB2 is unchanged at this age. Moreover, CDC42 inhibitor ML141 causes similar stereocilia development deficits plus PCP phenotypes, further supporting an important role of CDC42 in stereocilia development.

Stereocilia development is a multi-step, tightly controlled process (Tilney et al., 1992; Kaltenbach et al., 1994). In immature cochlear hair cells, there are multiple rows of elongated stereocilia on the apical surface, among which the shorter rows are eventually resorbed, leaving 3–4 rows of stereocilia grow to their final height in the mature mammalian cochlear hair cells (Kaltenbach et al., 1994). The underlying mechanism of shorter row stereocilia resorption largely remains unknown. Our present data suggest that CDC42 might play a role in this process. The extra fourth-row stereocilia in *Cdc42* cKO OHCs is possibly a result of reduced stereocilia resorption, which might be explained by altered actin polymerization and stabilization of stereocilia due to *Cdc42* inactivation. Similar reason might also account for the observed deficits in stereocilia length and width of *Cdc42* cKO cochlear hair cells.

Noticeably, our present data suggest that appropriate CDC42 activity is important for stereocilia development. It has been reported that in cultured cells, overexpression of constitutively active CDC42 mutant (Q61L) promotes the formation of filopodia (Kozma et al., 1995). In line with this, gain of CDC42 activity by disrupting ARHGAP1 (previously known as CDC42GAP) also promotes filopodia formation (Yang et al., 2006). However, our present data show that overexpression of CDC42 Q61L mutant in cochlear hair cells leads to complete loss of stereocilia. This is in sharp contrast to the reports in filopodia formation. It is possible that stereocilia development and/or maintenance is regulated so tightly that imbalance of this process would inevitably cause stereocilia deficits. Similar scenario is also observed in DIA1, whose dysfunction is associated with autosomal dominant sensorineural hearing loss DFNA1 (Lynch et al., 1997). Constitutive activation of DIA1 causes stereocilia disorganization as well as hearing loss in mice (Ueyama et al., 2016; Ninoyu et al., 2020).

Our present data show that treatment with CDC42 inhibitor results in more severe stereocilia phenotypes than hair cell-specific *Cdc42* inactivation. Noticeably, apparent PCP deficits are observed in cochlear culture treated with CDC42 inhibitor, but not in the hair cell-specific *Cdc42* cKO mice, suggesting that other cells such as supporting cells are involved in CDC42-mediated PCP regulation. This is consistent with previous reports that dysregulated PCP is observed in mice deleting *Cdc42* in both hair cells and supporting cells, but not in mice deleting *Cdc42* only in hair cells (Ueyama et al., 2014; Kirjavainen et al., 2015). In line with this, *in situ* hybridization reveals that *Cdc42* transcripts are expressed ubiquitously in the cochlea (Anttonen et al., 2012). The ubiquitous expression of *Cdc42* in the inner ear is also supported by RNAseq results of embryonic and adult mice (Cai et al., 2015; Scheffer et al., 2015; Liu et al., 2018). Taken together, the present data suggest that CDC42 regulates stereocilia development both in a cell autonomous and non-autonomous manner.

Loss of another Rho GTPase RAC1 has also been shown to cause stereocilia development deficits, such as stereocilia flattening, fragmentation, as well as altered PCP (Grimsley-Myers et al., 2009). Different stereocilia phenotypes observed in *Cdc42* and *Rac1* knockout mice suggest that these two Rho GTPases play important and non-complementary roles in stereocilia development. Guanine nucleotide exchange factor (GEF) ARHGEF6 specifically activates CDC42 and RAC1, and loss of ARHGEF6 causes stereocilia deficits (Zhu et al., 2018). Moreover, p21-activated kinase 1 (PAK1), a downstream effector of CDC42 and RAC1, is required for stereocilia development (Cheng et al., 2021). These studies highlight the essential role of Rho GTPases in stereocilia development. At present, the precise localization of these proteins in the stereocilia remains unknown, which prevents us from fully understanding the underlying mechanism. New imaging methods such as super-resolution microscopy definitely will help to address this question (Liu et al., 2019; Qi et al., 2019, 2020).

ETHICS STATEMENT

The animal study was reviewed and approved by the Animal Ethics Committee of Shandong University School of Life Sciences (Permit Number: SYDWLL-2020-31).

AUTHOR CONTRIBUTIONS

ZX: study concept and design. HD, HZ, YS, and XZ: acquisition of data. HD, ZC, YW, and ZX: analysis and interpretation of data. YW and ZX: supervision. HD, YW, and ZX: drafting the manuscript. All authors contributed to the article and approved the submitted version.

the National Natural Science Foundation of China (82071051 and 81771001), and the Shandong Provincial Natural Science Foundation (ZR2020ZD39 and ZR2020QC098).

ACKNOWLEDGMENTS

We thank Sen Wang, Xiaomin Zhao, and Haiyan Yu from the core facilities for life and environmental sciences, Shandong University for the technical support in SEM and confocal microscopy.

REFERENCES

Anttonen, T., Kirjavainen, A., Belevich, I., Laos, M., Richardson, W. D., Jokitalo, E., et al. (2012). Cdc42-dependent structural development of auditory supporting cells is required for wound healing at adulthood. *Sci. Rep.* 2:978. doi: 10.1038/srep00978

Avenarius, M. R., Krey, J. F., Dumont, R. A., Morgan, C. P., Benson, C. B., Vijayakumar, S., et al. (2017). Heterodimeric capping protein is required for stereocilia length and width regulation. *J. Cell Biol.* 216, 3861–3881. doi: 10.1083/jcb.201704171

Barr-Gillespie, P. G. (2015). Assembly of hair bundles, an amazing problem for cell biology. *Mol. Biol. Cell* 26, 2727–2732. doi: 10.1091/mbc.E14-04-0940

Belyantseva, I. A., Boger, E. T., and Friedman, T. B. (2003). Myosin XVa localizes to the tips of inner ear sensory cell stereocilia and is essential for staircase formation of the hair bundle. *Proc. Natl. Acad. Sci. U.S.A.* 100, 13958–13963. doi: 10.1073/pnas.2334417100

Beurg, M., Fettiplace, R., Nam, J. H., and Ricci, A. J. (2009). Localization of inner hair cell mechanotransducer channels using high-speed calcium imaging. *Nat. Neurosci.* 12, 553–558. doi: 10.1038/nn.2295

Cai, T., Jen, H. I., Kang, H., Klisch, T. J., Zoghbi, H. Y., and Groves, A. K. (2015). Characterization of the transcriptome of nascent hair cells and identification of direct targets of the Atoh1 transcription factor. *J. Neurosci.* 35, 5870–5883. doi: 10.1523/JNEUROSCI.5083-14.2015

Cao, H., Yin, X., Cao, Y., Jin, Y., Wang, S., Kong, Y., et al. (2013). FCHSD1 and FCHSD2 are expressed in hair cell stereocilia and cuticular plate and regulate actin polymerization in vitro. *PLoS One* 8:e56516. doi: 10.1371/journal.pone.0056516

Chen, F., Ma, L., Parrini, M. C., Mao, X., Lopez, M., Wu, C., et al. (2000). Cdc42 is required for PIP(2)-induced actin polymerization and early development but not for cell viability. *Curr. Biol.* 10, 758–765. doi: 10.1016/s0960-9822(00)00571-6

Cheng, C., Hou, Y., Zhang, Z., Wang, Y., Lu, L., Zhang, L., et al. (2021). Disruption of the autism-related gene Pak1 causes stereocilia disorganization, hair cell loss, and deafness in mice. *J. Genet. Genomics* 48, 324–332. doi: 10.1016/j.jgg.2021.03.010

Ciuman, R. R. (2011). Auditory and vestibular hair cell stereocilia: relationship between functionality and inner ear disease. *J. Laryngol. Otol.* 125, 991–1003. doi: 10.1017/S0022215111001459

Drummond, M. C., Barzik, M., Bird, J. E., Zhang, D. S., Lechene, C. P., Corey, D. P., et al. (2015). Live-cell imaging of actin dynamics reveals mechanisms of stereocilia length regulation in the inner ear. *Nat. Commun.* 6:6873. doi: 10.1038/ncomms7873

Du, H., Zou, L., Ren, R., Li, N., Li, J., Wang, Y., et al. (2020). Lack of PDZD7 long isoform disrupts ankle-link complex and causes hearing loss in mice. *FASEB J.* 34, 1136–1149. doi: 10.1096/fj.201901657RR

Ellwanger, D. C., Scheibinger, M., Dumont, R. A., Barr-Gillespie, P. G., and Heller, S. (2018). Transcriptional dynamics of hair-bundle morphogenesis revealed with Cell Trails. *Cell Rep.* 23, 2901–2914. doi: 10.1016/j.celrep.2018.05.002

Flock, A., and Cheung, H. C. (1977). Actin filaments in sensory hairs of inner ear receptor cells. *J. Cell Biol.* 75(2 Pt 1), 339–343.

Grimsley-Myers, C. M., Sipe, C. W., Geleoc, G. S., and Lu, X. (2009). The small GTPase Rac1 regulates auditory hair cell morphogenesis. *J. Neurosci.* 29, 15859–15869. doi: 10.1523/JNEUROSCI.3998-09.2009

Hart, M. J., Eva, A., Evans, T., Aaronson, S. A., and Cerione, R. A. (1991). Catalysis of guanine-nucleotide exchange on the Cdc42hs protein by the Dbl oncogene product. *Nature* 354, 311–314. doi: 10.1038/354311a0

Hudspeth, A. J., and Jacobs, R. (1979). Stereocilia mediate transduction in vertebrate hair cells. *Proc. Natl. Acad. Sci. U.S.A.* 76, 1506–1509.

Jones, C., Roper, V. C., Foucher, I., Qian, D., Banizs, B., Petit, C., et al. (2008). Ciliary proteins link basal body polarization to planar cell polarity regulation. *Nat. Genet.* 40, 69–77. doi: 10.1038/ng.2007.54

Kaltenbach, J. A., Falzarano, P. R., and Simpson, T. H. (1994). Postnatal development of the hamster cochlea. II. growth and differentiation of stereocilia bundles. *J. Comp. Neurol.* 350, 187–198. doi: 10.1002/cne.903500204

Kirjavainen, A., Laos, M., Anttonen, T., and Pirvola, U. (2015). The Rho GTPase Cdc42 regulates hair cell planar polarity and cellular patterning in the developing cochlea. *Biol. Open* 4, 516–526. doi: 10.1242/bio.20149753

Kozma, R., Ahmed, S., Best, A., and Lim, L. (1995). The Ras-related protein Cdc42hs and Bradykinin promote formation of peripheral actin microspikes and filopodia in Swiss 3T3 fibroblasts. *Mol. Cell. Biol.* 15, 1942–1952. doi: 10.1128/MCB.15.4.1942

Krey, J. F., and Barr-Gillespie, P. G. (2019). Molecular composition of vestibular hair bundles. *Cold Spring Harb. Perspect. Med.* 9:a033209. doi: 10.1101/cshperspect.a033209

Krey, J. F., Chatterjee, P., Dumont, R. A., O'Sullivan, M., Choi, D., Bird, J. E., et al. (2020). Mechanotransduction-dependent control of stereocilia dimensions and row identity in inner hair cells. *Curr. Biol.* 30, 442–454. doi: 10.1016/j.cub.2019.11.076

Li, S. H., Mecca, A., Kim, J., Caprara, G. A., Wagner, E. L., Du, T. T., et al. (2020). Myosin-VIIa is expressed in multiple isoforms and essential for tensioning the hair cell mechanotransduction complex. *Nat. Commun.* 11:2066. doi: 10.1038/s41467-020-15936-z

Lindeman, H. H., Ades, H. W., Bredberg, G., and Engstrom, H. (1971). The sensory hairs and the tectorial membrane in the development of the cat's organ of Corti. A scanning electron microscopic study. *Acta Otolaryngol.* 72, 229–242.

Liu, H. Z., Chen, L., Giffen, K. P., Stringham, S. T., Li, Y., Judge, P. D., et al. (2018). Cell-specific transcriptome analysis shows that adult Pillar and Deiters' cells express genes encoding machinery for specializations of cochlear hair cells. *Front. Mol. Neurosci.* 11:356. doi: 10.3389/fnmol.2018.00356

Liu, Y., Qi, J. Y., Chen, X., Tang, M. L., Chu, C. F., Zhu, W. J., et al. (2019). Critical role of spectrin in hearing development and deafness. *Sci. Adv.* 5:eaav7803. doi: 10.1126/sciadv.aav7803

Lynch, E. D., Lee, M. K., Morrow, J. E., Welcsh, P. L., Leon, P. E., and King, M. C. (1997). Nonsyndromic deafness DFNA1 associated with mutation of a human homolog of the Drosophila gene diaphanous. *Science* 278, 1315–1318.

Manor, U., Disanza, A., Grati, M., Andrade, L., Lin, H., Di Fiore, P. P., et al. (2011). Regulation of stereocilia length by myosin XVa and whirlin depends on the actin-regulatory protein Eps8. *Curr. Biol.* 21, 167–172. doi: 10.1016/j.cub.2010.12.046

Matei, V., Pauley, S., Kaing, S., Rowitch, D., Beisel, K. W., Morris, K., et al. (2005). Smaller inner ear sensory epithelia in Neurog 1 null mice are related to earlier hair cell cycle exit. *Dev. Dyn.* 234, 633–650. doi: 10.1002/dvdy.20551

McGrath, J., and Perrin, B. J. (2020). Cell biology: function guides form of auditory sensory cells. *Curr. Biol.* 30, R128–R130. doi: 10.1016/j.cub.2019.12.039

McGrath, J., Roy, P., and Perrin, B. J. (2017). Stereocilia morphogenesis and maintenance through regulation of actin stability. *Semin. Cell Dev. Biol.* 65, 88–95. doi: 10.1016/j.semcdb.2016.08.017

McGrath, J., Tung, C. Y., Liao, X., Belyantseva, I. A., Roy, P., Chakraborty, O., et al. (2021). Actin at stereocilia tips is regulated by mechanotransduction and ADF/cofilin. *Curr. Biol.* 31, 1141–1153. doi: 10.1016/j.cub.2020.12.006

Narayanan, P., Chatterton, P., Ikeda, A., Ikeda, S., Corey, D. P., Ervasti, J. M., et al. (2015). Length regulation of mechanosensitive stereocilia depends on very slow actin dynamics and filament-severing proteins. *Nat. Commun.* 6:6855. doi: 10.1038/Ncomms7855

Ninoyu, Y., Sakaguchi, H., Lin, C., Suzuki, T., Hirano, S., Hisa, Y., et al. (2020). The integrity of cochlear hair cells is established and maintained through the localization of Dia1 at apical junctional complexes and stereocilia. *Cell Death Dis.* 11:536. doi: 10.1038/s41419-020-02743-z

Qi, J. Y., Liu, Y., Chu, C. F., Chen, X., Zhu, W. J., Shu, Y. L., et al. (2019). A cytoskeleton structure revealed by super-resolution fluorescence imaging in inner ear hair cells. *Cell Discov.* 5:12. doi: 10.1038/s41421-018-0076-4

Qi, J. Y., Zhang, L. Y., Tan, F. Z., Liu, Y., Chu, C. F., Zhu, W. J., et al. (2020). Espin distribution as revealed by super-resolution microscopy of stereocilia. *Am. J. Transl. Res.* 12, 130–141.

Rohatgi, R., Ma, L., Miki, H., Lopez, M., Kirchhausen, T., Takenawa, T., et al. (1999). The interaction between N-WASP and the Arp2/3 complex links Cdc42-dependent signals to actin assembly. *Cell* 97, 221–231. doi: 10.1016/s0092-8674(00)80732-1

Scheffer, D. I., Shen, J., Corey, D. P., and Chen, Z. Y. (2015). Gene expression by mouse inner ear hair cells during development. *J. Neurosci.* 35, 6366–6380. doi: 10.1523/JNEUROSCI.5126-14.2015

Sit, S. T., and Manser, E. (2011). Rho GTPases and their role in organizing the actin cytoskeleton. *J. Cell Sci.* 124, 679–683. doi: 10.1242/jcs.064964

Surviladze, Z., Waller, A., Strouse, J. J., Bologa, C., Ursu, O., Salas, V., et al. (2010). "A potent and selective inhibitor of Cdc42 GTPase," in *Probe Reports from the NIH Molecular Libraries Program*, (Bethesda, MD: National Center for Biotechnology Information).

Tilney, L. G., Derosier, D. J., and Mulroy, M. J. (1980). The organization of actin filaments in the stereocilia of cochlear hair cells. *J. Cell Biol.* 86, 244–259.

Tilney, L. G., Tilney, M. S., and DeRosier, D. J. (1992). Actin filaments, stereocilia, and hair cells: how cells count and measure. *Annu. Rev. Cell Biol.* 8, 257–274. doi: 10.1146/annurev.cb.08.110192.001353

Ueyama, T., Ninoyu, Y., Nishio, S. Y., Miyoshi, T., Torii, H., Nishimura, K., et al. (2016). Constitutive activation of DIA1 (DIAPH1) via C-terminal truncation causes human sensorineural hearing loss. *EMBO Mol. Med.* 8, 1310–1324. doi: 10.15252/emmm.201606609

Ueyama, T., Sakaguchi, H., Nakamura, T., Goto, A., Morioka, S., Shimizu, A., et al. (2014). Maintenance of stereocilia and apical junctional complexes by Cdc42 in cochlear hair cells. *J. Cell Sci.* 127(Pt 9), 2040–2052. doi: 10.1242/jcs.143602

van Hengel, J., D'Hooge, P., Hooghe, B., Wu, X., Libbrecht, L., De Vos, R., et al. (2008). Continuous cell injury promotes hepatic tumorigenesis in cdc42-deficient mouse liver. *Gastroenterology* 134, 781–792. doi: 10.1053/j.gastro.2008.01.002

Velez-Ortega, A. C., and Frolenkov, G. I. (2019). Building and repairing the stereocilia cytoskeleton in mammalian auditory hair cells. *Hear. Res.* 376, 47–57. doi: 10.1016/j.heares.2018.12.012

Wang, Y., Li, J., Yao, X., Li, W., Du, H., Tang, M., et al. (2017). Loss of CIB2 causes profound hearing loss and abolishes mechanoelectrical transduction in mice. *Front. Mol. Neurosci.* 10:401. doi: 10.3389/fnmol.2017.00401

Yang, H., Xie, X., Deng, M., Chen, X., and Gan, L. (2010). Generation and characterization of Atoh1-Cre knock-in mouse line. *Genesis* 48, 407–413. doi: 10.1002/dvg.20633

Yang, L., Wang, L., and Zheng, Y. (2006). Gene targeting of Cdc42 and Cdc42GAP affirms the critical involvement of Cdc42 in filopodia induction, directed migration, and proliferation in primary mouse embryonic fibroblasts. *Mol. Biol. Cell* 17, 4675–4685. doi: 10.1091/mbc.e06-05-0466

Zampini, V., Ruttiger, L., Johnson, S. L., Franz, C., Furness, D. N., Waldhaus, J., et al. (2011). Eps8 regulates hair bundle length and functional maturation of mammalian auditory hair cells. *PLoS Biol.* 9:e1001048. doi: 10.1371/journal.pbio.1001048

Zhang, D. S., Piazza, V., Perrin, B. J., Rzadzinska, A. K., Poczatek, J. C., Wang, M., et al. (2012). Multi-isotope imaging mass spectrometry reveals slow protein turnover in hair-cell stereocilia. *Nature* 481, 520–524. doi: 10.1038/nature10745

Zhu, C., Cheng, C., Wang, Y., Muhammad, W., Liu, S., Zhu, W., et al. (2018). Loss of ARHGEF6 causes hair cell stereocilia deficits and hearing loss in mice. *Front. Mol. Neurosci.* 11:362. doi: 10.3389/fnmol.2018.00362

Zou, J., Zheng, T., Ren, C., Askew, C., Liu, X. P., Pan, B., et al. (2014). Deletion of PDZD7 disrupts the Usher syndrome type 2 protein complex in cochlear hair cells and causes hearing loss in mice. *Hum. Mol. Genet.* 23, 2374–2390. doi: 10.1093/hmg/ddt629

7

Spatiotemporal Developmental Upregulation of Prestin Correlates With the Severity and Location of Cyclodextrin-Induced Outer Hair Cell Loss and Hearing Loss

Dalian Ding, Haiyan Jiang, Senthilvelan Manohar, Xiaopeng Liu, Li Li, Guang-Di Chen and Richard Salvi*

Center for Hearing and Deafness, University at Buffalo, Buffalo, NY, United States

***Correspondence:**
Richard Salvi
salvi@buffalo.edu

2-Hyroxypropyl-beta-cyclodextrin (HPβCD) is being used to treat Niemann-Pick C1, a fatal neurodegenerative disease caused by abnormal cholesterol metabolism. HPβCD slows disease progression, but unfortunately causes severe, rapid onset hearing loss by destroying the outer hair cells (OHC). HPβCD-induced damage is believed to be related to the expression of prestin in OHCs. Because prestin is postnatally upregulated from the cochlear base toward the apex, we hypothesized that HPβCD ototoxicity would spread from the high-frequency base toward the low-frequency apex of the cochlea. Consistent with this hypothesis, cochlear hearing impairments and OHC loss rapidly spread from the high-frequency base toward the low-frequency apex of the cochlea when HPβCD administration shifted from postnatal day 3 (P3) to P28. HPβCD-induced histopathologies were initially confined to the OHCs, but between 4- and 6-weeks post-treatment, there was an unexpected, rapid and massive expansion of the lesion to include most inner hair cells (IHC), pillar cells (PC), peripheral auditory nerve fibers, and spiral ganglion neurons at location where OHCs were missing. The magnitude and spatial extent of HPβCD-induced OHC death was tightly correlated with the postnatal day when HPβCD was administered which coincided with the spatiotemporal upregulation of prestin in OHCs. A second, massive wave of degeneration involving IHCs, PC, auditory nerve fibers and spiral ganglion neurons abruptly emerged 4–6 weeks post-HPβCD treatment. This secondary wave of degeneration combined with the initial OHC loss results in a profound, irreversible hearing loss.

Keywords: cyclodextrin, prestin, Niemann-Pick C1, spiral ganglion neurons, outer hair cells, inner hair cells, otoacoustic emissions, compound action potential

---

Abbreviations: ANF, auditory nerve fibers; HPβCD, 2-hydroxylpropyl-beta-cyclodextrin; CAP, compound action potential; DPOAE, distortion product otoacoustic emission; IHC, inner hair cells; NF, nerve fiber; NPC1, Niemann-Pick Type C1; OHC, outer hair cells; PC, pillar cells; SGN, spiral ganglion neurons; SL, spiral limbus; WT, wild type.

INTRODUCTION

Cyclodextrins are widely used in many industries because they can encapsulate hydrophobic compounds within a hydrophobic shell (Okamura et al., 2002; Laza-Knoerr et al., 2010; Loftsson and Brewster, 2010). Consequently, cyclodextrins are often employed as excipients because they enhance the solubility, absorption, and stability of these compounds (Otero-Espinar et al., 2010), making them extremely useful for drug delivery (Davis and Brewster, 2004; Tang et al., 2006; Ren et al., 2010; Wu et al., 2013). At the doses normally employed commercially, cyclodextrins have negligible side effects (Marttin et al., 1998; Uchenna Agu et al., 2000; Stella and He, 2008) and are considered safe (FDA; Notices 000155, 000074, 000046).

Because cyclodextrins can remove lipids and cholesterol from cells, they are being evaluated as potential therapeutics to treat vascular, kidney, liver, and neurodegenerative diseases caused by the cellular accumulation of cholesterol (Lirussi et al., 2002; Walenbergh et al., 2015; Coisne et al., 2016; Zimmer et al., 2016; Mitrofanova et al., 2018; Bessell et al., 2019; Cho et al., 2019; Kim et al., 2020). 2-Hydroypropyl-beta-cyclodextrin (HPβCD) is currently being evaluated as an investigational new drug to treat Niemann-Pick Type C1 disease (NPC1) (ClinicalTrials.gov Identifier: NCT02534844), a fatal neurodegenerative disease caused by the buildup of unesterified cholesterol in brain (Kolodny, 2000; Ory, 2000; Newton et al., 2018). Unesterified cholesterol plays an important role in plasma membrane turnover, which in neurons, is estimated to be more than 20%/day (Dietschy and Turley, 2004). In the brain, inactivation of NPC1 leads to the sequestration of unesterified cholesterol in endosomes and lysosomes resulting in neurodegeneration (Aqul et al., 2011). Mutant *npc1*$^{-/-}$ mice, an animal model of NPC1 disease, develop severe pulmonary, hepatic and neurodegenerative disorders. However, when *npc1*$^{-/-}$ mice are treated with high systemic doses of HPβCD, the compound overcomes the cholesterol transport deficits allowing the release of excess sterols thereby alleviating symptoms (Liu et al., 2010; Ramirez et al., 2010; Taylor A. M. et al., 2012). Although HPβCD slows NPC1 neurodegeneration, the high therapeutic doses employed can cause hearing loss (Ward et al., 2010; Crumling et al., 2012; King et al., 2014; Cronin et al., 2015; Maarup et al., 2015; Liu et al., 2020). Cyclodextrin-induced hearing loss has an abrupt onset due to the rapid degeneration of outer hair cells (OHC; Crumling et al., 2012, 2017; Cronin et al., 2015; Takahashi et al., 2016). Over time, the inner hair cells (IHCs), spiral ganglion neurons (SGNs), and auditory nerve fibers (ANFs) eventually degenerate following high-dose cyclodextrin treatment, but the time course over which this occurs is unclear (Liu et al., 2020; Ding et al., 2021). Because HPβCD initially destroys only OHCs and because cholesterol modulates OHC electromotility mediated by prestin (Rajagopalan et al., 2007), it was assumed that this selective damage was related to the expression of the electromotile protein prestin located in the plasma membrane along the OHC lateral wall (Takahashi et al., 2016; Crumling et al., 2017). Because mutant mice with a non-electromotile version of prestin continued to be vulnerable to HPβCD ototoxicity; it was concluded that electromotility per se was not a critical factor in HPβCD ototoxicity (Zhou et al., 2018). On the other hand, OHCs in the middle and basal turn of prestin knockout mice were substantially less susceptible to HPβCD toxicity than wild type (WT) mice. Despite the absence of prestin, approximately 20% more OHCs were damaged by HPβCD in the knockout mice compared to saline controls (Takahashi et al., 2016). Moreover, there was still considerable OHC loss in the apical turn of prestin knockout mice. While these results indicate that prestin is important, other factors may contribute to cyclodextrin ototoxicity.

Prestin undergoes a developmental spatial and temporal upregulation in altricial mammals. In rodents, prestin expression in the OHC lateral wall progressively increases from postnatal day 0 (P0) reaching adult-like levels in the basal turn at approximately P9, in the middle turn around P11 and in the apical turn around P12 (Belyantseva et al., 2000; Jensen-Smith and Hallworth, 2007). In contrast, cholesterol expression in the OHC lateral wall decreases slightly from P3 to P21 (Jensen-Smith and Hallworth, 2007). If prestin expression is a key element in cyclodextrin ototoxicity, then high-dose HPβCD should only damage basal turn OHCs if the drug is administered in early postnatal life, but OHC damage should progressively increase and spread from the base to the apex of the cochlea from P0 to adulthood. To test this hypothesis, the developmental expression of prestin was evaluated in OHCs along the length of the cochlea and compared to the cochlear frequency-dependent functional deficits and time-dependent histopathological damage patterns in the cochlea. By carefully assessing the time course of cyclodextrin ototoxicity over several months, we were able to show that HPβCD, in addition to causing early onset OHC damage, also caused a large, secondary wave of damage to IHCs, ANFs and SGNs between 4- and 6-weeks after HPβCD treatment.

MATERIALS AND METHODS

Subjects

Sprague-Dawley rats (Charles River) were used for all experiments. In Experiment #1, the developmental upregulation of prestin was evaluated in the OHCs of postnatal day 5 (P5, $n = 4$), day 10 (P10, $n = 4$), day 15 (P15, $n = 4$) and day 28 (P28, $n = 4$) rats. In Experiments #2, P5 ($n = 6$), P10 ($n = 6$), P15 ($n = 6$), and P28 ($n = 6$) Sprague-Dawley rats were treated subcutaneously with a single dose of 4,000 mg/kg of HPβCD and a Control group ($n = 10$) was treated similarly with saline. The cochleae from these animals underwent histological analysis 8-weeks post-treatment ($n = 6$/group). DPOAEs and CAPs were measured from the P5 ($n = 6$), P10 ($n = 6$), and P15 ($n = 6$) groups 8-weeks after HPβCD treatment. DPOAEs ($n = 10$) and CAPs ($n = 8$) were also measured from the saline Control group. In Experiments #3, which was designed to assess the time-course of degeneration, the extent of hair cell, nerve fiber and SGN loss was evaluated in adult rats (~12 weeks old at time of HPβCD treatment) as a function of time after treatment with 4,000 mg/kg of HPβCD. Sprague-Dawley rats were evaluated 1-week ($n = 5$) and 4- ($n = 4$), 6- ($n = 6$) or 8-weeks ($n = 4$) post-treatment and the results compared to a saline Control group (n = 6) 8-weeks post-treatment.

HPβCD Treatment

2-Hyroxypropyl-beta-cyclodextrin was administered subcutaneously to rats at a dose of 4,000 mg/kg of HPβCD in sterile saline (volume: 0.2 ml for P5, P10, P15, and P28 rats and 1 ml for adult rats). This high 4,000 mg/kg dose was used in order to destroy OHCs over the length of the cochlea in order to assess the developmental upregulation of prestin from the base to apex of the cochlea. Rats in the Control group (n = 6) were subcutaneously injected with the same amount of sterile saline. One ear of each rat in the experimental group was used to prepare cochlear surface preparations; the other was used to prepare temporal bone sections. Animals were sacrificed for histological analysis at 1-week or 4-, 6- or 8-weeks after the saline or HPβCD treatments. All experimental procedures were approved by the Institutional Animal Care and Use Committee (HER05080Y) at the University at Buffalo in accordance with NIH guidelines.

Cochlear Preparations

Rats were anesthetized with ketamine (50 mg/kg, i.p.) and xylazine (6 mg/kg, i.p), decapitated and the bullae quickly removed. Openings were carefully made in the cochlear apex, round window, and the oval window and then the cochleae were perfused with 10% formalin in phosphate buffered saline (PBS) and immersed in the fixative overnight.

Cochleograms

One cochlea from each animal was stained with Ehrlich's hematoxylin solution as previously described (Johnson et al., 2017). Afterward, the samples were mounted as a flat surface preparation in glycerin on glass slides, coverslipped and examined with a light microscope (Zeiss Standard, 400X). IHCs, OHCs, and pillar cells (PCs) were counted along successive 0.12–0.24 mm intervals from the apex to the base of the cochlea by a second person blind to the experimental conditions. A hair cell or PC was counted as present if both the cuticular plate and cell nucleus were clearly visible and considered missing if either were absent. The percentages of missing IHCs, OHCs and PCs were determined for each animal based on lab norms and a cochleogram constructed showing the percentage of missing OHCs, IHCs, and PCs as a function of percent distance from the apex of the cochlea. Position in the cochlea was related to frequency using a rat tonotopic map (Müller, 1991). Mean percent OHC, IHC, and PC losses were computed over 5% intervals of the cochlea.

Immunolabeling

In Experiment 1, cochleae from postnatal rats were incubated for 24 h with a primary rabbit anti-SLC26A5 antibody (Millipore Sigma, AV44176, 1:100 dilution) and then incubated for 2 h in a fluorescently labeled (Alexa Fluor 555) goat anti-rabbit secondary antibody (Abcam, ab15008, 1:100 dilution). The specimens were then doubled-labeled with for 1 h with Alexa Fluor 488 conjugated phalloidin (1:200, Invitrogen 474685) to label the hair cell stereocilia and cuticular plate. Specimens were mounted on glass slide, cover slipped, and examined under a confocal microscope with appropriate filters as described previously (Ding et al., 2010).

Spiral Ganglion Neurons and Auditory Nerve Fibers

To determine if HPβCD resulted in degeneration of SGNs and NFs fibers in the habenula perforata, the temporal bones from rats in Experiment 3 were fixed with 0.25% glutaraldehyde in phosphate-buffered saline for 2 h and then treated with 2% osmium tetroxide for 2 h as described in earlier publications (Ding et al., 1999; Wang et al., 2003). The temporal bones were decalcified for 48 h (Decal, Baxter Scientific Immunoreactivity Products), dehydrated through a graded series of ethanol solutions ending at 100% and then embedded in Epon 812 resin. The Epon-embedded blocks were cut parallel to the axis of the cochlear modiolus at a thickness of 4 μm using an ultramicrotome (Reichert Supernova) equipped with glass knives. Serial sections were collected on glass slides, stained with toluidine blue and examined under a light microscope (Zeiss Axioskop). Specimens were photographed with a digital camera (SPOT Insight, Diagnostic Instruments Inc.) and processed with imaging software (SPOT Software, version 4.6; Adobe Photoshop 5.5). Sections cut tangential to the habenula perforata were used to count the number of fibers passing through each habenula perforata canal. For each experimental condition, the numbers of nerve fibers were counted from 10 habenula perforata canals located in the middle of the basal turn (~70%-distance-from-apex) of the cochlea of each animal. Measurements were obtained from each animal in the control group (n = 6) and each animal in the groups treated with 1,000, 2,000, 3,000, or 4,000 mg/kg HPβCD (n = 6/group) (Ding et al., 1999; Fu et al., 2012). Sections cut through the modiolus were used to count the number of SGNs in Rosenthal's canal in the middle of the basal turn (~70%-distance-from-apex) of the cochlea as described previously (Ding et al., 1998; McFadden et al., 1999; Fu et al., 2012). For each experimental condition, the number of SGNs in Rosenthal's canal was counted in each section; data were obtained from five separate sections in each animal (sections separated by 20 μm) and a mean value was computed for each animal. Mean numbers of SGNs per section were computed for each experimental group and the Control group (n = 6/group).

DPOAE and CAP

Our procedures for measuring DPOAEs and CAPs have been described in a recent publication (Liu et al., 2020). The rats in Experiment #2 that were treated with a single 4,000 mg/kg dose of HPβCD at P5, P10, or P15 and the saline Control group were evaluated 8-weeks post-treatment. The animals were anesthetized with ketamine (100 mg/kg, i.p.) and xylazine (20 mg/kg, i.p.), placed on a heating pad to maintain normal body temperature and DPOAEs were measured with an Extended-Bandwidth Acoustic Probe System (ER10X, Etymotic Research, Elk Grove Village, IL, United States) containing two loudspeakers and a low-noise microphone. Custom software was used to generate pairs of primary tones, f1 and f2, and the microphone was used to measure the primary tones and DPOAEs in the ear canal.

The higher frequency, f2, of the pair of tones was presented at a frequency 1.2 times greater than the lower frequency, f1 (i.e., f2/f1 = 1.2). The intensity of the lower frequency, L1, was set 10 dB greater than the intensity of the higher frequency, L2. The stimuli were presented for 90 ms at the rate of 5 Hz and repeated 32 times. The acoustic signal in the ear canal was recorded with the low-noise microphone, digitized (RME Babyface Pro, 192 kHz sampling rate, 24 bit A/D converter) and the intensity of f1, f2 and 2f1-f2 calculated using a fast Fourier transform (FFT). DPOAE input/output functions were constructed at f2 frequencies of 4, 8, 16, 24, 30, and 45 kHz by plotting the amplitude of 2f1-f2 at L2 intensities from 15 to 70 dB SPL in 5 dB SPL steps. DPOAEs were measured eight weeks after HPβCD treatment.

Our procedures for recording the CAP are described in a recent publication (Liu et al., 2020). Tone bursts were generated (5 ms duration, 1 ms rise/fall time, cosine2-gated, 2–60 kHz, TDT RX6 Multifunction Processor, 200 kHz sampling rate) and sent to a half-inch condenser microphone/sound source (ACO ½" microphone driven in reverse). The sound source, located within a speculum-like assembly was inserted in the ear canal. The sound source was calibrated with the aid of a ½" microphone (model 2540, Larson Davis), microphone preamplifier (Model 2221, Larson Davis) and A/D converter (RME Babyface Pro) connected to a personal computer and custom sound calibration software.

Rats were anesthetized (ketamine/xylazine cocktail; 100 mg/kg, i.p./30 mg/kg, i.p.), mounted in a custom head-holder, and placed on a temperature controlled heating blanket (Harvard Apparatus) The right cochlea was surgically opened and a recording electrode (Teflon-coated gold wire) was placed on the round window membrane and a silver chloride ground electrode placed in the neck muscle. The electrode output was amplified (1000X, DAM-50 amplifier, WPI), filtered (0.1 Hz–10 kHz), delivered to an A/D converter (100 kHz sampling rate, TDT RX6 Multifunction Processor) and averaged (100X) using custom data acquisition and filtering software (MATLAB 6.1) optimized to exclude the cochlear microphonic potential and isolate the CAP. CAP amplitude was defined as the voltage difference between the first negative peak (N1) and following positive peak (P1). CAP amplitude was plotted as a function of stimulus intensity level to construct CAP input/output functions at 4, 8, 16, 24, 30, and 45 kHz.

Analysis

GraphPad Prism (ver. 5) and/or Sigma Stat (ver. 3) software were used to plot and/or analyze the results as described below. HPβCD-induced losses of SGNs and ANFs were evaluated using a one-way ANOVA followed by Tukey's post-hoc comparison.

This research was approved by the University at Buffalo Institutional Animal Care and Use Committee and carried out in accordance with NIH Guidelines.

RESULTS

Prestin Is Developmentally Upregulated Along the Cochlear Tonotopic Axis in Rat OHCs

Prestin immunolabeling was used to identify the location and relative abundance of prestin in P5, P10, P15, and P28 rats. Strong prestin immunolabeling was only evident in OHCs in the basal turn of the cochlea at P5 (**Figures 1A–J**) and P10 (**Figures 1K–S**). However, prestin expression spread to OHCs in the middle

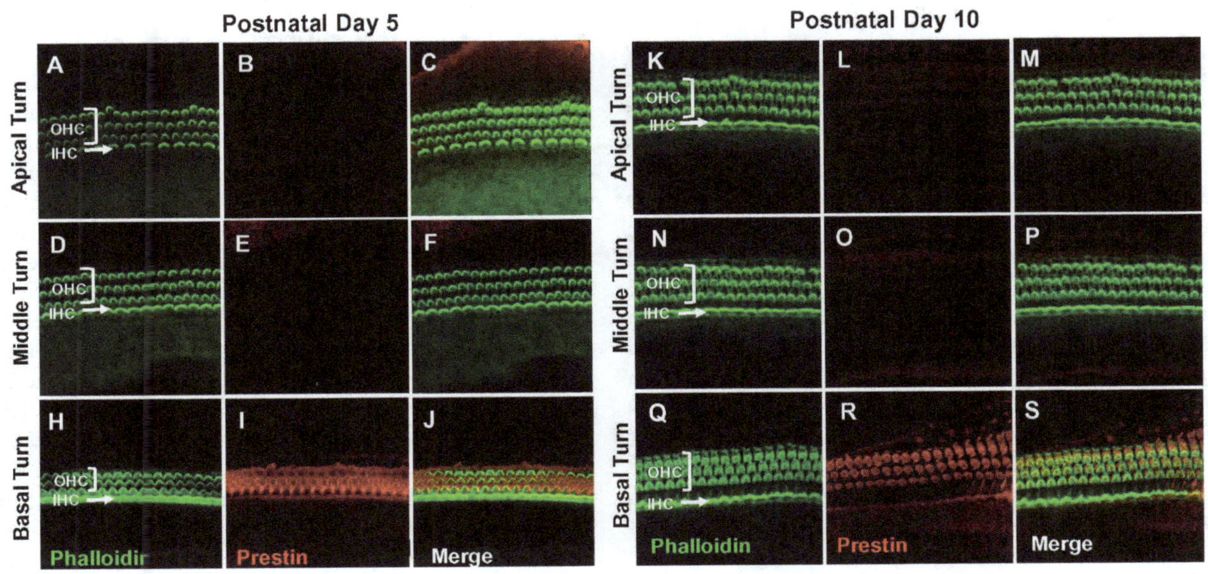

FIGURE 1 | Prestin is only expressed in the basal turn of normal rats on postnatal day 5 (P5) and day 10 (P10). Representative phalloidin-labeled images, prestin-labeled images and merged confocal images of cochlear surface preparations from the apical, middle and basal turn of normal P5 rats **(A–J)** and P10 rats **(K–S)**. **(I,R)** Note strong prestin immunolabeling in basal turn outer hair cells (OHCs), but absence of prestin labeling in inner hair cells (IHCs).

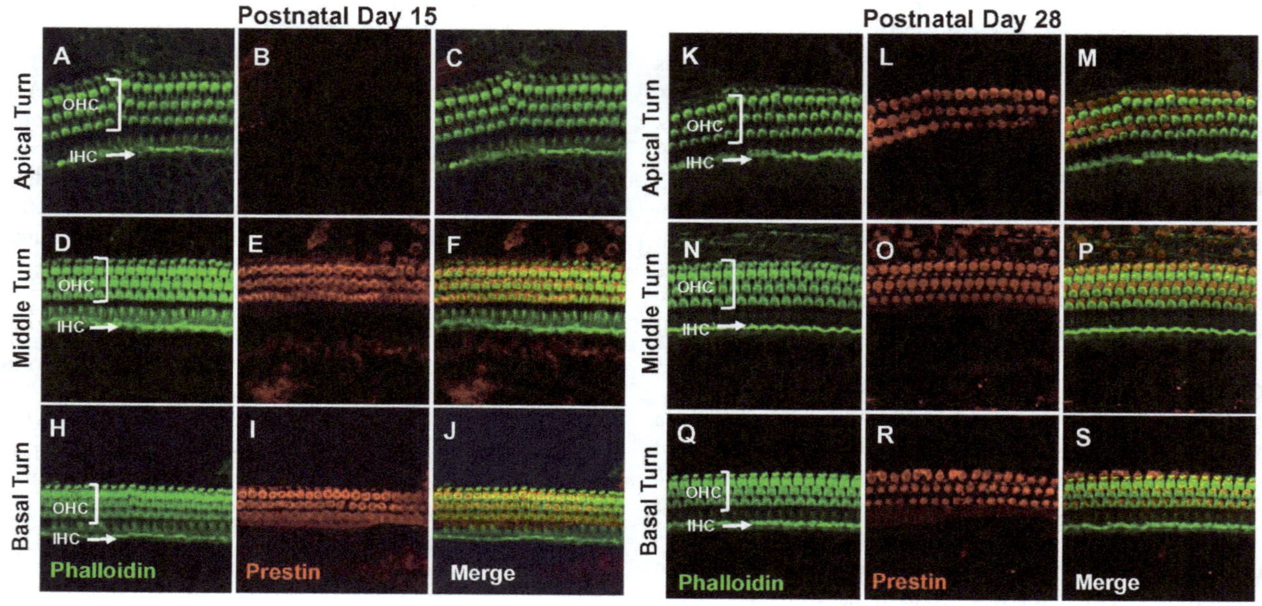

FIGURE 2 | Prestin labeling present in outer hair cells (OHCs) in basal and middle turn at P15 and labeling spreads to OHCs in apical turn at P28. Representative phalloidin-labeled, prestin-labeled and merged confocal images of cochlear surface preparations from the apical, middle and basal turn of normal P15 rats **(A–J)** and P28 rats **(K–S)**. **(I,R)** Note strong prestin immunolabeling in OHCs at P15 and P28, but absence of prestin labeling in inner hair cells IHCs.

turn at P15 (**Figures 2A–J**) and to OHCs in the apical turn at P28 (**Figures 2K–S**) consistent with previous reports related to the spatiotemporal developmentally upregulated expression of prestin in OHCs in rats and other rodents (Belyantseva et al., 2000; Jensen-Smith and Hallworth, 2007).

DPOAE Deficits Greater When HPβCD Administered at P15 Than P5

The exquisite sensitivity and frequency selectivity of the auditory system is dependent on the nonlinear, electromotile properties of OHCs, which contribute to the generation of distortion products that can be detected in the ear canal using DPOAEs (Brownell, 1990; Liberman et al., 2002). Thus, DPOAEs provide a non-invasive method for assessing OHC function. DPOAEs were evaluated 8-weeks after P5, P10, and P15 rats were treated with 4,000 mg/kg of HPβCD or in P5 rats treated with saline. To aid in the interpretation of the results, the mean (n = 10) DPOAE input/output functions of the Control group are presented with their 95% confidence intervals and compared to the mean (n = 6/group, +/−SEM) input/output functions obtained from the groups treated with HPβCD at P5, P10, or P15 HPβCD (**Figure 3**). The DPOAEs in the group treated with HPβCD at P15 were largely abolished at frequencies from 8 to 45 kHz and greatly reduced at 4 kHz. In contrast, the groups treated with HPβCD at P5 and P10 had DPOAE input/output functions at 4, 8, and 16 kHz that were completely normal (**Figures 3A–C**). The P5 DPOAE input/output function at 24 kHz was within normal limits whereas P10 DPOAE amplitudes were slightly below normal at high intensities (**Figure 3D**). P5 and P10 DPOAE amplitudes at 30 kHz were far below normal; however, the deficits were consistently less for P5 than P10 (**Figure 3E**). P5 and P10 DPOAE amplitudes were barely detectable except at L2 intensities greater than 60 dB SPL. Thus, HPβCD almost completely eliminated DPOAEs in the P15 group whereas in the P5 and P10 groups it only reduced DPOAE amplitudes at the high, but not the low frequencies.

CAP Deficits Greater When HPβCD Administered at P15 Than P5

Type I auditory nerve fibers make one to one synaptic contact with IHCs. Tone burst-evoked activation of IHCs results in the sudden release of neurotransmitter from the base of the IHC onto afferent terminals resulting in synchronous neural discharges that generate the CAP (Bourien et al., 2014). The CAP, which reflects the neural output of the cochlea relayed from the IHCs, was measured 8-weeks after the P5, P10, and P15 rats had been treated with 4,000 mg/kg of HPβCD and compared to measurements from rats in the saline Control. The CAP waveforms elicited by 80 dB SPL tone bursts presented at 8 kHz are shown in **Figure 4A**; results are presented for a representative rat in the saline Control group and rats treated with HPβCD at P5, P10, or P15. The CAP measurement were obtained 8-weeks post-treatment. Large N1 and N2 responses were present in the Control, P5 and P10 rats, whereas N1 and N2 response were absent in the P15 rat. To visualize the age-dependent effects of the HPβCD treatment, the mean (n = 8) CAP input/output functions of the Control group are presented with their 95% confidence intervals and the results compared to the mean (n = 6/group, +/−SEM) CAP input/output functions measured 8-weeks after the P5, P10, and P15 groups had been treated with 4,000 mg/kg HPβCD (**Figures 4B–G**). CAP

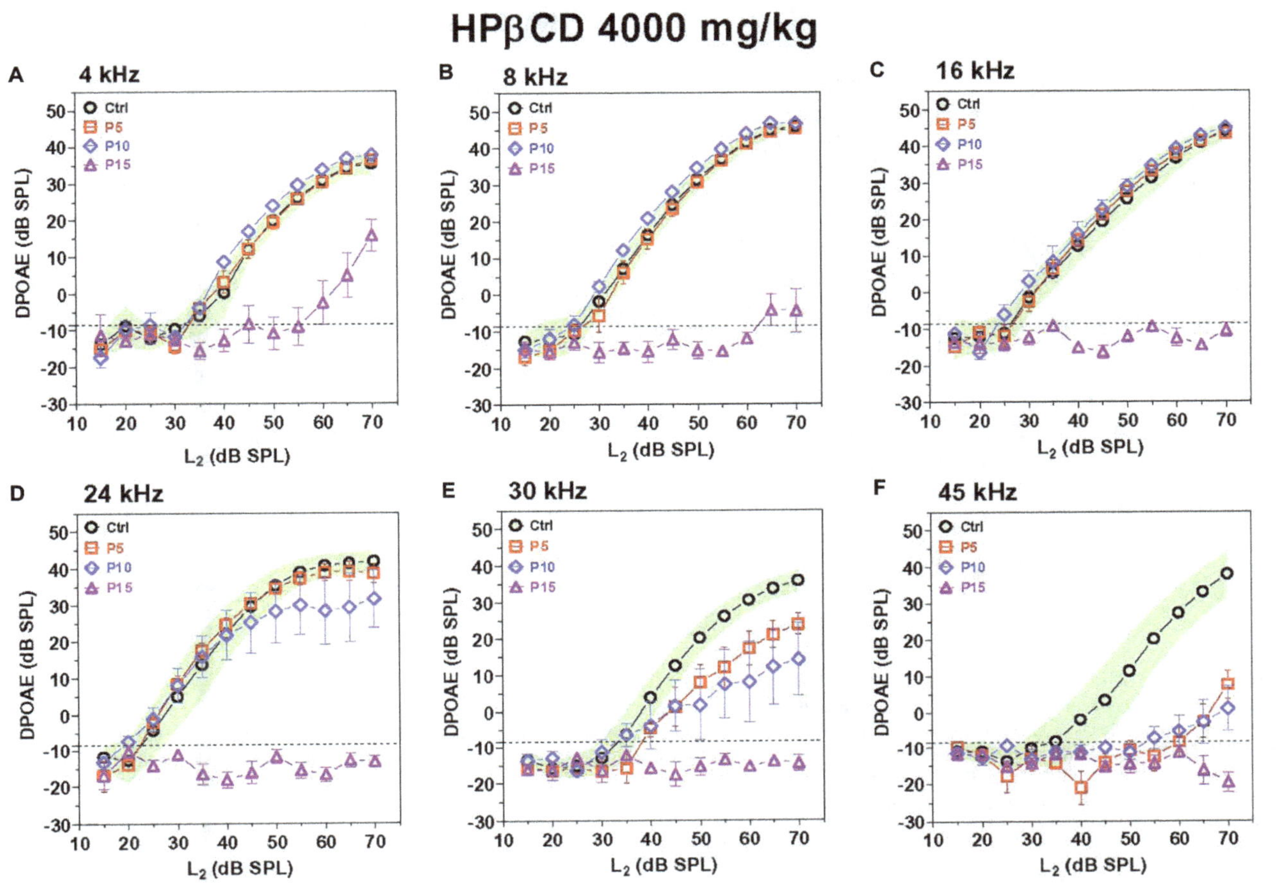

FIGURE 3 | DPOAE deficits are more severe in adulthood if HPβCD is administered to postnatal rats at P15 than P5 or P10. Mean DPOAE input/output functions measured in the adult Control group (*n* = 10, +/-95% confidence interval) compared to mean (+/–SEM, *n* = 6/group) DPOAE input/output functions measured in adults 8-weeks after the rats were treated with 4,000 mg/kg HPβCD at P5, P10 or P15. Data shown for **(A)** 4 kHz, **(B)** 8 kHz, **(C)** 16 kHz, **(D)** 24 kHz, **(E)** 30 kHz and **(F)** 45 kHz.

responses in the P15 group were largely abolished from 8 to 45 kHz; the CAP was present at 4 kHz, but the amplitude was greatly reduced (**Figure 4B**). In contrast, CAP responses in the P5 and P10 group were similar to the Control group from 4 to 24 kHz (**Figures 4B–E**), slightly reduced at 30 kHz (**Figure 4F**) and greatly reduced at 45 kHz compared to the Control group (**Figure 4G**). The deficits at 45 kHz were slightly greater at P10 than at P5 (**Figure 4G**). HPβCD was thus much more ototoxic when administered at P15 than P5 or P10 and the ototoxic effects were more severe at the high frequencies.

Cochlear Lesions Greater When HPβCD Administered at P28 Than P10 or P15

To determine if the cochlear histopathologies from HPβCD treatment were age-dependent, mean cochleograms ($n = 6$/group, +/-SEM) were prepared 8-weeks after the P5, P10, P15, and P28 rats had been treated with 4,000 mg/kg of HPβCD. The smallest cochlear pathologies occurred in the group treated with HPβCD at P5 (**Figure 5A**). The OHC losses in this group decreased from 100% at the base to less than 10% approximately 70% distance from the apex (DFA). Small (<25%) IHC and PC losses were present 90–100% DFA. The OHC losses in the P10 group were similar to those seen in the P5 group (**Figure 5B**), but the IHC and PC losses in the P10 group, which were more severe than at P5, approached 90% at the most basal location. The cochlear lesions were much more extensive and severe in the P15 group (**Figure 5C**). All of the OHCs were missing over the basal half of the cochlea followed by a decrease in OHC loss to less than 10% loss ~30% DFA. All of the IHCs and PCs were missing over the basal two-thirds of the cochlea; the loss decreased to less than 10% approximately 45% DFA. There was a further apical expansion of the lesion in the group treated with HPβCD at P28 (**Figure 5D**). The OHC lesion decreased from 100% over the basal two-thirds of the cochlea to ~30% at the extreme apex. Unlike the P15 group, the IHC and PC lesions in the P28 group hovered around 80% over the basal two-thirds of the cochlea followed by a gradual decline to less than 10% IHC and PC loss in the extreme apex. Thus, the OHC lesion was confined to the base of the cochlea when HPβCD was administered at P5 or P10 and the OHC lesion was only slightly greater at P10 than P5. The OHC lesion rapidly expanded toward the apex when the drug was

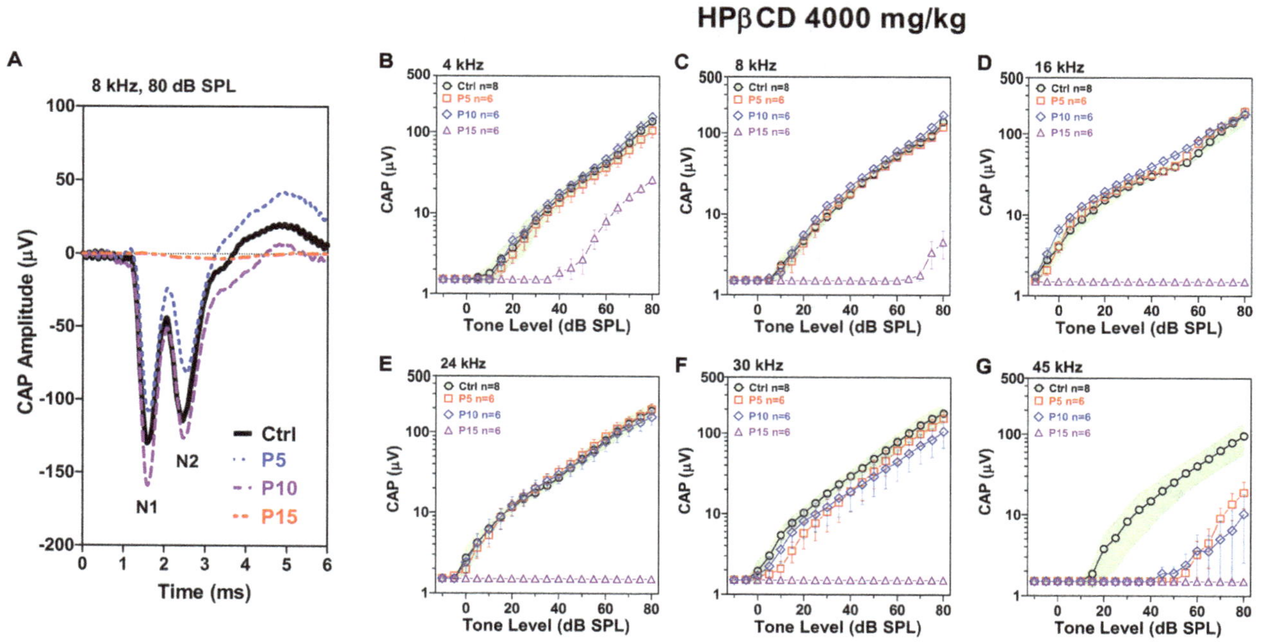

FIGURE 4 | Adult CAP deficits are more severe when HPβCD is administered to postnatal rats at P15 than P5 or P10. **(A)** Representative CAP waveforms elicited by 8 kHz tone bursts presented at 80 dB SPL. Note large reduction in CAP amplitude in adult rats when HBβCD was administered at P15 and nearly normal response when the drug was administered at P5 or P10. Mean (n = 8, +/-95% confidence interval) CAP input/output functions at **(B)** 4 kHz, **(C)** 8 kHz, **(D)** 16 kHz, **(E)** 24 kHz, **(F)** 30 kHz and **(G)** 45 kHz in Control rats compared to mean (+/–SEM, n = 6/group) input/output functions obtained 8-weeks after the rats were treated with 4000 mg/kg HPβCD at P5, P10 or P15. CAP amplitudes in the P5 and P10 group were much larger than those in the P15 group. At 45 kHz, CAP amplitudes in the P5 and P10 group were much smaller than in the Control group.

administered from P15 to P28 (**Figure 5E**), a pattern consistent with the developmental upregulation of prestin expression in rat OHCs (Belyantseva et al., 2000). HPβCD also caused extensive damage to IHCs and PCs, but the damage was restricted to cochlear locations where the drug also caused at least 30% or more OHC loss. IHC and PC damage was never observed at cochlear locations where nearly all the OHCs were present. The IHC lesion also rapidly expanded toward the apex when HPβCD was administered at P15 or P28 (**Figure 5F**).

Delayed Onset Between OHC Loss and IHC and PC Degeneration

2-Hyroxypropyl-beta-cyclodextrin was originally believed to only damage prestin-bearing OHCs (Crumling et al., 2012; Cronin et al., 2015; Takahashi et al., 2016). However, more recent work indicates that HPβCD also leads to the delayed destruction of IHCs and PCs (Liu et al., 2020). To determine when the IHCs and PCs degenerated, we treated adult rats with 4,000 mg/kg of HPβCD or saline and evaluated their cochleae from 1- to 8-weeks post-treatment. The mean cochleogram (n = 6) from the saline Control group showed no loss of OHCs, IHCs, or PCs 8-weeks post-treatment (**Figure 6A**) whereas massive OHC loss was evident over most of the cochlea 1-week after HPβCD treatment (**Figure 6B**). The magnitude and extent of the OHC lesion was roughly the same at 4-, 6-, and 8-weeks post-treatment (**Figures 6C–E**). There was little evidence of IHC or PC loss 1-week after HPβCD treatment. After 4-weeks, a mild IHC/PC lesion emerged near the base of the cochlea, but at 6-weeks post-treatment the IHC/PC lesion underwent a massive expansion to match the large OHC pathology (**Figure 6D**). A large IHC/PC lesion that followed the general contour of the OHC pathology was also present 8-weeks post-treatment. To illustrate the delayed, but rapid expansion of IHC lesion between 4- and 6-weeks, **Figure 6F** compares the mean IHC lesion at 1-, 4-, 6-, and 8-week(s) post-treatment. The massive IHC/PC lesions present at 6- and 8-weeks post-treatment were associated with a flattened sensory epithelium composed of large cuboidal cells (**Figures 7C,D**) that had replaced the highly stereotyped network of sensory cells and support cells that comprise the partially damaged (**Figure 7B**) or normal organ of Corti (**Figure 7A**).

Delayed Nerve Fiber and Spiral Ganglion Degeneration

Massive loss of hair cells and support cells often leads to the degeneration of nerve fibers that innervate the cochlea (McFadden et al., 2004). To determine if and when the nerve fibers were degenerating after administering 4,000 mg/kg of HPβCD, we counted the number of nerve fibers in the habenula perforata in the basal turn of the cochlea 1-, 4-, 6-, and 8-week(s) after treatment with 4,000 mg/kg of HPβCD. The habenula perforatae were densely packed with nerve fibers in the Control cochlea (**Figure 8A**) and there was only a slight hint of a reduction in fiber density at 1- and 4-weeks post-treatment

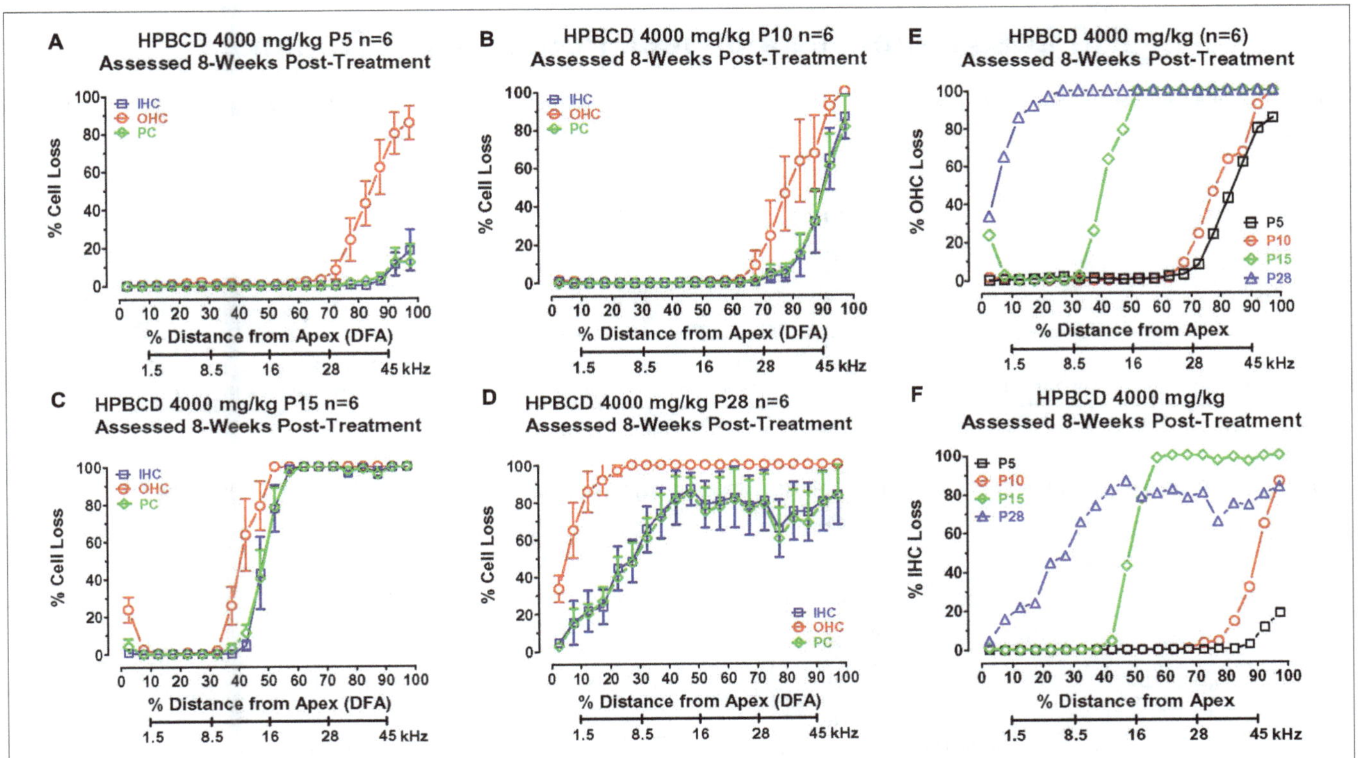

FIGURE 5 | Mean (+/−SEM, *n* = 6) cochleograms showing percent missing outer hair cells (OHCs), inner hair cells (IHCs), and pillar cells (PCs) plotted as function of percent distance from the apex (DFA). Frequency-place map of rat cochlea below abscissa (Müller, 1991). Data obtained 8-weeks after **(A)** P5, **(B)** P10, **(C)** P15, and **(D)** P28 rats were treated with 4,000 mg/kg of HPβCD. Large OHC lesion present 70–100% DFA at P5 and P10 **(A,B)**. OHC lesion spreads toward the apex from P15 **(C)** to P28 **(D)**. Minimal IHC and PC losses in base of cochlea at P5 **(A)**. IHC and PC losses increase dramatically and spread from the base toward the apex of the cochlea from P10 to P28. Comparison of mean (*n* = 6/group) **(E)** OHC loss and **(F)** IHC loss when HPβCD administered at P5, P10, P15 or P28. Note rapid expansion of OHC and IHC losses from P5 to P28.

(**Figures 8B,C**); however, there was a massive reduction in fiber density in the habenula perforatae at 6- and 8-weeks post-treatment (**Figures 8D,E**). The mean (n = 6/group, +SEM) number of nerve fibers per habenula perforata was approximately 116 (n = 6 rats) in the saline Control group (**Figure 8F**). The mean (n = 6 rats/group) numbers of nerve fibers decreased to 106, 99, 28, and 5, respectively when rats were evaluated at 1-week or 4-, 6-, or 8-week(s) after treatment with 4,000 mg/kg HPβCD. The numbers of nerve fibers in the 6- and 8-weeks groups were significantly less than those in the Control group [one-way analysis of variance (F (4, 25) = 62.47, $p < 0.0001$, Tukey's multiple comparison, $p < 0.05$].

The nerve fiber loss in the habenula perforatae was accompanied by a corresponding loss of SGNs. Rosenthal's canal in the middle of the basal turn of the cochlea was packed with SGNs in the saline Control group together with IHCs and OHCs in the organ of Corti adjacent to the spiral limbus (SL) (**Figure 9A**). The OHCs were missing 1-week after treatment with 4,000 mg/kg of HPβCD, but numerous SGNs were still present in Rosenthal's canal (**Figure 9B**). The modest reduction of SGNs in Rosenthal's canal at 4-weeks post-treatment was followed by a massive loss at 6-weeks post-treatment (**Figure 9D**) and a nearly complete loss at 8-weeks post-treatment (**Figure 9E**). Despite the massive loss of hair cells, SGNs and collapse of the organ of Corti, the SL appeared relatively normal (**Figure 9D**). The loss of SGNs was quantified in the different groups in the middle of the basal turn. The mean (n = 6, +SEM) number of SGNs per Rosenthal's canal was approximately 49 in both the saline Control group and the group evaluated 1-week after treatment with 4,000 mg/kg HPβCD (**Figure 9F**). The mean (n = 6 rats/group, +SEM) number decreased slightly to 43 at 4-weeks post-treatment followed by a dramatic reduction to 14 at 6-weeks and nearly a complete loss of SGNs at 8-weeks post-treatment. The numbers of SGNs in the 6- and 8-weeks groups were significantly less than in the Control group (one-way analysis of variance (F (4, 25) = 179.9, $p < 0.0001$, Tukey's multiple comparison, $p < 0.05$).

DISCUSSION

Prestin Upregulation Determines Spread of High-Frequency Auditory Impairment

2-Hyroxypropyl-beta-cyclodextrin-induced hearing loss is associated with the rapid destruction of OHCs (Crumling et al., 2012, 2017; Cronin et al., 2015; Ding et al., 2020, 2021). This rapid destruction of OHCs can be tracked non-invasively by

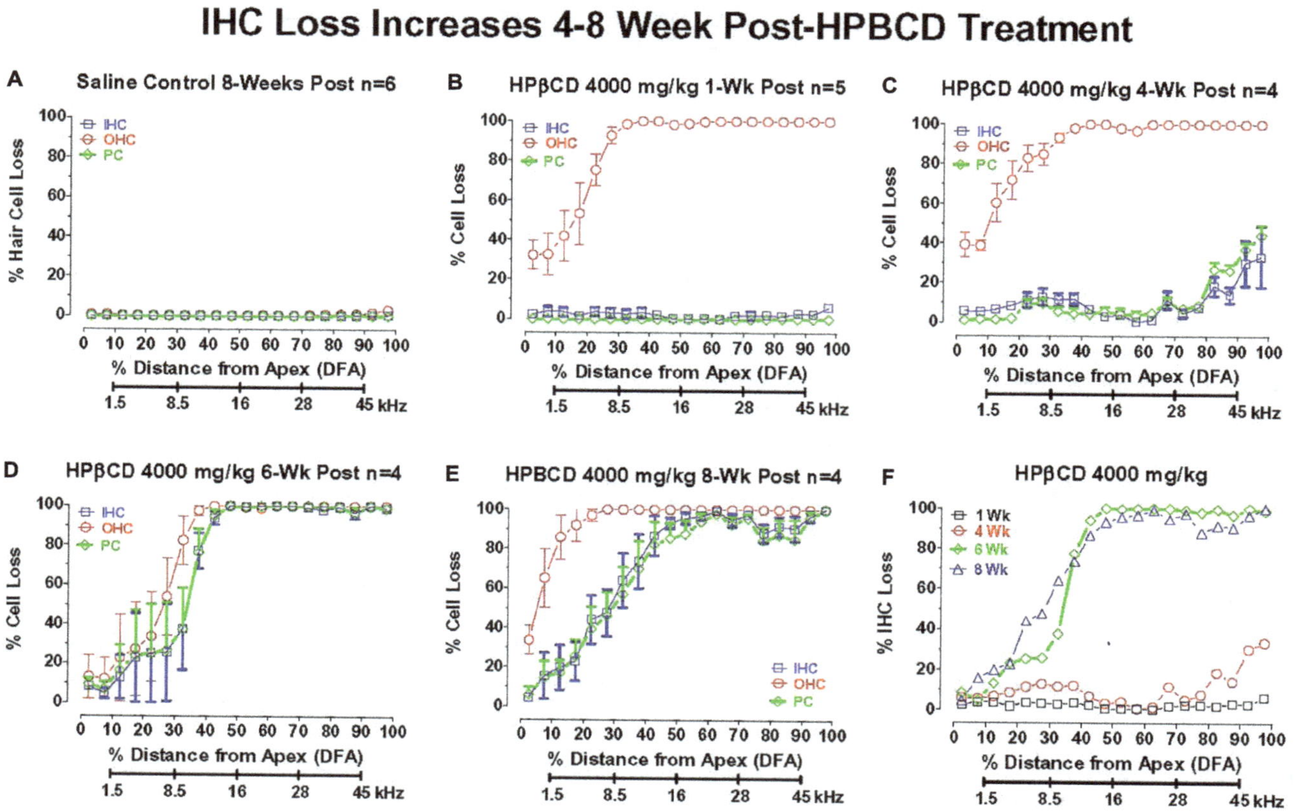

FIGURE 6 | Inner hair cell (IHC) and pillar cell (PC) losses dramatically increase in adult rats 4–8 week after 4,000 mg/kg HPβCD treatment. Mean (+/–SEM) cochleograms showing percent missing OHCs, IHCs and pillar cells (PC) plotted as function of percent distance from the apex (DFA) in adult rats. Rat cochlear frequency-place map shown below abscissa (Müller, 1991). **(A)** Mean (*n* = 6) data from saline Control group 8-weeks post-treatment (*n* = 6). Mean cochleograms obtained from adult rats treated with 4,000 mg/kg HPβCD and evaluated **(B)** 1-week post-treatment (*n* = 5), **(C)** 4-weeks post-treatment (*n* = 4) **(D)** 6-weeks post-treatment (*n* = 4), and **(E)** 8-weeks post-treatment (*n* = 4). Massive OHC loss 1-week after 4,000 mg/kg treatment, but no IHC and PC loss **(B)**, but massive IHC and PC loss occurs 6- to 8-weeks post-treatment **(D,E)**. **(F)** Mean cochleogram showing percent IHC loss as a function of percent distance from the apex (DFA) of the cochlea; cochlear frequency-place map shown on the abscissa. Note large increase in IHC loss between 4- and 6-weeks post-treatment.

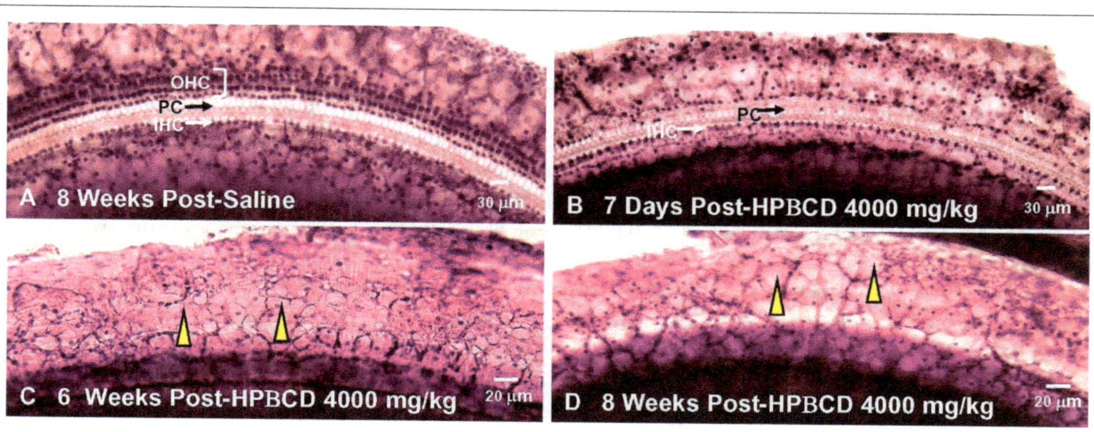

FIGURE 7 | Massive inner hair cell (IHC) and pillar cells(PC) loss occurs 6–8 weeks after treatment with 4,000 mg/kg HPβCD. Representative photomicrographs of hematoxylin and eosin stained cochlear surface preparation from middle of the basal turn (60–80% distance from apex) of the cochlea. Representative photomicrograph shown for **(A)** 8-weeks after saline treatment and **(B)** 1-week, **(C)** 6-weeks, and **(D)** 8-weeks after treatment with 4,000 mg/kg of HPβCD. **(A)** Three orderly rows of outer hair cells (OHC), single row of inner hair cells (IHC) and pillar cells present in saline controls. **(B)** IHCs and PCs present, but most OHCs missing 1-week after treatment with 4,000 mg/kg HPβCD. **(C,D)** Massive OHC, IHC and PC loss results in flattened sensory epithelium that is replaced by many large, cuboidal cells (yellow arrowhead).

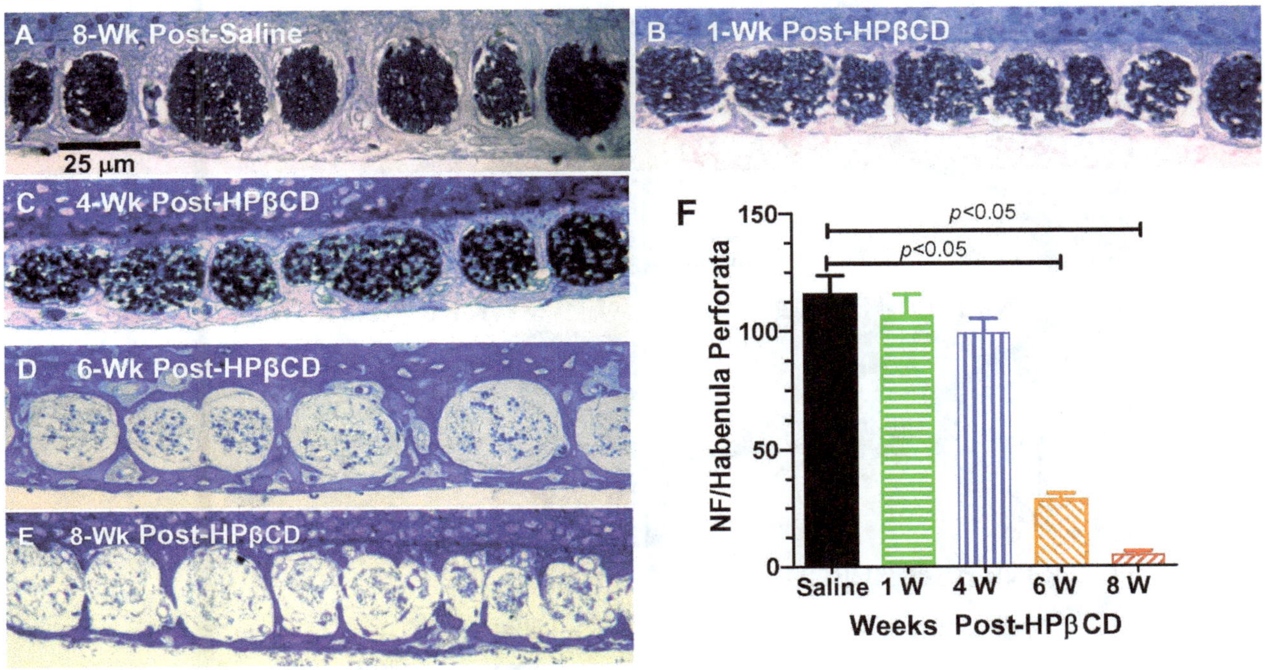

FIGURE 8 | Massive loss of nerve fibers occurs in habenula perforata 6- to 8-weeks following 4,000 mg/kg treatment with HPβCD. Representative photomicrograph of methylene blue-stained 4 micron sections taken tangent to the habenula perforata in the middle of the basal turn from an adult rat in the **(A)** saline Control group 8-weeks post-treatment and from adult rats treated with 4,000 mg/kg HPβCD and evaluated **(B)** 1-week, **(C)** 4-weeks, **(D–E)** 6- and 8-weeks post-treatment. Nerve fibers densely packed in habenula perforata of **(A)** saline control; nerve fiber packing density slightly reduced at 1- and 4-week post-treatment followed by a massive reduction in nerve fiber density 6- and 8-weeks post-treatment **(C,D)**. **(F)** Mean numbers (+SEM, n = rats/group) of nerve fibers per habenula perforata in saline Control group and groups treated with 4,000 mg/kg HPβCD and evaluated 1-, 4-, 6- or 8-weeks post-treatment.

serially measuring DPOAEs. In adult rats, the 4,000 mg/kg dose of HPβCD completely eliminated the DPOAE 2-days post-treatment (Liu et al., 2020). Although several mechanisms have been suggested (Crumling et al., 2017), selective cyclodextrin ototoxicity is believed to be correlated with prestin expression in OHCs because knockout mice missing this protein are more resistant to cyclodextrin damage than wild type mice (Takahashi et al., 2016) or mutant mice with a non-electromotile form of prestin (Zhou et al., 2018).

In order to investigate the developmental upregulation of prestin in OHCs from base to apex, we employed a high 4,000 mg/kg dose of HPβCD that would destroy OHCs over the entire length of the rat cochlea (Liu et al., 2020). The functional deficits observed in our postnatal rats treated with HPβCD were closely correlated with the temporal and spatial upregulation of prestin in OHCs indicating that prestin, or some other unknown factor associated with its expression, is critically important for initiating cyclodextrin-induced OHC loss. If HPβCD was administered to rats at P5 or P10, when prestin was absent from OHCs in the apical and middle turn, then low- and mid-frequency DPOAEs and CAPs measured 8-weeks post-treatment were normal, i.e., the absence of prestin in OHCs when HPβCD was administered prevented cyclodextrin ototoxicity at the low- and mid-frequencies. Prestin was already present in basal turn OHCs at P5 and P10 and when rats were treated with HPβCD at these ages, high-frequency DPOAEs and CAPs measured 8-weeks post-treatment were greatly depressed. When HPβCD was administered to rats at P15, when prestin was also expressed in middle-turn OHCs, then mid-frequency DPOAEs and CAPs measured 8-weeks post-treatment were also depressed. Thus, the developmental spatiotemporal upregulation of prestin in OHCs determined when the OHC loss and cochlear hearing loss spread from high to low frequencies.

The postnatal time at which HPβCD was administered together with the spatiotemporal expression of prestin determined the location and breadth of the HPβCD-induced OHC lesion (**Figure 5F**). The OHC lesion was confined to the high-frequency, basal third of the cochlea when HPβCD was administered at P5 or P10, consistent with the presence of prestin in the base of the cochlea. However, the OHC lesion expanded to cover the basal two-thirds of the cochlea when cyclodextrin was administered at P15, at which time prestin expression had expanded from the base to the middle turn of the cochlea. Importantly, prestin was expressed in the apical turn, as well as middle and basal turns, at P28. Only then did the OHC lesions appear in the most apical region of the cochlea. Thus, the expansion of the OHC lesion toward the apex of the cochlea was closely correlated with the developmental base to apex upregulation of prestin, which finally appeared in the cochlear apex at P28. Our apical turn results might account for the lack of OHC loss in the apex of the cochlea of WT mice treated with 8000 mg/kg of HPβCD on P21 (Takahashi et al., 2016). The

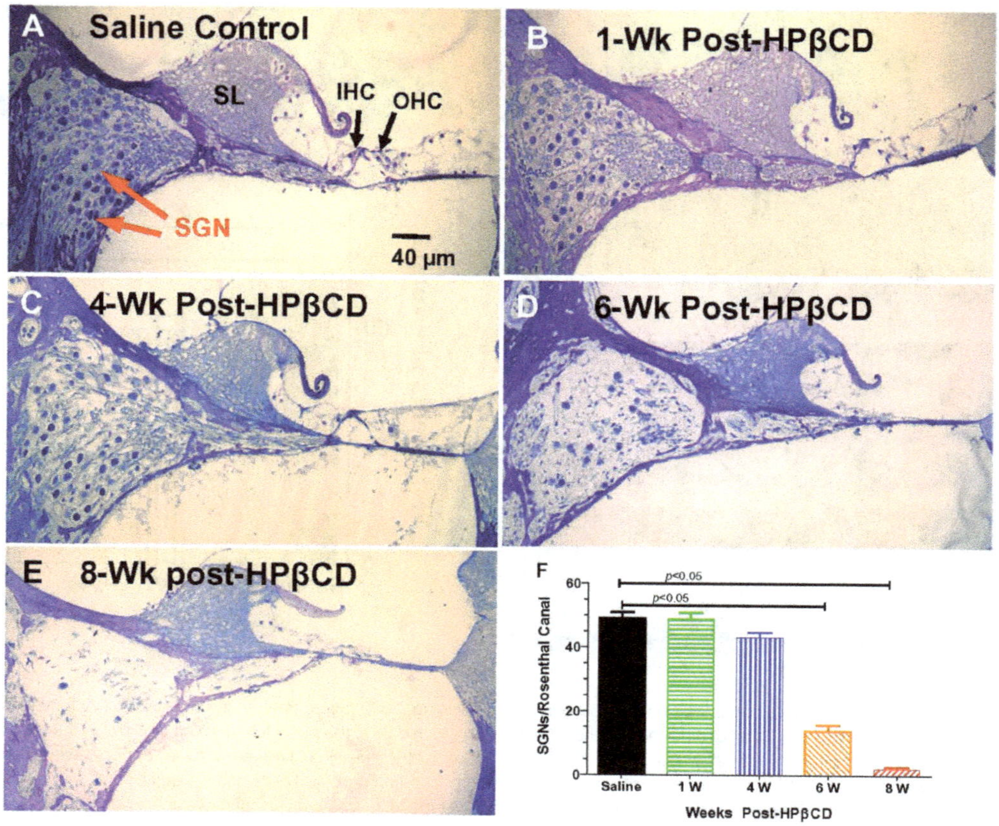

FIGURE 9 | Massive loss of spiral ganglion neurons (SGN) in Rosenthal's canal 6- to 8-weeks following 4,000 mg/kg treatment with HPβCD. Thin sections (4 μm) through the modiolus in the middle of the basal turn of the cochlea. **(A)** Saline control showing inner hair cell (IHC), outer hair cells (OHC), and spiral limbus (SL). Rosenthal's canal filled with SGNs. **(B–E)** Sections from adult rats treated with 4,000 mg/kg of HPβCD and evaluated 1-, 4-, 6- and 8-weeks post-treatment: Numbers of SGNs in Rosenthal's canal **(B)** normal at 1-week post-treatment, **(C)** slightly reduced at 4-weeks post-treatment and greatly reduced at **(D)** 6-weeks and **(E)** 8-weeks post-treatment. **(F)** Mean (*n* = 6, +SEM) numbers of SGNs in Rosenthal's canal in the saline Control group versus the groups treated with 4,000 mg/kg HPβCD and evaluated 1-, 4-, 6- and 8-weeks post-treatment. Numbers of SGNs in HPβCD-treated groups evaluated at 6- and 8-weeks post-treatment were significantly less than in the saline Control group.

absence of OHC damage in the apex of the WT mouse cochlea is most likely due to the fact that prestin was expressed at such a low level on P21 that HPβCD was unable to damage OHCs in the most apical portion of the cochlea.

Mechanisms of HPβCD OHC Damage

Several different mechanisms could contribute to the cyclodextrin-induced OHC death (Crumling et al., 2012, 2017), but interactions between cholesterol and prestin have garnered the most attention. Prestin is expressed in the lateral wall of mature OHCs and has also been reported in the cytoplasm of vestibular hair cells although its cytoplasmic expression has not been independently verified (Belyantseva et al., 2000; Adler et al., 2003). Systemic administration of cyclodextrin, however, does not damage adult vestibular hair cells (Ding et al., 2020, 2021), nor does it damage postnatal OHCs lacking prestin. Prestin is heavily expressed along the OHC lateral wall, adjacent to the actin-spectrin cortical lattice and subsurface cisternae (Jensen-Smith and Hallworth, 2007; Legendre et al., 2008). Prestin appears to interact with cholesterol (Takahashi et al., 2016) and experimental manipulations of cholesterol affect OHC stiffness, electromotility, the lateral mobility of prestin in the membrane and prestin function (Nguyen and Brownell, 1998; Rajagopalan et al., 2007; Kamar et al., 2012). Imaging studies have revealed high levels of cholesterol staining at the apical and basal poles of normal OHCs. In contrast, low-levels of cholesterol are present along the lateral wall of OHCs in WT mice whereas cholesterol labeling is more abundant in the lateral wall of prestin knockout mice (Nguyen and Brownell, 1998; Rajagopalan et al., 2007; Brownell et al., 2011; Takahashi et al., 2016). Treatment of isolated OHCs with cyclodextrin often leads to rapid cell death associated with rupture of the cell's membrane. In contrast, OHCs in prestin knockout mice are largely resistant to cyclodextrin (Rajagopalan et al., 2007; Takahashi et al., 2016). In cochlear organotypic cultures, HPβCD-induced OHC death was initiated by the extrinsic caspase-8 apoptotic pathway that is triggered by ligands that bind to death receptors on the cell's membrane (Salvesen, 2002; Cheng et al., 2005; Ding et al., 2020). Because of the low-abundance of cholesterol in the lateral wall of normal OHCs, further cyclodextrin-induced depletion of cholesterol from this region likely leads to the breakdown of the plasma membrane in the lateral wall of OHCs leading to rapid onset of caspase-8 mediated cell death (Garofalo et al., 2003; Schonfelder et al., 2006). Caspase-8 inhibitors could be used to test this hypothesis (Wang et al., 2004; Bozzo et al., 2006).

Time Course of IHC, PC, and SGN Degeneration

Much of the previous literature on HPβCD ototoxicity in mice has focused on its early, selective destruction of OHCs with little evidence of damage to IHCs, ANFs, or SGNs (Crumling et al., 2012, 2017; Takahashi et al., 2016; Zhou et al., 2018). However, recent studies from our lab have revealed that HPβCD unexpectedly causes massive, delayed degeneration of rat IHCs, PCs, ANFs, SGNs, and much of the organ of Corti (Ding et al., 2020; Liu et al., 2020). The abrupt onset of this massive secondary loss of IHCs, ANFs, and SGNs differs from the progressive loss of SGNs seen after most other ototoxic drug insults or traumatic noise exposures (Koitchev et al., 1982; Bichler et al., 1983; Yagi et al., 2000; Lin et al., 2011). The abrupt onset of this second wave of degeneration may have been missed in previous mouse studies because the bulk of the damage occurred well beyond the time period when degeneration of OHCs and IHCs typically occurs. From our previous studies, it was unclear exactly when the IHC, ANF, and SGN damage occurred. Our results indicate that this secondary degenerative process occurs suddenly, starting in the base of the cochlea 4-weeks post-treatment and expanding to virtually all of the cochlea by 8-weeks post-treatment (**Figures 5, 8, 9**). The sudden increase in these IHC, ANF and SGN pathologies occurred between 4- and 6-weeks post-treatment. We are unaware of any ototoxicity studies showing an abrupt, massive upsurge of IHC, ANF and SGN damage more than a month after the initial damage to OHCs occurs. In some cases nearly 100% of the IHCs and PCs were missing in regions with complete OHC loss (**Figure 6**), but in other cases only ~80% had degenerated (**Figure 5**). Additional studies are needed to determine if all the IHCs, support cells and SGNs eventually degenerate with longer survival times or if the degenerative processes are essentially complete by 8-weeks post-treatment. Although high doses of HPβCD are highly ototoxic, studies have shown that very little of the drug actually crosses the blood-brain barrier when it is administered systemically (Ramirez et al., 2011 Pontikis et al., 2013; Vecsernyes et al., 2014). Therefore, the levels of HPβCD in the cochlea would be expected to be low unless the blood-labyrinth barrier was uniquely permeable to HPβCD or if the drug disrupted the blood-labyrinth barrier. Systemically administered HPβCD is rapidly cleared from the body within a few hours; however, its effects on cholesterol synthesis may be long lasting (Aqul et al., 2011) raising the possibility of more prolonged degenerative effects.

2-Hyroxypropyl-beta-cyclodextrin-induced OHC degeneration occurs rapidly within hours after intracerebral administration and within 1 day after subcutaneous dosing (Crumling et al., 2017). The acute damage to OHCs has been repeatedly observed (**Figure 6**; Crumling et al., 2012; Cronin et al., 2015; Takahashi et al., 2016; Ding et al., 2020). In contrast, the onset of IHC, PC, ANF and SGN degeneration did not begin until 4-weeks post-treatment, but during the following two weeks there was a large increase in the magnitude and apical expansion of the lesion (**Figures 6F**, **8F**, **9F**; Liu et al., 2020; Ding et al., 2021). The PC losses were highly correlated with the IHC lesions suggesting that the survival of these two structures depended on some common factor such as loss of neurotrophic support (Mueller et al., 2002; Pickles and Chir, 2002; Fritzsch et al., 2004). Reintroducing one or more neurotrophic factors into the cochlea at specific times following HPβCD treatment could aid in identification of specific neurotrophic factors that enhance the survival of IHCs, PCs, ANFs or SGNs (Atkinson et al., 2012; Chen et al., 2018;

A P5 HPBCD: Damage Early or Late

Cochear Location	Apex	Middle	Base
Prestin			X
Frequency	Low <20 kHz	Mid 20-40 kHz	High >40 kHz
OHC Loss			Early
DPOAE Loss			Early
CAP Loss			Early
IHC/ANF/SGN Loss			Late
CAP Loss			Late

B P10 HPBCD: Damage Early or Late

Cochear Location	Apex	Middle	Base
Prestin		X	X
Frequency	Low <20 kHz	Mid 20-40 kHz	High >40 kHz
OHC Loss		Early	Early
DPOAE Loss		Early	Early
CAP Loss		Early	Early
IHC/ANF/SGN Loss		Late	Late
CAP Loss		Late	Late

C P15 HPBCD: Damage Early or Late

Cochear Location	Apex	Middle	Base
Prestin	X	X	X
Frequency	Low <20 kHz	Mid 20-40 kHz	High >40 kHz
OHC Loss	Early	Early	Early
DPOAE Loss	Early	Early	Early
CAP Loss	Early	Early	Early
IHC/ANF/SGN Loss	Late	Late	Late
CAP Loss	Late	Late	Late

FIGURE 10 | Schematics in panels **(A–C)** showing the approximate location of prestin in outer hair cells (OHCs) in the base, middle, and apex of the cochlea on postnatal day 5, 10, and 15 (P5, P10, and P15) when HPβCD was administered. Each panel shows the approximate cochlear location and frequency of the loss and/or damage to OHCs, distortion product otoacoustic emissions (DPOAEs), the compound action potential (CAP), inner hair cells (IHCs), auditory nerve fibers (ANFs), and spiral ganglion neurons (SGNs) approximately 1-week (Early phase) and approximately 8-weeks (Late phase) after HPβCD treatment. The least damage/loss occurs when HPβCD is administered at P5 when prestin is mainly expressed in the base of the cochlea. The greatest damage/loss occurs when HPβCD is administered at P15 when prestin is expressed over most of the cochlea. CAP loss is observed in the early phase because the OHC and DPOAE losses affect the input to the IHCs. CAP losses are exacerbated during the late phase because of the additional loss of IHCs, ANFs and SGNs.

Leake et al., 2019; Ma et al., 2019). Cholesterol depletion is known to disrupt intercellular communication and tight junctions and lead to anoikis-like cell death (Lambert et al., 2007; Park et al., 2009; Zhang et al., 2018), disruption of the reticular lamina and/or dedifferentiation of the organ of Corti (Favre and Sans, 1991; Kiernan et al., 2005; Oesterle and Campbell, 2009; Taylor R. R. et al., 2012). In order to account for the delayed degeneration of these structures, HPβCD would need to induce long-lasting changes in sterol homeostasis.

The early, massive loss of OHCs could lead to chronic cochlear neuroinflammation associated with release of toxic substances from dying cells or the subsequent invasion and/or upregulation of phagocytic cells (macrophages/microglia) (Wood and Zuo, 2017). Chronic macrophage/microglia activation begins around 4-weeks after intense noise exposure (Baizer et al., 2015). The proinflammatory molecules which these immune cells release (Dheen et al., 2007) could contribute to the delayed HPβCD-induced IHC, PC, ANF, and SGN degeneration. This hypothesis could be tested by administering therapeutic compounds that suppress neuroinflammation (Lee et al., 2016; Tillinger et al., 2018). Finally, if the secondary wave of IHC, ANF, and SGN degeneration is caused by an inflammatory storm initiated by the massive degeneration of OHCs, then HPβCD-induced damage to these structures would be expected to be minimal in animals in which the OHCs have been already be eliminated by genetic or other manipulations. However, if this secondary wave of degeneration is due to long term disruption of cholesterol homeostasis, then HPβCD would be expected to cause delayed damage (second wave) to IHCs, ANFs and SGNs in animals with missing OHCs.

Synthesis

Figure 10 is a schematic that attempts to synthesize and integrate the general findings of the current study as well as the results from earlier reports (Ding et al., 2020, 2021; Liu et al., 2020). At P5, prestin is most heavily expressed in the base of the cochlea (**Figure 10A**). When HPβCD is administered at P5, it initially (early phase 1-week post-treatment) destroys only the OHCs in the base of the cochlea eliminating or greatly reducing high frequency DPOAEs. Because of OHC amplification, the input to the IHCs is reduced during the early phase of damage thereby increasing the threshold and reducing the CAP amplitude that is initiated by IHC neurotransmitter release (Dallos and Harris, 1978). Between 4- and 8-weeks after HPβCD treatment, the IHCs, ANFs, and SGNs abruptly die off during the late phase of degeneration; this further exacerbates the CAP loss. If HPβCD is administered at P10 when prestin expression in OHCs expands further toward the middle of the cochlea (**Figure 10B**), the OHC, DPOAE, and CAP losses expand further toward the apex and to lower frequencies during the early phase of damage (1-week post-treatment). During the late phase, the IHCs, ANFs, SGNs suddenly die off and CAP losses are exacerbated. Now the losses include both high- and mid-frequencies. If HPβCD is administered at P15 or later when prestin in OHCs is expressed throughout the cochlea (**Figure 10C**), the OHC, DPOAE, and CAP losses expand toward the apex and lower frequencies during the early phase of damage. During the late phase, the IHCs, ANFs, and SGNs also die off and CAP losses are further exacerbated. Thus, the greatest and most widespread damage from HPβCD occurs after prestin expression has reached adult levels.

Clinical Implications

2-Hyroxypropyl-beta-cyclodextrin ameliorates many of the clinical disorders associated with NPC1 and slows the progression of the disease, but a major side effect is rapid onset sensorineural hearing loss that spreads from high to low frequencies (Ward et al., 2010; Crumling et al., 2012; King et al., 2014; Cronin et al., 2015; Maarup et al., 2015). The initial reports in animals suggested that the HPβCD-induced hearing loss was caused by early damage to the OHCs consistent with the results presented here, but recent results indicate that there is massive, delayed damage to IHCs, ANFs and SGNs that occurs between 4 and 8-weeks post-treatment (**Figures 6**, **8**, **9**; Liu et al., 2020; Ding et al., 2021). This second, delayed wave of degeneration implies that HPβCD ototoxicity is worse than previously believed. The clinical consequences of IHC and SGN degeneration is that it greatly reduces the benefits of hearing aids and cochlear implants for patients receiving HPβCD treatments. Given that the delayed degeneration of IHCs, ANFs, and SGNs occurs over a well-defined 4- to 8-week time window following HBβCD treatment, researchers could use this animal model to test out various therapeutic interventions to prevent the secondary degeneration of the remaining IHC, ANFs and SGNs using antioxidants, neurotrophins or a cocktail of the two (Rybak and Whitworth, 2005; Atkinson et al., 2012; Leake et al., 2019; Chen et al., 2020). The optimal time for delivering these therapies would seem to be from approximately 7-days after HPβCD treatment to 8-weeks post-treatment and possibly longer.

ETHICS STATEMENT

The animal study was reviewed and approved by University at Buffalo Institutional Animal Care and Use Committee and carried out in accordance with NIH Guidelines.

AUTHOR CONTRIBUTIONS

DD: conceptualization, investigation, methodology, data curation, formal analysis, visualization, writing, and revision. HJ: investigation, methodology, and data curation. SM: conceptualization, methodology, and revision. XL: methodology and software development. LL: investigation, formal analysis, and visualization. G-DC: conceptualization, investigation, methodology, data curation, formal analysis, visualization, and revision. RS: conceptualization, formal analysis, visualization, writing, revision, project administration, and funding acquisition. All authors contributed to the article and approved the submitted version.

REFERENCES

Adler, H. J., Belyantseva, I. A., Merritt, R. C., Frolenkov, G. I. Jr., Dougherty, G. W., and Kachar, B. (2003). Expression of prestin, a membrane motor protein, in the mammalian auditory and vestibular periphery. *Hear. Res.* 184, 27–40. doi: 10.1016/s0378-5955(03)00192-8

Aqul, A., Liu, B., Ramirez, C. M., Pieper, A. A., Estill, S. J., Burns, D. K., et al. (2011). Unesterified cholesterol accumulation in late endosomes/lysosomes causes neurodegeneration and is prevented by driving cholesterol export from this compartment. *J. Neurosci.* 31, 9404–9413. doi: 10.1523/jneurosci.1317-11.2011

Atkinson, P. J., Wise, A. K. Flynn, B. O., Nayagam, B. A., Hume, C. R., O'Leary, S. J., et al. (2012). Neurotrophin gene therapy for sustained neural preservation after deafness. *PLoS One* 7:e52338. doi: 10.1371/journal.pone.0052338

Baizer, J. S., Wong, K. M., Manohar, S., Hayes, S. H., Ding, D., Dingman, R., et al. (2015). Effects of acoustic trauma on the auditory system of the rat: the role of microglia. *Neuroscience* 303, 299–311. doi: 10.1016/j.neuroscience.2015.07.004

Belyantseva, I. A., Adler, H. J., Curi, R., Frolenkov, G. I., and Kachar, B. (2000). Expression and localization of prestin and the sugar transporter GLUT-5 during development of electromotility in cochlear outer hair cells. *J. Neurosci.* 20:RC116.

Bessell, E., Fuller, N. R., Markovic, T. P., Burk, J., Picone, T., Hendy, C., et al. (2019). Effects of alpha-cyclodextrin on cholesterol control and compound K on glycaemic control in people with pre-diabetes: protocol for a phase III randomized controlled trial. *Clin. Obes.* 9:e12324.

Bichler, E., Spoendlin, H., and Rauchegger, H. (1983). Degeneration of cochlear neurons after amikacin intoxication in the rat. *Arch. Otorhinolaryngol.* 237, 201–208. doi: 10.1007/bf00453725

Bourien, J., Tang, Y., Batrel, C., Huet, A., Lenoir, M., Ladrech, S., et al. (2014). Contribution of auditory nerve fibers to compound action potential of the auditory nerve. *J. Neurophysiol.* 112, 1025–1039. doi: 10.1152/jn.00738.2013

Bozzo, C., Sabbatini, M., Tiberio, R., Piffanelli, V., Santoro, C., and Cannas, M. (2006). Activation of caspase-8 triggers anoikis in human neuroblastoma cells. *Neurosci. Res.* 56, 145–153. doi: 10.1016/j.neures.2006.06.008

Brownell, W. E. (1990). Outer hair cell electromotility and otoacoustic emissions. *Ear Hear.* 11, 82–92. doi: 10.1097/00003446-199004000-00003

Brownell, W. E., Jacob, S., Hakizimana, P., Ulfendahl, M., and Fridberger, A. (2011). Membrane cholesterol modulates cochlear electromechanics. *Pflugers Arch.* 461, 677–686. doi: 10.1007/s00424-011-0942-5

Chen, G. D., Daszynski, D. M., Ding, D., Jiang, H., Woolman, T., Blessing, K., et al. (2020). Novel oral multifunctional antioxidant prevents noise-induced hearing loss and hair cell loss. *Hear. Res.* 388:107880. doi: 10.1016/j.heares.2019.107880

Chen, H., Xing, Y., Xia, L., Chen, Z., Yin, S., and Wang, J. (2018). AAV-mediated NT-3 overexpression protects cochleae against noise-induced synaptopathy. *Gene Ther.* 25, 251–259. doi: 10.1038/s41434-018-0012-0

Cheng, A. G., Cunningham, L. L., and Rubel, E. W. (2005). Mechanisms of hair cell death and protection. *Curr. Opin. Otolaryngol. Head Neck Surg.* 13, 343–348. doi: 10.1097/01.moo.0000186799.45377.63

Cho, Y. Y., Kwon, O. H. Park, M. K., Kim, T. W., and Chung, S. (2019). Elevated cellular cholesterol in familial Alzheimer's presenilin 1 mutation is associated with lipid raft localization of beta-amyloid precursor protein. *PLoS One* 14:e0210535. doi: 10.1371/journal.pone.0210535

Coisne, C., Tilloy, S., Monflier, E., Wils, D., Fenart, L., and Gosselet, F. (2016). Cyclodextrins as emerging therapeutic tools in the treatment of cholesterol-associated vascular and neurodegenerative diseases. *Molecules* 21:1748. doi: 10.3390/molecules21121748

Cronin, S., Lin, A., Thompson, K., Hoenerhoff, M., and Duncan, R. K. (2015). Hearing loss and otopathology following systemic and intracerebroventricular delivery of 2-hydroxypropyl-beta-cyclodextrin. *J. Assoc. Res. Otolaryngol.* 16, 599–611. doi: 10.1007/s10162-015-0528-6

Crumling, M. A., King, K. A., and Duncan, R. K. (2017). Cyclodextrins and iatrogenic hearing loss: new drugs with significant risk. *Front. Cell. Neurosci.* 11:355. doi: 10.3389/fncel.2017.00355

Crumling, M. A., Liu, L., Thomas, P. V., Benson, J., Kanicki, A., Kabara, L., et al. (2012). Hearing loss and hair cell death in mice given the cholesterol-chelating agent hydroxypropyl-beta-cyclodextrin. *PLoS One* 7:e53280. doi: 10.1371/journal.pone.0053280

Dallos, P., and Harris, D. (1978). Properties of auditory nerve responses in absence of outer hair cells. *J. Neurophysiol.* 41, 365–383. doi: 10.1152/jn.1978.41.2.365

Davis, M. E., and Brewster, M. E. (2004). Cyclodextrin-based pharmaceutics: past, present and future. *Nat. Rev. Drug Discov.* 3, 1023–1035. doi: 10.1038/nrd1576

Dheen, S. T., Kaur, C., and Ling, E. A. (2007). Microglial activation and its implications in the brain diseases. *Curr. Med. Chem.* 14, 1189–1197. doi: 10.2174/092986707780597961

Dietschy, J. M., and Turley, S. D. (2004). Thematic review series: brain lipids. cholesterol metabolism in the central nervous system during early development and in the mature animal. *J. Lipid Res.* 45, 1375–1397. doi: 10.1194/jlr.r400004-jlr200

Ding, D. L., Wang, J., Salvi, R., Henderson, D., Hu, B. H., McFadden, S. L., et al. (1999). Selective loss of inner hair cells and type-I ganglion neurons in carboplatin-treated chinchillas. Mechanisms of damage and protection. *Ann. N. Y. Acad. Sci.* 884, 152–170. doi: 10.1111/j.1749-6632.1999.tb08640.x

Ding, D., Jiang, H., and Salvi, R. (2021). Cochlear spiral ganglion neuron degeneration following cyclodextrin-induced hearing loss. *Hear. Res.* 400:108125. doi: 10.1016/j.heares.2020.108125

Ding, D., Jiang, H., and Salvi, R. J. (2010). Mechanisms of rapid sensory hair-cell death following co-administration of gentamicin and ethacrynic acid. *Hear. Res.* 259, 16–23. doi: 10.1016/j.heares.2009.08.008

Ding, D., Manohar, S., Jiang, H., and Salvi, R. (2020). Hydroxypropyl-beta-cyclodextrin causes massive damage to the developing auditory and vestibular system. *Hear. Res.* 396:108073. doi: 10.1016/j.heares.2020.108073

Ding, D., Wang, J., Zheng, X.-Y., and Salvi, R. J. (1998). Early damage of spiral ganglion caused by carboplatin in chinchilla. *J. Audiol. Speech Pathol.* 6, 65–67.

Favre, D., and Sans, A. (1991). Dedifferentiation phenomena after denervation of mammalian adult vestibular receptors. *Neuroreport* 2, 501–504. doi: 10.1097/00001756-199109000-00001

Fritzsch, B., Tessarollo, L., Coppola, E., and Reichardt, L. F. (2004). Neurotrophins in the ear: their roles in sensory neuron survival and fiber guidance. *Prog. Brain Res.* 146, 265–278. doi: 10.1016/s0079-6123(03)46017-2

Fu, Y., Ding, D., Jiang, H., and Salvi, R. (2012). Ouabain-induced cochlear degeneration in rat. *Neurotox. Res.* 22, 158–169. doi: 10.1007/s12640-012-9320-0

Garofalo, T., Misasi, R., Mattei, V., Giammarioli, A. M., Malorni, W., Pontieri, G. M., et al. (2003). Association of the death-inducing signaling complex with microdomains after triggering through CD95/Fas. Evidence for caspase-8-ganglioside interaction in T cells. *J. Biol. Chem.* 278, 8309–8315. doi: 10.1074/jbc.m207618200

Jensen-Smith, H., and Hallworth, R. (2007). Lateral wall protein content mediates alterations in cochlear outer hair cell mechanics before and after hearing onset. *Cell Motil. Cytoskeleton* 64, 705–717. doi: 10.1002/cm.20217

Johnson, K. R., Tian, C., Gagnon, L. H., Jiang, H., Ding, D., and Salvi, R. (2017). Effects of Cdh23 single nucleotide substitutions on age-related hearing loss in C57BL/6 and 129S1/Sv mice and comparisons with congenic strains. *Sci. Rep.* 7:44450.

Kamar, R. I., Organ-Darling, L. E., and Raphael, R. M. (2012). Membrane cholesterol strongly influences confined diffusion of prestin. *Biophys. J.* 103, 1627–1636. doi: 10.1016/j.bpj.2012.07.052

Kiernan, A. E., Cordes, R., Kopan, R., Gossler, A., and Gridley, T. (2005). The Notch ligands DLL1 and JAG2 act synergistically to regulate hair cell development in the mammalian inner ear. *Development* 132, 4353–4362. doi: 10.1242/dev.02002

Kim, H., Han, J., and Park, J. H. (2020). Cyclodextrin polymer improves atherosclerosis therapy and reduces ototoxicity. *J. Control Release* 319, 77–86. doi: 10.1016/j.jconrel.2019.12.021

King, K. A., Gordon-Salant, S., Yanjanin, N., Zalewski, C., Houser, A., Porter, F. D., et al. (2014). Auditory phenotype of Niemann-Pick disease, type C1. *Ear Hear.* 35, 110–117. doi: 10.1097/aud.0b013e3182a362b8

Koitchev, K., Guilhaume, A., Cazals, Y., and Aran, J. M. (1982). Spiral ganglion changes after massive aminoglycoside treatment in the guinea pig. Counts and ultrastructure. *Acta Otolaryngol.* 94, 431–438. doi: 10.3109/00016488209128931

Kolodny, E. H. (2000). Niemann-Pick disease. *Curr. Opin. Hematol.* 7, 48–52.

Lambert, D., O'Neill, C. A., and Padfield, P. J. (2007). Methyl-beta-cyclodextrin increases permeability of Caco-2 cell monolayers by displacing specific claudins from cholesterol rich domains associated with tight junctions. *Cell. Physiol. Biochem.* 20, 495–506. doi: 10.1159/000107533

Laza-Knoerr, A. L., Gref, R., and Couvreur, P. (2010). Cyclodextrins for drug delivery. *J. Drug Target* 18, 645–656.

Leake, P. A., Rebscher, S. J., Dore, C., and Akil, O. (2019). AAV-mediated neurotrophin gene therapy promotes improved survival of cochlear spiral ganglion neurons in neonatally deafened cats: comparison of AAV2-hBDNF and AAV5-hGDNF. *J. Assoc. Res. Otolaryngol.* 20, 341–361. doi: 10.1007/s10162-019-00723-5

Lee, J. N., Kim, S. G., Lim, J. Y., Dutta, R. K., Kim, S. J., Choe, S. K., et al. (2016). 3-Aminotriazole protects from CoCl2-induced ototoxicity by inhibiting the generation of reactive oxygen species and proinflammatory cytokines in mice. *Arch. Toxicol.* 90, 781–791. doi: 10.1007/s00204-015-1506-9

Legendre, K., Safieddine, S., Kussel-Andermann, P., Petit, C., and El-Amraoui, A. (2008). alphaII-betaV spectrin bridges the plasma membrane and cortical lattice in the lateral wall of the auditory outer hair cells. *J. Cell Sci.* 121(Pt 20), 3347–3356. doi: 10.1242/jcs.028134

Liberman, M. C., Gao, J., He, D. Z., Wu, X., Jia, S., and Zuo, J. (2002). Prestin is required for electromotility of the outer hair cell and for the cochlear amplifier. *Nature* 419, 300–304. doi: 10.1038/nature01059

Lin, H. W., Furman, A. C., Kujawa, S. G., and Liberman, M. C. (2011). Primary neural degeneration in the Guinea pig cochlea after reversible noise-induced threshold shift. *J. Assoc. Res. Otolaryngol.* 12, 605–616. doi: 10.1007/s10162-011-0277-0

Lirussi, F., Beccarello, A., Zanette, G., Monte, A. De, Donadon, V., Velussi, M., et al. (2002). Silybin-beta-cyclodextrin in the treatment of patients with diabetes mellitus and alcoholic liver disease. Efficacy study of a new preparation of an anti-oxidant agent. *Diabetes Nutr. Metab.* 15, 222–231.

Liu, B., Ramirez, C. M., Miller, A. M., Repa, J. J., Turley, S. D., and Dietschy, J. M. (2010). Cyclodextrin overcomes the transport defect in nearly every organ of NPC1 mice leading to excretion of sequestered cholesterol as bile acid. *J. Lipid Res.* 51, 933–944. doi: 10.1194/jlr.m000257

Liu, X., Ding, D., Chen, G. D., Li, L., Jiang, H., and Salvi, R. (2020). 2-hydroxypropyl-beta-cyclodextrin ototoxicity in adult rats: rapid onset and massive destruction of both inner and outer hair cells above a critical dose. *Neurotox. Res.* 38, 808–823. doi: 10.1007/s12640-020-00252-7

Loftsson, T., and Brewster, M. E. (2010). Pharmaceutical applications of cyclodextrins: basic science and product development. *J. Pharm. Pharmacol.* 62, 1607–1621. doi: 10.1111/j.2042-7158.2010.01030.x

Ma, Y., Wise, A. K., Shepherd, R. K., and Richardson, R. T. (2019). New molecular therapies for the treatment of hearing loss. *Pharmacol. Ther.* 200, 190–209. doi: 10.1016/j.pharmthera.2019.05.003

Maarup, T. J., Chen, A. H., Porter, F. D., Farhat, N. Y., Ory, D. S., Sidhu, R., et al. (2015). Intrathecal 2-hydroxypropyl-beta-cyclodextrin in a single patient with Niemann-Pick C1. *Mol. Genet. Metab.* 116, 75–79. doi: 10.1016/j.ymgme.2015.07.001

Marttin, E., Verhoef, J. C., and Merkus, F. W. (1998). Efficacy, safety and mechanism of cyclodextrins as absorption enhancers in nasal delivery of peptide and protein drugs. *J. Drug Target* 6, 17–36. doi: 10.3109/10611869808997878

McFadden, S. L., Ding, D., Burkard, R. F., Jiang, H., Reaume, A. G., Flood, D. G., et al. (1999). Cu/Zn SOD deficiency potentiates hearing loss and cochlear pathology in aged 129,CD-1 mice. *J. Comp. Neurol.* 413, 101–112. doi: 10.1002/(sici)1096-9861(19991011)413:1<101::aid-cne7>3.0.co;2-l

McFadden, S. L., Ding, D., Jiang, H., and Salvi, R. J. (2004). Time course of efferent fiber and spiral ganglion cell degeneration following complete hair cell loss in the chinchilla. *Brain Res.* 997, 40–51. doi: 10.1016/j.brainres.2003.10.031

Mitrofanova, A., Molina, J., Santos, J. Varona, Guzman, J., Morales, X. A., Ducasa, G. M., et al. (2018). Hydroxypropyl-beta-cyclodextrin protects from kidney disease in experimental Alport syndrome and focal segmental glomerulosclerosis. *Kidney Int.* 94, 1151–1159. doi: 10.1016/j.kint.2018.06.031

Mueller, K. L., Jacques, B. E., and Kelley, M. W. (2002). Fibroblast growth factor signaling regulates pillar cell development in the organ of corti. *J. Neurosci.* 22, 9368–9377. doi: 10.1523/jneurosci.22-21-09368.2002

Müller, M. (1991). Frequency representation in the rat cochlea. *Hear. Res.* 51, 247–254. doi: 10.1016/0378-5955(91)90041-7

Newton, J., Milstien, S., and Spiegel, S. (2018). Niemann-Pick type C disease: the atypical sphingolipidosis. *Adv. Biol. Regul.* 70, 82–88. doi: 10.1016/j.jbior.2018.08.001

Nguyen, T. V., and Brownell, W. E. (1998). Contribution of membrane cholesterol to outer hair cell lateral wall stiffness. *Otolaryngol. Head Neck Surg.* 119, 14–20. doi: 10.1016/s0194-5998(98)70167-6

Oesterle, E. C., and Campbell, S. (2009). Supporting cell characteristics in long-deafened aged mouse ears. *J. Assoc. Res. Otolaryngol.* 10, 525–544. doi: 10.1007/s10162-009-0183-x

Okamura, W. H., Zhu, G. D., Hill, D. K., Thomas, R. J., Ringe, K., Borchardt, D. B., et al. (2002). Synthesis and NMR studies of (13)C-labeled vitamin D metabolites. *J. Org. Chem.* 67, 1637–1650.

Ory, D. S. (2000). Niemann-Pick type C: a disorder of cellular cholesterol trafficking. *Biochim. Biophys. Acta* 1529, 331–339. doi: 10.1016/s1388-1981(00)00158-x

Otero-Espinar, F. J., Luzardo-Alvarez, A., and Blanco-Mendez, J. (2010). Cyclodextrins: more than pharmaceutical excipients. *Mini Rev. Med. Chem.* 10, 715–725. doi: 10.2174/138955710791572479

Park, E. K., Park, M. J., Lee, S. H., Li, Y. C., Kim, J., Lee, J. S., et al. (2009). Cholesterol depletion induces anoikis-like apoptosis via FAK down-regulation and caveolae internalization. *J. Pathol.* 218, 337–349. doi: 10.1002/path.2531

Pickles, J. O., and Chir, B. (2002). Roles of fibroblast growth factors in the inner ear. *Audiol. Neurootol.* 7, 36–39. doi: 10.1159/000046861

Pontikis, C. C., Davidson, C. D., Walkley, S. U., Platt, F. M., and Begley, D. J. (2013). Cyclodextrin alleviates neuronal storage of cholesterol in Niemann-Pick C disease without evidence of detectable blood-brain barrier permeability. *J. Inherit. Metab. Dis.* 36, 491–498. doi: 10.1007/s10545-012-9583-x

Rajagopalan, L., Greeson, J. N., Xia, A., Liu, H., Sturm, A., Raphael, R. M., et al. (2007). Tuning of the outer hair cell motor by membrane cholesterol. *J. Biol. Chem.* 282, 36659–36670. doi: 10.1074/jbc.m705078200

Ramirez, C. M., Liu, B., Aqul, A., Taylor, A. M., Repa, J. J., Turley, S. D., et al. (2011). Quantitative role of LAL, NPC2, and NPC1 in lysosomal cholesterol processing defined by genetic and pharmacological manipulations. *J. Lipid Res.* 52, 688–698. doi: 10.1194/jlr.m013789

Ramirez, C. M., Liu, B., Taylor, A. M., Repa, J. J., Burns, D. K., Weinberg, A. G., et al. (2010). Weekly cyclodextrin administration normalizes cholesterol metabolism in nearly every organ of the Niemann-Pick type C1 mouse and markedly prolongs life. *Pediatr. Res.* 68, 309–315. doi: 10.1203/pdr.0b013e3181ee4dd2

Ren, L. L., Wu, Y., Han, D., Zhao, L. D., Sun, Q. M., Guo, W. W., et al. (2010). Math1 gene transfer based on the delivery system of quaternized chitosan/Na-carboxymethyl-beta-cyclodextrin nanoparticles. *J. Nanosci. Nanotechnol.* 10, 7262–7265. doi: 10.1166/jnn.2010.2822

Rybak, L. P., and Whitworth, C. A. (2005). Ototoxicity: therapeutic opportunities. *Drug Discov. Today* 10, 1313–1321. doi: 10.1016/s1359-6446(05)03552-x

Salvesen, G. S. (2002). Caspases and apoptosis. *Essays Biochem.* 38, 9–19.

Schonfelder, U., Radestock, A., Elsner, P., and Hipler, U. C. (2006). Cyclodextrin-induced apoptosis in human keratinocytes is caspase-8 dependent and accompanied by mitochondrial cytochrome c release. *Exp. Dermatol.* 15, 883–890. doi: 10.1111/j.1600-0625.2006.00481.x

Stella, V. J., and He, Q. (2008). Cyclodextrins. *Toxicol. Pathol.* 36, 30–42.

Takahashi, S., Homma, K., Zhou, Y., Nishimura, S., Duan, C., Chen, J., et al. (2016). Susceptibility of outer hair cells to cholesterol chelator 2-hydroxypropyl-beta-cyclodextrine is prestin-dependent. *Sci. Rep.* 6:21973.

Tang, G. P., Guo, H. Y., Alexis, F., Wang, X., Zeng, S., Lim, T. M., et al. (2006). Low molecular weight polyethylenimines linked by beta-cyclodextrin for gene transfer into the nervous system. *J. Gene Med.* 8, 736–744. doi: 10.1002/jgm.874

Taylor, A. M., Liu, B., Mari, Y., Liu, B., and Repa, J. J. (2012). Cyclodextrin mediates rapid changes in lipid balance in Npc1-/- mice without carrying cholesterol through the bloodstream. *J. Lipid Res.* 53, 2331–2342. doi: 10.1194/jlr.m028241

Taylor, R. R., Jagger, D. J., and Forge, A. (2012). Defining the cellular environment in the organ of Corti following extensive hair cell loss: a basis for future sensory cell replacement in the Cochlea. *PLoS One* 7:e30577. doi: 10.1371/journal.pone.0030577

Tillinger, J. A., Gupta, C., Ila, K., Ahmed, J., Mittal, J., Van De Water, T.R., et al. (2018). l-N-acetylcysteine protects outer hair cells against TNFalpha initiated ototoxicity in vitro. *Acta Otolaryngol.* 138, 676–684. doi: 10.1080/00016489.2018.1440086

Uchenna Agu, R., Jorissen, M., Willems, T., Van den Mooter, G., Kinget, R., Verbeke, N., et al. (2000). Safety assessment of selected cyclodextrins – effect on ciliary activity using a human cell suspension culture model exhibiting in vitro ciliogenesis. *Int. J. Pharm.* 193, 219–226. doi: 10.1016/s0378-5173(99)00342-7

Vecsernyes, M., Fenyvesi, F., Bacskay, I., Deli, M. A., Szente, L., and Fenyvesi, E. (2014). Cyclodextrins, blood-brain barrier, and treatment of neurological diseases. *Arch. Med. Res.* 45, 711–729. doi: 10.1016/j.arcmed.2014.11.020

Walenbergh, S. M., Houben, T., Hendrikx, T., Jeurissen, M. L., van Gorp, P. J., Vaes, N., et al. (2015). Weekly treatment of 2-hydroxypropyl-beta-cyclodextrin improves intracellular cholesterol levels in LDL receptor knockout mice. *Int. J. Mol. Sci.* 16, 21056–21069. doi: 10.3390/ijms160921056

Wang, J., Ding, D., and Salvi, R. J. (2003). Carboplatin-induced early cochlear lesion in chinchillas. *Hear. Res.* 181, 65–72. doi: 10.1016/s0378-5955(03)00176-x

Wang, J., Ladrech, S., Pujol, R., Brabet, P., Van De Water, T. R., and Puel, J. L. (2004). Caspase inhibitors, but not c-Jun NH2-terminal kinase inhibitor treatment, prevent cisplatin-induced hearing loss. *Cancer Res.* 64, 9217–9224. doi: 10.1158/0008-5472.can-04-1581

Ward, S., O'Donnell, P., Fernandez, S., and Vite, C. H. (2010). 2-hydroxypropyl-beta-cyclodextrin raises hearing threshold in normal cats and in cats with Niemann-Pick type C disease. *Pediatr. Res.* 68, 52–56. doi: 10.1203/pdr.0b013e3181df4623

Wood, M. B., and Zuo, J. (2017). The contribution of immune infiltrates to ototoxicity and cochlear hair cell loss. *Front. Cell. Neurosci.* 11:106. doi: 10.3389/fncel.2017.00106

Wu, N., Li, M., Chen, Z. T., Zhang, X. B., Liu, H. Z., Li, Z., et al. (2013). In vivo delivery of Atoh1 gene to rat cochlea using a dendrimer-based nanocarrier. *J. Biomed. Nanotechnol.* 9, 1736–1745. doi: 10.1166/jbn.2013.1684

Yagi, M., Kanzaki, S., Kawamoto, K., Shin, B., Shah, P. P., Magal, E., et al. (2000). Spiral ganglion neurons are protected from degeneration by GDNF gene therapy. *J. Assoc. Res. Otolaryngol.* 1, 315–325.

Zhang, J., Sun, H., Salvi, R., and Ding, D. (2018). Paraquat initially damages cochlear support cells leading to anoikis-like hair cell death. *Hear. Res.* 364, 129–141. doi: 10.1016/j.heares.2018.03.014

Zhou, Y., Takahashi, S., Homma, K., Duan, C., Zheng, J., Cheatham, M. A., et al. (2018). The susceptibility of cochlear outer hair cells to cyclodextrin is not related to their electromotile activity. *Acta Neuropathol. Commun.* 6:98.

Zimmer, S., Grebe, A., Bakke, S. S., Bode, N., Halvorsen, B., Ulas, T., et al. (2016). Cyclodextrin promotes atherosclerosis regression via macrophage reprogramming. *Sci. Transl. Med.* 8:333ra50. doi: 10.1126/scitranslmed.aad6100

8

Single-Cell Sequencing Applications in the Inner Ear

Mingxuan Wu[1†], Mingyu Xia[1†], Wenyan Li[1] and Huawei Li[1,2,3,4*]*

[1] ENT Institute and Department of Otorhinolaryngology, Eye and ENT Hospital, State Key Laboratory of Medical Neurobiology and MOE Frontiers Center for Brain Science, Fudan University, Shanghai, China, [2] Institutes of Biomedical Sciences, Fudan University, Shanghai, China, [3] NHC Key Laboratory of Hearing Medicine, Fudan University, Shanghai, China, [4] The Institutes of Brain Science and The Collaborative Innovation Center for Brain Science, Fudan University, Shanghai, China

***Correspondence:**
Wenyan Li
wenyan_li2000@126.com
Huawei Li
hwli@shmu.edu.cn

[†] These authors have contributed equally to this work

Genomics studies face specific challenges in the inner ear due to the multiple types and limited amounts of inner ear cells that are arranged in a very delicate structure. However, advances in single-cell sequencing (SCS) technology have made it possible to analyze gene expression variations across different cell types as well as within specific cell groups that were previously considered to be homogeneous. In this review, we summarize recent advances in inner ear research brought about by the use of SCS that have delineated tissue heterogeneity, identified unknown cell subtypes, discovered novel cell markers, and revealed dynamic signaling pathways during development. SCS opens up new avenues for inner ear research, and the potential of the technology is only beginning to be explored.

Keywords: single cell sequencing, hair cell, inner ear, supporting cell, spiral ganglion neuron

INTRODUCTION

The inner ear is one of the most intricate parts of the body, located within the petrous portion of the temporal bone with its attendant sensory structures responsible for auditory and balance function (Groves and Fekete, 2012). The cochlea is the auditory portion of the membranous labyrinth, while the vestibular organ collects motion, equilibrium, and spatial orientation information. Previous studies have defined some crucial signaling pathways – such as FGF, Notch, and Wnt – and genes – such as *Pax2* and *Atoh1* – that play essential roles in the development and maintenance of the inner ear (Scheffer et al., 2015; Zhong et al., 2019). Each region of the sensory epithelium is composed of highly heterogeneous populations of cells depending on the physiological and anatomical criteria of that region (Szarama et al., 2012; Jeng et al., 2020; Ono et al., 2020; Yao et al., 2020), and this highlights the importance of examining the expression of a large number of genes at the single cell level.

Previous genetic studies have mainly focused on analyzing bulk tissue samples composed of millions of cells, and thus have only looked at the average expression of specific transcripts, which is dependent on the expression level of each gene as well as the populations of different cell subtype. Over the past centuries, major advances have been made in genomic studies, and single cell sequencing (SCS) has emerged as a powerful tool for studying the contributions from individual cells (Knouse et al., 2014; Cao et al., 2019; Pijuan-Sala et al., 2019). In this review, we will briefly show the developmental history and utilization of SCS technology in basic research, and we will summarize its utility in inner ear research that has improved our knowledge of inner ear cellular heterogeneity, inner ear development, genetic deafness, and hair cell (HC) regeneration.

THE DEVELOPMENT AND THE ADVANTAGES OF SCS TECHNOLOGY

With the advent of next-generation sequencing, SCS technology has been developed and adopted to obtain genomic, transcriptomic, and epigenomic information from single cells (Tang X. et al., 2019). The data are collected following single cell isolation, capture, and lysis, nucleic acid extraction and amplification, and high-throughput sequencing, as shown in **Figure 1A**. Tang et al. (2009) modified the previously reported single-cell transcriptome amplification method and analyzed the transcriptomes of individual blastomeres, and this marked the beginning of single-cell omics. Later, Navin et al. (2011) flow-sorted nuclei and investigated copy number variations in liver tumor subpopulations. Further, Smart-Seq was developed as a robust method for improving read coverage and for enhancing the detailed analyses of alternative transcript isoforms and the identification of single-nucleotide polymorphisms (Ramskold et al., 2012).

The SCS procedures have been continuously updated and modified over the past decade. Advances in single-cell isolation have greatly expanded the fields of research, as cells of various tissue could be isolated and captured by different method. Magnetic-activated cell sorting (MACS), flow-activated cell sorting (FACS), and microfluidic platforms enable high throughput study, while laser capture microdissection (LCM) technology preserves original spatial information which may be of great importance under some circumstances. In addition, numerous methods have been developed for single cell genome, transcriptome, and epigenome study, as shown in **Figure 1B**. Coverage, sensitivity, efficiency as well as accuracy of these methods differ from each other because of distinct amplification process. Characteristics and suitable applications of different methods are summarized as shown in **Tables 1–4**.

Furthermore, researchers can now go beyond single-omics studies and can integrate multiple omics in a single cell. For example, the combination of DNA and RNA sequencing by DR-seq (DNA-mRNA sequencing) (Dey et al., 2015) or G&T-seq (genome and transcriptome sequencing) (Macaulay et al., 2015) from the same cell can reveal genomic variations between individual cells, thus explaining changes at the transcription level. Techniques that analyze the epigenome and transcriptome of the same cell have been used to reveal the regulatory role of methylation and chromatin accessibility in gene expression (Angermueller et al., 2016; Hu et al., 2016; Clark et al., 2018), and Hou et al. (2016) have developed scTrio-seq (single-cell triple omics sequencing) that simultaneously obtains genome, DNA methylome, and transcriptome information from a single cell.

There has been an explosion of studies utilizing SCS in recent years due to its remarkable ability compared with traditional sequencing technology to detect new genes that might be missed by bulk sample sequencing and to discern previously unknown cell types (Proserpio and Lonnberg, 2016). In addition, SCS visualization of cell fate transition and possible cell origin has allowed the reconstruction of cell lineage trajectories of many important life activities in cells (Pijuan-Sala et al., 2019), and SCS has proven to be of great importance for illustrating new mechanism of tumorigenesis and metastasis and thus improving the diagnosis and treatment of cancer (Navin et al., 2011). In embryonic organ development, SCS provides genetic information at different stages, thus helping to identify master genes and regulatory signaling pathways in early embryonic development (Tang et al., 2010; Biase et al., 2014) and during the development of the cerebral cortex (Pollen et al., 2014), kidney (Wang P. et al., 2018), lung epithelium (Treutlein et al., 2014), etc. SCS has also promoted the identification of new species of microorganisms and clarified the molecular evolutionary mechanisms and kinetics of infection by obtaining genetic information at the single-cell level (McLean et al., 2013; Combe et al., 2015; Guo et al., 2017b). In studies of the immune system, where the cell subtypes are highly heterogeneous and are even more diversified after gene recombination, SCS has revealed single cell gene-expression networks in immune responses, therefore deepening our understanding of complex immune mechanisms and laying the foundation for advances in immunotherapy (Bossel Ben-Moshe et al., 2019; Rao et al., 2020). In reproduction and heredity studies, SCS is able to detect the dynamic genetic profiles of single germ cells (Hou et al., 2013; Chen et al., 2018; Wang M. et al., 2018) and embryonic cells (Wagner et al., 2018), which is significant for understanding germ cell genesis, alternative splicing patterns, and the key regulators of these processes. SCS also shows promise in reproductive disorders by improving prenatal and preimplantation genetic diagnosis (Li et al., 2017). SCS has also stimulated stem cell research, and embryonic stem cells and induced pluripotent stem cells have been traced by SCS to identify the regulators of embryonic and organ primordium outgrowth (Ealy et al., 2016). Various tissue-specific stem cells have also been explored with SCS, including hematopoietic stem cells (Kowalczyk et al., 2015), intestinal epithelium stem cells (Grun et al., 2015), lung epithelium stem cells (Ikonomou et al., 2020), neural stem cells (Llorens-Bobadilla et al., 2015), and germline stem cells (Guo F. et al., 2015). The single cell genetic patterns provide us with a more comprehensive means of evaluating the dynamic regulatory networks of progenitor cells *in vivo*, and this has helped to clarify the developmental process and has led to modifications of *in vitro* induction protocols. Broad applications of SCS in diverse fields of basic research are summarized in **Figure 1C**.

SINGLE-CELL SEQUENCING IN INNER EAR CELL HETEROGENEITY

Hair cells in the inner ear function in transducing the sound waves into electric signals (Hilding, 1953; Zwislocki, 1975; Balak et al., 1990); while SCs function in supporting the HCs and providing the potential pool for HC regeneration (Corwin and Cotanche, 1988; Balak et al., 1990). Damage from a variety of sources can impair HC function, including mutations in deafness genes, ototoxic drugs, aging, chronic cochlear infections, and noise overexposure (Wright, 1973; Cotanche et al., 1987; Hashino et al., 1991; Jiang et al., 2018). As shown in **Figure 2**, SCS enables the analysis of vast amounts of genetic data simultaneously at single-cell resolution with unbiased cell clustering, thus leading to

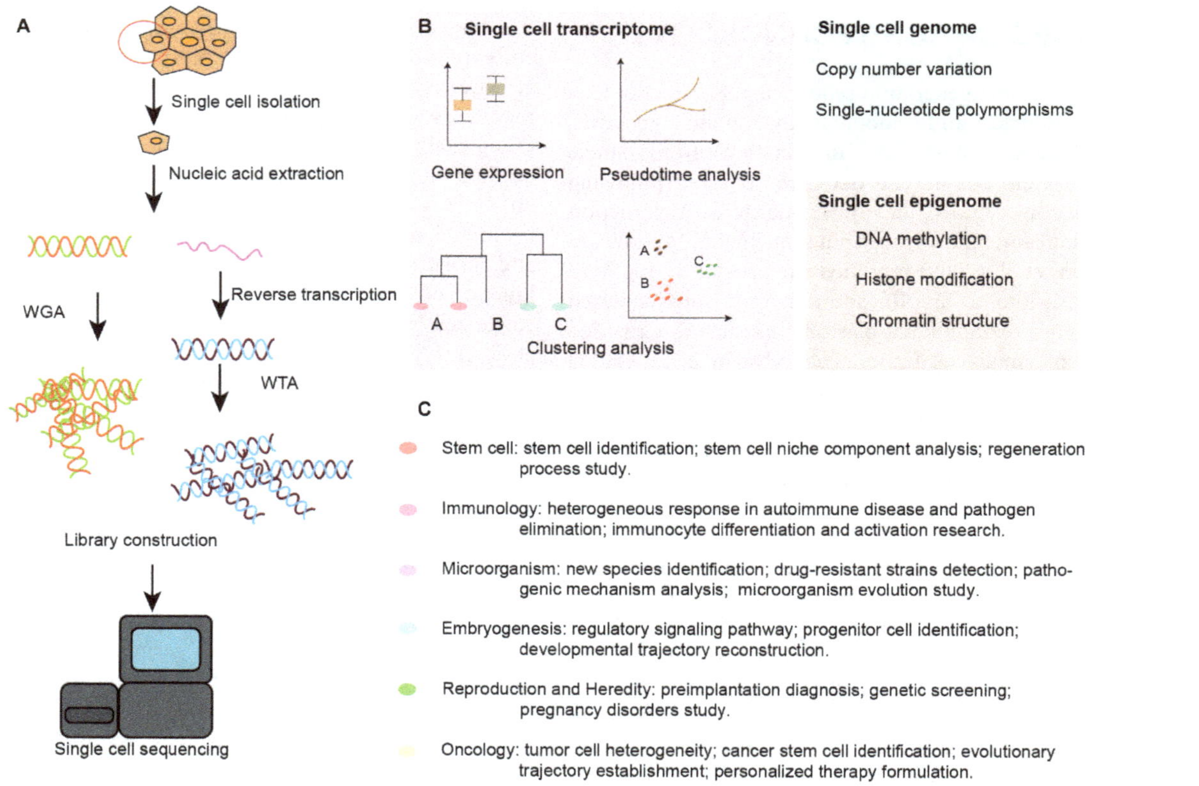

FIGURE 1 | Overview of SCS workflow and applications in the inner ear. **(A)** Schematic strategy of SCS workflow. After dissociation of the organ or tissue of interest to live single cell, cells are then captured by various methods and lysed to release RNA and DNA fragment, the former is reversed transcribed to synthesized cDNA. DNA fragment or cDNA must be amplified to generate sequencing library. Next-generation sequencing is subsequently performed to generate the readouts that can be assigned to single cells via cell-specific barcodes. **(B)** Analysis of single cell transcriptome, genome and epigenome data. **(C)** Diverse fields of basic research that have been impacted by SCS technologies. WGA, whole genome amplification; WTA, whole transcriptome amplification.

the identification of novel markers for inner ear resident cells and new cell subtypes of type II extrastriolar HCs, cochlear supporting cells (SCs), neuromast SCs, and spiral ganglion neurons (SGNs) (Burns et al., 2015; Shrestha et al., 2018).

Heterogeneity of the Sensory Epithelium

Based on single cell transcriptional profiles of postnatal day (P)1 mouse utricular epithelium, Burns et al. (2015) used known markers to identify three major groups [*Gata2*, *Lmx1a*, *Slc26a4*, and *Cldn8* in transitional epithelial cells (TECs); *Otog*, *Otoa*, *Jag1*, *Hes1*, and *Slc1a3* in SCs; *Myo7a*, *Pou4f3*, *Otof*, *Calb2*, and *Ptprq* in HCs] and subdivided them into seven subclusters following principal component analysis-based reduction. TECs contained one cluster, whereas SCs comprised two clusters and HCs consisted of four clusters. In unbiased trajectory analysis, HC.i appeared to be in a transitional state between SC.ii and HC.iii–iv, which is consistent with a study confirming the development of HCs from SCs (Wang et al., 2015). Surprisingly, HC.ii was assigned between TECs and HC.iii–iv, which suggested novel TEC-like progenitor cells located outside the sensory epithelium. In addition, striolar HCs and SCs seem to be distinct cell subtypes compared with their counterparts in the extrastriolar region (Wang et al., 2015; Li et al., 2016). Striolar HCs express high levels of oncomodulin and clusterin, while striolar SCs distinctly express the otolithic membrane glycoprotein beta-tectorin, the transcription factor Gata3, and the retinoic acid-inactivating protein Cyp26b1. In addition, P1 striolar SCs have a greater propensity to regenerate into HCs in response to Notch inhibition. Together, these results indicate that the striola is a molecularly distinct region within the utricle. Another study analyzed single utricular HC data from P1, P12, and P100 mice and identified *Spp1* as a specific marker for Type I HCs and *Mapt* and *Anxa4* as markers for Type II HCs (McInturff et al., 2018). In addition, Ellwanger et al. (2018) identified two classes of type II extrastriolar HCs based on the discrepant expression of *ATP2B2*, *CCDC50*, *MYO1H*, *TMC2*, and *TNNC2* (Ellwanger et al., 2018).

Burns et al. (2015) adopted a similar process to analyze the single cell transcriptomes of P1 cochlear epithelium tissue and identified four major clusters of cells – HCs, SCs, medial non-sensory cells (NSC.i) and lateral non-sensory cells (NSC.ii). *Rasd2*, *Anxa4*, and *Pcp4* were found to be novel markers for HCs, and *Cdh4* and *Mia1* were identified as medial SC markers and *Cntn1* as a lateral SC marker. Although genetic heterogeneity within the clusters indicated possible cell subtypes, definitive conclusion was not available in Burns's study because of the limited sample size, and this highlights the importance of the

TABLE 1 | Comparison of single-cell isolation methods.

Item	Advantage	Disadvantage	References
Serial dilution	Simple operation, low cost	Low throughput, cell loss, difficulty in filtering target cells	Gross et al., 2015
Manual pipetting	Simple operation, low cost	Low throughput	Gross et al., 2015
Robotic micromanipulation	Precise separation	Low efficiency, dependence on apparatus, mechanical damage	Guo et al., 2017a
MACS	High throughput, high accuracy	Mechanical damage, requirement for high cell abundance	Guo and Cairns, 2019
FACS	High throughput, high accuracy	Mechanical damage, requirement for high cell abundance and fluorescence intensity	Shapiro et al., 2013
LCM	High accuracy, conservation of spatial information	Low efficiency, high cost, likely contamination form adjacent cells	Nichterwitz et al., 2016
Microfluidic platforms	High throughput, high accuracy, available commercial platform	Dependence on homogeneous cell size	Macosko et al., 2015

MACS, magnetic-activated cell sorting; FACS, flow-activated cell sorting; LCM, laser capture microdissection.

TABLE 2 | Comparison of single-cell DNA sequencing technologies.

Item	Coverage	Characteristics	Application	References
DOP-PCR	Low	Exponential amplification, simple operation, fast speed, sequence-dependent bias, high allele dropout rate	CNV	Arneson et al., 2008; Huang et al., 2015
MDA	Medium	Exponential amplification, high replication fidelity, sequence-dependent bias, normalization ineffective	SNV	Spits et al., 2006
MALBAC	High	Linear amplification, high accuracy for CNV detection, low false negative rate for SNV detection	CNV and SNV	Zong et al., 2012

DOP-PCR, degenerate oligonucleotide–primed polymerase chain reaction; MDA, multiple displacement amplification; MALBAC, multiple annealing and looping-based amplification cycles; CNV, copy number variation; SNV, single-nucleotide polymorphisms.

TABLE 3 | Comparison of single-cell RNA sequencing technologies.

Item	Coverage	Characteristics	References
Smart-seq/seq2	Full length	High sensitivity, low efficiency	Ramskold et al., 2012; Picelli et al., 2014
Quarz-seq/seq2	Full length	High sensitivity, high reproducibility	Sasagawa et al., 2013, 2018
CEL- seq/seq2	Full length	High accuracy, sequence-dependent bias	Hashimshony et al., 2012, 2016
Drop-seq	3′-end	High efficiency, low cost, highly parallel analysis	Macosko et al., 2015
inDROP-seq	3′-end	High throughput, low efficiency	Klein et al., 2015
STRT-seq	5′-end	High accuracy, sequence-dependent bias	Islam et al., 2012
MARS-seq	3′-end	High sensitivity, high accuracy	Jaitin et al., 2014
Cyto-seq	3′-end	Direct analysis of complex samples, relatively expensive and time-consuming	Fan et al., 2015

TABLE 4 | Comparison of single-cell epigenome technologies.

Item	Application	Characteristics	References
scRRBS-seq	DNA methylation	Low throughput, low coverage rate	Guo H. et al., 2015
scBS-seq	DNA methylation	Low throughput, low coverage rate	Smallwood et al., 2014
scCGI-seq	DNA methylation	Low throughput, high coverage rate	Han et al., 2017
scChIL-seq	Histone modification	Low throughput, high coverage rate	Harada et al., 2019
scCUT&tag	Histone modification	High throughput, low coverage rate	Kaya-Okur et al., 2019
scChIC-seq	Histone modification	Low throughput, low coverage rate	Ku et al., 2019
scATAC-seq	Chromatin structure	High throughput, high coverage rate	Buenrostro et al., 2015

power of sequencing (Burns et al., 2015; McInturff et al., 2018). Hoa et al. (2020) collected single cell transcriptomes of cochlear SCs and categorized adult cochlear SCs into two subclusters that differentially expressed *S100a6*, *Pla2g7*, *Tuba1b*, and *Spry2*. *S100a6* and *Pla2g7* were identified as medial SC markers, and *Tuba1b* and *Spry2* were identified as lateral SC markers.

Comparisons of gene expression between inner HCs (IHCs) and outer HCs (OHCs) provide a deeper understanding of these cells' unique functions. Using AUC rankings, *Ocm* and *Sri* were identified as the top two most upregulated genes in OHCs, both of which are associated with calcium regulation (Ranum et al., 2019). Expressed predominantly by OHCs, *Ocm* encodes Oncomodulin, a calcium-buffering protein that is essential for mechanoelectric transduction and electromotility amplification (Simmons et al., 2010). *Sri* encodes sorcin, a regulator of calcium-based excitation-contraction (Fowler et al., 2008). OHCs express Ca2+ release channels/ryanodine receptors in a pattern similar to cardiac myocytes, which raises the possibility that Ca2+ plays a similar role in regulating OHC motility (Grant et al., 2006). The

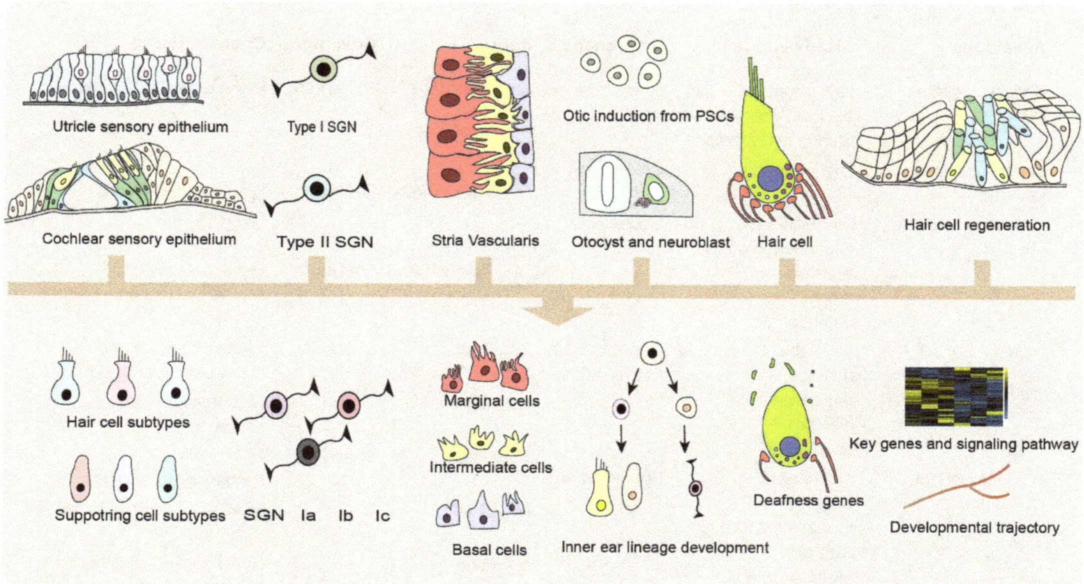

FIGURE 2 | Applications of SCS in basic research. Applications of single cell sequencing (SCS) in the inner ear enable recognition of previously unknown cell subtype and novel marker genes of hair cells (HCs), supporting cells (SCs), spiral ganglion neurons (SGNs), and cells in the stria vascularis (SV), identification of unappreciated exons and splicing diversity of genetic deafness and reconstruction of developmental trajectory and regeneration process.

expression of other components required for calcium-mediated excitation-contraction in the OHC transcriptome is consistent with this hypothesis and suggests a unique requirement for the tight regulation of calcium in these cells (Ranum et al., 2019).

Compared with mammals, non-mammalian vertebrates constantly regenerate sensory HCs in lateral line organs in order to replace senescent or injured cells, and this occurs through SC proliferation and differentiation (Steiner et al., 2014; Romero-Carvajal et al., 2015; Chen et al., 2017; Zhang et al., 2018, 2019). Regular RNA-Seq has been extensively used in analyzing the proliferation and differentiation ability of SCs (Waqas et al., 2016a; Cheng et al., 2017; Zhang et al., 2017; You et al., 2018), and scRNA-seq was used to identify quiescent and activated stem cell populations and their spatial arrangements in zebrafish neuromasts (Lush et al., 2019). The SC subtypes included central SCs (*Lfng*, *Ebf3a*, *Gata2a/b*, and *Slc1a3a/Glasta*), anterior-posterior (A/P) SCs (*Cx44.2*, *Fap*, *Fgf10a*, and *Hmx2*), dorsal-ventral (D/V) amplifying SCs (*Sost*, *Fsta*, *Srrt/Ars*, *Six2b*, and *Adcyap1b*), and dividing/differentiating SCs (*Dld*, *Her4.1*, *Pcna*, and *Atoh1b*). Dividing/differentiating SCs were considered to be an HC progenitors cluster in the HC lineage with young HCs and mature HCs, which were marked by *Atoh1b* and *Tekt3*, respectively. Mantle cells had enriched expression of *Cldne*, *Crb3b*, *Cripl*, and *Cts12*. The authors then mapped the amplifying divisions to D/V poles and the differentiating divisions to the center and thus identified distinct locations of two SC lineages, while cells in the A/P poles were relatively quiescent. Along this timeline, cells lose their expression of SC and stem cell genes and take on HC-specific markers. Genes related to translation, cell cycle regulation, and Notch signaling (*Dla*, *Dlb*, *Dlc*, *Dld*) were downregulated, suggesting their roles in early developmental stages rather than subsequent differentiation stages.

Heterogeneity of Cochlear SGNs

After mechanical stimulation of auditory HCs, sound information is conveyed to the dendrites of SGNs via synaptic vesicles containing the neurotransmitter glutamate (Eybalin et al., 1996; Yan et al., 2018; Guo et al., 2019; Liu et al., 2019). The perception of auditory information – including sound frequency, intensity, timbre, and pitch – is a complex process that appears to be associated with SGN diversity (Pfeiffer and Kiang, 1965; Sachs et al., 1974; Liberman, 1982; Temchin, 1988). Based on recent studies of SGN single-cell transcriptomes, three novel subclasses of type I neurons have been identified (Petitpre et al., 2018; Shrestha et al., 2018; Sun et al., 2018). The clustering of type I SGN subtypes in the three studies used almost identical gene sets and obtained similar transcriptional profiles, but the authors named the three subtypes differently. Genes were found to enriched in each subtype, including *CALB2*, *Trim54*, *Rxrg* in type Ia neurons; *CALB1*, *Runx1*, and *Ttn* in type Ib neurons; and *Pou4f1*, *Lypd1*, *Grm8*, *Kcnc2*, *Lypd1*, and *Runx1* in type Ic neurons (Petitpre et al., 2018; Shrestha et al., 2018; Sun et al., 2018). Shrestha et al. (2018) examined genes involved in synaptic transmission and electrophysiological properties. The expression of AMPA-type glutamate receptor subunit *Grik4*, metabotropic receptor subunit *Grm8*, and dopamine receptor subunit *Drd1* were highly increased in Ic SGNs, and the cholinergic receptor subunits *Chrna1* and *Chrna4* were enriched in Ia SGNs. As for the genes encoding K^+ channel subunits, *Kcnq4* was detected in Ia SGNs, while *Kcnd2* and *Kcnip2* were expressed in Ib SGNs and *Kcnj9* was expressed in Ic SGNs. *Cacna1b*, *Cacna1h*, and

Cacna2d1 are voltage-gated Ca^{2+} channels that were enriched in Ia SGNs. The leaky sodium channel *Nalcn* was detected tin Ib and Ic SGNs, and the voltage-gated sodium channel subunit *Scn2b* was expressed in an increasing gradient from Ia to Ic SGNs. Based on a previous study that SGNs projecting to different positions along the basolateral surface of IHCs differ in spontaneous firing rate (SR) (Liberman, 1982), Shrestha assumed that type Ia SGNs that projected onto the pillar side of the IHC and formed synapses with small ribbons corresponded to high-SR fibers, that Ib SGNs on the middle of the basolateral surface with medium ribbons corresponded to medium-SR fibers, and that Ic SGNs that projected onto the modiolar side with small ribbons corresponded to low-SR fibers (Shrestha et al., 2018). In addition, enriched gene sets for mitochondrial function and neurofilament formation in type Ia SGNs were consistent with increased mitochondrial content and fiber thickness in high-SR neurons (Sun et al., 2018). They also found tonotopic differences in functionally relevant genes within these subpopulations. *Efna1*, for example, was condensed in the middle and base compared with the apex within Ib SGNs and was enriched in Ia and Ic SGNs at the base (Shrestha et al., 2018). The transcriptional profiles and anatomical arrangements, combined with their electrophysiological properties, suggested that the heterogeneous neural populations were involved in encoding of sound intensities and for maintaining of hearing discrimination in noisy environments (Petitpre et al., 2018). This diversity of cochlear neurons is established at birth, followed by refinement over the first postnatal week that requires intact HC mechanotransduction activity (Shrestha et al., 2018; Sun et al., 2018).

Heterogeneity of the Stria Vascularis

Hair cell mechanotransduction requires high-K^+ endolymph and positive endocochlear potential (EP), both of which are generated by the stria vascularis (SV), a non-sensory epithelial tissue located on the lateral side of the cochlear duct (Wangemann, 2002; Patuzzi, 2011). Marginal cells (MCs), intermediate cells (ICs), and basal cells (BCs) have been identified in the SV and are indispensable for endolymph ionic homeostasis and EP maintenance.

Korrapati et al. (2019) performed single cell RNA-seq and single nucleus RNA-seq to investigate SV cell populations. Known markers, including *Kcne1* and *Kcnq1* for MCs, *Cd44* and *Met* for ICs, *Cldn11* and *Tjp1* for BCs, and *Slc26a4* for spindle/root cells, were used to define cell identities after unbiased clustering. Gene ontology (GO) analysis showed that MCs had enriched expression of genes involved in positive regulation of K^+ transport, Ca^{2+}-transporting ATPase activity, and G-protein–coupled receptor complex formation, that ICs exhibited high expression of H^+-transporting ATPase activity, neutrophil degranulation, and interleukin-28 receptor complex formation, and that BCs expressed genes involved in rhodopsin expression regulation and platelet alpha granule lumen. The transcriptional profiles of the SV cell populations suggested roles for MCs and ICs in ion homeostasis maintenance and possible interactions between SV cells (ICs and BCs) and the immune system. In addition, novel markers, including *Abcg1* and *Heyl* in MCs, *Nrp2* and *Kcnj13* in ICs, *Sox8* and *Nr2f2* in BCs, and *P2rx2* and *Kcnj16* in spindle/root cells were discovered and confirmed by smFISH (single molecule fluorescence *in situ* hybridization).

SINGLE-CELL SEQUENCING IN INNER EAR DEVELOPMENT

Generation of the entire otic lineage from non-neural ectoderm (NNE) through pre- placodal ectoderm (PPE) and the posterior placode fates remains elusive, but *in vitro* studies have contributed to understanding the molecular mechanism of early otic lineage formation. Ealy et al. (2016) used human embryonic stem cells and induced pluripotent stem cells to test conditions for stepwise induction of NNE to the otic lineage, and the process was monitored by SCS. They successfully developed a protocol that combined BMP, Wnt, and FGF signaling regulations with retinoic acid treatment to generate a lineage that chronologically expressed markers of NNE (*Dlx3*, *Dlx5*, *Dlx6*, *Tfap2a*, *Tfap2c*, *Gata3*, and *Gata2*), PPE (*Eya1*, *Eya2*, *Six1*, and *Six4*), and ultimately of the otic lineage (*Myosin7a*, *Foxi3*, *Fbxo2*, *Pax2*, and *Pax8*). This breakthrough showed the potential of applying SCS in the refinement of the cell guidance protocol.

The otocyst is regarded as the origin for almost all cells of the inner ear, including sensory epithelial cells and neurons. Durruthy-Durruthy et al. (2014) conducted scRNA-seq of cells from mouse otocysts and neuroblasts at embryonic day (E)10.5, which is the developmental stage at which delaminating and migrating neuroblast cells coexist. Clusters identified by known markers included early neuroblasts (by *Neurog1* and *Fgf3*), post-delaminated neuroblasts (by *Isl1*, *Neurod1*, and *Eya1*), ventral otocysts (by *Lfng*, *Sox2*, *Pax2*, and *Gli1*), and dorsal otocysts (by *Bmp4*, *Dlx5*, *Gata2*, and *Oc90*). Because neuroblasts are committed to their lineage, repressed Shh and Wnt signaling was observed, as shown by downregulation of Shh pathway genes (*Smo* and *Ptc2* and *Gli3*) and Wnt pathway genes (*Fzd2*, *Fzd7*, *Fzd8*, and *Axin2*). Fgf signaling was also downregulated and Fgf gene (*Fgf8* and *Fgf10*) and *Fgfr1* expression was decreased and *Fgfr1* antagonist *Spry2* expression was increased along the axis of development. However, Notch signaling showed a bimodal distribution, and expression of *Dll1*, *Jag1*, *Notch2*, *Hes1*, *Hes5*, and *Hey2* declined while expression of *Jag2* and *Hey1* increased toward the later stages. In addition, two distinct cell populations were identified within the late neuroblasts that expressed *Foxg1* and *Jag2* asymmetrically, which implied the separation of cochlear and vestibular ganglion neurons (Lu et al., 2011; He et al., 2019, 2020). In the otocysts, Notch signaling was mapped to the dorso-anterior side (*Notch2*) and ventro-anterior side (*Hes1*, *Hey1*, and *Hey2*), and the Shh receptor gene *Ptc2* and effector gene *Gli3* were expressed in cells located in the ventral part of otocysts. A small group of cells in the ventral otocyst cell cluster were identified as potential prosensory predecessors due to their enriched expression of prosensory markers (*Sox2*, *Jag1*, and *Lfng*) and weak expression of the early neuroblast marker *Neurog1*. Signaling pathway analysis of this subcluster revealed active Notch (*Hey1*,

Hey2, *Hes1*, *Hes5*, *Dll1*, *Jag1*, and *Notch2*) and Shh signaling (*Gli2*, *Gli3*, and *Smo*) activity and autonomously regulated Fgf signaling (*Fgf3*, *Fgf10*, *Spry1*, and *Spry2*), indicating the complexity of the signals that need to be integrated to induce the prosensory lineage. *Fbxo2* and *Otol1* were otic-specific candidate genes in the heterogeneous area that gives rise to the prosensory domains.

The endolymphatic sac forms at E10 and is the earliest structure to arise from the otocyst, and it is important in fluid resorption during inner ear development (Morsli et al., 1998; Raft et al., 2014). The major cell types in the endolymphatic sac are ribosome-rich cells (RRCs) and mitochondria-rich cells (MRCs) (Dahlmann and von During, 1995). Honda et al. (2017) conducted single-cell RNA-seq of the mouse endolymphatic sac from E12.5 to P30. Early RRCs predominantly expressed genes involved in proteins secretion (*Dmkn*, *Clu*, *Igsf1*, and *Cyr61*), while mature RRCs expressed genes related to innate immunity (*Lcn2*, *Slpi*, and *Serping1*). In contrast, MRCs expressed high levels of genes related to ion transport (*Slc26a4*, *Atp6v1b1*, *Clcnkb*, *Slc4a9*, *Kcnma1*, and *Slc34a2*). These results confirmed that embryonic endolymphatic sac fluid resorption is carried out by MRCs and is dependent on the anion exchanger SLC26A4.

After cell fate commitment, primitive cells undergo a series of changes in gene expression and cellular morphology to become mature cells. McInturff et al. (2018) identified new markers for utricular HCs (*Spp1* for Type I HCs and *Mapt* and *Anxa4* for Type II HCs), and they traced these genes to study the temporal and spatial development of utricular HCs. They found that type I HCs develop from the posterior-medial side to the anterior-lateral side and that type II HCs initially develop in the striolar region and extend to the periphery. Marked by *Spp1*, 90% of type I HCs arise between E11.5 and E14.5, while almost all type II HCs develop postnatally.

In HCs, hair bundle assembly and protrusion are prerequisites for their mechanotransduction function (Ó Maoiléidigh and Ricci, 2019). Although four stages of developing bundles have been defined according to their structural pattern as pre-growth, initial growth, widening, and secondary growth (Tilney et al., 1992), the molecular basis for this division has remained poorly understood. Using SCS, Zhu et al. (2019) found that utricle hair bundle assembly and growth requires regulation of local Ca^{2+} concentrations. The Ca^{2+} regulator *Calb2* and the calcium pump *Atp2b2* were shown to be important for stereocilia growth because the highest level of *Calb2* protein occurred at the onset of the secondary growth and *Aatatp2b2* protein expression peaked during stereocilia widening (Ellwanger et al., 2018). It has been confirmed that HCs use existing monomeric actin to build hair bundles without significant upregulation of actin gene transcription (Tilney and Tilney, 1988). Zhu et al. (2019) reported the use of single-cell proteomics analysis combined with single-cell RNA-seq to study the utricles of E15 chickens. The authors found previously unannotated proteins that were abundant in different populations, such as GSTO1, GPX2, CRABP1, and AK1 in HCs and TMSB4X and AGR3 in SCs. Single cell proteomics revealed that the actin monomer binding protein thymosin b4 (TMSB4X) was abundant in SCs and that its expression decreased as progenitor cells developed into HCs. Comparative single-cell RNA-seq analysis showed that *Tmsb4x* transcripts were downregulated when transcription of *Atoh1* was activated, which suggested that existing monomeric actin is made available for hair bundle assembly through the degradation of *Tmsb4x*.

SINGLE-CELL SEQUENCING IN DEAFNESS

Numerous variants in genes related to deafness have been identified, thus illustrating the heterogeneous genetic background of deafness (Shearer et al., 2014). Ranum et al. (2019) used single cell full-length reverse transcriptional analysis with long-read sequencing to identify novel exons and to reveal the unappreciated splicing diversity among deafness-associated genes. They analyzed 12 deafness-associated genes and detected 20 unannotated exons, including exon 1B of *Cabp2* and exons 1B, 22B, 9B, and 31B of *Cacna1d*. Their work showed that the heterogeneity and complexity of genetic deafness is greater than previously believed and suggested that current genetic tests for deafness are incomplete.

Single-cell sequencing technology can also be used to demonstrate the mechanism by which genetic changes lead to specific phenotypes. For example, chromodomain helicase DNA binding protein 7 (*Chd7*) has been shown to be involved in early inner ear development (E8.5–E10.5) by regulating ATP-dependent nucleosome remodeling (Adams et al., 2007; Bouazoune and Kingston, 2012), and single cell transcriptomes of E10.5 mouse otocysts showed that loss of *Chd7* leads to the misexpression of neurogenic genes (*Neurog1* and *Neurod1*), the ventral-associated gene *Lfng*, and Notch genes (*Hey1* and *Hey2*) in dorsal otic cells (Durruthy-Durruthy et al., 2018). This indicated that *Chd7* mutant dorsal otic cells aberrantly adopt mixed dorsal and neurogenic fates, probably because of additional Notch signals. Type II transmembrane serine protease (*Tmprss3*) is another gene that is required for normal hearing, and mutations in *Tmprss3* cause rapid cochlear HC loss between P12 and P14 (Fasquelle et al., 2011). Single cell RNA-seq of inner ear organoid cells revealed elevated expression of apoptosis genes and genes associated with the extracellular matrix in *Tmprss3*-knockout hair cells, while *Kcnma1* (which encodes the α subunits of a Ca2+-activated K+ channel), Ca2+-binding protein genes (*Myl1*, *Pvalb*, *Cib2*, *Mylpf*, and *Tnnc2*), and the Ca2+regulator gene *Sln* were downregulated, suggesting the important role for *Tmprss3* in cellular homeostasis (Tang P. C. et al., 2019).

SINGLE-CELL SEQUENCING IN HC REGENERATION

In mammals, the loss of cochlear HCs leads to permanent hearing impairment because these cells only exhibit very limited spontaneous regeneration capacity and only within the first postnatal week, and such regeneration occurs via the mitotic proliferation or transdifferentiation of SCs (Ni et al., 2016; Waqas et al., 2016b; Wu et al., 2016; He et al., 2017; McGovern et al., 2019). Researchers have focused on the genes involved in cell cycle progression in adult cochlear SC transcriptional profiles generated by SCS and found that lateral SCs (pillar and Deiters' cells) express some of the transcripts that are enriched in Lgr5 + neonatal SCs, including *Cdkn1b*, *Cks1b*, *Mcm3*, *Mdm2*, and *Shc3*, while genes involved in G1/S transition are more preferentially expressed in adult cochlear SCs (Hoa et al., 2020). GO molecular function and cellular component analysis indicated that the inability of adult cochlear SCs to reenter the cell cycle was related to cyclin-dependent protein serine/threonine kinase activity and condensed chromatin at the centromere.

Overexpression of *Atoh1* can induce SCs to differentiate into ectopic HCs (Zheng and Gao, 2000; Gubbels et al., 2008; Lewis et al., 2012). In work by Yamashita et al. (2018), the *Atoh1*-overexpression transgene was driven by *Fgfr3* (in Deiters' cells and Pillar cells) in mouse cochleae after tamoxifen-mediated induction at P12, and single-cell transcriptomes were obtained at P12, P26, and P33. *Atoh1*-induced HCs were divided into three groups based on their developmental stages, from initial HCs cells to mature HCs. Along the regeneration trajectory, the expression of HC markers (*Myo6*, *Rasd2*, *Chrna9*, *Pvalb*, *Pou4f3*, and *Chrna10*) increased. *Atoh1* and *Pou4f3* were considered to be key reprogramming factors, while other transcription factors, including *Barhl1* and *Lhx3*, improved the conversion efficiency. In addition, the authors found that *Isl1* boosted the efficiency *Atoh1*-mediated SC to HC conversion.

The Notch and Wnt pathways and their interactions were investigated in HC regeneration, and it was shown that Notch signaling downregulation after HC ablation led to the disinhibition of Wnt signaling and the induction of HC regeneration (Romero-Carvajal et al., 2015). The Fgf pathway is downregulated after HC loss in neuromasts (Jiang et al., 2014). To get deeper insights into the mechanism of HC regeneration driven by these three important signaling pathways, scRNA-seq showed that *fgf3* in zebrafish is only expressed in central SCs under normal conditions and is downregulated when the overlying HCs die (Lush et al., 2019). Moreover, *fgf3-null* mutant zebrafish neuromast cells showed that the Wnt inhibitor *sost* was downregulated and the Wnt target gene *wnt10a* was upregulated, indicating that Wnt signaling is activated in *fgf3*-null mutants. The authors demonstrated that loss of *fgf3* in central SCs led to increased HC regeneration independent of Notch signaling likely through fgfr1a and fgfr2 receptors.

CONCLUSION AND FUTURE DIRECTION

Over the past decade, SCS technologies have emerged as powerful tools for dissecting cellular heterogeneity and for reconstructing developmental lineages in various tissues, and the application of SCS has brought gene expression studies in inner ear cells to an unprecedented level. SCS provides unbiased research methods for analyzing single cell gene-expression characteristics and global cell heterogeneity in the sensory epithelium, the non-sensory epithelium, and the SGNs, thus allowing the identification of novel marker genes and unknown cell subtypes. AUC ranking and GO analysis point to diverse physiological properties among different cell populations and illustrate the different biological functions of each cell type. The use of SCS in the developing inner ear has revealed dynamic transcriptional profiles, varying signaling pathways, and constantly changing cellular states along the developmental axis, and this has led to the reconstruction of cell lineage progression and the discovery of key regulators of these processes. In addition, SCS supports research into the pathogenic mechanisms of deafness and HC regeneration. With the help of full-length sequencing, the identification of unannotated exons and isoforms of deafness-related genes has expanded our knowledge of the genetic basis of deafness and provides a foundation for new advances in gene therapy.

Despite the wide application of SCS methods in inner ear research, SCS technologies still require further development to reduce background noise, amplification errors, and costs and to improve coverage and sequencing depth. Single-cell isolation methods also need improvement in order to avoid genetic changes during dissociation. Thus, there is great room for improvement and development in SCS technologies. We anticipate that the future application of single-cell profiling in the inner ear will shed substantial light on the cellular heterogeneity involved in inner ear development and hearing and balance functions and will improve the accuracy of regenerative therapies. The potential of SCS technology remains to be fully explored, and single-cell sequencing technologies are likely to yield new discoveries in inner ear research in the future.

AUTHOR CONTRIBUTIONS

HL and WL designed this systematic review article and present a synthesis of previous researches on Single-cell sequencing in the inner ear. MW and MX went through all the related manuscript. MW, MX, WL, and HL wrote the manuscript. All the authors contributed to the article and approved the submitted version.

REFERENCES

Adams, M. E., Hurd, E. A., Beyer, L. A., Swiderski, D. L., Raphael, Y., and Martin, D. M. (2007). Defects in vestibular sensory epithelia and innervation in mice with loss of Chd7 function: implications for human CHARGE syndrome. *J. Comp. Neurol.* 504, 519–532. doi: 10.1002/cne.21460

Angermueller, C., Clark, S. J., Lee, H. J., Macaulay, I. C., Teng, M. J., Hu, T. X., et al. (2016). Parallel single-cell sequencing links transcriptional and epigenetic heterogeneity. *Nat. Methods* 13, 229–232. doi: 10.1038/nmeth.3728

Arneson, N., Hughes, S., Houlston, R., and Done, S. (2008). Whole-genome amplification by degenerate oligonucleotide primed PCR (DOP-PCR). *CSH Protoc.* 2008:dbrot4919.

Balak, K. J., Corwin, J. T., and Jones, J. E. (1990). Regenerated Hair-cells can originate from supporting cell progeny - evidence from phototoxicity and laser ablation experiments in the lateral line system. *J. Neurosci.* 10, 2502–2512. doi: 10.1523/jneurosci.10-08-02502.1990

Biase, F. H., Cao, X., and Zhong, S. (2014). Cell fate inclination within 2-cell and 4-cell mouse embryos revealed by single-cell RNA sequencing. *Genome Res.* 24, 1787–1796. doi: 10.1101/gr.177725.114

Bossel Ben-Moshe, N., Hen-Avivi, S., Levitin, N., Yehezkel, D., Oosting, M., Joosten, L. A. B., et al. (2019). Predicting bacterial infection outcomes using single cell RNA-sequencing analysis of human immune cells. *Nat. Commun.* 10:3266.

Bouazoune, K., and Kingston, R. E. (2012). Chromatin remodeling by the CHD7 protein is impaired by mutations that cause human developmental disorders. *Proc. Natl. Acad. Sci. U.S.A.* 109, 19238–19243. doi: 10.1073/pnas.1213825109

Buenrostro, J. D., Wu, B., Litzenburger, U. M., Ruff, D., Gonzales, M. L., Snyder, M. P., et al. (2015). Single-cell chromatin accessibility reveals principles of regulatory variation. *Nature* 523, 486–490. doi: 10.1038/nature14590

Burns, J. C., Kelly, M. C., Hoa, M., Morell, R. J., and Kelley, M. W. (2015). Single-cell RNA-Seq resolves cellular complexity in sensory organs from the neonatal inner ear. *Nat. Commun.* 6:8557.

Cao, J., Spielmann, M., Qiu, X., Huang, X., Ibrahim, D. M., Hill, A. J., et al. (2019). The single-cell transcriptional landscape of mammalian organogenesis. *Nature* 566, 496–502. doi: 10.1038/s41586-019-0969-x

Chen, Y., Lu, X. L., Guo, L., Ni, W. L., Zhang, Y. P., Zhao, L. P., et al. (2017). Hedgehog signaling promotes the proliferation and subsequent hair cell formation of progenitor cells in the neonatal mouse cochlea. *Front. Mol. Neurosci.* 10:426. doi: 10.3389/fnmol.2017.00426

Chen, Y., Zheng, Y., Gao, Y., Lin, Z., Yang, S., Wang, T., et al. (2018). Single-cell RNA-seq uncovers dynamic processes and critical regulators in mouse spermatogenesis. *Cell Res.* 28, 879–896. doi: 10.1038/s41422-018-0074-y

Cheng, C., Guo, L., Lu, L., Xu, X. C., Zhang, S. S., Gao, J. Y., et al. (2017). Characterization of the transcriptomes of Lgr5+hair cell progenitors and Lgr5-supporting cells in the mouse cochlea. *Front. Mol. Neurosci.* 10:122. doi: 10.3389/fnmol.2017.00122

Clark, S. J., Argelaguet, R., Kapourani, C. A., Stubbs, T. M., Lee, H. J., Alda-Catalinas, C., et al. (2018). scNMT-seq enables joint profiling of chromatin accessibility DNA methylation and transcription in single cells. *Nat. Commun.* 9:781.

Combe, M., Garijo, R., Geller, R., Cuevas, J. M., and Sanjuan, R. (2015). Single-cell analysis of RNA virus infection identifies multiple genetically diverse viral genomes within single infectious units. *Cell Host Microbe* 18, 424–432. doi: 10.1016/j.chom.2015.09.009

Corwin, J. T., and Cotanche, D. A. (1988). Regeneration of sensory hair cells after acoustic trauma. *Science* 240, 1772–1774. doi: 10.1126/science.3381100

Cotanche, D. A., Saunders, J. C., and Tilney, L. G. (1987). Hair cell damage produced by acoustic trauma in the chick cochlea. *Hear. Res.* 25, 267–286. doi: 10.1016/0378-5955(87)90098-0

Dahlmann, A., and von During, M. (1995). The endolymphatic duct and sac of the rat: a histological, ultrastructural, and immunocytochemical investigation. *Cell Tissue Res.* 282, 277–289. doi: 10.1007/bf00319118

Dey, S. S., Kester, L., Spanjaard, B., Bienko, M., and Van Oudenaarden, A. (2015). Integrated genome and transcriptome sequencing of the same cell. *Nat. Biotechnol.* 33, 285–289. doi: 10.1038/nbt.3129

Durruthy-Durruthy, R., Gottlieb, A., Hartman, B. H., Waldhaus, J., Laske, R. D., Altman, R., et al. (2014). Reconstruction of the mouse otocyst and early neuroblast lineage at single-cell resolution. *Cell* 157, 964–978. doi: 10.1016/j.cell.2014.03.036

Durruthy-Durruthy, R., Sperry, E. D., Bowen, M. E., Attardi, L. D., Heller, S., and Martin, D. M. (2018). Single cell transcriptomics reveal abnormalities in neurosensory patterning of the Chd7 mutant mouse ear. *Front. Genet.* 9:473. doi: 10.3389/fgene.2018.00473

Ealy, M., Ellwanger, D. C., Kosaric, N., Stapper, A. P., and Heller, S. (2016). Single-cell analysis delineates a trajectory toward the human early otic lineage. *Proc. Natl. Acad. Sci. U.S.A.* 113, 8508–8513. doi: 10.1073/pnas.1605537113

Ellwanger, D. C., Scheibinger, M., Dumont, R. A., Barr-Gillespie, P. G., and Heller, S. (2018). Transcriptional dynamics of hair-bundle morphogenesis revealed with celltrails. *Cell Rep.* 23, 2901.e2913–2914.e2913.

Eybalin, M., Norenberg, M. D., and Renard, N. (1996). Glutamine synthetase and glutamate metabolism in the guinea pig cochlea. *Hear. Res.* 101, 93–101. doi: 10.1016/s0378-5955(96)00136-0

Fan, H. C., Fu, G. K., and Fodor, S. P. A. (2015). Combinatorial labeling of single cells for gene expression cytometry. *Science* 9:347.

Fasquelle, L., Scott, H. S., Lenoir, M., Wang, J., Rebillard, G., Gaboyard, S., et al. (2011). Tmprss3, a transmembrane serine protease deficient in human DFNB8/10 deafness, is critical for cochlear hair cell survival at the onset of hearing. *J. Biol. Chem.* 286, 17383–17397. doi: 10.1074/jbc.m110.190652

Fowler, M. R., Colotti, G., Chiancone, E., Smith, G. L., and Fearon, I. M. (2008). Sorcin modulates cardiac L-type Ca2+ current by functional interaction with the alpha1C subunit in rabbits. *Exp. Physiol.* 93, 1233–1238. doi: 10.1113/expphysiol.2008.043497

Grant, L., Slapnick, S., Kennedy, H., and Hackney, C. (2006). Ryanodine receptor localisation in the mammalian cochlea: an ultrastructural study. *Hear. Res.* 219, 101–109. doi: 10.1016/j.heares.2006.06.002

Gross, A., Schoendube, J., Zimmermann, S., Steeb, M., Zengerle, R., and Koltay, P. (2015). Technologies for Single-Cell Isolation. *Int. J. Mol. Sci.* 16, 16897–16919.

Groves, A. K., and Fekete, D. M. (2012). Shaping sound in space: the regulation of inner ear patterning. *Development* 139, 245–257. doi: 10.1242/dev.067074

Grun, D., Lyubimova, A., Kester, L., Wiebrands, K., Basak, O., Sasaki, N., et al. (2015). Single-cell messenger RNA sequencing reveals rare intestinal cell types. *Nature* 525, 251–255. doi: 10.1038/nature14966

Gubbels, S. P., Woessner, D. W., Mitchell, J. C., Ricci, A. J., and Brigande, J. V. (2008). Functional auditory hair cells produced in the mammalian cochlea by in utero gene transfer. *Nature* 455, 537–541. doi: 10.1038/nature07265

Guo, F., Li, L., Li, J., Wu, X., Hu, B., Zhu, P., et al. (2017a). Single-cell multi-omics sequencing of mouse early embryos and embryonic stem cells. *Cell Res.* 27, 967–988. doi: 10.1038/cr.2017.82

Guo, F., Li, S., Caglar, M. U., Mao, Z., Liu, W., Woodman, A., et al. (2017b). Single-cell virology: on-chip investigation of viral infection dynamics. *Cell Rep.* 21, 1692–1704. doi: 10.1016/j.celrep.2017.10.051

Guo, F., Yan, L. Y., Guo, H. S., Li, L., Hu, B. Q., Zhao, Y. Y., et al. (2015). The transcriptome and DNA methylome landscapes of human primordial germ cells. *Cell* 161, 1437–1452. doi: 10.1016/j.cell.2015.05.015

Guo, H., Zhu, P., Guo, F., Li, X., Wu, X., Fan, X., et al. (2015). Profiling DNA methylome landscapes of mammalian cells with single-cell reduced-representation bisulfite sequencing. *Nat. Protoc.* 10, 645–659. doi: 10.1038/nprot.2015.039

Guo, J., and Cairns, B. R. (2019). Isolation and enrichment of spermatogonial stem cells from human testis tissues. *Curr. Protoc. Stem. Cell Biol.* 49:e77. doi: 10.1002/cpsc.77

Guo, R. R., Ma, X. F., Liao, M. H., Liu, Y., Hu, Y. N., Qian, X. Y., et al. (2019). Development and application of cochlear implant-based electric-acoustic stimulation of spiral ganglion neurons. *ACS Biomater. Sci. Eng.* 5, 6735–6741. doi: 10.1021/acsbiomaterials.9b01265

Han, L., Wu, H. J., Zhu, H., Kim, K. Y., Marjani, S. L., Riester, M., et al. (2017). Bisulfite-independent analysis of CpG island methylation enables genome-scale stratification of single cells. *Nucleic Acids Res.* 45:e77.

Harada, A., Maehara, K., Handa, T., Arimura, Y., Nogami, J., Hayashi-Takanaka, Y., et al. (2019). A chromatin integration labelling method enables epigenomic profiling with lower input. *Nat. Cell Biol.* 21, 287–296. doi: 10.1038/s41556-018-0248-3

Hashimshony, T., Senderovich, N., Avital, G., Klochendler, A., De Leeuw, Y., Anavy, L., et al. (2016). CEL-Seq2: sensitive highly-multiplexed single-cell RNA-Seq. *Genome Biol.* 17:77.

Hashimshony, T., Wagner, F., Sher, N., and Yanai, I. (2012). CEL-Seq: single-cell RNA-Seq by multiplexed linear amplification. *Cell Rep.* 2, 666–673. doi: 10.1016/j.celrep.2012.08.003

Hashino, E., Tanaka, Y., and Sokabe, M. (1991). Hair cell damage and recovery following chronic application of kanamycin in the chick cochlea. *Hear. Res.* 52, 356–368. doi: 10.1016/0378-5955(91)90025-5

He, Y. Z., Lu, X. L., Qian, F. P., Liu, D., Chai, R. J., and Li, H. W. (2017). Insm1a is required for zebrafish posterior lateral line development. *Front. Mol. Neurosci.* 10:241. doi: 10.3389/fnmol.2017.00241

He, Z. H., Fang, Q. J., Li, H., Shao, B. W., Zhang, Y., Zhang, Y. H., et al. (2019). The role of FOXG1 in the postnatal development and survival of mouse cochlear hair cells. *Neuropharmacology* 144, 43–57. doi: 10.1016/j.neuropharm.2018.10.021

He, Z. H., Zou, S. Y., Li, M., Liao, F. L., Wu, X., Sun, H. Y., et al. (2020). The nuclear transcription factor FoxG1 affects the sensitivity of mimetic aging hair cells to inflammation by regulating autophagy pathways. *Redox Biol.* 28:101364. doi: 10.1016/j.redox.2019.101364

Hilding, A. C. (1953). The tectorial membrane in the theory of hearing - the significance of the tectorial membrane in the transmission of sound vibrations to the hair cells and a theory of the mechanism of tone location in the cochlea. *Acta Oto Laryngol.* 43, 490–490.

Hoa, M., Olszewski, R., Li, X., Taukulis, I., Gu, S., Detorres, A., et al. (2020). Characterizing adult cochlear supporting cell transcriptional diversity using single-cell RNA-Seq: validation in the adult mouse and translational implications for the adult human cochlea. *Front. Mol. Neurosci.* 13:13. doi: 10.3389/fnmol.2020.00013

Honda, K., Kim, S. H., Kelly, M. C., Burns, J. C., Constance, L., Li, X., et al. (2017). Molecular architecture underlying fluid absorption by the developing inner ear. *Elife* 6:e26851.

Hou, Y., Fan, W., Yan, L., Li, R., Lian, Y., Huang, J., et al. (2013). Genome analyses of single human oocytes. *Cell* 155, 1492–1506. doi: 10.1016/j.cell.2013.11.040

Hou, Y., Guo, H., Cao, C., Li, X., Hu, B., Zhu, P., et al. (2016). Single-cell triple omics sequencing reveals genetic, epigenetic, and transcriptomic heterogeneity in hepatocellular carcinomas. *Cell Res.* 26, 304–319. doi: 10.1038/cr.2016.23

Hu, Y., Huang, K., An, Q., Du, G., Hu, G., Xue, J., et al. (2016). Simultaneous profiling of transcriptome and DNA methylome from a single cell. *Genome Biol.* 17:88.

Huang, L., Ma, F., Chapman, A., Lu, S., and Xie, X. S. (2015). Single-cell whole-genome amplification and sequencing: methodology and applications. *Annu. Rev. Genomics Hum. Genet.* 16, 79–102.

Ikonomou, L., Herriges, M. J., Lewandowski, S. L., Marsland, R., Villacorta-Martin, C., Caballero, I. S., et al. (2020). The in vivo genetic program of murine primordial lung epithelial progenitors. *Nat. Commun.* 11:635. doi: 10.1038/s41467-020-14348-3

Islam, S., Kjallquist, U., Moliner, A., Zajac, P., Fan, J. B., Lonnerberg, P., et al. (2012). Highly multiplexed and strand-specific single-cell RNA 5' end sequencing. *Nat. Protoc.* 7, 813–828. doi: 10.1038/nprot.2012.022

Jaitin, D. A., Kenigsberg, E., Keren-Shaul, H., Elefant, N., Paul, F., Zaretsky, I., et al. (2014). Massively parallel single-Cell RNA-Seq for marker-free decomposition of tissues into cell types. *Science* 343, 776–779. doi: 10.1126/science.1247651

Jeng, J. Y., Ceriani, F., Hendry, A., Johnson, S. L., Yen, P., Simmons, D. D., et al. (2020). Hair cell maturation is differentially regulated along the tonotopic axis of the mammalian cochlea. *J. Physiol.* 598, 151–170. doi: 10.1113/jp279012

Jiang, L., Romero-Carvajal, A., Haug, J. S., Seidel, C. W., and Piotrowski, T. (2014). Gene-expression analysis of hair cell regeneration in the zebrafish lateral line. *Proc. Natl. Acad. Sci. U.S.A.* 111, E1383–E1392.

Jiang, L., Xu, J., Jin, R., Bai, H., Zhang, M., Yang, S., et al. (2018). Transcriptomic analysis of chicken cochleae after gentamicin damage and the involvement of four signaling pathways (Notch, FGF, Wnt and BMP) in hair cell regeneration. *Hear. Res.* 361, 66–79. doi: 10.1016/j.heares.2018.01.004

Kaya-Okur, H. S., Wu, S. J., Codomo, C. A., Pledger, E. S., Bryson, T. D., Henikoff, J. G., et al. (2019). CUT&Tag for efficient epigenomic profiling of small samples and single cells. *Nat. Commun.* 10:1930.

Klein, A. M., Mazutis, L., Akartuna, I., Tallapragada, N., Veres, A., Li, V., et al. (2015). Droplet barcoding for single-cell transcriptomics applied to embryonic stem cells. *Cell* 161, 1187–1201. doi: 10.1016/j.cell.2015.04.044

Knouse, K. A., Wu, J., Whittaker, C. A., and Amon, A. (2014). Single cell sequencing reveals low levels of aneuploidy across mammalian tissues. *Proc. Natl. Acad. Sci. U.S.A.* 111, 13409–13414. doi: 10.1073/pnas.1415287111

Korrapati, S., Taukulis, I., Olszewski, R., Pyle, M., Gu, S., Singh, R., et al. (2019). Single cell and single nucleus RNA-Seq reveal cellular heterogeneity and homeostatic regulatory networks in adult mouse stria vascularis. *Front. Mol. Neurosci.* 12:316. doi: 10.3389/fnmol.2019.00316

Kowalczyk, M. S., Tirosh, I., Heck, D., Rao, T. N., Dixit, A., Haas, B. J., et al. (2015). Single-cell RNA-seq reveals changes in cell cycle and differentiation programs upon aging of hematopoietic stem cells. *Genome Res.* 25, 1860–1872. doi: 10.1101/gr.192237.115

Ku, W. L., Nakamura, K., Gao, W., Cui, K., Hu, G., Tang, Q., et al. (2019). Single-cell chromatin immunocleavage sequencing (scChIC-seq) to profile histone modification. *Nat. Methods* 16, 323–325. doi: 10.1038/s41592-019-0361-7

Lewis, R. M., Hume, C. R., and Stone, J. S. (2012). Atoh1 expression and function during auditory hair cell regeneration in post-hatch chickens. *Hear. Res.* 289, 74–85. doi: 10.1016/j.heares.2012.04.008

Li, W., Ma, Y., Yu, S., Sun, N., Wang, L., Chen, D., et al. (2017). The mutation-free embryo for in vitro fertilization selected by MALBAC-PGD resulted in a healthy live birth from a family carrying PKD 1 mutation. *J. Assist. Reprod. Genet.* 34, 1653–1658. doi: 10.1007/s10815-017-1018-z

Li, W. Y., You, D., Chen, Y., Chai, R. J., and Li, H. W. (2016). Regeneration of hair cells in the mammalian vestibular system. *Front. Med.* 10:143–151. doi: 10.1007/s11684-016-0451-1

Liberman, M. C. (1982). Single-neuron labeling in the cat auditory nerve. *Science* 216, 1239–1241. doi: 10.1126/science.7079757

Liu, W. W., Xu, X. C., Fan, Z. M., Sun, G. Y., Han, Y. C., Zhang, D. G., et al. (2019). Wnt signaling activates TP53-induced glycolysis and apoptosis regulator and protects against cisplatin-induced spiral ganglion neuron damage in the mouse cochlea. *Antioxid. Redox Signal.* 30, 1389–1410. doi: 10.1089/ars.2017.7288

Llorens-Bobadilla, E., Zhao, S., Baser, A., Saiz-Castro, G., Zwadlo, K., and Martin-Villalba, A. (2015). Single-cell transcriptomics reveals a population of dormant neural stem cells that become activated upon brain injury. *Cell Stem Cell* 17, 329–340. doi: 10.1016/j.stem.2015.07.002

Lu, C. C., Appler, J. M., Houseman, E. A., and Goodrich, L. V. (2011). Developmental profiling of spiral ganglion neurons reveals insights into auditory circuit assembly. *J. Neurosci.* 31, 10903–10918. doi: 10.1523/jneurosci.2358-11.2011

Lush, M. E., Diaz, D. C., Koenecke, N., Baek, S., Boldt, H., St Peter, M. K., et al. (2019). scRNA-Seq reveals distinct stem cell populations that drive hair cell regeneration after loss of Fgf and Notch signaling. *Elife* 8:e44431.

Macaulay, I. C., Haerty, W., Kumar, P., Li, Y. I., Hu, T. X., Teng, M. J., et al. (2015). G&T-seq: parallel sequencing of single-cell genomes and transcriptomes. *Nat. Methods* 12, 519–522.

Macosko, E. Z., Basu, A., Satija, R., Nemesh, J., Shekhar, K., Goldman, M., et al. (2015). Highly parallel genome-wide expression profiling of individual cells using nanoliter droplets. *Cell* 161, 1202–1214. doi: 10.1016/j.cell.2015.05.002

McGovern, M. M., Randle, M. R., Cuppini, C. L., Graves, K. A., and Cox, B. C. (2019). Multiple supporting cell subtypes are capable of spontaneous hair cell regeneration in the neonatal mouse cochlea. *Development* 146:dev171009. doi: 10.1242/dev.171009

McInturff, S., Burns, J. C., and Kelley, M. W. (2018). Characterization of spatial and temporal development of Type I and Type II hair cells in the mouse utricle using new cell-type-specific markers. *Biol. Open* 7:bio038083. doi: 10.1242/bio.038083

McLean, J. S., Lombardo, M. J., Badger, J. H., Edlund, A., Novotny, M., Yee-Greenbaum, J., et al. (2013). Candidate phylum TM6 genome recovered from a hospital sink biofilm provides genomic insights into this uncultivated phylum. *Proc. Natl. Acad. Sci. U.S.A.* 110, E2390–E2399.

Morsli, H., Choo, D., Ryan, A., Johnson, R., and Wu, D. K. (1998). Development of the mouse inner ear and origin of its sensory organs. *J. Neurosci.* 18, 3327–3335. doi: 10.1523/jneurosci.18-09-03327.1998

Navin, N., Kendall, J., Troge, J., Andrews, P., Rodgers, L., Mcindoo, J., et al. (2011). Tumour evolution inferred by single-cell sequencing. *Nature* 472, 90–94. doi: 10.1038/nature09807

Ni, W. L., Zeng, S., Li, W. Y., Chen, Y., Zhang, S. S., Tang, M. L., et al. (2016). Wnt activation followed by Notch inhibition promotes mitotic hair cell regeneration in the postnatal mouse cochlea. *Oncotarget* 7, 66754–66768. doi: 10.18632/oncotarget.11479

Nichterwitz, S., Chen, G., Aguila Benitez, J., Yilmaz, M., Storvall, H., Cao, M., et al. (2016). Laser capture microscopy coupled with Smart-seq2 for precise spatial transcriptomic profiling. *Nat. Commun.* 7:12139.

Ó Maoiléidigh, D., and Ricci, A. J. (2019). A bundle of mechanisms: inner-ear hair-cell mechanotransduction. *Trends Neurosci.* 42, 221–236. doi: 10.1016/j.tins.2018.12.006

Ono, K., Keller, J., Lopez Ramirez, O., Gonzalez Garrido, A., Zobeiri, O. A., Chang, H. H. V., et al. (2020). Retinoic acid degradation shapes zonal development of vestibular organs and sensitivity to transient linear accelerations. *Nat. Commun.* 11:63.

Patuzzi, R. (2011). Ion flow in stria vascularis and the production and regulation of cochlear endolymph and the endolymphatic potential. *Hear. Res.* 277, 4–19. doi: 10.1016/j.heares.2011.01.010

Petitpre, C., Wu, H. H., Sharma, A., Tokarska, A., Fontanet, P., Wang, Y. Q., et al. (2018). Neuronal heterogeneity and stereotyped connectivity in the auditory afferent system. *Nat. Commun.* 9:3691.

Pfeiffer, R. R., and Kiang, N. Y. (1965). Spike discharge patterns of spontaneous and continuously stimulated activity in the cochlear nucleus of anesthetized cats. *Biophys. J.* 5, 301–316. doi: 10.1016/s0006-3495(65)86718-2

Picelli, S., Faridani, O. R., Bjorklund, A. K., Winberg, G., Sagasser, S., and Sandberg, R. (2014). Full-length RNA-seq from single cells using Smart-seq2. *Nat. Protoc.* 9, 171–181. doi: 10.1038/nprot.2014.006

Pijuan-Sala, B., Griffiths, J. A., Guibentif, C., Hiscock, T. W., Jawaid, W., Calero-Nieto, F. J., et al. (2019). A single-cell molecular map of mouse gastrulation and early organogenesis. *Nature* 566, 490–495. doi: 10.1038/s41586-019-0933-9

Pollen, A. A., Nowakowski, T. J., Shuga, J., Wang, X., Leyrat, A. A., Lui, J. H., et al. (2014). Low-coverage single-cell mRNA sequencing reveals cellular heterogeneity and activated signaling pathways in developing cerebral cortex. *Nat. Biotechnol.* 32, 1053–1058. doi: 10.1038/nbt.2967

Proserpio, V., and Lonnberg, T. (2016). Single-cell technologies are revolutionizing the approach to rare cells. *Immunol. Cell Biol.* 94, 225–229. doi: 10.1038/icb.2015.106

Raft, S., Andrade, L. R., Shao, D., Akiyama, H., Henkemeyer, M., and Wu, D. K. (2014). Ephrin-B2 governs morphogenesis of endolymphatic sac and duct epithelia in the mouse inner ear. *Dev. Biol.* 390, 51–67. doi: 10.1016/j.ydbio.2014.02.019

Ramskold, D., Luo, S., Wang, Y. C., Li, R., Deng, Q., Faridani, O. R., et al. (2012). Full-length mRNA-Seq from single-cell levels of RNA and individual circulating tumor cells. *Nat. Biotechnol.* 30, 777–782. doi: 10.1038/nbt.2282

Ranum, P. T., Goodwin, A. T., Yoshimura, H., Kolbe, D. L., Walls, W. D., Koh, J. Y., et al. (2019). Insights into the Biology of Hearing and Deafness Revealed by Single-Cell RNA Sequencing. *Cell Rep.* 26, 3160.e3–3171.e3.

Rao, D. A., Arazi, A., Wofsy, D., and Diamond, B. (2020). Design and application of single-cell RNA sequencing to study kidney immune cells in lupus nephritis. *Nat. Rev. Nephrol.* 16, 238–250. doi: 10.1038/s41581-019-0232-6

Romero-Carvajal, A., Navajas Acedo, J., Jiang, L., Kozlovskaja-Gumbriene, A., Alexander, R., Li, H., et al. (2015). Regeneration of sensory hair cells requires localized interactions between the notch and Wnt pathways. *Dev. Cell* 34, 267–282. doi: 10.1016/j.devcel.2015.05.025

Sachs, M. B., Young, E. D., and Lewis, R. H. (1974). Discharge patterns of single fibers in the pigeon auditory nerve. *Brain Res.* 70, 431–447. doi: 10.1016/0006-8993(74)90253-4

Sasagawa, Y., Danno, H., Takada, H., Ebisawa, M., Tanaka, K., Hayashi, T., et al. (2018). Quartz-Seq2: a high-throughput single-cell RNA-sequencing method that effectively uses limited sequence reads. *Genome Biol.* 19:29.

Sasagawa, Y., Nikaido, I., Hayashi, T., Danno, H., Uno, K. D., Imai, T., et al. (2013). Quartz-Seq: a highly reproducible and sensitive single-cell RNA sequencing method, reveals non-genetic gene-expression heterogeneity. *Genome Biol.* 14:R31.

Scheffer, D. I., Shen, J., Corey, D. P., and Chen, Z. Y. (2015). Gene expression by mouse inner ear hair cells during development. *J. Neurosci.* 35, 6366–6380. doi: 10.1523/jneurosci.5126-14.2015

Shapiro, E., Biezuner, T., and Linnarsson, S. (2013). Single-cell sequencing-based technologies will revolutionize whole-organism science. *Nat. Rev. Genet.* 14, 618–630. doi: 10.1038/nrg3542

Shearer, A. E., Eppsteiner, R. W., Booth, K. T., Ephraim, S. S., Gurrola, J. II, Simpson, A., et al. (2014). Utilizing ethnic-specific differences in minor allele frequency to recategorize reported pathogenic deafness variants. *Am. J. Hum. Genet.* 95, 445–453. doi: 10.1016/j.ajhg.2014.09.001

Shrestha, B. R., Chia, C., Wu, L., Kujawa, S. G., Liberman, M. C., and Goodrich, L. V. (2018). Sensory neuron diversity in the inner ear is shaped by activity. *Cell* 174, 1229.e17–1246.e17.

Simmons, D. D., Tong, B., Schrader, A. D., and Hornak, A. J. (2010). Oncomodulin identifies different hair cell types in the mammalian inner ear. *J. Comp. Neurol.* 518, 3785–3802. doi: 10.1002/cne.22424

Smallwood, S. A., Lee, H. J., Angermueller, C., Krueger, F., Saadeh, H., Peat, J., et al. (2014). Single-cell genome-wide bisulfite sequencing for assessing epigenetic heterogeneity. *Nat. Methods* 11, 817–820. doi: 10.1038/nmeth.3035

Spits, C., Le Caignec, C., De Rycke, M., Van Haute, L., Van Steirteghem, A., Liebaers, I., et al. (2006). Whole-genome multiple displacement amplification from single cells. *Nat. Protoc.* 1, 1965–1970. doi: 10.1038/nprot.2006.326

Steiner, A. B., Kim, T., Cabot, V., and Hudspeth, A. J. (2014). Dynamic gene expression by putative hair-cell progenitors during regeneration in the zebrafish lateral line. *Proc. Natl. Acad. Sci. U.S.A.* 111, E1393–E1401.

Sun, S. H., Babola, T., Pregernig, G., So, K. S., Nguyen, M., Su, S. S. M., et al. (2018). Hair cell mechanotransduction regulates spontaneous activity and spiral ganglion subtype specification in the auditory system. *Cell* 174, 1247.e15–1263.e15.

Szarama, K. B., Gavara, N., Petralia, R. S., Kelley, M. W., and Chadwick, R. S. (2012). Cytoskeletal changes in actin and microtubules underlie the developing surface mechanical properties of sensory and supporting cells in the mouse cochlea. *Development* 139, 2187–2197. doi: 10.1242/dev.073734

Tang, F., Barbacioru, C., Bao, S., Lee, C., Nordman, E., Wang, X., et al. (2010). Tracing the derivation of embryonic stem cells from the inner cell mass by single-cell RNA-Seq analysis. *Cell Stem Cell* 6, 468–478. doi: 10.1016/j.stem.2010.03.015

Tang, F., Barbacioru, C., Wang, Y., Nordman, E., Lee, C., Xu, N., et al. (2009). mRNA-Seq whole-transcriptome analysis of a single cell. *Nat. Methods* 6, 377–382. doi: 10.1038/nmeth.1315

Tang, P. C., Alex, A. L., Nie, J., Lee, J., Roth, A. A., Booth, K. T., et al. (2019). Defective Tmprss3-associated hair cell degeneration in inner ear organoids. *Stem Cell Rep.* 13, 147–162. doi: 10.1016/j.stemcr.2019.05.014

Tang, X., Huang, Y., Lei, J., Luo, H., and Zhu, X. (2019). The single-cell sequencing: new developments and medical applications. *Cell Biosci.* 9:53.

Temchin, A. N. (1988). Unusual discharge patterns of single fibers in the pigeon's auditory nerve. *J. Comp. Physiol. A* 163, 99–115. doi: 10.1007/bf00612001

Tilney, L. G., and Tilney, M. S. (1988). The actin filament content of hair cells of the bird cochlea is nearly constant even though the length, width, and number of stereocilia vary depending on the hair cell location. *J. Cell Biol.* 107, 2563–2574. doi: 10.1083/jcb.107.6.2563

Tilney, L. G., Tilney, M. S., and Derosier, D. J. (1992). Actin filaments, stereocilia, and hair cells: how cells count and measure. *Annu. Rev. Cell Biol.* 8, 257–274. doi: 10.1146/annurev.cb.08.110192.001353

Treutlein, B., Brownfield, D. G., Wu, A. R., Neff, N. F., Mantalas, G. L., Espinoza, F. H., et al. (2014). Reconstructing lineage hierarchies of the distal lung epithelium using single-cell RNA-seq. *Nature* 509, 371–375. doi: 10.1038/nature13173

Wagner, D. E., Weinreb, C., Collins, Z. M., Briggs, J. A., Megason, S. G., and Klein, A. M. (2018). Single-cell mapping of gene expression landscapes and lineage in the zebrafish embryo. *Science* 360, 981–987. doi: 10.1126/science.aar4362

Wang, M., Liu, X., Chang, G., Chen, Y., An, G., Yan, L., et al. (2018). Single-cell RNA sequencing analysis reveals sequential cell fate transition during human spermatogenesis. *Cell Stem Cell* 23, 599.e594–614.e594.

Wang, P., Chen, Y. D., Yong, J., Cui, Y. L., Wang, R., Wen, L., et al. (2018). Dissecting the global dynamic molecular profiles of human fetal kidney development by single-Cell RNA sequencing. *Cell Rep.* 24, 3554.e3–3567.e3.

Wang, T., Chai, R., Kim, G. S., Pham, N., Jansson, L., Nguyen, D. H., et al. (2015). Lgr5+ cells regenerate hair cells via proliferation and direct transdifferentiation in damaged neonatal mouse utricle. *Nat. Commun.* 6:6613.

Wangemann, P. (2002). K+ cycling and the endocochlear potential. *Hear. Res.* 165, 1–9. doi: 10.1016/s0378-5955(02)00279-4

Waqas, M., Guo, L., Zhang, S. S., Chen, Y., Zhang, X. L., Wang, L., et al. (2016a). Characterization of Lgr5+progenitor cell transcriptomes in the apical and basal turns of the mouse cochlea. *Oncotarget* 7, 41123–41141. doi: 10.18632/oncotarget.8636

Waqas, M., Zhang, S. S., He, Z. H., Tang, M. L., and Chai, R. J. (2016b). Role of Wnt and notch signaling in regulating hair cell regeneration in the cochlea. *Front. Med.* 10:237–249. doi: 10.1007/s11684-016-0464-9

Wright, M. I. (1973). Ototoxicity: a consideration of routes and mechanisms of hair cell damage associated with certain antibiotics and diuretics. *Proc. R Soc. Med.* 66, 189–193. doi: 10.1177/003591577306600241

Wu, J. F., Li, W. Y., Lin, C., Chen, Y., Cheng, C., Sun, S., et al. (2016). Co-regulation of the Notch and Wnt signaling pathways promotes supporting cell proliferation and hair cell regeneration in mouse utricles. *Sci. Rep.* 6:29418.

Yamashita, T., Zheng, F., Finkelstein, D., Kellard, Z., Robert, C., Rosencrance, C. D., et al. (2018). High-resolution transcriptional dissection of in vivo Atoh1-mediated hair cell conversion in mature cochleae identifies Isl1 as a coreprogramming factor. *PLoS Genet.* 14:e1007552. doi: 10.1371/journal.pgen.1007552

Yan, W. Q., Liu, W. W., Qi, J. Y., Fang, Q. J., Fan, Z. M., Sun, G. Y., et al. (2018). A Three-dimensional culture system with matrigel promotes purified spiral ganglion neuron survival and function in vitro. *Mol. Neurobiol.* 55, 2070–2084. doi: 10.1007/s12035-017 0471-0

Yao, Q., Wang, L., Mittal, R., Yan, D., Richmond, M. T., Denyer, S., et al. (2020). Transcriptomic analyses of inner ear sensory epithelia in Zebrafish. *Anat. Rec.* 303, 527–543. doi: 10.1002/ar.24331

You, D., Guo, L., Li, W. Y., Sun, S., Chen, Y., Chai, R. J., et al. (2018). Characterization of Wnt and notch-responsive Lgr5+hair cell progenitors in the striolar region of the neonatal mouse utricle. *Front. Mol. Neurosci.* 11:137. doi: 10.3389/fnmol.2018.00137

Zhang, S., Liu, D., Dong, Y., Zhang, Z., Zhang, Y., Zhou, H., et al. (2019). Frizzled-9+ supporting cells are progenitors for the generation of hair cells in the postnatal mouse cochlea. *Front. Mol. Neurosci.* 12:184. doi: 10.3389/fnmol.2019.00184

Zhang, S. S., Zhang, Y., Yu, P. F., Hu, Y., Zhou, H., Guo, L. N., et al. (2017). Characterization of Lgr5+progenitor cell transcriptomes after neomycin injury in the neonatal mouse cochlea. *Front. Mol. Neurosci.* 10:213. doi: 10.3389/fnmol.2017.00213

Zhang, Y. P., Guo, L., Lu, X. L., Cheng, C., Sun, S., Li, W., et al. (2018). Characterization of Lgr6+cells as an enriched population of hair cell progenitors compared to Lgr5+cells for hair cell generation in the neonatal mouse cochlea. *Front. Mol. Neurosci.* 11:147. doi: 10.3389/fnmol.2018.00147

Zheng, J. L., and Gao, W. Q. (2000). Overexpression of Math1 induces robust production of extra hair cells in postnatal rat inner ears. *Nat. Neurosci.* 3, 580–586. doi: 10.1038/75753

Zhong, C., Fu, Y., Pan, W., Yu, J., and Wang, J. (2019). Atoh1 and other related key regulators in the development of auditory sensory epithelium in the mammalian inner ear: function and interplay. *Dev. Biol.* 446, 133–141. doi: 10.1016/j.ydbio.2018.12.025

Zhu, Y., Scheibinger, M., Ellwanger, D. C., Krey, J. F., Choi, D., Kelly, R. T., et al. (2019). Single-cell proteomics reveals changes in expression during hair-cell development. *Elife* 8:e50777.

Zong, C., Lu, S., Chapman, A. R., and Xie, X. S. (2012). Genome-wide detection of single-nucleotide and copy-number variations of a single human cell. *Science* 338, 1622–1626. doi: 10.1126/science.1229164

Zwislocki, J. J. (1975). Phase opposition between inner and outer hair cells and auditory sound analysis. *Audiology* 14, 443–455. doi: 10.3109/00206097509071755

High Resolution and Labeling Free Studying the 3D Microstructure of the Pars Tensa-Annulus Unit of Mice

Jian-Ping Wu[1,2†‡], Xiaojie Yang[2†‡], Yilin Wang[3], Ben Swift[4†], Robert Adamson[5], Yongchang Zheng[6†], Rongli Zhang[7], Wen Zhong[8] and Fangyi Chen[2,9*†]*

[1] Academy of Advanced Interdisciplinary Studies, Southern University of Science and Technology, Shenzhen, China, [2] Department of Biomedical Engineering, Southern University of Science and Technology, Shenzhen, China, [3] Core Research Facilities, Southern University of Science and Technology, Shenzhen, China, [4] College of Computing, Australian National University, Canberra, ACT, Australia, [5] School of Biomedical Engineering, Electrical and Computer Engineering, Dalhousie University, Halifax, NS, Canada, [6] Peking Union Medical College Hospital, Chinese Academy of Medical Sciences and Peking Union Medical College, Beijing, China, [7] Guangdong Provincial People's Hospital, Guangdong Academy of Medical Science, School of Medicine, South China University of Technology, Guangzhou, China, [8] School of Mechanical Engineering and Automation, Xihua University, Chengdu, China, [9] Department of Biology, Brain Research Centre, Southern University of Science and Technology, Shenzhen, China

***Correspondence:**
Jian-Ping Wu
jianpingliwu@outlook.com
Fangyi Chen
chenfy@sustech.edu.cn

†ORCID:
Jian-Ping Wu
orcid.org/0000-0003-4725-2398
Xiaojie Yang
orcid.org/0000-0003-0551-6252
Ben Swift
orcid.org/0000-0003-2138-5969
Yongchang Zheng
orcid.org/0000-0002-5916-2392
Fangyi Chen
orcid.org/0000-0002-5024-6215

‡These authors have contributed equally to this work

Hearing loss is a serious illness affecting people's normal life enormously. The acoustic properties of a tympanic membrane play an important role in hearing, and highly depend on its geometry, composition, microstructure and connection to the surrounding annulus. While the conical geometry of the tympanic membrane is critical to the sound propagation in the auditory system, it presents significant challenges to the study of the 3D microstructure of the tympanic membrane using traditional 2D imaging techniques. To date, most of our knowledge about the 3D microstructure and composition of tympanic membranes is built from 2D microscopic studies, which precludes an accurate understanding of the 3D microstructure, acoustic behaviors and biology of the tissue. Although the tympanic membrane has been reported to contain elastic fibers, the morphological characteristic of the elastic fibers and the spatial arrangement of the elastic fibers with the predominant collagen fibers have not been shown in images. We have developed a 3D imaging technique for the three-dimensional examination of the microstructure of the full thickness of the tympanic membranes in mice without requiring tissue dehydration and stain. We have also used this imaging technique to study the 3D arrangement of the collagen and elastic fibrillar network with the capillaries and cells in the pars tensa-annulus unit at a status close to the native. The most striking findings in the study are the discovery of the 3D form of the elastic and collagen network, and the close spatial relationships between the elastic fibers and the elongated fibroblasts in the tympanic membranes. The 3D imaging technique has enabled to show the 3D waveform contour of the collagen and elastic scaffold in the conical tympanic membrane. Given the close relationship among the acoustic properties, composition, 3D microstructure and geometry of tympanic membranes, the findings may advance the understanding of the structure—acoustic functionality of the tympanic membrane. The knowledge will also be very helpful in the development of advanced cellular therapeutic technologies and 3D printing techniques to restore damaged tympanic membranes to a status close to the native.

Keywords: tympanic membrane, pars tensa-annulus unit, 3D microstructure, collagen, elastic fibres

INTRODUCTION

The tympanic membrane (TM) receives and converts sound-pressure waves over a broad frequency spectrum from the external environment into mechanical vibrations, which are conducted through the ossicular chain resulting in movement of perilymph and neural transduction in the hair cells of cochlea (Decraemer et al., 1991; Caminos et al., 2018). Damage, perforation and degeneration of the TM due to injury, otitis media and aging are leading causes of hearing impairment and deafness, with obvious impacts on an individual's life quality.

In mammals, the TM appears as a shallow conical dish with the apex toward the medial side. It consists of two distinctive parts known as the pars flaccida and pars tensa (Lim, 1968, 1970, 1995), as shown in **Figure 1A**. Across the thickness, a TM comprises three distinctive layers; the external epidermal layer, the fibrous lamina propria and internal mucosal layer (Igarashi and Kawamata, 1993; Lim, 1995). The fibrous lamina propria, which is composed predominantly of collagen fibers, largely determines the shape and mechanical behaviors of the TM (Secondi, 1951; Funnell and Laszlo, 1982; Lim, 1995; Stenfeldt et al., 2006). The lamina propria of the pars flaccida is made of loose collagen (Lim, 1995). In contrast, the lamina propria within the pars tensa consists of collagen fibers organized into radial and circumferential arrays, respectively, in the lateral and medial side of the TM (Uno, 2000; Fay et al., 2006; Jackson et al., 2008; Liu et al., 2016). Despite extensive research, the unique arrangement of the collagen fibers in the physiology of TMs remains exclusive. TMs also contain a small fraction of elastic fibers (Chole and Kodama, 1989; Lim, 1995; Volandri et al., 2011) but the microstructural features of the elastic fibers and the spatial relationship of the elastic fibers with the cells, collagen fibers and capillaries have not yet been shown in images.

While physically coupling to the manubrium of the malleus in the ossicular chain and anchoring itself on the cartilaginous annulus of the bony tympanic ring attached to the bulla, the pars tensa makes up the majority of the TM (De Greef et al., 2016). The morphology, composition and microstructure of the pars tensa as well as its connection to the annulus are considered to play a crucial role in the acoustic function of TMs (De Greef et al., 2014; Kozin et al., 2016). Although the conical shape of TMs is critical to the sound propagation of the TMs (Decraemer et al., 1991; Fay et al., 2006), it creates significant impediment to study the 3D microstructure and composition of the TMs using conventional 2D microscopy.

Various technologies have been developed to study the morphology, composition and microstructure of TMs. Conventional histology is routinely used in identifying the pathological changes of TMs at a cellular level (Stenfeldt et al., 2006). However, the use of traditional optical microscopy with insufficient imaging resolution restricts the application of the technique from revealing the ultrastructure of the collagen fibers and subtle microstructural change of TMs beyond a subcellular level. Alternatively, the electron microscopy (EM) has superior imaging resolution for tracing the ultrastructure of the TMs (Igarashi and Kawamata, 1993; Lim, 1995; Uno, 2000) but it requires an extreme imaging environment, which could denaturize the form of the TMs and potentially introduce artifacts. Besides, none of these technologies is capable of imaging the microstructure and composition of the brittle and conical TMs. To date, knowledge about the composition and 3D microstructure of TMs has primarily been built from studies using 2D imaging technologies. This has prevented deep understanding of the 3D microstructure, acoustic properties and biology of TMs.

Multiphoton microscopy (MPM) offers submicron imaging resolution for studying three-dimensionally the intrinsic microstructure of biological tissues without tissue stain, dehydration and sectioning (He et al., 2013c; Pang et al., 2017; Wu et al., 2017). MPM harnesses non-linear optical imaging technologies that detect the photons emitted from featured molecular compounds under the laser excitation at the near-infrared spectrum. This guarantees that the emitted photons only occur at the focal plane for 3D imaging the microstructure of biological tissues without a pinhole. Second harmonic generation (SHG) and two-photon fluorescence (TPF) imaging are the two primary imaging modalities used in modern MPM. The SHG signals arise from non-absorptive tissue-light interaction of substances possessing a non-centrosymmetrical and crystallized molecular structure (Prockop and Kivirikko, 1995), such as collagen, which produces a large quantity of SHG signals under two-photon excitation for SHG imaging without photobleaching (Campagnola and Loew, 2003; Cox et al., 2003; Chen et al., 2012; Wu et al., 2017).

In comparison, TPF utilizes two-photon excitation to generate the endogenous fluorescence of tissues (Cahalan et al., 2002; Koch et al., 2014). One of the important applications of TPF in biology is to study the elastic fibers of tissues through the autofluorescence emission of the fluorophores presenting in the elastin under two-photon excitation (König et al., 2005; Mansfield et al., 2009; He et al., 2013b,c, 2014). By comprising a central core of elastin attached by microfibrils, elastic fibers endow the tissues with the elasticity required to recover quickly from deformation to eliminate fatigue damages, while also influence the biological function and physiology of the tissues (Montes, 1996; Debelle and Tamburro, 1999). Elastin is well present in cell membranes, the walls of blood vessels and extracellular matrix (ECM) of many tissues such as lungs, skin, tendons and cartilage (Curran et al., 1993; Li et al., 1998; He et al., 2013a,b; Pang et al., 2017). Therefore, TPF is an ideal tool for visualizing cells and capillaries without tissue dehydration and stain (Zheng et al., 2011). Numerous studies have applied SHG and TPF for examining the spatial network of collagen with the elastic fibers and cells without tissue dehydration and stain (Zoumi et al., 2004; Mansfield et al., 2009; He et al., 2013a,b,c; Pang et al., 2017).

Using SHG and TPF, we have developed a 3D imaging technique for label-free imaging of the 3D microstructure of hydrated and full-thickness TMs in mice. The study has led to reveal the intrinsic collagen structure and the spatial arrangement of the collagen with the elastic fibers, fibroblasts, vimentin positive cells, capillaries and chondrocytes in the pars tensa-annulus unit. The high-resolution images of the collagen fibers have also provided the opportunity to perform quantitative analysis of the orientation of the collagen fibers

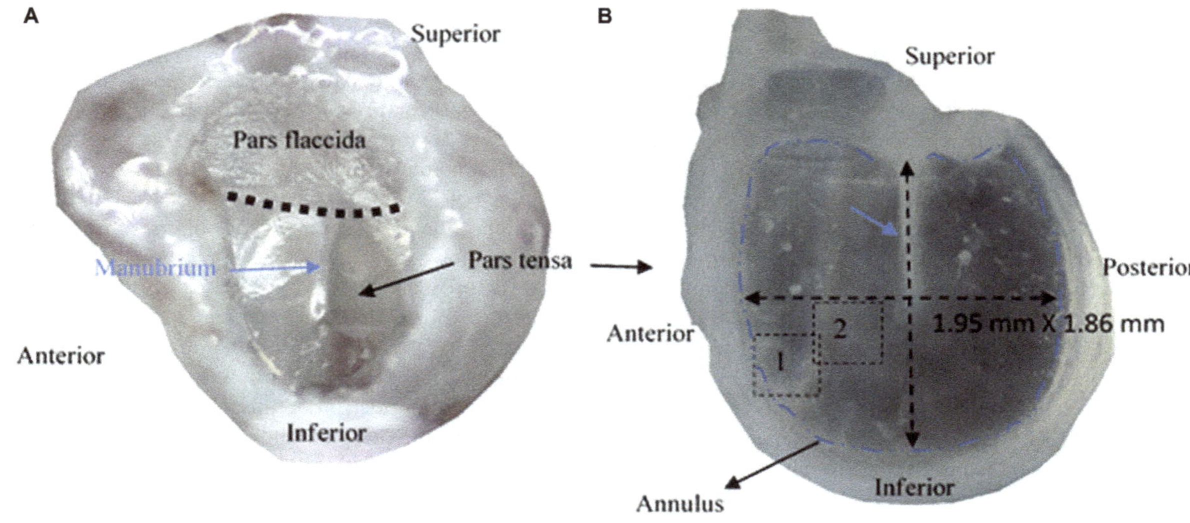

FIGURE 1 | Photographs of tympanic membranes of mice. **(A)** A tympanic membrane of a mouse is typically made of pars flaccida and pars tensa. **(B)** The pars tensa attached with the anulus was extracted for studying the 3D microstructure using multiphoton microscopy.

comprising the pars tensa for a consistent description of the collagen orientation.

We believe this is the first study that has characterized simultaneously the elastic fibrillar network and the intrinsic microstructure of the collagen with the elastic fibers, cells and capillaries in the pars tensa-annulus unit at a status close to the native. This study has advanced our knowledge about the 3D microstructure and composition of the pars tensa-annulus unit and the connection between the pars tensa and annulus. The knowledge will be useful to the understanding of the acoustic function and biology of TMs, and development of advanced cellular therapy and 3D printing technologies to restore perforated TMs to an extension close to the native.

MATERIALS AND METHODS

Samples

Ex vivo mouse TM samples used in this study were donated by other unrelated research in accordance with approvals from the Animal Ethics Committee at Southern University of Science and Technology, Shenzhen, China. A total of five bullae with a normal appearance were harvested from five C57 mice (two females, three males) of 10–12 weeks old. The bullae were washed thoroughly with neutral phosphate buffered solution (PBS) and fixed in 4% paraformaldehyde for 24 hours before being decalcified in 10% ethylene diamine tetra acetic acid (EDTA) (Phygene Biotechnology, Fuzhou, China) for 48 hours. After washing the bullae with neutral PBS, with the aid of a stereoscope, the TMs were dissected from the bullae with the cartilaginous annulus attached (**Figure 1**) before the epidermal and mucosal layers of the TMs were carefully removed from the TMs using a surgical knife and tweezers. Only the lamina propria without visible fiber broken under the stereoscope was used as the sample.

After cleaning with PBS, the samples were carefully placed on a glass slide with the medial side up and coated a drop of PBS before covered with a coverslip for SHG and TPF imaging. During imaging, the tissues were kept in a hydrated status.

Imaging Acquisition and Thickness Measurement of Collagen Fibers and Fibrils

An Olympus FVMPE-RS upright MPM (Olympus, Japan) with an apochromatic 25 × /NA 1.05 water-immersion objective lens offering a 2.0 mm working distance (Olympus, Japan) was used in this study. The MPM is equipped with a femtosecond-pulsed Ti:Sa laser (Mai Tai DeepSee, Spectral-Physics, United States) with a tunable wavelength range from 690 to 1,300 nm.

The SHG and TPF imaging were performed by tuning the excitation laser at 890 nm and fitting a filter cube (Chroma Technology, China) with a 475 nm dichroic mirror, a green barrier filter of 495–540 nm and a violet barrier filter of 410–455 nm. In this configuration, the emission light was split into two independent imaging channels for acquiring green-fluorescence and SHG image stacks through the photomultiplier tubes (PMT). The resultant green fluorescence channel at the emission wavelength of 495–540 nm was assigned for TPF imaging. The violet imaging channel was set up in a reflectance mode and used for acquiring SHG images at 445 nm, which is exactly half the wavelength of the excitation.

For studying the collagen and elastic fibers within the pars tensa-annulus unit, the SHG and TPF imaging stacks were acquired simultaneously at pixel resolution of 1,024 × 1,024 over the field of the view of about 509 μm × 509 μm. High magnification SHG imaging stacks at the field of the view of

127 μm × 127 μm were also acquired at the pars tensa (the dashed square shown in **Figure 4A**) to verify that the coast collagen fibers or bundles constituting the pars tensa were composed of the subclass collagen fibrils (e.g., **Figure 7**). The imaging step used to acquire the imaging stacks was set at 0.5 μm.

The gray level intensity distribution graphs of the thickness of the collagen fibers and fibrils comprising the pars tensa were plotted, as shown in **Figure 8**. The full width at half maximum (FWAHM) intensity was used to determine the thickness of the collagen fibers and fibrils.

Reconstructing 3D and Maximum Brightness Images

ImageJ (Rasband, 1997-2014) was used to reconstruct the SHG and TPF imaging stacks into 3D images to study the microstructure of the pars tensa-annulus unit (e.g., **Figures 2, 3**) and the tissue near the center of the TMs (**Figure 5**). For further studying the subtle internal features within the tissues, imaging stacks representing the microstructure of the full thickness tissues have also been optically subdivided into several smaller imaging stacks to reconstruct the maximum brightness images (MBI), as shown in **Figures 4, 6**. Here, an MBI is built by combining the pixels with the maximum intensity within a series of 2D images along the lateral-medial axis of the TM. Therefore, it represents a view of all the data in the 2D imaging series as if the imaging sequence were combined into a single image containing only the in-focus data.

Quantify the Orientation of Collagen Constituting the Pars Tensa

Quantitative imaging analysis of the orientation of the collagen fibers comprising the pars tensa allows for greater consistency in describing the orientation characteristics over the subjective visual inspection. OrientationJ in ImageJ (Rezakhaniha et al., 2012) was used to quantify the orientation and coherency features of the collagen fibers constituting the pars tensa across the thickness from the lateral to medial direction. OreintationJ applies structural tensors to measure the gray level of pixels in the local neighborhood to determine the isotropic or anisotropic features in the image (Jähne, 1993; Jahne, 1997; Wu et al., 2017). Pixels with a high value indicate anisotropic features, whilst pixels with a low value represent isotropic features.

The SHG imaging stacks contain the spatial information of the collagen fibers comprising the pars tensa from the lateral to medial side. Therefore, OrientationJ has enabled quantifying (three-dimensionally) the orientation of the collagen fibers comprising the pars tensa across its thickness. Because the collagen scaffold in the pars tensa has a conical shape and the wall of the cone has a waveform contour (black arrows, **Figures 2, 3**), the collagen scaffold was subdivided into five regions of interest (ROI) (white boxes, **Figure 9A**) to conduct the fiber orientation and coherency analysis. The fiber orientation is shown in degrees from −90° to 90° in relation to the x axis (**Figure 9A**). The coherency has a value between zero and one. A value of one indicates the fibers are highly coherent whilst a value of zero indicates the fibers are extremely incoherent.

Fast Fourier transform (FFT) is a well-known mathematic procedure for efficiently identifying of the isotropic or anisotropic features in an image. FFT converts data in the spatial domain into the frequency domain, which makes it possible to efficiently identify the features in an image. FFT has also been used to objectively describe the orientation of the collagen fibers comprising the pars tensa (e.g., **Figure 9C**).

RESULTS

3D Microstructure of the Tympanic Membrane-Annulus Unit

Figures 2, 3 are representative 3D images of SHG (green) and TPF (red), showing the typical 3D collagen (green) and elastic (red) fibrillar network with the capillaries and cells (red) in the pars tensa-annulus (at region 1 of **Figure 1B**). The 3D TPF images (red) mainly illustrate the elastic fibrillar network (orange arrows in **Figure 2E**), the fibroblasts (black arrow heads in **Figures 2E,F**), capillaries (double white arrows in **Figures 2B,F**) and annulus chondrocytes in the pars tensa-annulus unit. **Figures 2C,F** dedicate the 3D composition of the collagen network (green) with the fibroblasts, capillaries and chondrocytes in the pars tensa-annulus unit. Unfortunately, the elastic fibers in the pars tensa are buried in the predominant collagen fibers in the merged images.

Collagen Network

The typical 3D collagen network of the pars tensa-annulus unit is shown in **Figures 2A,D**. At the lateral side (**Figure 2A**), the collagen fibers comprising the pars tensa orient three-dimensionally in a primary direction radial toward the TM center. The radial fibers become thinner and thinner as they run toward the TM center. At the medial side (**Figure 2B**), the collagen fibers orient predominantly in a circumferential direction. These circumferential collagen fibers (green) originate from the annulus (**Figure 2F**). Nevertheless, the radial and circumferential fibers appear to braid with each other to form the 3D collagenous network of the pars tensa, whilst some oblique and parabolic collagen fibers (white arrows in **Figures 2A,C,D,F, 3B, 4A,B**) are observed among the predominated radial and circumferential fibers.

It is worth noting that the 3D collagen scaffold of the pars tensa demonstrates a waveform contour (long back arrows, **Figures 2A,C,D, 3A**). The capillary network (double white arrows in **Figures 2B,F**) is contained within the medial side of the pars tensa (**Figures 2F, 3A**) to conform to the contour of the collagen scaffold (green, **Figures 3A,C**).

Elastic Fibers, Capillary and Cells

Without tissue stain, the TPF images (red) document the elastic fibers (orange arrows in **Figure 2E**, white arrow heads in **Figures 4D–F,J–L**), spindle fibroblasts (black arrow heads, **Figures 2E,F**), the capillary network (double white arrows, **Figure 2B**), vimentin positive cells (blue arrows, **Figures 4D–F,J–L**) and annulus chondrocytes (black arrow in **Figure 4J**) in the pars tensa-annulus unit. The spindle shape fibroblasts

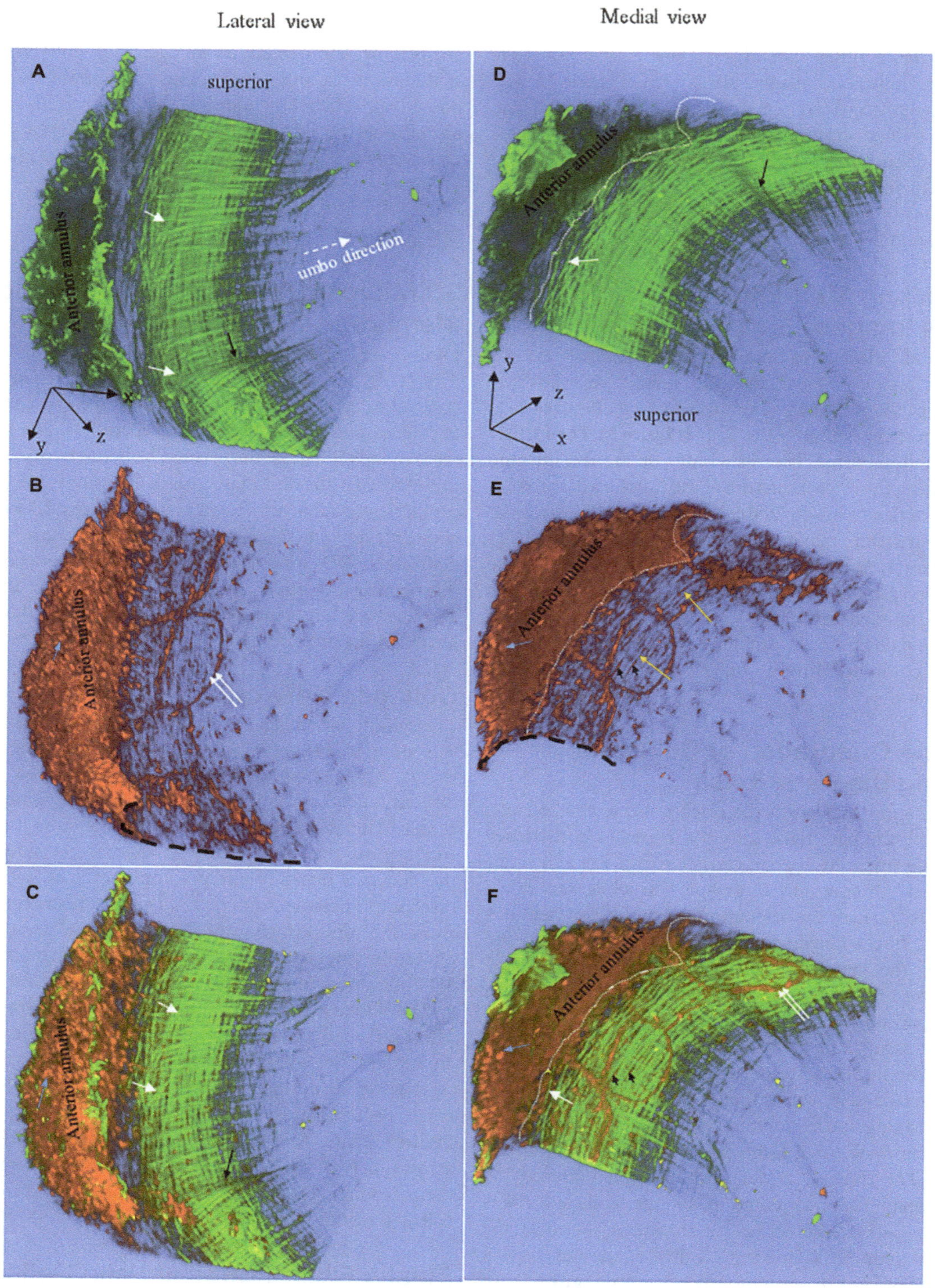

FIGURE 2 | Representative 3D images of the anterior pars tensa-annulus unit reconstructed from SHG (green) and TPF (red) image stacks. **(A,D)** The lateral and medial view of the 3D collagen network. **(B,E)** The lateral and medial view of the 3D microstructure of the capillaries (double white arrows), elastic fibers (orange arrows), fibroblasts (black arrowheads) and annulus chondrocytes (blue arrows). **(C,F)** The merged images dedicate the 3D microstructure arrangement of the collagen network (green) with capillaries (double white arrows), fibroblasts (black arrowheads) and annulus chondrocytes (blue arrows). The 3D collagen network of the pars tensa notably exhibits a waveform contour [black arrows, panels **(A,C)**]. The white dash line draws approximately the boundary between the pars tensa and annulus. Field of the view: 509 × 509 μm^2.

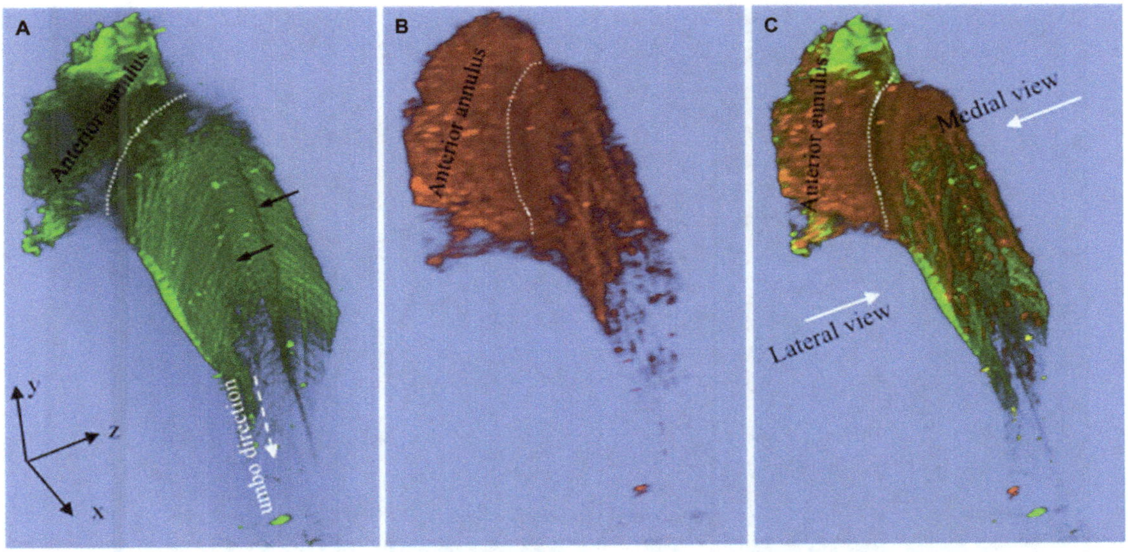

FIGURE 3 | (A) The superior view of the 3D collagen scaffold (green) of the anterior pars tensa-annulus unit. The collagen scaffold in the pars tensa has a notable waveform contour (black arrows). **(B)** The corresponding TPF shows the capillary network and annulus chondrocytes of the parse tensa-annulus unit. **(C)** The merged image shows the capillary network (red) runs along the medial side and conforms to the collagen network (green). Field of the view: 509 × 509 μm^2.

(black arrow heads, in **Figure 2E**) and circumferential elastic fibers (orange arrows) are within the pars tensa and connected into series compliant to the circumferential collagen fibers (**Figure 4L**). The capillaries (double white arrows, **Figures 4E,K**) were seen to contain hemoglobin (hollow arrows, **Figures 4D–F,K**). The TM annulus is a fibrocartilage tissue so that it contains massive chondrocytes.

The elastic fibers in the pars tensa can be seen in more detail in **Figures 4D–F,J,K**. As shown, the elastic fibers orient in both the radial (yellow arrowheads, **Figures 4D,J**) and circumferential (white arrowheads) direction. **Figure 4L** further confirms the co-existence of collagen (green) and elastic fibers in the pars tensa at the circumferential (white arrowheads) and radial direction (yellow arrowheads).

The 3D Microstructure of the Pars Tensa Near the Tympanic Membrane Center

As shown in **Figures 5A,B**, as approaching the TM center (region 2, **Figure 1B**), the collagen network becomes much thinner, resembling "a waving collagenous flag" composed of fine collagen fibers running in the radial (white arrowheads, in **Figure 5A**) and circumferential (white arrows, **Figure 5A**) direction. The corresponding TPF images (**Figures 5B,E**) reveal the fine elastic fibers (white arrows), blood vessels (oval arrows) and vimentin positive cells in various shapes (hollow arrows). The integration of the 3D collagen network (green) with the vimentin positive cells, blood vessels and elastic fibers are shown in **Figures 5C,F**. Clearly, the tissues near the TM center contain more vimentin positive cells than those near the annulus.

The more detailed morphological characteristics of the micro components of the tissue near the TM center are shown in **Figure 6**. As confirmed in **Figure 6A**, the radial collagen fibers (blue arrowheads, **Figures 6A,C**) run continuously toward the TM center while they braid frequently with the circumferential fiber (blue arrows, **Figures 6A,C**). The corresponding TPF image (red, **Figure 6B**) shows in more detail the morphology of the blood vessels (oval arrow), fine radial (white arrows) and circumferential (blue arrows) elastic fibers, vimentin positive cells (hollow arrows) and the nucleus of the vimentin positive cells (diamond arrows). **Figure 6D** is an enlarged image from region 1 in **Figure 6C** that shows the detailed colocalization of the fine collagen fibers (green) with the elastic fibers (white arrows), vimentin positive cells (hollow arrows and the nucleus of vimentin positive cells (diamond arrows).

Collagen Fibers and Fibrils

High magnification SHG images (**Figure 7**) acquired at the dashed square in **Figure 4A** have verified that the thick collagen fibers (double headed arrows) at the periphery of the pars tensa are made of the subclass collagen fibrils (white and black arrows). As shown in **Figure 8**, the collagen fibers are 5.49 ± 1.98 μm thick and the collagen fibrils are 1.16 ± 0.28 μm thick. The collagen fibrils orient in the radial and circumferential direction approximately compliant with the collagen fibers.

Microstructural Integration of Pars Tensa and Annulus

The spatial microstructural integration between the pars tensa and annulus is shown in **Figures 2C,F**, **3C** while the detailed connection mechanism between the two parts is shown in **Figures 4A,D,G** (indicated by *). The oblique and circumferential collagen fibers (white arrows, **Figure 4A**) are originated from the fibrocartilage annulus containing dense round chondrocytes (red, **Figure 4G**) and they are continued into the collagen network of

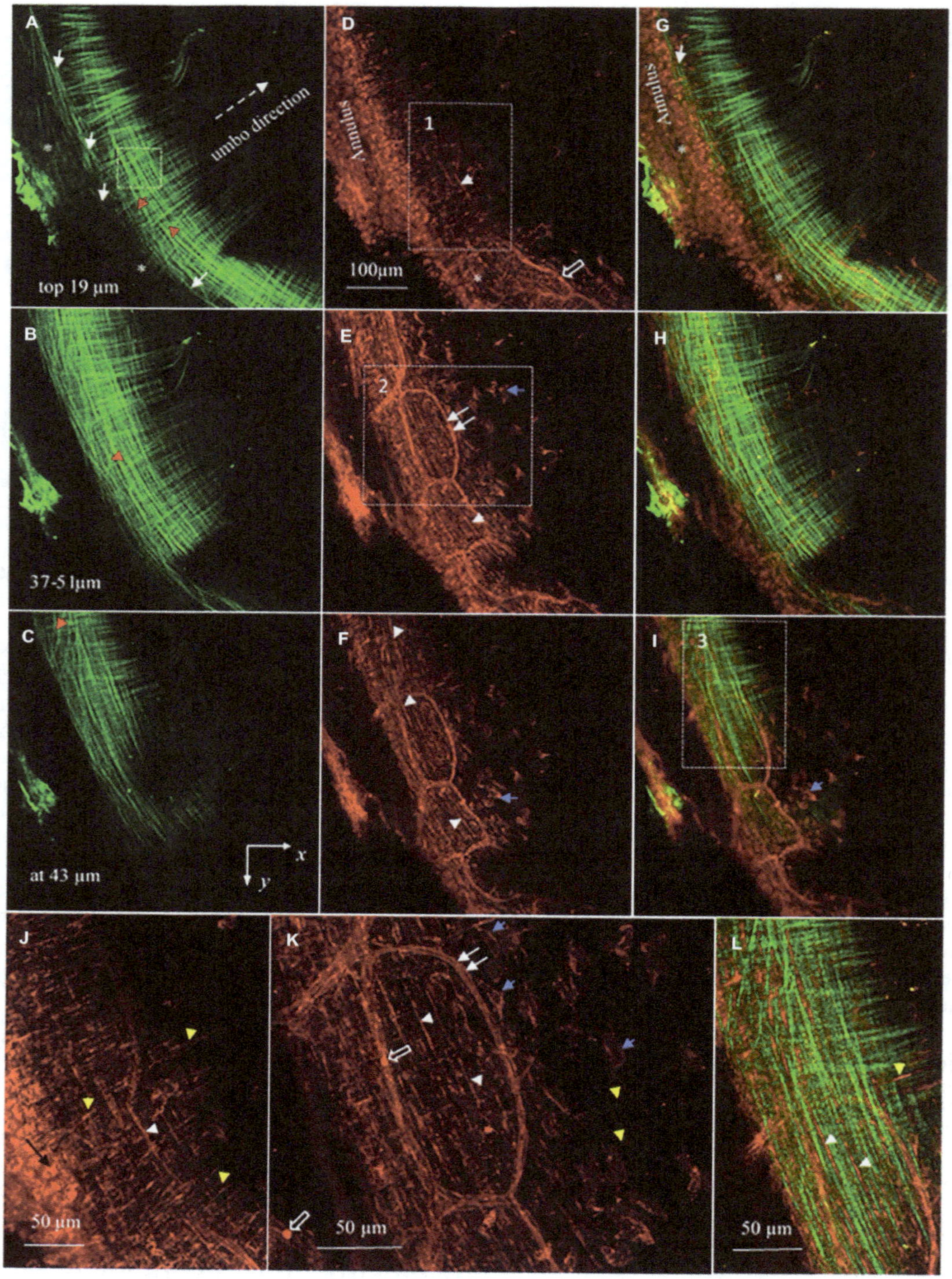

FIGURE 4 | Maximum brightness images of the pars tensa annulus unit. **(A–C)** Maximum brightness images of SHG at different depths across the thickness of the pars tensa-annulus unit confirm that the collagen fibers constituting the parse tensa orient predominantly in the radial and circumferential direction, and the pars tensa and annulus are connected by collagen [* and white arrows, panels **(A,G)**]. Nevertheless, oblique and parabolic collagen fibers (red arrowheads) exist among the predominant radial and circumferential fibers. **(D–F)** The corresponding MBIs from TPF show the elastic fibers (white arrowheads), capillaries (double white arrows) with the hemoglobin (hollow arrow), vimentin positive cells (blue arrows) and annulus chondrocytes in the pars tensa-annulus unit. **(G–I)** The merged images highlight the integration of the collagen (green) with the chondrocytes, capillaries and vimentin cells (blue arrows) in the pars tensa-annulus unit. **(J)** An enlarged image extracted from region 1 in panel **(D)** showing in more detail the radial (yellow arrowheads) and circumferential (white arrowheads) elastic fibers and chondrocytes (black arrow) in the pars tensa–annulus unit. **(K)** An enlarged image extracted from region 2 in panel **(E)** showing in more detail the skeleton

(Continued)

FIGURE 4 | (Continued)
of vimentin positive cells (blue arrows), radial (yellow arrow heads) and circumferential (white arrow heads) elastic fibers and capillaries (double white arrows) with the hemoglobin (hollow arrows). **(L)** An enlarged image extracted from region 3 in panel **(I)** confirms that the pars tensa contains both the collagen fibers (green) and elastic fibers (white and yellow arrowheads) in the radial and circumferential direction.

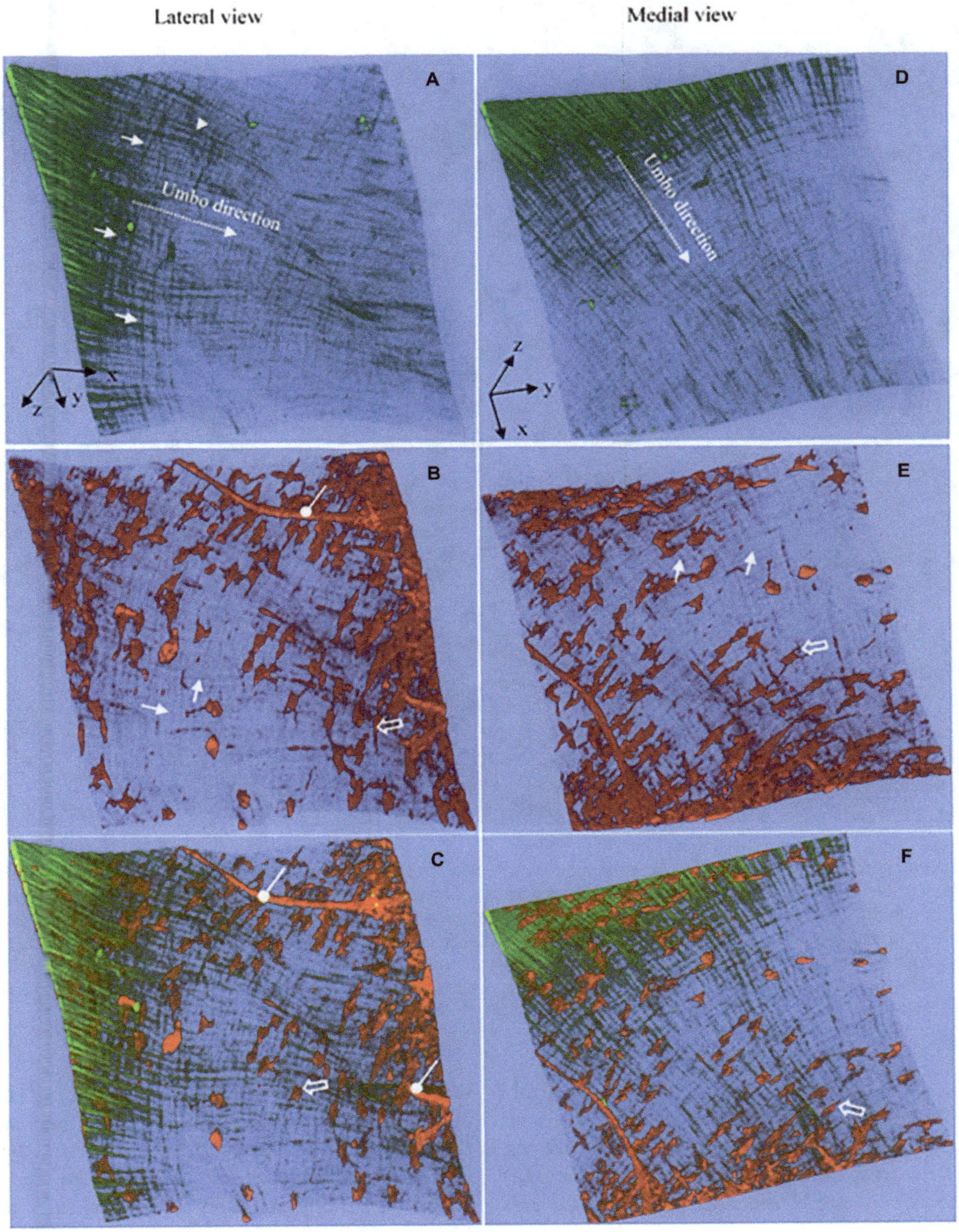

FIGURE 5 | Representative 3D images reconstructed from the SHG and TPF imaging stacks of the pars tensa near the TM center. **(A,D)** The 3D collagen framework of the pars tensa near the TM center. **(B,E)** The corresponding TPF images show the capillaries (oval arrows), vimentin positive cells in various shapes (hollow arrow) and elastic fibers (white arrows) running in the radial and circumferential direction. **(C,F)** The merged images highlight the colocalization of the collagen (green) with the elastic fibers, vimentin positive cells and capillaries. The collagen fibers become progressively thinner approaching to the TM center so that the collagen network (green) appears as "a wave collagen flag" scattered with the vimentin positive cells and capillaries. Field of the view: 509 × 509 μm^2.

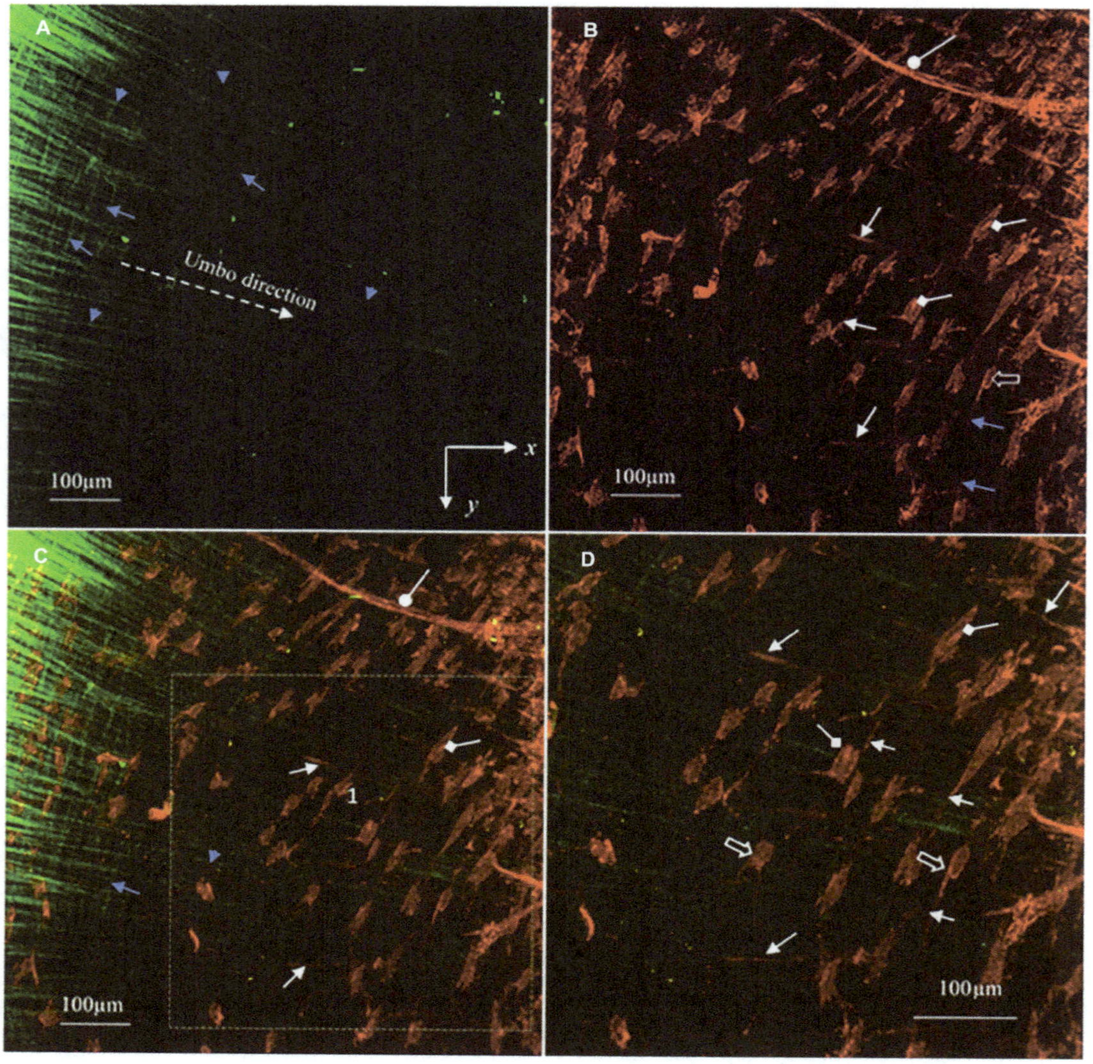

FIGURE 6 | MBIs reconstructed from the image stacks in **Figure 5** show in more detail the characteristics of the collagen (green), elastic fibers (white arrows), vimentin positive cells (hollow arrows), cell nuclei (diamond arrows) and capillaries (oval arrows) of the pars tensa near the TM center. **(A)** The collagen fibers gradually become finer approaching the TM center. **(B)** The corresponding TPF image shows the elastic fibers (white arrows), capillaries (oval arrow) and vimentin positive cells (hollow arrow) with the nuclei (diamond arrow). **(C)** The merged image dedicates the composition of the collagen fibers (green) with the cells, capillaries and elastic fibers. **(D)** An enlarged image extracted from region 1 of panel **(C)** highlight the characteristics of the fine collagen fibrils (green), elastic fibers (white arrows), vimentin positive cells (hollow arrow) and the cell nuclei (diamond arrow) of the pars tensa near the TM center. There is an apparent increase of the population of the vimentin positive cells near the TM center.

the pars tensa. The radial collagen fibers of the pars tensa firmly connect to the oblique and parabolic/circumferential collagen fibers at the border with the annulus (* and white arrows, **Figures 4A,G**). The corresponding TPF images (**Figures 4D,J**) confirm the connection of the elastic fibers between the pars tensa and annulus.

Quantitative Analysis of the Orientation of the Collagen Fibers

The quantitative analysis on the orientation of the collagen fibers comprising the pars tensa (**Figure 9A**) confirms that from the lateral to medial direction of the TMs the collagen fibers orient into two distinctive direction (long dashed arrows indicated in **Figure 9B**). This is consistent with the visual observations that across the thickness of the pars tensa the collagen fibers change from the radial orientation to the circumferential orientation. The FFT analysis also indicates that the collagen fibers comprising the pars tensa are largely oriented in two distinct directions approximately perpendicular to each other (double headed arrows in **Figure 9C**).

The coherency analysis (**Figure 9D**) shows that the collagen fibers comprising the pars tensa have a low coherency value below 0.2. This is consistent with the fact that the radial collagen fibers run approximately toward the TM center while

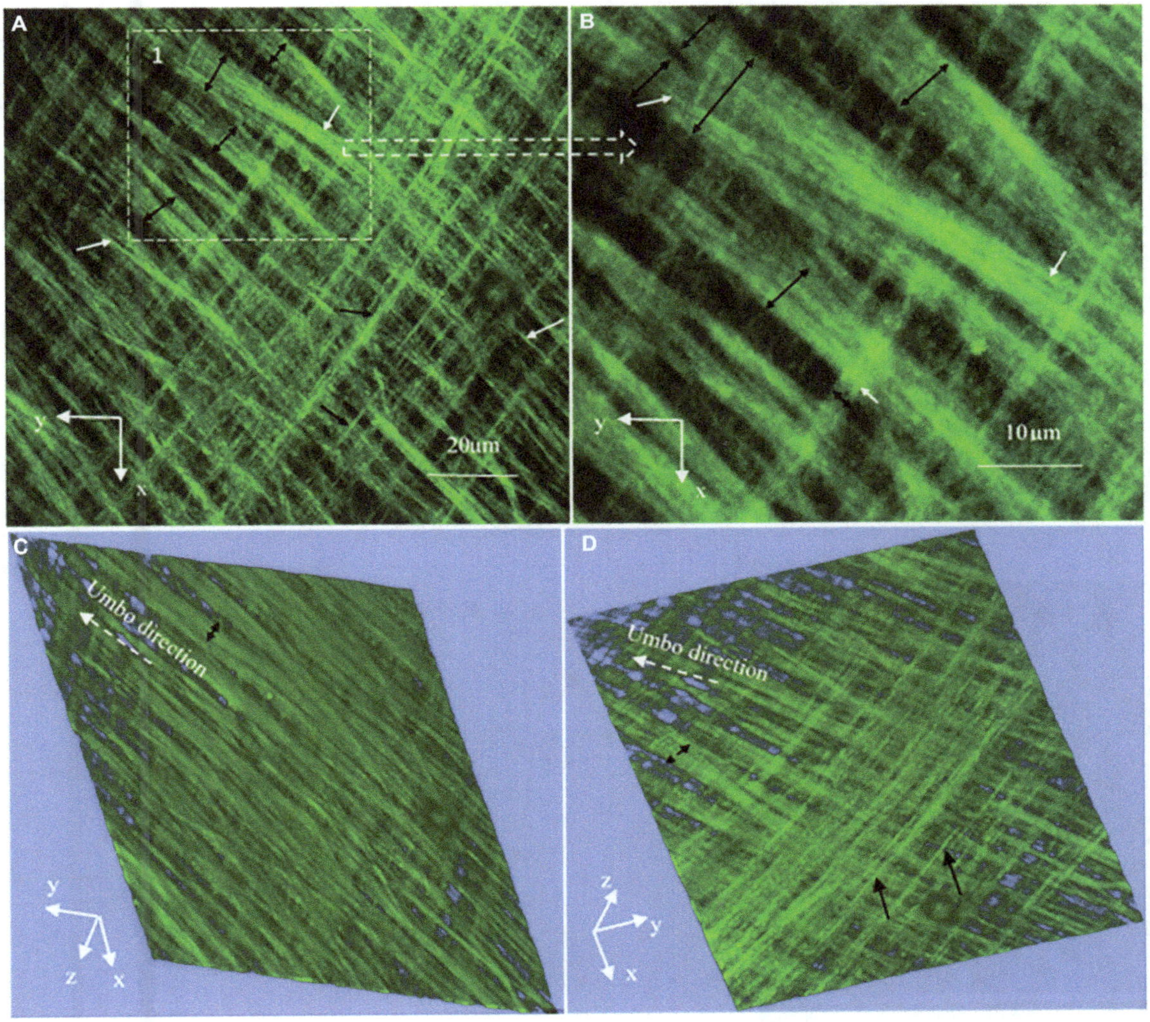

FIGURE 7 | High magnification SHG images (at a 127 × 127 μm^2 field of the view) at the periphery of the TM pars tensa (approximately at region 1 in **Figure 4A**). **(A)** The high magnification observations verify that the thick collagen fibers (double headed black arrows) of the periphery of the pars tensa are composed of the subclass collagen fibrils in the corresponding radial (white arrows) and circumferential (black arrows) direction. **(B)** An enlarged image extracted from region 1 of panel **(A)** shows in more detail that the collagen fibers (black double headed arrows) comprise the subclass collagen fibrils (white arrows). **(B,C)** The corresponding 3D images in the lateral **(C)** and medial **(D)** direction.

the circumferential collagen fibers align approximately around the TM center. While the fibers in the two directions intensively braid with each other, neither the radial nor the circumferential fibers align parallel, resulting in the low coherency value. Also, the small portion of oblique and parabolic collagen fibers in the pars tensa has also contributed to the low coherency value.

DISCUSSION

Perforation or pathology of TMs is a serious medical condition leading to conductive hearing impairment and deafness if left untreated. Despite great efforts and advances in the research and development of collagen scaffold-based tissues engineering, 3D printing technologies and surgical interventions in the repairs of TMs, the outcomes are not yet satisfactory. This may be attributed to a lack of deep and accurate understanding about the 3D microstructure, composition and biology of the TMs at a close status to the native.

In this study, we demonstrated a 3D imaging technique for acquiring and examining the intrinsic 3D microstructure and composition of the lamina propria of hydrated mouse TMs in a full thickness. The study has brought new insights into the characteristics of the 3D microstructure and composition of the pars tensa-annulus unit. This information will be very useful for the development of cellular therapy and 3D printing technologies for regenerating a perforation or damaged TM.

Due to the close relationship between the microstructure and acoustic properties of TMs, the knowledge provided by this study will increase the understanding of the acoustic behavior and

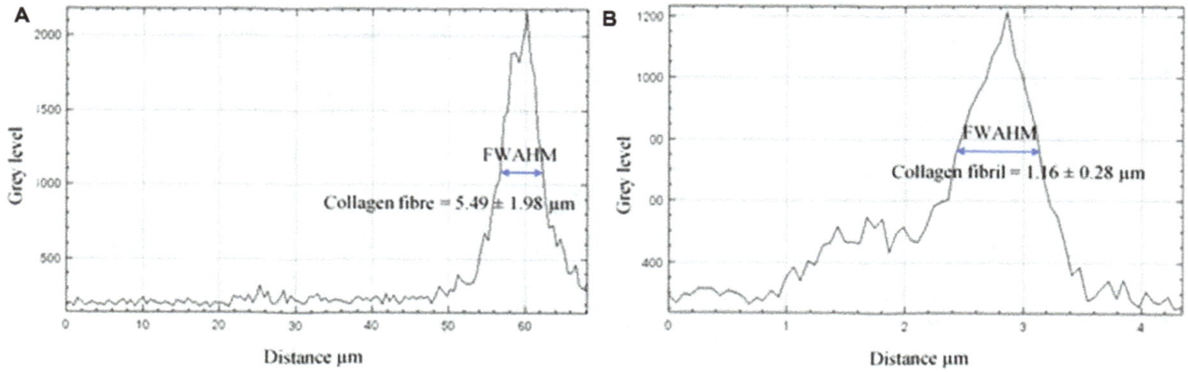

FIGURE 8 | The gray level intensity distribution graphs across the collagen fibers and fibrils. **(A)** The FWAHM and gray level intensity distribution graph across the thickness of the collagen fibers were used to measure the thickness of the collagen fibers comprising the pars tensa. **(B)** The FWAHM and gray level intensity distribution graph across the thickness of the collagen fibrils were used to measure the thickness of the collagen fibrils.

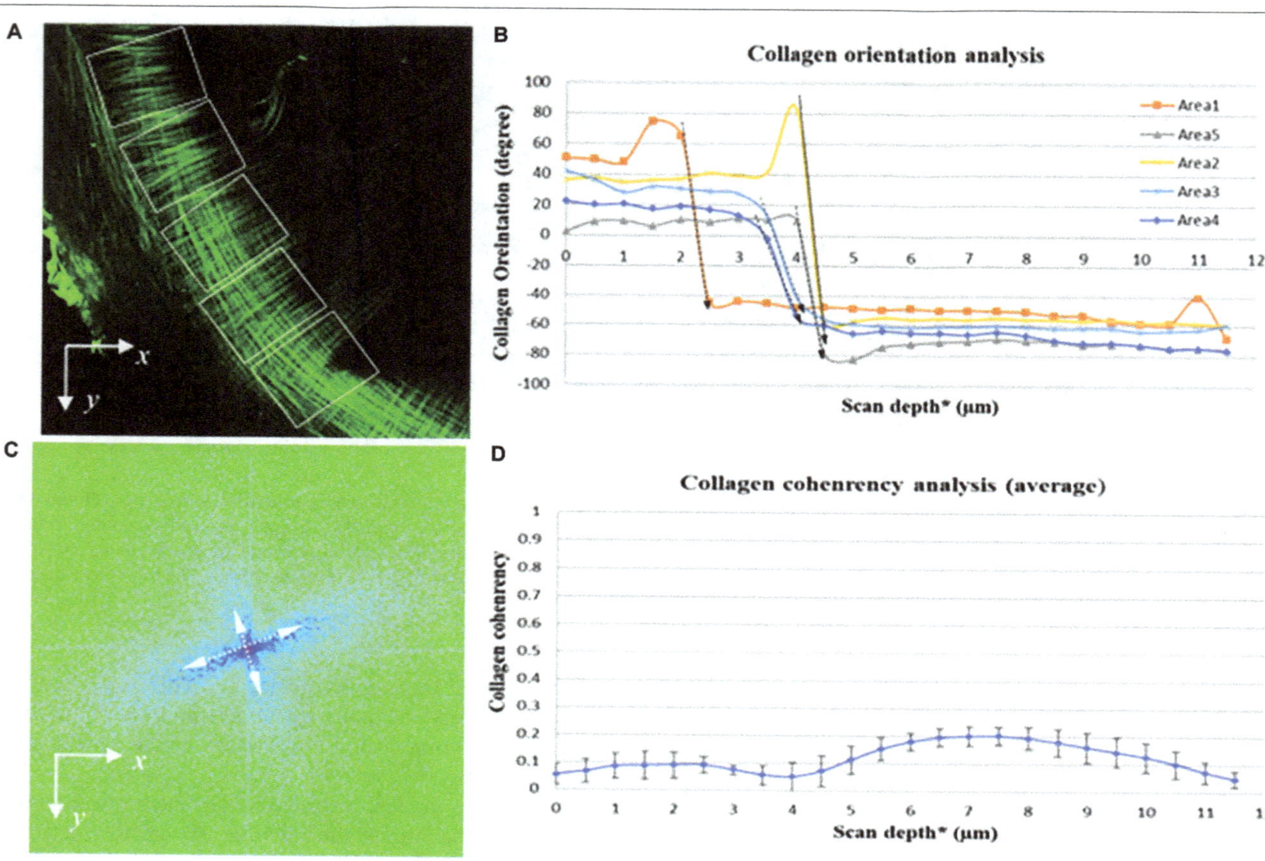

FIGURE 9 | Quantitative imaging analysis of the orientation and coherency of the collagen fibers in the pars tensa from the lateral to medial side. **(A)** SHG images were divided into five regions of interest (dashed boxes) to quantify the orientation and coherency of the collagen fibers comprising the parse tensa from the lateral to medial side. **(B)** Collagen orientation analysis confirms across the TM thickness the collagen fibers comprising the pars tensa sharply change their orientation (dash arrows highlight). **(C)** FFT analysis confirms that the collagen fibers composing the pars tensa orient into two distinctive directions approximately perpendicular to each other. **(D)** The coherency analysis shows that the collagen fibers comprising the pars tensa have a very low coherency value just below 0.2. *The collagen scaffold in the pars tensa is in a shallow conical shape so that the scan depth has been used in the orientation and coherency analysis of the collagen fibers but the entire scan depth does not equal to the thickness of the pars tensa.

physiology of the TM. Also, the 3D imaging technique developed will offer a useful tool for studies of the disruption of the 3D microstructure and composition of TMs during otitis media and aging to the alteration of the acoustic function.

Collagen is the most abundant protein of the ECM of TMs determining the acoustic characteristics of the TMs. The microstructure and concentration of the collagen have a significant influence over the shape, mechanical properties and health status of the TMs (Fay et al., 2006). Using a 3D imaging technique that does not require tissue dehydration and sectioning, it has been confirmed in this study that the collagen fibers of the pars tensa form a 3D collagenous network constituted primarily of the radial fibers and circumferential fibers in the lateral and medial side respectively, with some oblique and parabolic collagen fibers among the predominant radial and circumferential fibers. This study has also confirmed that the thick collagen fibers at the periphery of TMs bordering the fibrocartilaginous annulus are made of the subclass collagen fibrils, and become finer toward the TM center. The findings are consistent with the previous studies (Secondi, 1951; Lim, 1968, 1970, 1995; Uno, 2000).

Although we have not examined the orientation and characteristics of the collagen fibers in respect to their influence on the acoustic properties of TMs, some studies have indicated that the radial and circumferential collagen fibers play individual roles in the sound transmission and acoustic behavior of the TMs (Fay et al., 2006). Therefore, the spatial orientation and characteristics of the collagen fibers in the pars tensa and the connection features of the collagen between the pars tensa and annulus revealed by this study will help studies and understanding of the sound propagation mechanism in TMs.

Relatively to the collagen, research on the elastin in the TMs is underrepresented in the literature (Lim, 1995). To our knowledge, there is not yet a study showing the form of the elastic fibers and the 3D characteristics of the elastic fibers with the collagen fibers, cells and capillaries in TMs. TPF imaging has been used by a number of studies for high resolution and label-free visualizing the 3D microstructure of the elastic fibers with cells in tissues (Zipfel et al., 2003; He et al., 2013b; Wu et al., 2020). The most striking discovery in this study is the 3D architecture of the elastic fibers with the collagen, and the close physical connection of the elastic fibers with the spindle fibroblasts in the pars tensa (**Figures 2B,E**). The close physical connection of elastic fibers with fibroblasts has also been found in studies of tendons (Pang et al., 2017), and has been suggested to be a possible way mediating the mechanotransduction between the fibroblasts and ECM of the tissue. Therefore, this study will open potential for studying the mechanism of hearing loss.

As a crucial building block of cellular membranes, blood vessel walls and ECM of many biological tissues, elastic fibers provide the tissues with the essential elasticity to recover quickly from dynamic strain while they also influence the physiology and disease states of many tissues (He et al., 2013b). Collagen is well known for its great tensile strength to keep and maintain the static shape of tissues while elastic fibers endow tissues with recoil properties to recover rapidly from dynamic deformation. Therefore, the coexistence and 3D morphological characteristics of the collagen and elastic fibers in the pars tensa may have important implications in studies of the acoustic behaviors and health status of TMs. The deterioration or absence of elastic fibers may lead to abnormal fatigue to accelerate the degradation of the acoustic properties of the TMs. Thus, the discovery of the elastic fibers as a coexisting fibrillar element to the predominant collagen fibers in the ECM of the pars tensa will increase the understanding of the biomechanics of TMs and degeneration mechanism of TMs with aging.

There are some factors that prevented observing sharply the elastic fibers and fibroblasts in the unstained status of the TMs using TPF, for accurately quantifying the orientation features of the elastic fibers. Firstly, the excitation efficiency for TPF decays dramatically with the increase of the excitation wavelength (Zheng et al., 2011; Wu et al., 2020). When the excitation wavelength increases from 600 to 700 nm, the excitation efficiency of the TPF drops by a factor of 10 (Zheng et al., 2011; Wu et al., 2020). In this study, the excitation laser available for the TPF imaging was at the near-infrared range and set at 890 nm. As a result, there was a significant decrease in the excitation efficiency of the TPF, and the intensity of the autofluorescence of the elastic fibers and fibroblasts in the images. Secondly, the MMP used in this study is only configured with a 25 X/NA 1.05 water immersion objective lens. The magnification power and numerical aperture of the objective lens is not high enough to reveal the skinning fibroblasts and elastic fibers in the TMs. Either the previous studies (Pang et al., 2017) or this present study (e.g., **Figures 4J–L**) have shown that the use of high magnification observations is crucial to discover the elastic fibers among massive volume of collagen fibers. Moreover, the fibroblasts, elastic and collagen fibrils are intensively tangled and integrated in the TMs, while the volume of the elastic fibers and fibroblasts is much less than that of the predominant collagen fibers. The elastic fibers and fibroblasts are buried in the larger volume of the collagen matrix, which makes them difficulty to be seen at low magnification observations (e.g., **Figures 2C,F**).

However, more recent studies have shown that the use of short wavelength excitation lasers at a visible range of 520 nm can improve greatly the excitation efficiency and signal to noise ratio in TPF imaging of unstained tissues (Wu et al., 2020). Therefore, future studies, using advanced multiphoton microscopy integrated short wavelength excitation laser and objective lenses with high magnification powers and numerical aperture, will lead to increase the visibility of the elastic fibers and fibroblasts among the abundant collagen fibers in TMs, allowing simultaneously quantifying the orientation characteristics of the collagen, elastic fibers and fibroblasts, and developing more sophisticated auto classification systems for scoring the physical conditions of TMs.

In addition, this study has found that the tissues near the TM center or umbo contain more vimentin positive cells than those near the annulus. This may explain why tissue cultures harvested from the umbo regions are more proliferative in the regrowth of vimentin positive cells than those from the annulus containing round chondrocytes (Liew et al., 2017). This is an important finding that could have implications for improving the efficacy of cellular therapeutic techniques for TM repairs.

Visualization of cells and tissue structure using high resolution imaging techniques is highly desirable in medical clinics and research because it provides a way to visually inspect the morphology of the cells for briefly determining the cell types and tissue health status. In this study, we reported the cells visualized by the 3D imaging technique using a visual inspection of the cell morphological characteristics. Therefore, it is crucial to carry out a study in future to accurately examine the phenotypes of the cells documented by the 3D imaging technique using advanced immunohistological and genetic tools.

ETHICS STATEMENT

Ex vivo mouse TM samples used in this study were donated by other unrelated research in accordance with approvals from the Animal Ethics Committee at Southern University of Science and Technology, Shenzhen, China.

AUTHOR CONTRIBUTIONS

J-PW: conceptual design, supervision, data analysis and interpretation, and writing and revision of the manuscript. XY: sample preparation, imaging, experiment, and data analysis and writing the manuscript. YW and RZ: imaging. BS: quantitative imaging analysis, discussions, and critical revisions of the manuscript. RA, WZ, and YZ: discussion and revision of the manuscript. FC: conceptual design, supervision, and writing and revision of the manuscript. All authors contributed to the article and approved the submitted version.

REFERENCES

Cahalan, M. D., Parker, I., Wei, S. H., and Miller, M. J. (2002). Two-photon tissue imaging: seeing the immune system in a fresh light. *Nat. Rev. Immunol.* 2, 872–880. doi: 10.1038/nri935

Caminos, L., Garcia-Manrique, J., Lima-Rodriguez, A., and Gonzalez-Herrera, A. (2018). Analysis of the mechanical properties of the human tympanic membrane and its influence on the dynamic behaviour of the human hearing system. *Appl. Bionics Biomech.* 2018:1736957. doi: 10.1155/2018/1736957

Campagnola, P. J., and Loew, L. M. (2003). Second-harmonic imaging microscopy for visualizing biomolecular arrays in cells, tissues and organisms. *Nat. Biotechnol.* 21, 1356–1360. doi: 10.1038/nbt894

Chen, X., Nadiarynkh, O., Plotnikov, S., and Campagnola, P. J. (2012). Second harmonic generation microscopy for quantitative analysis of collagen fibrillar structure. *Nat. Protoc.* 7, 654–669. doi: 10.1038/nprot.2012.009

Chole, R. A., and Kodama, K. (1989). Comparative histology of the tympanic membrane and its relationship to cholesteatoma. *Ann. Otol. Rhinol. Laryngol.* 98, 761–766. doi: 10.1177/000348948909801002

Cox, G., Kable, E., Jones, A., Fraser, I., Manconi, F., and Gorrell, M. D. (2003). 3-Dimensional imaging of collagen using second harmonic generation. *J. Struct. Biol.* 141, 53–62. doi: 10.1016/S1047-8477(02)00576-2

Curran, M. E., Atkinson, D. L., Ewart, A. K., Morris, C. A., Leppert, M. F., and Keating, M. T. (1993). The elastin gene is disrupted by a translocation associated with supravalvular aortic stenosis. *Cell* 73, 159–168. doi: 10.1016/0092-8674(93)90168-P

De Greef, D., Aernouts, J., Aerts, J., Cheng, J. T., Horwitz, R., Rosowski, J. J., et al. (2014). Viscoelastic properties of the human tympanic membrane studied with stroboscopic holography and finite element modeling. *Hear. Res.* 312, 69–80. doi: 10.1016/j.heares.2014.03.002

De Greef, D., Goyens, J., Pintelon, I., Bogers, J. P., Van Rompaey, V., Hamans, E., et al. (2016). On the connection between the tympanic membrane and the malleus. *Hear. Res.* 340, 50–59. doi: 10.1016/j.heares.2015.12.002

Debelle, L., and Tamburro, A. M. (1999). Elastin: molecular description and function. *Int. J. Biochem. Cell Biol.* 31, 261–272. doi: 10.1016/S1357-2725(98)00098-3

Decraemer, W. F., Dirckx, J. J. J., and Funnell, W. R. J. (1991). Shape and derived geometrical parameters of the adult, human tympanic membrane measured with a phase-shift moiré interferometer. *Hear. Res.* 51, 107–121. doi: 10.1016/0378-5955(91)90010-7

Fay, J. P., Puria, S., and Steele, C. R. (2006). The discordant eardrum. *Proc. Natl. Acad. Sci. U.S.A.* 103, 19743–19748. doi: 10.1073/pnas.0603898104

Funnell, W. R. J., and Laszlo, C. A. (1982). A critical review of experimental observations on ear-drum structure and function. *ORL* 44, 181–205. doi: 10.1159/000275593

He, B., Wu, J. P., Chim, S. M., Xu, J., and Kirk, T. B. (2013c). Microstructural analysis of collagen and elastin fibres in the kangaroo articular cartilage reveals a structural divergence depending on its local mechanical environment. *Osteoarthr. Cartil. OARS Osteoarthr. Res. Soc.* 21:782. doi: 10.1016/j.joca.2013.02.660

He, B., Wu, J. P., Chen, H., Kirk, T., and Xu, J. (2013b). Elastin fibers display a versatile microfibril network in articular cartilage depending on the mechanical microenvironments. *J. Orthopaedic Res.* 31, 1345–1453. doi: 10.1002/jor.22384

He, B., Wu, J., Xu, J., Day, R., and Kirk, T. B. (2013a). Microstructural and compositional features of the fibrous and hyaline cartilage on the medical tibial plateau imply a unique role for the hopping locomotion of kangaroos. *PLoS One* 8:e74303. doi: 10.1371/journal.pone.0074303

He, B., Wu, J. P., Kirk, T. B., Carrino, J. A., Xiang, C., and Xu, J. (2014). High-resolution measurements of the multilayer ultra-structure of articular cartilage and their translational potential. *Arthritis Res. Ther.* 16:205. doi: 10.1186/ar4506

Igarashi, Y., and Kawamata, S. (1993). The fine structure of the guinea pig tympanic membrane with special reference to the fiber arrangement. *Acta Oto-Laryngologica* 113, 140–142. doi: 10.3109/00016489309128141

Jackson, R. P., Chlebicki, C., Krasieva, T. B., and Puria, S. (2008). "Multiphoton microscopy imaging of collagen fiber layers and orientation in the tympanic membrane," in *Proceedings of the SPIE*, Bellingham, WA. doi: 10.1117/12.774353

Jähne, B. (1993). *Spatio-Temporal Image Processing: Theory and Scientific Applications*. Berlin: Springer Science & Business Media. doi: 10.1007/3-540-57418-2

Jahne, B. (1997). *Practical Handbook on Image Processing for Scientific Applications*. New York, NY: CRC Press.

Koch, R. G., Tsamis, A., D'amore, A., Wagner, W. R., Watkins, S. C., Gleason, T. G., et al. (2014). A custom image-based analysis tool for quantifying elastin and collagen micro-architecture in the wall of the human aorta from multi-photon microscopy. *J. Biomech.* 47, 935–943. doi: 10.1016/j.jbiomech.2014.01.027

König, K., Schenke-Layland, K., Riemann, I., and Stock, U. A. (2005). Multiphoton autofluorescence imaging of intratissue elastic fibers. *Biomaterials* 26, 495–500. doi: \doi{10.1016/j.jbiomech.2014.01.027}

Kozin, E. D., Black, N. L., Cheng, J. T., Cotler, M. J., Mckenna, M. J., Lee, D. J., et al. (2016). Design, fabrication, and in vitro testing of novel three-dimensionally printed tympanic membrane grafts. *Hear. Res.* 340, 191–203. doi: 10.1016/j.heares.2016.03.005

Li, D. Y., Brooke, B., Davis, E. C., Mecham, R. P., Sorensen, L. K., Boak, B. B., et al. (1998). Elastin is an essential determinant of arterial morphogenesis. *Nature* 393, 276–280. doi: 10.1038/30522

Liew, L. J., Day, R. M., and Dilley, R. J. (2017). Tympanic membrane organ culture using cell culture well inserts engrafted with tympanic membrane tissue explants. *BioTechniques* 62, 109–114. doi: 10.2144/000114523

Lim, D. J. (1968). Tympanic membrane. Electron microscopic observation. I: pars tensa. *Acta Otolaryngol.* 66, 181–198. doi: 10.3109/00016486809126286

Lim, D. J. (1970). Human tympanic membrane. *Acta Oto-Laryngologica* 70, 176–186. doi: 10.3109/00016487009181875

Lim, D. J. (1995). Structure and function of the tympanic membrane: a review. *Acta Otorhinolaryngol. Belg.* 49, 101–115.

Liu, J., Agrawal, S. K., Ladak H. M., and Wan, W. (2016). Fiber arrangement in the rat tympanic membrane. *Anat. Record* 299, 1531–1539. doi: 10.1002/ar.23461

Mansfield, J., Yu, J., Attenburrow, D., Moger, J., Tirlapur, U., Urban, J., et al. (2009). The elastin network: its relationship with collagen and cells in articular cartilage as visualized by multiphoton microscopy. *J. Anat.* 215, 682–691. doi: 10.1111/j.1469-7580.2009.01149.x

Montes, G. S. (1996). Structural biology of the fibres of the collagenous and elastic systems. *Cell Biol. Int.* 20, 15–27. doi: 10.1006/cbir.1996.0004

Pang, X., Wu, J.-P., Allison, G. T., Xu, J., Rubenson, J., Zheng, M.-H., et al. (2017). Three dimensional microstructural network of elastin, collagen, and cells in Achilles tendons. *J. Orthopaedic Res.* 35, 1203–1214. doi: 10.1002/jor.23240

Prockop, D. J., and Kivirikko, K. J. (1995). Collagens: molecular biology, diseases and potentials for therapy. *Annu. Rev. Biochem.* 64, 403–434. doi: 10.1146/annurev.bi.64.070195.002155

Rasband, W. S. (1997-2014). *ImageJ, U.S. National Institutes of Healthy.* Available online at: http://imagej.nih.gov/ij/

Rezakhaniha, R., Agianniotis, A., Schrauwen, J. T. C., Griffa, A., Sage, D., Bouten, C., et al. (2012) Experimental investigation of collagen waviness and orientation in the arterial adventitia using confocal laser scanning microscopy. *Biomech. Model. Mechanobiol.* 11, 461–473. doi: 10.1007/s10237-011-0325-z

Secondi, U. (1951). Structure and function of the lamina propria of the tympanic membrane in various mammals. *A.M.A. Arch. Otolaryngol.* 53, 170–181. doi: 10.1001/archotol.1951.03750020044006

Stenfeldt, K., Johansson, C., and Hellström, S. (2006). The collagen structure of the tympanic membrane: collagen types I, II, and III in the healthy tympanic membrane, during healing of a perforation, and during infection. *Arch. Otolaryngol. Head Neck Surg.* 132, 293–298. doi: 10.1001/archotol.132.3.293

Uno, Y. (2000). The attachment structure of the guinea pig tympanic membrane. *Auris Nasus Larynx* 27, 45–50. doi: 10.1016/S0385-8146(99)00040-1

Volandri, G., Puccio, F. D., Forte, P., and Carmignani, C. (2011). Biomechanics of the tympanic membrane. *J. Biomech.* 44, 1219–1236. doi: 10.1016/j.jbiomech.2010.12.023

Wu, J.-P., Swift, B. J., Becker, T., Squelch, A., Wang, A., Zheng, Y.-C., et al. (2017). High-resolution study of the 3D collagen fibrillary matrix of Achilles tendons without tissue labelling and dehydrating. *J. Microscopy* 266, 273–287. doi: 10.1111/jmi.12537

Wu, T., Liao, J., Yu, J., Gao, Y., Li, H., Wu, J., et al. (2020). In vivo label-free two-photon excitation autofluorescence microscopy of microvasculature using a 520 nm femtosecond fiber laser. *Opt. Lett.* 45, 2704–2707. doi: 10.1364/OL.394242

Zheng, W., Li, D., Zeng, Y., Luo, Y., and Qu, J. Y. (2011). Two-photon excited hemoglobin fluorescence. *Biomed. Optics Exp.* 2, 71–79. doi: 10.1364/BOE.2.000071

Zipfel, W. R., Williams, R. M., and Webb, W. W. (2003). Nonlinear magic: multiphoton microscopy in the biosciences. *Nat. Biotechnol.* 21, 1369–1377. doi: 10.1038/nbt899

Zoumi, A., Lu, X., Kassab, G. S., and Tromberg, B. J. (2004). Imaging coronary artery microstructure using second-harmonic and two-photon fluorescence microscopy. *Biophys. J.* 87, 2778–2786. doi: 10.1529/biophysj.104.042887

10

Auditory Neuropathy as the Initial Phenotype for Patients With *ATP1A3* c.2452 G > A: Genotype–Phenotype Study and CI Management

Wenjia Wang[1,2], Jin Li[1,2], Lan Lan[1,2], Linyi Xie[1,2], Fen Xiong[1,2], Jing Guan[1,2], Hongyang Wang[1,2] and Qiuju Wang[1,2]**

[1] *College of Otolaryngology, Head and Neck Surgery, Institute of Otolaryngology, Chinese PLA General Hospital, Beijing, China,*
[2] *National Clinical Research Center for Otolaryngologic Diseases, Beijing, China*

Correspondence:
Hongyang Wang
whyx301@foxmail.com
Qiuju Wang
wqcr301@vip.sina.com

Objective: The objective of this study is to analyze the genotype–phenotype correlation of patients with auditory neuropathy (AN), which is a clinical condition featuring normal cochlear responses and abnormal neural responses, and *ATP1A3* c.2452 G > A (p.E818K), which has been generally recognized as a genetic cause of cerebellar ataxia, areflexia, pes cavus, optic atrophy, and sensorineural hearing loss (CAPOS) syndrome.

Methods: Four patients diagnosed as AN by clinical evaluation and otoacoustic emission and auditory brainstem responses were recruited and analyzed by next-generation sequencing to identify candidate disease-causing variants. Sanger sequencing was performed on the patients and their parents to verify the results, and short tandem repeat-based testing was conducted to confirm the biological relationship between the parents and the patients. Furthermore, cochlear implantation (CI) was performed in one AN patient to reconstruct hearing.

Results: Four subjects with AN were identified to share a *de novo* variant, p.E818K in the *ATP1A3* gene. Except for the AN phenotype, patients 1 and 2 exhibited varying degrees of neurological symptoms, implying that they can be diagnosed as CAPOS syndrome. During the 15 years follow-up of patient 1, we observed delayed neurological events and progressive bilateral sensorineural hearing loss in pure tone threshold (pure tone audiometry, PTA). Patient 2 underwent CI on his left ear, and the result was poor. The other two patients (patient 3 and patient 4, who were 8 and 6 years old, respectively) denied any neurological symptoms.

Conclusion: *ATP1A3* p.E818K has rarely been documented in the Chinese AN population. Our study confirms that p.E818K in the *ATP1A3* gene is a multiethnic cause of AN in Chinese individuals. Our study further demonstrates the significance of genetic testing for this specific mutation for identifying the special subtype of AN with somewhat favorable CI outcome and offers a more accurate genetic counseling about the specific *de novo* mutation.

Keywords: auditory neuropathy (AN), *ATP1A3*, *de novo*, CAPOS syndrome, cochlear implantation (CI)

INTRODUCTION

Auditory neuropathy (AN) is a kind of hearing disorder involving different lesion sites beyond the outer hair cells (OHCs), ranging from the inner hair cells (IHCs) and synapses to auditory nerve and higher auditory centers (Rance and Starr, 2015; Moser and Starr, 2016). AN features impaired or absent response in auditory brainstem responses (ABR) and the presence of cochlear microphonics and/or detectable otoacoustic emission (OAE), showing evidence of intact outer hair cell function. Varying degrees of hearing loss are present in subjects with AN; however, their speech recognition rates are generally poor, disproportionate to the degree of hearing loss (Harrison et al., 2015; Rance and Starr, 2015; Moser and Starr, 2016). A variety of etiologies can trigger AN, generally considered to be hypoxia, infection, kernicterus cytotoxic oncologic drugs, and genetic factors (Harrison et al., 2015).

Considering postlingual-onset AN, many syndromic forms that cause sensory and motor neuropathy have been documented, including Charcot-Marie-Tooth disease, Friedreich's ataxia, deafness-dystonia-optic neuropathy (DDON) syndrome, autosomal dominant optic atrophy (ADOA), and AUNX1 due to *AIFM1* gene mutations in apoptosis-inducing factor (Han et al., 2017). Han et al. (2017) explored the molecular etiology of three unrelated Korean subjects manifesting AN with postlingual onset, identified a mutation in c.2452 G > A (p.E818K) of *ATP1A3* gene, and demonstrated *ATP1A3* gene to be an important and prevalent causative gene for progressive AN with postlingual onset. *ATP1A3* gene has thus been said to occur frequently *de novo* in both Caucasians and Koreans (Han et al., 2017). However, p.E818K in the *ATP1A3* gene has rarely been documented in the Chinese population.

In this study, we reported four Chinese AN patients carrying a *de novo* variant, p.E818K mutation of *ATP1A3* gene, identified through next generation sequencing (NGS). *ATP1A3* p.E818K has been generally recognized as a genetic cause of cerebellar ataxia, areflexia, pes cavus, optic atrophy, and sensorineural hearing loss (CAPOS) syndrome. A genotype-phenotype correlation study of *ATP1A3* was performed, and one AN patient underwent cochlear implantation (CI) to reconstruct hearing.

MATERIALS AND METHODS

Ethics Statement

The study was approved by the Committee of Medical Ethics of Chinese PLA General Hospital. Written informed consent was obtained from participants.

Subject Recruitment and Clinical Evaluations

Four AN patients at the Institute of Otolaryngology, Chinese PLA General Hospital were recruited and underwent genetic testing. The diagnostic criteria were as follows: ABR had no obvious differentiation waveform and the OAE and/or the cochlear microphonic (CM) potential could be normally extracted. Medical evidence of hearing loss, tinnitus, and other clinical abnormalities of either affected or unaffected family members was identified. Pure tone threshold (pure tone audiometry, PTA), speech discrimination score (SDS), ABR, OAE, and electrocochleogram (ECochG) were carried out to evaluate auditory status. In general, low frequencies were primarily affected; thus, we focused on the low-frequency data and calculated the PTA as the average of the thresholds of 250–1,000 Hz to avoid bias in the assessment of the degree of AN hearing loss. High-resolution computed tomography (CT) scans of the temporal bone and MRI of the internal auditory canal were performed to exclude other possible neuropathic or anatomical disorders. For patients who exhibited neurological symptoms, we carried out neurological examinations to evaluate those symptoms.

Genetic Techniques

Next generation sequencing, including whole genome sequencing and targeted genes capture and sequencing, was performed on the four probands, Sanger sequencing was performed on the patients and their parents to verify any candidate gene variations as previously described. Variation interpretation (evaluation of the pathogenicity) was based on the standards and guidelines of the American College of Medical Genetics and Genomics and the Association for Molecular Pathology (ACMG and AMP). Short tandem repeat (STR)-based testing was conducted to confirm the biological relationship between the parents and the patients (Wang et al., 2018).

RESULTS

General Clinical Information

A total of four AN cases with *ATP1A3* variants were recruited in this study. Details on the patients in this report were collated. Clinical and audiological data were collected retrospectively. Audiological details were outlined in **Figure 1** and **Supplementary Figure 1**.

Detailed Medical History and Clinical Phenotype of Four Auditory Neuropathy Subjects

Patient 1 was a 24-year-old male (**Figure 2A**). He exhibited dystonia and ataxia at a very early age after having a fever. At age 5, he started to suffer from visual disturbance, and at age 7, his hearing level of both ears started to deteriorate. He was diagnosed as optic atrophy at Beijing Tongren Hospital at age 8. At age 9, he was diagnosed with AN at our hospital. His sensorineural hearing loss (SNHL) matched AN, with a detectable OAE response and disappearance of the ABR response (**Figures 1C,D,F**), and ratios of -SP/AP were more than 0.4 in both ears (**Figure 1G**). His pattern visual evoked potential (P-VEP) amplitude was already reduced, indicating amblyopia found in him. Imaging tests demonstrated anatomically intact auditory nerves (**Figure 2G**). Somatosensory evoked potentials (SSEPs) showed prolonged latency of the bilateral tibial nerve,

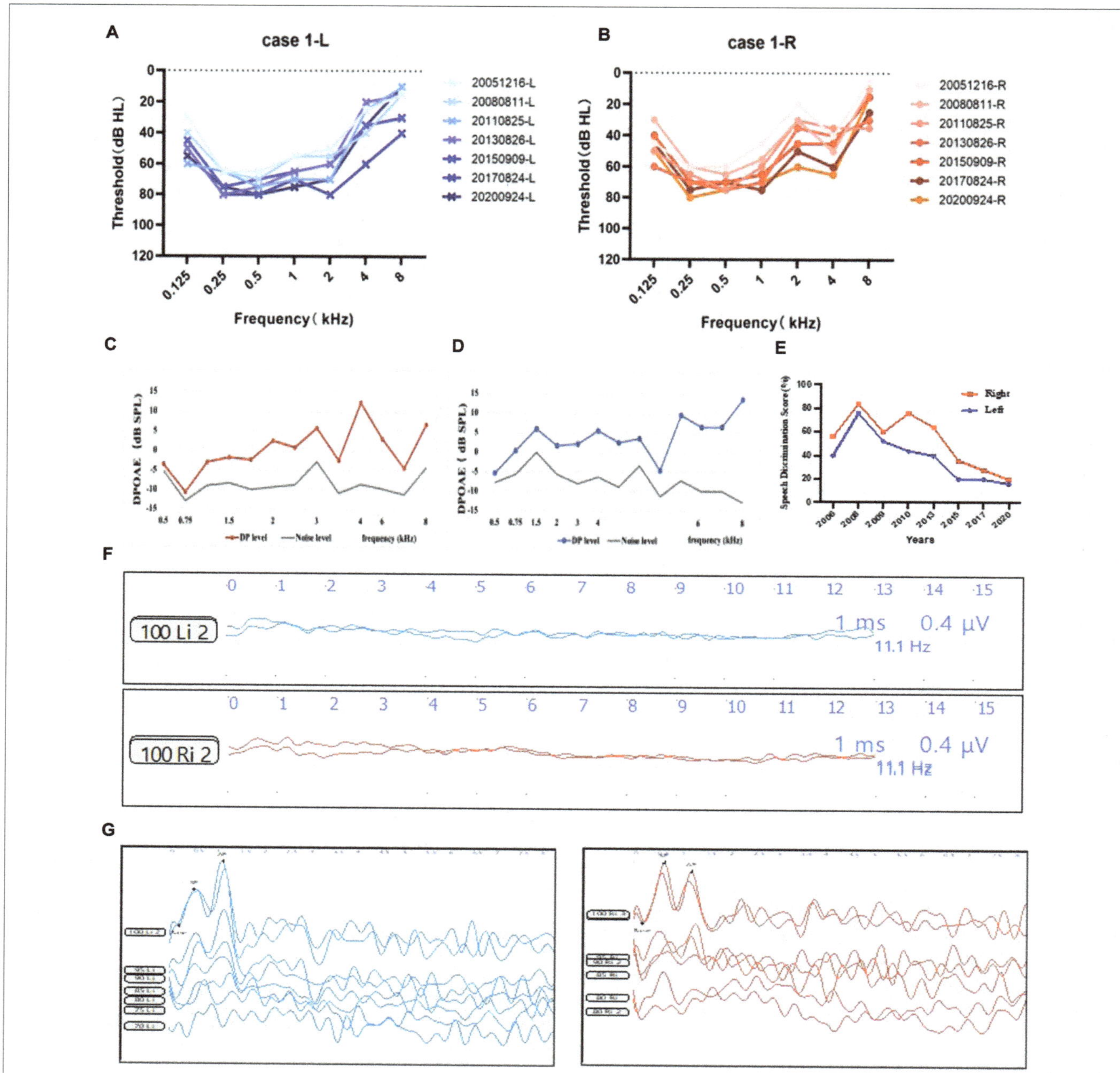

FIGURE 1 | Audiological phenotype of subject 1. **(A,B)** PTA of the subject 1. Audiograms of patient 1 from 2005 to 2020 displaying moderate to severe sensorineural hearing loss, predominantly affecting the low frequencies and progressively deteriorated overtime. Blue, left ear; red, right ear. **(C,D)** Observed DPOAE responses from the right and the left ear. Red line, DPOAE level from the right ear; blue line, DPOAE level from the left ear; gray line, noise level. **(E)** SDS results from 2006 to 2020 showing decreased speech discrimination score. Blue, left ear; red, right ear. **(F)** Absent ABR waveforms at 90 dB nHL stimulus on both ears. **(G)** ECochG shows the mean ratios of -SP/AP were larger than 0.4 from both ears. Blue, left ear; red, right ear. Abbreviations: PTA, pure tone audiometry; SDS, speech discrimination score; DPOAE, distortion product optoacoustic emission; ABR, auditory brainstem response; CM, cochlear microphonic.

suggesting abnormal tibial nerve conduction. Electromyographic (EMG) signals of the upper and lower limbs did not display abnormalities. The amplitude-integrated EEG (aEEG) detected minor dysfunction. Through 15 years of follow-up from 2005 to 2020, we observed that his eyesight deteriorated over time, as did his hearing level and speech discrimination score (**Figures 1A,B,E**).

Patient 2 was a 22-year-old male patient (**Figure 2B**). He had a fever and took gentamicin at the age of 2, and he presented with bilateral hearing loss at the age of 7. His SNHL deteriorated over

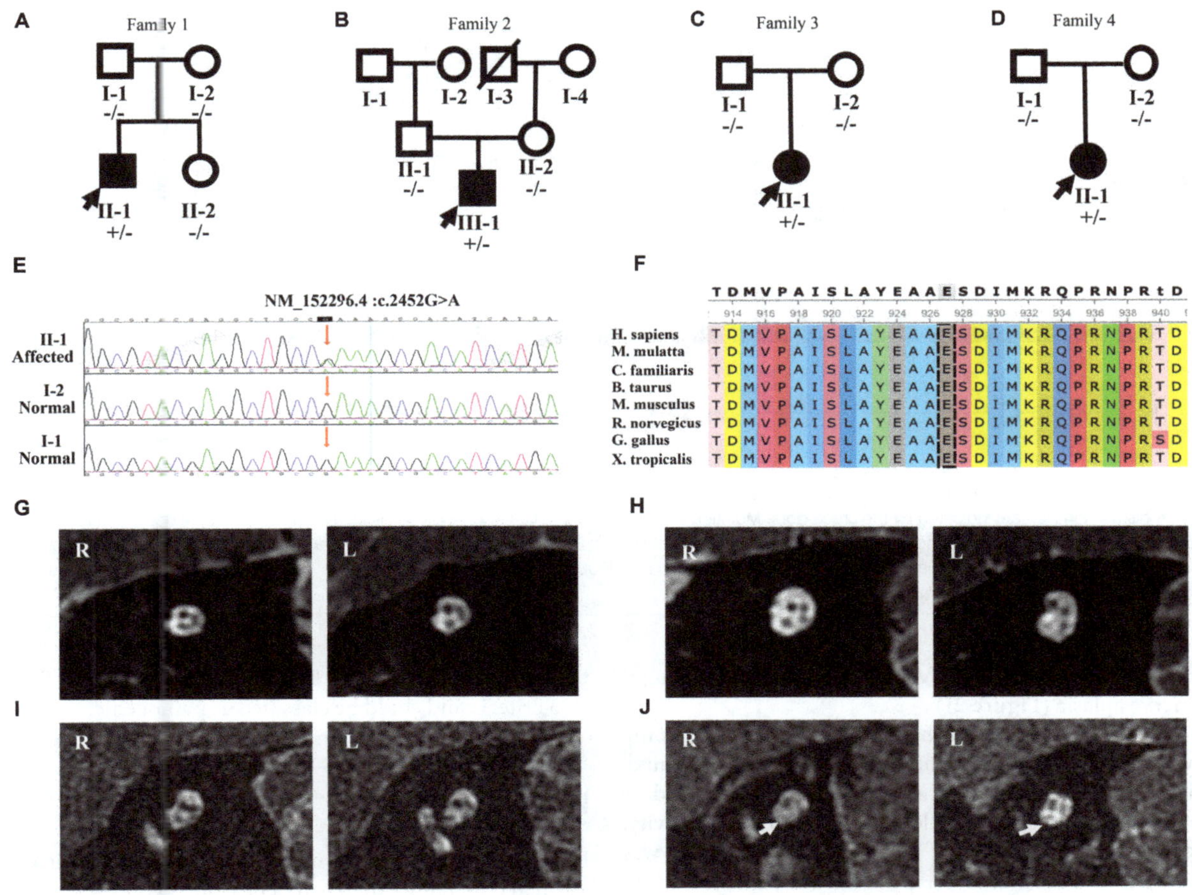

FIGURE 2 | Mutation analysis and MRI results of four patients with the p.E818K mutation. **(A–C)**, and **(D)** Pedigree of four families. Filled symbols denote affected individuals, whereas unfilled symbols denote the unaffected. A slash (/) indicates a deceased person. Minus sign (-/-) represents homozygosity for the wild-type allele, and plus-minus sign (±) represents heterozygosity for the mutant allele. Probands are indicated by arrows. **(E)** Sanger sequencing chromatograms of four pedigrees confirmed that all four subjects shared one common heterozygous mutation, c.2452 G > A (arrow) leading to p.E818K amino acid change, whereas their parents are normal. **(F)** Protein conservation of no. 818 amino acid among vertebrate species (*H. sapiens*, *M. mulatta*, *C. familiaris*, *B. taurus*, *M. musculus*, *R. norvegicus*, *G. gallus*, and *X. tropicalis*). No. 818 amino acid is highly conserved. **(G–I)**, and **(J)** MRI results showing bilateral internal auditory canals (IACs) of patients 1, 2, 3, and 4, respectively. The oblique sagittal image through the bilateral IACs of patient 4 **(J)** demonstrates absent bilateral cochlear nerves (white arrows).

time, accelerating from 13 to 14 years old. Along with bilateral tinnitus, he experienced alalia as well as fatigue. However, he denied other neurologic episodes and could even ride a bicycle, although his eyesight began to decline at the age of 12. His threshold of 40 Hz AERP was 90 dB HL in both ears. Both CT scan and MRI of the internal auditory canal showed only normal findings (**Figure 2H**). He underwent CI on the left ear at our hospital in 2013, yet his speech perception did not improve much in 1-year follow-up period. In addition, he exhibited facial muscle twitching when the cochlear implant was used in louder environment.

Patient 3 was an 8-year-old girl (**Figure 2C**). She did not exhibit abnormal hearing function until the age of 7, when she suffered from a fever. Three days after her fever, she experienced hearing loss accompanied by poor speech discrimination. Her symptoms did not improve with the administration of Ginaton as well as other neurotrophic drugs, such as vitamin B12. Her PTA showed an upward sloping configuration, with an average threshold being 70 dB HL in the left ear and 61 dB HL in the right ear (**Supplementary Figure 1A**). In contrast, her reduction in speech recognition was drastic, being 8% in the left ear and 4% in the right ear. Her SNHL was entirely compatible with AN, considering a detectable OAE response without ABR response (**Supplementary Figures 1C,E**). CT scan showed no abnormality, and MRI of the internal auditory canal confirmed that she had intact cochlear nerve (**Figure 2I**). With no obvious neurological condition exhibited, she was diagnosed with bilateral AN.

Patient 4 was a 6-year-old girl (**Figure 2D**). Her syndrome of hearing loss accompanied by tinnitus appeared at age 4. Unable to benefit from the hearing aids at age 5, she came to our clinic for help. Her PTA showed an upward sloping configuration (**Supplementary Figure 1B**). She was diagnosed with AN with no neurological symptoms found

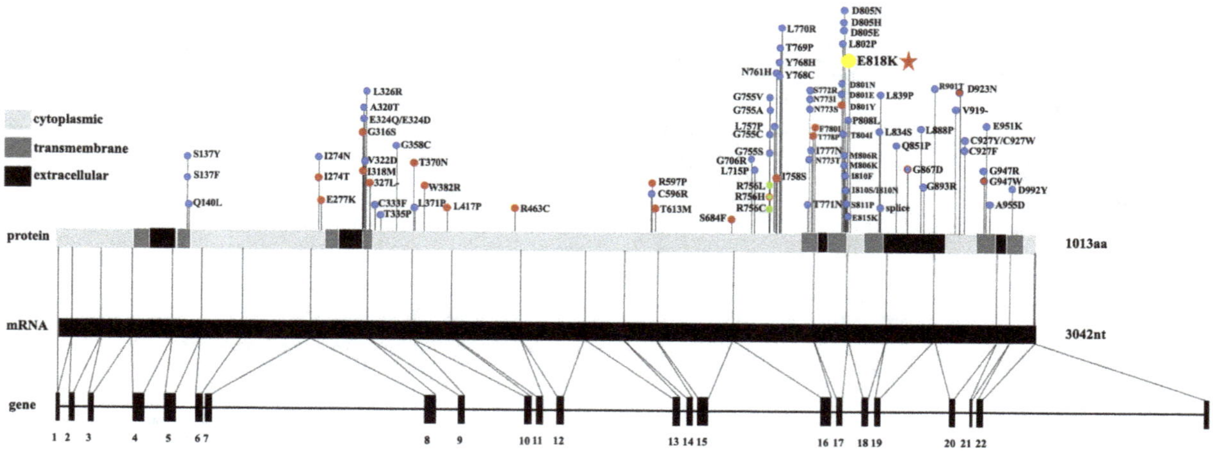

FIGURE 3 | The location of AHC-causing (blue dots), RDP-causing (red dots), and CAPOS-causing (yellow dots) mutations in *ATP1A3*, mRNA, and protein. Three rare polymorphisms identified are indicated by the green dots. Mutation shared between different phenotypes is located at D923N (blue dot with a red dot inside), G867N (red dot with a blue dot inside), and R756H (red dot with a green dot inside). Different regions (cytoplasmic, transmembrane, and extracellular) of the protein are listed on the left. Abbreviations: AHC, alternating hemiplegia of childhood; CAPOS, cerebellar ataxia, areflexia, pes cavus, optic atrophy, and sensorineural hearing loss; RDP, rapid-onset dystonia Parkinsonism.

(**Supplementary Figures 1D,F**). MRI result showed bilateral cochlear nerve aplasia (**Figure 2J**).

All the four probands passed the newborn hearing screening test successfully, suggesting that their SNHL was not congenital. Furthermore, they presented with the presence of OAEs and/or CMs, indicating preserved cochlear outer hair cell activity. However, the ABR, a sign of neural dyssynchrony, was grossly abnormal. In addition, a poor SDS was observed in all four patients, especially in noisy environments, and was disproportionate to the level of hearing loss.

Molecular Genetic Testing and Delineation of the Causative Variant From the Four Subjects

We performed NGS, including targeted genes capture and whole genome capture, in four probands with sporadic AN and identified the most convincing causative variant that has previously been described (Kim et al., 2015). Candidate variants were validated by standard Sanger sequencing. All four AN subjects shared one heterozygous missense variant, c.2452 G > A (p.E818K) in the *ATP1A3* gene (NM_152296.4, NP_689509.1, OMIM *182350), which was located on chromosome 19q13.2 and classified as "pathogenic" according to CLINVAR [1] (Landrum et al., 2016). Unaffected parents showed no variation in *ATP1A3*, indicating a *de novo* occurrence of an autosomal dominant variant, p.E818K, in all four families (**Figure 2E**). Evolutionary conservation analysis revealed that this variant was highly conserved throughout evolution among species (**Figure 2F**). STR-based testing was conducted, confirming the biological relationship between the parents and the cases and indicating that the *ATP1A3* mutation was *de novo* in nature, which strongly supports the pathogenicity. According to the ACMG guidelines, p. E818K variant met the PS2, PS3, PS4, PM2, PP1_Strong, and PP3 criteria and could be classified as pathogenic.

[1] https://www.ncbi.nlm.nih.gov/clinvar/

DISCUSSION

Hearing loss is the most common sensorineural disorder. It is estimated that more than half of hearing loss cases are attributable to genetic factors (He Y. et al., 2017; Wang et al., 2017; Zhu et al., 2018; Fang et al., 2019; He Z. et al., 2019; Fu et al., 2021), while the other half of hearing loss could be caused by aging, chronic infections, infectious diseases, ototoxic drugs, and noise exposure (Liu L. et al., 2016; He Z. et al., 2017; Cheng et al., 2019; Gao et al., 2019; Tan et al., 2019; Zhang et al., 2019; Zhong et al., 2020). The functions of these hearing loss genes play an essential role in the development and function of hair cells and synaptic transmission of spiral ganglion neurons (Qi et al., 2020; Qian et al., 2020; Zhang et al., 2020, 2021; Cheng et al., 2021; Lv et al., 2021). Thus, hearing loss is often induced by loss of sensory hair cells (Liu Y. et al., 2019; Qi et al., 2019; Han et al., 2020; He et al., 2020, 2021; Chen et al., 2021) and spiral ganglion neurons (Guo et al., 2016, 2019, 2020, 2021; Liu W. et al., 2019; Hu et al., 2021; Liu W. et al., 2021) in the inner ear cochlea. AN is a hearing disorder with functional outer hair cells and disrupted function of inner hair cells and/or the auditory nerve itself. Han et al. (2017) first proposed that p.E818K in *ATP1A3* gene, which encodes the NKAα3 subunit of Na, K-ATPases, can cause AN in Caucasians and Koreans, implying that *ATP1A3* serves as a global contributor to AN (**Supplementary Table 1**). In our study, four AN cases were tested with p.E818K in the *ATP1A3* gene. The incidence of p.E818K accounting for AN in Chinese individuals is still under investigation. Nevertheless, we found that the p.E818K mutation accounts for a high proportion of AN with postlingual onset, not only in Koreans and Caucasians but also in Chinese individuals.

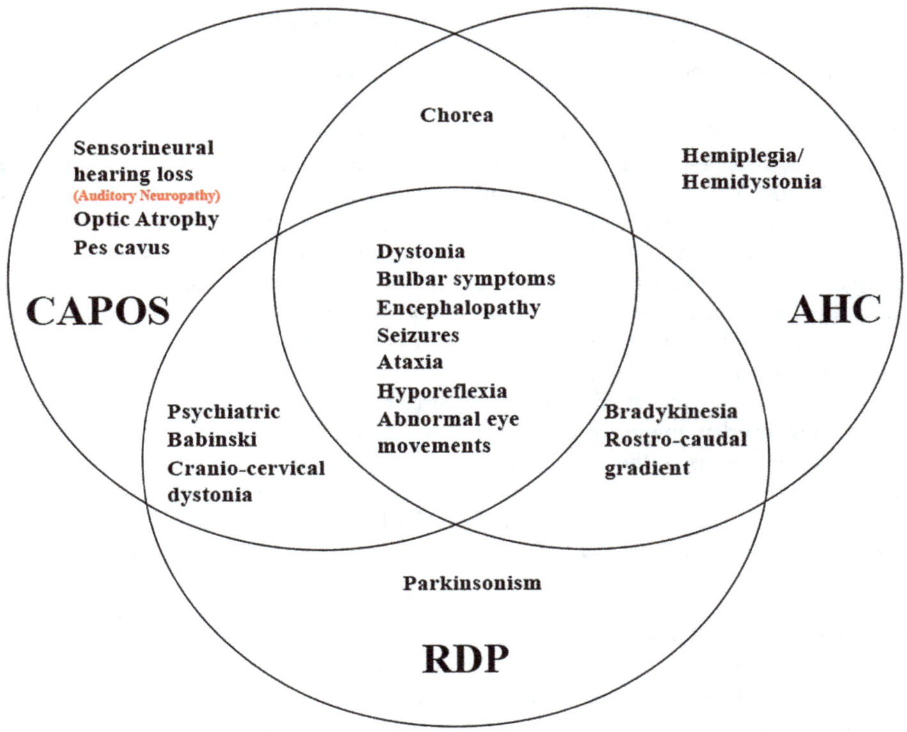

FIGURE 4 | Unique and shared features between AHC, RDP, and CAPOS phenotypes. Auditory neuropathy is either a symptom of CAPOS or a new phenotype of *ATP1A3* gene.

ATP1A3 p.E818K has been regarded as a causal mutation of CAPOS syndrome since identified in 2014 (Carecchio et al., 2018), long after the initial description in 1996 (Nicolaides et al., 1996). CAPOS syndrome is a rare disorder, with fewer than 100 CAPOS patients worldwide, and is sporadically reported (Demos et al., 2014; Rosewich et al., 2014; Heimer et al., 2015; Potic et al., 2015; Maas et al., 2016; Duat Rodriguez et al., 2017). Growing evidence shows that sensorineural hearing loss in CAPOS syndrome is AN, which may progress slowly over time. The typical CAPOS phenotype is characterized by acute neurological deterioration manifesting in infancy and triggered by stressful episodes, such as a febrile illness (Paquay et al., 2018). Meticulous history as well as comprehensive neurologic examination should be performed on postlingual-onset AN subjects, to detect any episode of visual disturbance and ataxia associated with CAPOS syndrome triggered by a fever that might otherwise go unnoticed. CAPOS syndrome patients initially have cochlear apical turns, manifested in a low-frequency loss in PTA. However, neuronal distribution of NKAα3 is also observed in middle and basal turns of the cochlea (Paquay et al., 2018), indicating that mid and high frequencies may also be involved. Through 15 years follow-up, we detected progressing hearing defects involving all frequencies, predominantly the low frequencies in patient 1. It is worth continuing the follow-up periods for patients with p.E818K to detect changes in PTA over time, to clarify the significance of the p.E818K mutation in AN.

In previous study, Demos et al. (2014) reported follow-up of three patients with *ATP1A3* p.E818K. All the patients showed slow progression of all symptoms with no further acute episodes. Demos et al. (2014) further reported two Caucasian families with *ATP1A3* p.E818K. In the first family, all affected suffered from acute episodic ataxic encephalopathy and/or weakness triggered by a febrile illness onset in infancy or early childhood. Recovery was not as desirable after these episodes, when variable neurologic abnormalities was lingering. All affected individuals eventually had optic atrophy and sensorineural hearing loss. One patient exhibited mild cognitive dysfunction at age 10 years. In the second family, the affected mother and her two children presented with recurrent acute episodes of neurologic disorders associated with febrile illnesses beginning in the first years of life. Features included weakness, ataxia, and a progressive decline in hearing and vision. In our study, patient 1 exhibited dystonia and ataxia at a very early age after having a fever. He exhibited optic atrophy and auditory neuropathy at an early age, which were slowly progressive over time. Follow-up period was needed for every patient to further clarify whether there was a slow progression of all symptoms, be it neurological disorders or visual and hearing impairment.

The *ATP1A3* gene has also been reported in two other clinical entities, alternating hemiplegia of childhood (AHC, AHC2, OMIM #614820) and rapid-onset dystonia Parkinsonism (RDP, DYT12, OMIM #128235) (Blanco and Mercer, 1998;

Starr et al., 2005; Rodacker et al., 2006; Blanco-Arias et al., 2009). Mutation sites are distributed across the entire coding region of *ATP1A3* in RDP and AHC (**Supplementary Table 1**; Clausen et al., 2017). Interestingly, all CAPOS patients reported without exception share a common mutation, p.E818K in the *ATP1A3* gene. Also, p.E818K is seemingly tightly coupled with CAPOS syndrome and has never been reported in other two disorders (Han et al., 2017; **Figure 3**). There is no report of hearing or visual impairment in AHC and RDP, which is vastly different from CAPOS syndrome (**Figure 4**; Tranebjærg et al., 2018a). However, those three entities present with an expanding phenotypic spectrum and are more often reported to share somewhat overlapping neurological phenotypes. In addition, atypical phenotypes due to *ATP1A3* gene mutations have recently been identified (Gropman et al., 2020; Guo et al., 2020). It becomes gradually clear that these overlapping phenotypes may be a series of *ATP1A3*-related symptoms, rather than allelic disorders (Carecchio et al., 2018). Moreover, the expression timing of neurological deficits of the mutation varies and has still not been fully characterized until now (Han et al., 2017). In our study, it was not very hard to observe the latency of occurrence of numerous symptoms in patients 1 and 2. Notably, patients 3 and 4 denied all neurological episodes. Continuation of the follow-up periods for these four patients is therefore necessary for the discovery of other delayed neurological symptoms. Nevertheless, whether AN is simply a symptom of CAPOS or a completely new phenotype of the *ATP1A3* gene remains to be seen.

Early diagnosis of hearing loss and timely prevention of sensory deprivation are of vital importance and confer lifelong benefits to CAPOS patients, especially for those with visual interference. The 818 position is previously confirmed located at the cytoplasmic end of transmembrane helix 6 of NKAα3, forming a salt bridge with the backbone carbonyl of Arg930, which is a residue known to stabilize the C-terminus. Tranebjærg et al. (2018b) have evaluated functional impact of Glu818Lys to the C-terminal structure and demonstrated that Glu818Lys leads to low affinity for extracellular sodium and a high rate of sodium release from the third ion-binding portion; therefore, it disrupts the function of the NKAα3 subunit of Na, K-ATPases, which is a key regulator of regaining the resting potential of the membrane after excitatory activity in the auditory pathway. In the auditory pathway, NKAα3 is expressed in the membranes of type I afferent terminals contacting the inner hair cells, spiral ganglion, and medial efferent terminals that contact the outer hair cells (Erichsen et al., 1996; McLean et al., 2009; Bottger et al., 2011), providing evidence that CI in those patients could generate likely preferable outcomes. One example of CI having an ideal outcome is CI in AN together with ADOA (OMIM #165500) owing to *OPA1* variations (Santarelli et al., 2008; Huang et al., 2009; Moser and Starr, 2016). The expression site of *OPA1* significantly overlaps with that of NKAα3, being it in the hair cells as well as in the neuronal fibers innervating the inner hair cells, ganglion cells of the cochlea, and vestibular organs (Bette et al., 2007).

Auditory neuropathy with *ATP1A3* mutation are generally considered to have ideal CI results. However, CI produces dubious outcomes in some reported cases. Tranebjaerg et al. (Fang et al., 2019) stated that four CAPOS patients received CI, two of whom gained significant benefits and the other two was relatively poor. In contrast, Atilgan et al. (2019) documented a much more beneficial effect of CI in a patient with CAPOS syndrome as compared to patients with SNHL. These findings could be explained by the fact that the *ATP1A3* gene is expressed not only in synapse but also in postsynaptic spiral ganglion cells (SGNs). If the lesion is mainly at the synapse, good CI results can be expected, similar to those in *OPA1* variants (Han et al., 2017), whereas CI is less useful with lesions dominantly at the SGNs. In fact, in most postsynaptic AN, CI has a dubious outcome (**Supplementary Table 2**). An example is CI in the SGNs (Fasquelle et al., 2011; Eppsteiner et al., 2012; Atilgan et al., 2019). CI performed earlier in *TMPRSS3* generated a preferable outcome, while the outcomes in later implantees were not as favorable (Chung et al., 2014). Patients who benefit most from CI were reported to be relatively younger (Han et al., 2017; Tranebjærg et al., 2018b), yet an accurate CI efficacy estimation with age and other possible impact factors taken into consideration is still awaiting discussion. Chaudhry et al. (2020) summarized 25 postsynaptic CI results, with 22 displaying modest to significant benefit, and demonstrated that CI behaves variably but generally good in postsynaptic AN. Moreover, the best functional outcome of CI observed at the short-term follow-up may decrease over time. Although earlier electrical stimulation of SGNs may attenuate the degeneration of the neurons, progressive degeneration of SGNs could possibly occur due to a disrupted function of NKAα3 (Han et al., 2017). In our study, patient 2 underwent CI on his left ear, but the result was hardly desirable. One possible explanation is that his age by the time he received surgery and the duration of his hearing loss are too long to ensure SGN activities. Moreover, the result of CI may be in relation with the characteristic of the PTA of the patients. Therefore, a continuous follow-up period for CI performance in those patients is warranted, to better determine if the current benefits from CI decreases over time.

The identification of p.E818K in *ATP1A3* has implications for future risk calculation and genetic counseling. In CAPOS families with an autosomal dominant inheritance pattern, the chance of offspring carrying pathogenic mutations is 50%, with varying degrees of penetrance. In addition, all reported CAPOS patients had unaffected siblings without exception, revealing that all pedigrees of CAPOS syndrome are sporadic cases. It is still unclear why *de novo* variants frequently occur in *ATP1A3*. The age of the father has been reported to be a strong impactor of *de novo* mutations (Niederberger, 2013). However, that study failed to explain all *de novo* cases. A genetic context in *ATP1A3* that favors the occurrence of *de novo* variants may account for this phenomenon, awaiting further clarification.

Here, four AN patients were identified with p.E818K mutation in the gene *ATP1A3*, causing progressive AN with postlingual onset and varying degrees of syndromic features. Our study confirms that *ATP1A3* in Chinese individuals is undoubtedly an important genetic cause of progressive AN with postlingual onset. Genetic testing for this specific mutation site allows for identification of a special subtype of AN with somewhat preferable CI results, as well as accurate genetic counseling.

ETHICS STATEMENT

The studies involving human participants were reviewed and approved by Committee of Medical Ethics of Chinese PLA General Hospital. Written informed consent to participate in this study was provided by the participants' legal guardian/next of kin. Written informed consent was obtained from the individual(s), and minor(s)' legal guardian/next of kin, for the publication of any potentially identifiable images or data included in this article.

AUTHOR CONTRIBUTIONS

HW and WW conceived and designed the experiments and wrote the manuscript. HW, WW, JL, LX, LL, and FX performed the experiments. HW analyzed the data. JL, LL, LX, and FX contributed to the reagents, materials, and analysis tools. HW, JG, and QW critically read and discussed the manuscript. All authors contributed to the article and approved the submitted version.

SUPPLEMENTARY MATERIAL

Supplementary Figure 1 | Audiological phenotype of subject 3 and 4. **(A,B)** PTA of subjects 3 and 4. Blue, left ear; red, right ear. **(C,D)** Observed DPOAE responses from the right and the left ear. Red line, DPOAE level from the right ear; blue line, DPOAE level from the left ear; gray line, noise level from both ears. **(E,F)** Absent ABR waveforms at 90 dB nHL stimulus on both ears of subjects 3 and 4. Blue, left ear; red, right ear.

Supplementary Table 1 | *ATP1A3* genotypes as they correlate with RDP, AHC, and CAPOS phenotypes.

Supplementary Table 2 | Postsynaptic auditory neuropathies and their CI outcomes.

REFERENCES

Atilgan, A., Yuksel, M., and Ciprut, A. (2019). Cochlear implantation in a case of auditory neuropathy spectrum disorder with CAPOS syndrome. *Med. Med. J.* 34, 318–323. doi: 10.5222/MMJ.2019.53503

Bette, S., Zimmermann, U., Wissinger, B., and Knipper, M. (2007). OPA1, the disease gene for optic atrophy type Kjer, is expressed in the inner ear. *Histochem. Cell Biol.* 128, 421–430. doi: 10.1007/s00418-007-0321-7

Blanco, G., and Mercer, R. (1998). Isozymes of the Na-K-ATPase: heterogeneity in structure, diversity in function. *Am. J. Physiol.* 275, F633–F650. doi: 10.1152/ajprenal.1998.275.5.F633

Blanco-Arias, P., Einholm, A., Mamsa, H., Concheiro, C., Gutiérrez-de-Terán, H., Romero, J., et al. (2009). Mutation of ATP1A3 underscores the crucial role of sodium affinity in the pathophysiology of rapid-onset dystonia-parkinsonism. *Hum. Mol. Genet.* 18, 2370–2377. doi: 10.1093/hmg/ddp170

Bottger, P., Tracz, Z., Heuck, A., Nissen, P., Romero-Ramos, M., and Lykke-Hartmann, K. (2011). Distribution of Na/K-ATPase alpha 3 isoform, a sodium-potassium P-type pump associated with rapid-onset of dystonia parkinsonism (RDP) in the adult mouse brain. *J. Comp. Neurol.* 519, 376–404. doi: 10.1002/cne.22524

Carecchio, M., Zorzi, G., Ragona, F., Zibordi, F., and Nardocci, N. (2018). ATP1A3-related disorders: an update. *Eur. J. Paediatr. Neurol.* 22, 257–263. doi: 10.1016/j.ejpn.2017.12.009

Chaudhry, D., Chaudhry, A., Muzaffar, J., Monksfield, P., and Bance, M. (2020). Cochlear implantation outcomes in post synaptic auditory neuropathies: a systematic review and narrative synthesis. *J. Int. Adv. Otol.* 16, 411–431. doi: 10.5152/iao.2020.9035

Chen, Y., Gu, Y., Li, Y., Li, G. L., Chai, R., Li, W., et al. (2021). Generation of mature and functional hair cells by co-expression of Gfi1, Pou4f3, and Atoh1 in the postnatal mouse cochlea. *Cell Rep.* 35:109016. doi: 10.1016/j.celrep.2021.109016

Cheng, C., Hou, Y., Zhang, Z., Wang, Y., Lu, L., Zhang, L., et al. (2021). Disruption of the autism-related gene Pak1 causes stereocilia disorganization, hair cell loss, and deafness in mice. *J. Genet. Genomics* 48, 324–332. doi: 10.1016/j.jgg.2021.03.010

Cheng, C., Wang, Y., Guo, L., Lu, X., Zhu, W., Muhammad, W., et al. (2019). Age-related transcriptome changes in Sox2+ supporting cells in the mouse cochlea. *Stem Cell Res. Ther.* 10:365. doi: 10.1186/s13287-019-1437-0

Chung, J., Park, S., Chang, S., Chung, T., Lee, K., Kim, A., et al. (2014). A novel mutation of TMPRSS3 related to milder auditory phenotype in Korean postlingual deafness: a possible future implication for a personalized auditory rehabilitation. *J. Mol. Med. (Berlin, Germany)* 92, 651–663. doi: 10.1007/s00109-014-1128-3

Clausen, M., Hilbers, F., and Poulsen, H. (2017). The structure and function of the Na,K-ATPase isoforms in health and disease. *Front. Physiol.* 8:371. doi: 10.3389/fphys.2017.00371

Demos, M., van Karnebeek, C., Ross, C., Adam, S., Shen, Y., Zhan, S., et al. (2014). A novel recurrent mutation in ATP1A3 causes CAPOS syndrome. *Orphanet J. Rare Dis.* 9:15. doi: 10.1186/1750-1172-9-15

Duat Rodriguez, A., Prochazkova, M., Santos Santos, S., Rubio Cabezas, O., Cantarin Extremera, V., and Gonzalez-Gutierrez-Solana, L. (2017). Early diagnosis of CAPOS syndrome before acute-onset ataxia-review of the literature and a new family. *Pediatr. Neurol.* 71, 60–64. doi: 10.1016/j.pediatrneurol.2017.01.009

Eppsteiner, R., Shearer, A., Hildebrand, M., Deluca, A., Ji, H., Dunn, C., et al. (2012). Prediction of cochlear implant performance by genetic mutation: the spiral ganglion hypothesis. *Hear. Res.* 292, 51–58. doi: 10.1016/j.heares.2012.08.007

Erichsen, S., Zuo, J., Curtis, L., Rarey, K., and Hultcrantz, M. (1996). Na,K-ATPase alpha- and beta-isoforms in the developing cochlea of the mouse. *Hear. Res.* 100, 143–149. doi: 10.1016/0378-5955(96)00105-0

Fang, Q., Zhang, Y., Da, P., Shao, B., Pan, H., He, Z., et al. (2019). Deletion of Limk1 and Limk2 in mice does not alter cochlear development or auditory function. *Sci. Rep.* 9:3357. doi: 10.1038/s41598-019-39769-z

Fasquelle, L., Scott, H., Lenoir, M., Wang, J., Rebillard, G., Gaboyard, S., et al. (2011). Tmprss3, a transmembrane serine protease deficient in human DFNB8/10 deafness, is critical for cochlear hair cell survival at the onset of hearing. *J. Biol. Chem.* 286, 17383–17397. doi: 10.1074/jbc.M110.190652

Fu, X., An, Y., Wang, H., Li, P., Lin, J., Yuan, J., et al. (2021). Deficiency of Klc2 induces low-frequency sensorineural hearing loss in C57BL/6 J mice and human. *Mol. Neurobiol.* doi: 10.21203/rs.3.rs-277106/v1

Gao, S., Cheng, C., Wang, M., Jiang, P., Zhang, L., Wang, Y., et al. (2019). Blebbistatin inhibits neomycin-induced apoptosis in hair cell-like HEI-OC-1 cells and in cochlear hair cells. *Front. Cell Neurosci.* 13:590. doi: 10.3389/fncel.2019.00590

Gropman, A., Uittenbogaard, M., Brantner, C., Wang, Y., Wong, L., and Chiaramello, A. (2020). Molecular genetic and mitochondrial metabolic analyses confirm the suspected mitochondrial etiology in a pediatric patient with an atypical form of alternating hemiplegia of childhood. *Mol. Genet. Metab. Rep.* 24:100609. doi: 10.1016/j.ymgmr.2020.100609

Guo, R., Li, J., Chen, C., Xiao, M., Liao, M., Hu, Y., et al. (2021). Biomimetic 3D bacterial cellulose-graphene foam hybrid scaffold regulates neural stem cell proliferation and differentiation. *Colloids Surf. B Biointerfaces* 200:111590. doi: 10.1016/j.colsurfb.2021.111590

Guo, R., Ma, X., Liao, M., Liu, Y., Hu, Y., Qian, X., et al. (2019). Development and application of cochlear implant-based electric-acoustic stimulation of spiral ganglion neurons. *ACS Biomater. Sci. Eng.* 5, 6735–6741. doi: 10.1021/acsbiomaterials.9b01265

Guo, R., Xiao, M., Zhao, W., Zhou, S., Hu, Y., Liao, M., et al. (2020). 2D Ti3C2TxMXene couples electrical stimulation to promote proliferation and neural differentiation of neural stem cells. *Acta Biomater.* S1742-7061(20)30749-2. doi: 10.1016/j.actbio.2020.12.035

Guo, R., Zhang, S., Xiao, M., Qian, F., He, Z., Li, D., et al. (2016). Accelerating bioelectric functional development of neural stem cells by graphene coupling: implications for neural interfacing with conductive materials. *Biomaterials* 106, 193–204. doi: 10.1016/j.biomaterials.2016.08.019

Han, K., Oh, D., Lee, S., Lee, C., Han, J., Kim, M., et al. (2017). ATP1A3 mutations can cause progressive auditory neuropathy: a new gene of auditory synaptopathy. *Sci. Rep.* 7:16504. doi: 10.1038/s41598-017-16676-9

Han, S., Xu, Y., Sun, J., Liu, Y., Zhao, Y., Tao, W., et al. (2020). Isolation and analysis of extracellular vesicles in a Morpho butterfly wing-integrated microvortex biochip. *Biosens. Bioelectron.* 154:112073. doi: 10.1016/j.bios.2020.112073

Harrison, R. V., Gordon, K. A., Papsin, B. C., Negandhi, J., and James, A. L. (2015). Auditory neuropathy spectrum disorder (ANSD) and cochlear implantation. *Int. J. Pediatr. Otorhinolaryngol.* 79, 1980–1987. doi: 10.1016/j.ijporl.2015.10.006

He, Y., Lu, X., Qian, F., Liu, D., Chai, R., and Li, H. (2017). Insm1a is required for zebrafish posterior lateral line development. *Front. Mol. Neurosci.* 10:241. doi: 10.3389/fnmol.2017.00241

He, Z., Fang, Q., Li, H., Shao, B., Zhang, Y., Zhang, Y., et al. (2019). The role of FOXG1 in the postnatal development and survival of mouse cochlear hair cells. *Neuropharmacology* 144, 43–57. doi: 10.1016/j.neuropharm.2018.10.021

He, Z., Guo, L., Shu, Y., Fang, Q., Zhou, H., Liu, Y., et al. (2017). Autophagy protects auditory hair cells against neomycin-induced damage. *Autophagy* 13, 1884–1904. doi: 10.1080/15548627.2017.1359449

He, Z. H., Li, M., Fang, Q. J., Liao, F. L., Zou, S. Y., Wu, X., et al. (2021). FOXG1 promotes aging inner ear hair cell survival through activation of the autophagy pathway. *Autophagy* 1–22. doi: 10.1080/15548627.2021.1916194

He, Z. H., Zou, S. Y., Li, M., Liao, F. L., Wu, X., Sun, H. Y., et al. (2020). The nuclear transcription factor FoxG1 affects the sensitivity of mimetic aging hair cells to inflammation by regulating autophagy pathways. *Redox Biol.* 28:101364. doi: 10.1016/j.redox.2019.101364

Heimer, G., Sadaka, Y., Israelian, L., Feiglin, A., Ruggieri, A., Marshall, C., et al. (2015). CAOS-episodic cerebellar ataxia, areflexia, optic atrophy, and sensorineural hearing loss: a third allelic disorder of the ATP1A3 gene. *J. Child Neurol.* 30, 1749–1756. doi: 10.1177/0883073815579708

Hu, Y., Li, D., Wei, H., Zhou, S., Chen, W., Yan, X., et al. (2021). Neurite extension and orientation of spiral ganglion neurons can be directed by superparamagnetic iron oxide nanoparticles in a magnetic field. *Int. J. Nanomed.* 16, 4515–4526. doi: 10.2147/IJN.S313673

Huang, T., Santarelli, R., and Starr, A. (2009). Mutation of OPA1 gene causes deafness by affecting function of auditory nerve terminals. *Brain Res.* 1300, 97–104. doi: 10.1016/j.brainres.2009.08.083

Kim, N., Kim, A., Park, K., Kim, S., Kim, M., Nam, J., et al. (2015). Whole-exome sequencing reveals diverse modes of inheritance in sporadic mild to moderate sensorineural hearing loss in a pediatric population. *Genet. Med.* 17, 901–911. doi: 10.1038/gim.2014.213

Landrum, M., Lee, J., Benson, M., Brown, G., Chao, C., Chitipiralla, S., et al. (2016). ClinVar: public archive of interpretations of clinically relevant variants. *Nucleic Acids Res.* 44, D862–D868. doi: 10.1093/nar/gkv1222

Liu, L., Chen, Y., Qi, J., Zhang, Y., He, Y., Ni, W., et al. (2016). Wnt activation protects against neomycin-induced hair cell damage in the mouse cochlea. *Cell Death Dis.* 7:e2136. doi: 10.1038/cddis.2016.35

Liu, W., Xu, L., Wang, X., Zhang, D., Sun, G., Wang, M., et al. (2021). PRDX1 activates autophagy via the PTEN-AKT signaling pathway to protect against cisplatin-induced spiral ganglion neuron damage. *Autophagy* 5, 1–23. doi: 10.1080/15548627.2021.1905466

Liu, W., Xu, X., Fan, Z., Sun, G., Han, Y., Zhang, D., et al. (2019). Wnt signaling activates TP53-induced glycolysis and apoptosis regulator and protects against cisplatin-induced spiral ganglion neuron damage in the mouse cochlea. *Antioxid. Redox Signal.* 30, 1389–1410. doi: 10.1089/ars.2017.7288

Liu, Y., Qi, J., Chen, X., Tang, M., Chu, C., Zhu, W., et al. (2019). Critical role of spectrin in hearing development and deafness. *Sci. Adv.* 5:eaav7803. doi: 10.1126/sciadv.aav7803

Lv, J., Fu, X., Li, Y., Hong, G., Li, P., Lin, J., et al. (2021). Deletion of Kcnj16 in mice does not alter auditory function. *Front. Cell Dev. Biol.* 9:630361. doi: 10.3389/fcell.2021.630361

Maas, R., Schieving, J., Schouten, M., Kamsteeg, E., and van de Warrenburg, B. (2016). The genetic homogeneity of CAPOS syndrome: four new patients with the c.2452G>A (p.Glu818Lys) mutation in the ATP1A3 gene. *Pediatr. Neurol.* 59, 71–75.e1. doi: 10.1016/j.pediatrneurol.2016.02.010

McLean, W., Smith, K., Glowatzki, E., and Pyott, S. (2009). Distribution of the Na,K-ATPase alpha subunit in the rat spiral ganglion and organ of corti. *J. Assoc. Res. Otolaryngol.* 10, 37–49. doi: 10.1007/s10162-008-0152-9

Moser, T., and Starr, A. (2016). Auditory neuropathy–neural and synaptic mechanisms. *Nat. Rev. Neurol.* 12, 135–149. doi: 10.1038/nrneurol.2016.10

Nicolaides, P., Appleton, R., and Fryer, A. (1996). Cerebellar ataxia, areflexia, pes cavus, optic atrophy, and sensorineural hearing loss (CAPOS): a new syndrome. *J. Med. Genet.* 33, 419–421. doi: 10.1136/jmg.33.5.419

Niederberger, C. (2013). Re: rate of De Novo mutations and the importance of father's age to disease risk. *J. Urol.* 189:655. doi: 10.1016/j.juro.2012.10.098

Paquay, S., Wiame, E., Deggouj, N., Boschi, A., De Siati, R., Sznajer, Y., et al. (2018). Childhood hearing loss is a key feature of CAPOS syndrome: a case report. *Int. J. Pediatr. Otorhinolaryngol.* 104, 191–194. doi: 10.1016/j.ijporl.2017.11.022

Potic, A., Nmezi, B., and Padiath, Q. (2015). CAPOS syndrome and hemiplegic migraine in a novel pedigree with the specific ATP1A3 mutation. *J. Neurol. Sci.* 358, 453–456. doi: 10.1016/j.jns.2015.10.002

Qi, J., Liu, Y., Chu, C., Chen, X., Zhu, W., Shu, Y., et al. (2019). A cytoskeleton structure revealed by super-resolution fluorescence imaging in inner ear hair cells. *Cell Discov.* 5:12. doi: 10.1038/s41421-018-0076-4

Qi, J., Zhang, L., Tan, F., Liu, Y., Chu, C., Zhu, W., et al. (2020). Espin distribution as revealed by super-resolution microscopy of stereocilia. *Am. J. Transl. Res.* 12, 130–141.

Qian, F., Wang, X., Yin, Z., Xie, G., Yuan, H., Liu, D., et al. (2020). The slc4a2b gene is required for hair cell development in zebrafish. *Aging (Albany NY)* 12, 18804–18821. doi: 10.18632/aging.103840

Rance, G., and Starr, A. (2015). Pathophysiological mechanisms and functional hearing consequences of auditory neuropathy. *Brain* 138, 3141–3158. doi: 10.1093/brain/awv270

Rodacker, V., Toustrup-Jensen, M., and Vilsen, B. (2006). Mutations Phe785Leu and Thr618Met in Na+,K+-ATPase, associated with familial rapid-onset dystonia parkinsonism, interfere with Na+ interaction by distinct mechanisms. *J. Biol. Chem.* 281, 18539–18548. doi: 10.1074/jbc.M601780200

Rosewich, H., Weise, D., Ohlenbusch, A., Gärtner, J., and Brockmann, K. (2014). Phenotypic overlap of alternating hemiplegia of childhood and CAPOS syndrome. *Neurology* 83, 861–863. doi: 10.1212/WNL.0000000000000735

Santarelli, R., Cama, E., Scimemi, P., Dal Monte, E., Genovese, E., and Arslan, E. (2008). Audiological and electrocochleography findings in hearing-impaired children with connexin 26 mutations and otoacoustic emissions. *Eur. Arch. Otorhinolaryngol.* 265, 43–51. doi: 10.1007/s00405-007-0412-z

Starr, P., Rau, G., Davis, V., Marks, W., Ostrem, J., Simmons, D., et al. (2005). Spontaneous pallidal neuronal activity in human dystonia: comparison with Parkinson's disease and normal macaque. *J. Neurophysiol.* 93, 3165–3176. doi: 10.1152/jn.00971.2004

Tan, F., Chu, C., Qi, J., Li, W., You, D., Li, K., et al. (2019). AAV-ie enables safe and efficient gene transfer to inner ear cells. *Nat. Commun.* 10:3733. doi: 10.1038/s41467-019-11687-8

Tranebjærg, L., Strenzke, N., Lindholm, S., Rendtorff, N., Poulsen, H., Khandelia, H., et al. (2018a). The CAPOS mutation in ATP1A3 alters Na/K-ATPase function and results in auditory neuropathy which has implications for management. *Hum. Genet.* 137, 279–280. doi: 10.1007/s00439-018-1870-7

Tranebjærg, L., Strenzke, N., Lindholm, S., Rendtorff, N., Poulsen, H., Khandelia, H., et al. (2018b). The CAPOS mutation in ATP1A3 alters Na/K-ATPase function and results in auditory neuropathy which has implications for management. *Hum. Genet.* 137, 111–127. doi: 10.1007/s00439-017-1862-z

Wang, H., Guan, J., Lan, L., Yu, L., Xie, L., Liu, X., et al. (2018). A novel de novo mutation of ACTG1 in two sporadic non-syndromic hearing loss cases. *Sci. China Life Sci.* 61, 729–732. doi: 10.1007/s11427-017-9165-2

Wang, Y., Li, J., Yao, X., Li, W., Du, H., Tang, M., et al. (2017). Loss of CIB2 causes profound hearing loss and abolishes mechanoelectrical transduction in mice. *Front. Mol. Neurosci.* 10:401. doi: 10.3389/fnmol.2017.00401

Zhang, S., Dong, Y., Qiang, R., Zhang, Y., Zhang, X., Chen, Y., et al. (2021). Characterization of Strip1 expression in mouse cochlear hair cells. *Front. Genet.* 12:625867. doi: 10.3389/fgene.2021.625867

Zhang, S., Zhang, Y., Dong, Y., Guo, L., Zhang, Z., Shao, B., et al. (2020). Knockdown of Foxg1 in supporting cells increases the trans-differentiation of supporting cells into hair cells in the neonatal mouse cochlea. *Cell. Mol. Life Sci.* 77, 1401–1419. doi: 10.1007/s00018-019-03291-2

Zhang, Y., Li, W., He, Z., Wang, Y., Shao, B., Cheng, C., et al. (2019). Pre-treatment with Fasudil prevents neomycin-induced hair cell damage by reducing the accumulation of reactive oxygen species. *Front. Mol. Neurosci.* 12:264. doi: 10.3389/fnmol.2019.00264

Zhong, Z., Fu, X., Li, H., Chen, J., Wang, M., Gao, S., et al. (2020). Citicoline protects auditory hair cells against neomycin-induced damage. *Front. Cell Dev. Biol.* 8:712. doi: 10.3389/fcell.2020.00712

Zhu, C., Cheng, C., Wang, Y., Muhammad, W., Liu, S., Zhu, W., et al. (2018). Loss of ARHGEF6 causes hair cell stereocilia deficits and hearing loss in mice. *Front. Molecul. Neurosci.* 11:362. doi: 10.3389/fnmol.2018.00362

11

Atrial Natriuretic Peptide Promotes Neurite Outgrowth and Survival of Cochlear Spiral Ganglion Neurons *in vitro* Through NPR-A/ cGMP/PKG Signaling

Fei Sun[1†], Ke Zhou[2†], Ke-yong Tian[1†], Xin-yu Zhang[1], Wei Liu[1], Jie Wang[3], Cui-ping Zhong[4], Jian-hua Qiu[1] and Ding-jun Zha[1*]*

[1] Department of Otolaryngology-Head and Neck Surgery, Xijing Hospital, Fourth Military Medical University, Xi'an, China, [2] Department of Laboratory Medicine, Institute of Clinical Laboratory Medicine of PLA, Xijing Hospital, Fourth Military Medical University, Xi'an, China, [3] Department of Otolaryngology-Head and Neck Surgery, The Affiliated Children Hospital of Xi'an Jiaotong University, Xi'an, China, [4] Department of Otolaryngology-Head and Neck Surgery, The 940th Hospital of Joint Logistics Support Force of PLA, Lanzhou, China

***Correspondence:**
Ding-jun Zha
zhadjun@fmmu.edu.cn
Jian-hua Qiu
qiujh@fmmu.edu.cn

[†] These authors have contributed equally to this work

Sensorineural hearing loss (SNHL) is a dominant public health issue affecting millions of people around the globe, which is correlated with the irreversible deterioration of the hair cells and spiral ganglion neurons (SGNs) within the cochlea. Strategies using bioactive molecules that regulate neurite regeneration and neuronal survival to reestablish connections between auditory epithelium or implanted electrodes and SGN neurites would become attractive therapeutic candidates for SNHL. As an intracellular second messenger, cyclic guanosine-3',5'-monophosphate (cGMP) can be synthesized through activation of particulate guanylate cyclase-coupled natriuretic peptide receptors (NPRs) by natriuretic peptides, which in turn modulates multiple aspects of neuronal functions including neuronal development and neuronal survival. As a cardiac-derived hormone, atrial natriuretic peptide (ANP), and its specific receptors (NPR-A and NPR-C) are broadly expressed in the nervous system where they might be involved in the maintenance of diverse neural functions. Despite former literatures and our reports indicating the existence of ANP and its receptors within the inner ear, particularly in the spiral ganglion, their potential regulatory mechanisms underlying functional properties of auditory neurons are still incompletely understood. Our recently published investigation revealed that ANP could promote the neurite outgrowth of SGNs by activating NPR-A/cGMP/PKG cascade in a dose-dependent manner. In the present research, the influence of ANP and its receptor-mediated downstream signaling pathways on neurite outgrowth, neurite attraction, and neuronal survival of SGNs *in vitro* was evaluated by employing cultures of organotypic explant and dissociated neuron from postnatal rats. Our data indicated that ANP could support and attract neurite outgrowth of SGNs and possess a high capacity to improve neuronal survival of SGNs against glutamate-induced excitotoxicity by triggering the NPR-A/cGMP/PKG pathway. The neuroregenerative and neuroprotective effects of ANP/NPRA/cGMP/PKG-dependent signaling on SGNs would represent an attractive therapeutic candidate for hearing impairment.

Keywords: sensorineural hearing loss, spiral ganglion neuron, atrial natriuretic peptide, natriuretic peptide receptors, cGMP, neurite outgrowth, neuroprotection

INTRODUCTION

Hearing loss has become a global health and economic problem affecting approximately 20% of the world's population (one in five people) suffering from different degrees of sensory disorder, while more than 430 million people experience disabling hearing loss, according to the first World Report on Hearing recently announced by the World Health Organization[1]. As a major type of hearing loss sensorineural hearing loss (SNHL) can be caused by various insults such as acoustic trauma, ototoxic drugs, infections, aging, genetic mutations, and tumor (He et al., 2017; McLean et al., 2017; Zhu et al., 2018; Fang et al., 2019; Jiang et al., 2020; Qian et al., 2020; Lv et al., 2021), resulting in irreversible deterioration of sensory cells, e.g., the cochlear hair cells (HCs) (He et al., 2016; Liu et al., 2016; Li A. et al., 2018; Xia et al., 2019; Zhang S. et al., 2019; Zhang et al., 2020c) and auditory neurons (Guo et al., 2016; Yan et al., 2018; Liu W. et al., 2019; Guo et al., 2020, 2021). The cochlear HCs in the organ of Corti are mechanosensory cells which convert mechanical sound waves into primary acoustic signals (Wang et al., 2017; Zhu et al., 2018; Liu Y. et al., 2019; Qi et al., 2019, 2020). The spiral ganglion neurons (SGNs) are the cochlear primary afferent neurons which perform a crucial function in hearing by conducting auditory information from the sensory HCs to the auditory center within the brain (Nayagam et al., 2011). Because the regenerative capacity of HCs and SGNs in the mature mammalian cochlea is very limited (Cox et al., 2014; Lu et al., 2017; Cheng et al., 2019; Tan et al., 2019; Zhang et al., 2020a,b), irreversible death of cochlear HCs followed by a progressive degeneration of SGNs ultimately causes permanent hearing loss (He et al., 2019; Ding et al., 2020; He et al., 2020; Roccio et al., 2020; Zhou et al., 2020).

Over a longer period, various strategies have been developed in an attempt to treat or at least prevent further progression of SNHL. Unfortunately, the therapeutic efficacy for patients with hearing impairment is still unsatisfactory. Novel therapeutics based on genetic and cell transplantation techniques appear to be a promising approach to restoring hearing function, including substitution or regeneration of HCs and/or SGNs by means of stem and progenitor cells transplantation (Li D. et al., 2019; Li G. et al., 2019; Tang et al., 2019; Zhao et al., 2019; Fang et al., 2020; Xia et al., 2020; Yang et al., 2020), as well as *in situ* reprogramming of adjacent supporting cells or glial cells into functional HCs or neurons (Chen et al., 2017; Cheng et al., 2017; McLean et al., 2017; Zhang et al., 2017; Noda et al., 2018; You et al., 2018; Zhang et al., 2018; Zhang Y. et al., 2019; Li et al., 2020; Waqas et al., 2020; Zhang et al., 2020c). Moreover, transplantation of stem/progenitor cells into the human cochlea is technically demanding and is accompanied by the possible risks of developing tumors (Nishimura et al., 2012). Currently, auditory prosthesis such as cochlear implants (CIs) are a favorable solution for patients with profound SNHL, which can substitute for the missing HCs to directly stimulate the surviving neurons from the auditory nerve (Ma et al., 2019). The effectiveness of such neural prosthetic devices relies not only on the integrated interface where the implant's electrodes make contact with peripheral neurites of SGNs but also on the number of functional auditory neurons being stimulated. In order to optimize the outcome of cochlear implantation, some biological approaches are attempted to preserve the residual auditory neurons from degeneration after the loss of auditory HCs or to promote regeneration and outgrowth of neurites from SGNs toward the electrode array (Kwiatkowska et al., 2016; Li et al., 2017; Guo et al., 2019). Consequently, new strategies using bioactive molecules that facilitate neurite regeneration and neuronal survival to reestablish the synaptic connections between the auditory sensory epithelium or implanted electrode array and SGNs neurites would become attractive therapeutic candidates for hearing impairment.

Cyclic guanosine-3',5'-monophosphate (cGMP) acts as an important secondary messenger which mediates various biological functions through three effector molecules comprising cGMP-dependent protein kinases (PKG, also known as cGK), cGMP-gated ion channels, and cGMP-regulated isoforms of phosphodiesterases. The pathway involving cGMP may offer a unique signaling mechanism in modulating neuronal development and synaptic plasticity associated with neurite outgrowth and pathfinding, neuronal survival, neuronal excitability, and the sensory transduction cascades associated with vision and olfaction (Zhao and Ma, 2009; Zhao et al., 2009). Under the physiology condition, cGMP can be catalyzed by two categories of molecularly distinct guanylate cyclases (GCs), including soluble GC which recognizes its ligand nitric oxide and particulate GC-coupled receptors that are specifically activated by natriuretic peptides (NPs). Specifically, the transmembrane GC-coupled natriuretic peptide receptors (NPRs), NPR-A and NPR-B, interact with three NPs, in turn leading to the activation of the intracellular GC domain and synthesis of cGMP. Owing to the absence of GC activity, the clearance receptor NPR-C can remove circulating NPs through ligand binding, internalization, and degradation (Potter et al., 2009).

Atrial natriuretic peptide (ANP) is a cardiac-derived hormone predominantly synthesized and secreted by the cardiac atria, which dynamically regulates blood pressure through decreasing

[1]https://www.who.int/activities/highlighting-priorities-for-ear-and-hearing-care

water and sodium loads in the circulatory system. Through binding to its specific receptors on the cell surface, NPR-A (also known as NPR1 or GC-A) and NPR-C, ANP exerts a fundamental role in the modulation of cardiovascular homeostasis (Potter et al., 2009). ANP, brain NP (BNP), and C-type NP (CNP) are structurally related peptides belonging to members of the NP family that are widely distributed in the mammalian central nervous system (CNS) (Cao and Yang, 2008; Mahinrad et al., 2016), especially in peripheral sensory organs such as the dorsal root, trigeminal, retinal, and cochlear ganglia (Lamprecht and Meyer zum Gottesberge, 1988; Furuta et al., 1995; Abdelalim and Tooyama, 2010; Xu et al., 2010; Loo et al., 2012; Abdelalim et al., 2013; Vilotti et al., 2013; Fitzakerley and Trachte, 2018). Recent research has shown the involvement of the BNP/NPR-A signaling pathway in the modulation of nociceptive processing for pain (Zhang et al., 2010) and itch responses (Solinski et al., 2019). Besides, cGMP signaling elicited by the CNP/NPR-B pathway regulates neurite outgrowth and pathfinding of sensory ganglion neurons within DRG (Schmidt et al., 2002, 2007; Kishimoto et al., 2008; Schmidt et al., 2009; Zhao et al., 2009; Xia et al., 2013; Ter-Avetisyan et al., 2014; Schmidt et al., 2016; Dumoulin et al., 2018a,b; Schmidt et al., 2018; Ter-Avetisyan et al., 2018; Tröster et al., 2018) and cochlear spiral ganglion (SG) (Lu et al., 2011, 2014; Ter-Avetisyan et al., 2014, 2018; Wolter et al., 2018; Schmidt and Fritzsch, 2019) during development. Additionally, all three NPs possess neuroprotective ability on retinal and central neurons through GC-coupled NPR stimulation (Fiscus et al., 2001; Cheng Chew et al., 2003; Kuribayashi et al., 2006; Ma et al., 2010; Colini Baldeschi et al., 2018). All these clues indicate that NPs and their receptors could probably be associated with the maintenance of various aspects of neuronal functions.

The existence of ANP and receptors in the sensory and secretory compartments of the mammalian inner ear has been systematically elucidated in a great number of literatures (Lamprecht and Meyer zum Gottesberge, 1988; Meyer and Lamprecht, 1989; Gottesberge et al., 1991; Koch et al., 1992; Yoon and Hellström, 1992; Yoon and Anniko, 1994; Furuta et al., 1995; Meyer Zum Gottesberge et al., 1995; Krause et al., 1997; Suzuki et al., 1998; Seebacher et al., 1999; Yoon et al., 2012; Sun et al., 2013, 2014; Yoon et al., 2015; Sun et al., 2020), while recent works also show that ANP receptors are distributed in rat cochlear SG and modiolus of the guinea pig (Lamprecht and Meyer zum Gottesberge, 1988; Furuta et al., 1995). However, the distribution patterns and potential functions of ANP and its receptors in the neural elements of the inner ear remain unclear. In our previous studies, the expression patterns of ANP and its receptors were investigated in the cochlear SG, which provided direct evidence for the presence and synthesis of ANP and its receptors in the neural region of the cochlea (Sun et al., 2013, 2014). We recently demonstrated that ANP might promote neurite outgrowth of cochlear SGNs by triggering the NPR-A/cGMP/PKG pathway in a dose-dependent manner (Sun et al., 2020). In the current study, the influence of ANP on neurite outgrowth, neurite attraction, and neuronal survival of rat SGNs was evaluated by employing organotypic explant and dissociated neuron cultures *in vitro*. All these findings demonstrated that ANP may promote neurite outgrowth and neuronal survival of SGNs by activating the NPR-A/cGMP/PKG pathway, not via interaction with the NPR-C pathway. ANP may perform a vital role in the normal neuritogenesis of cochlear auditory neurons during development of the inner ear and may enhance neurite regeneration and neuronal viability of SGNs, thus representing a potential therapeutic candidate for hearing impairment.

MATERIALS AND METHODS

Animals and Tissue Preparation

All experimental procedures have been permitted by the Animal Care Committee of the Fourth Military Medical University, China. Animals used for the study were provided by the Laboratory Animal Center of the Fourth Military Medical University. Sprague-Dawley rats of postnatal day 3 (P3) and P7 were used for analyses. For the preparation of cochlear sections and cultures, the rat pups were sacrificed by rapid decapitation, and their skulls were opened midsagitally. All cochleae were promptly separated from the temporal bone under a dissecting microscope, rinsed with ice-cold Hank's Balanced Salt Solution (HBSS; Thermo Fisher Scientific), and collected for further use. A schematic summary of the protocol and timeline for SG explant or dissociated SGN cultures used in this study is illustrated in **Figure 1**.

Immunofluorescent Analysis of ANP and Its Receptors on Cochlear Sections

For cochlear cryosections, cochleae extracted from P7 rats were superfused with fresh 4% paraformaldehyde solution through the round and oval windows and further immersed in an identical fixative solution overnight at 4°C. The cochlear tissues were decalcified for 2 days in 5% EDTA followed by dehydration in 30% sucrose overnight at 4°C. After being embedded in Tissue-Tek OCT compound (Sakura Finetek) at −20°C, tissues were oriented to obtain mid-modiolar cross sections and then cut on a cryostat microtome into 12-μm-thick sections. Cryosections were then placed onto poly-L-lysine-coated slides and allowed to dry overnight at room temperature (RT) before performance of immunofluorescence staining.

For immunohistochemistry, the cochlear sections were rinsed with phosphate-buffered saline (PBS) and incubated in a blocking and permeabilizing solution composed of 5% bovine serum albumin (BSA; Sigma-Aldrich) and 0.1% Triton X-100 dissolved in PBS for 40 min at 37°C. All slides were immersed into the antibody solution (1% BSA and 0.1% Triton X-100 in PBS) supplemented with the following primary antibodies at a concentration of 1:500 at 4°C overnight: monoclonal mouse anti-β-III tubulin (TUJ1) antibody (Abcam, #ab78078), polyclonal rabbit anti-ANP antibody (Thermo Fisher Scientific, #PA5-29559), polyclonal rabbit anti-NPR-A antibody (Thermo Fisher Scientific, #PA5-29049), and polyclonal rabbit anti-NPR-C antibody (Thermo Fisher Scientific, #PA5-96947). Immunolabeling was further visualized with Alexa Fluor 488-conjugated donkey anti-mouse IgG (1:500; Thermo Fisher Scientific, #A-21202) and Alexa Fluor 594-conjugated donkey anti-rabbit IgG (1:500; Thermo Fisher Scientific, #A-21207)

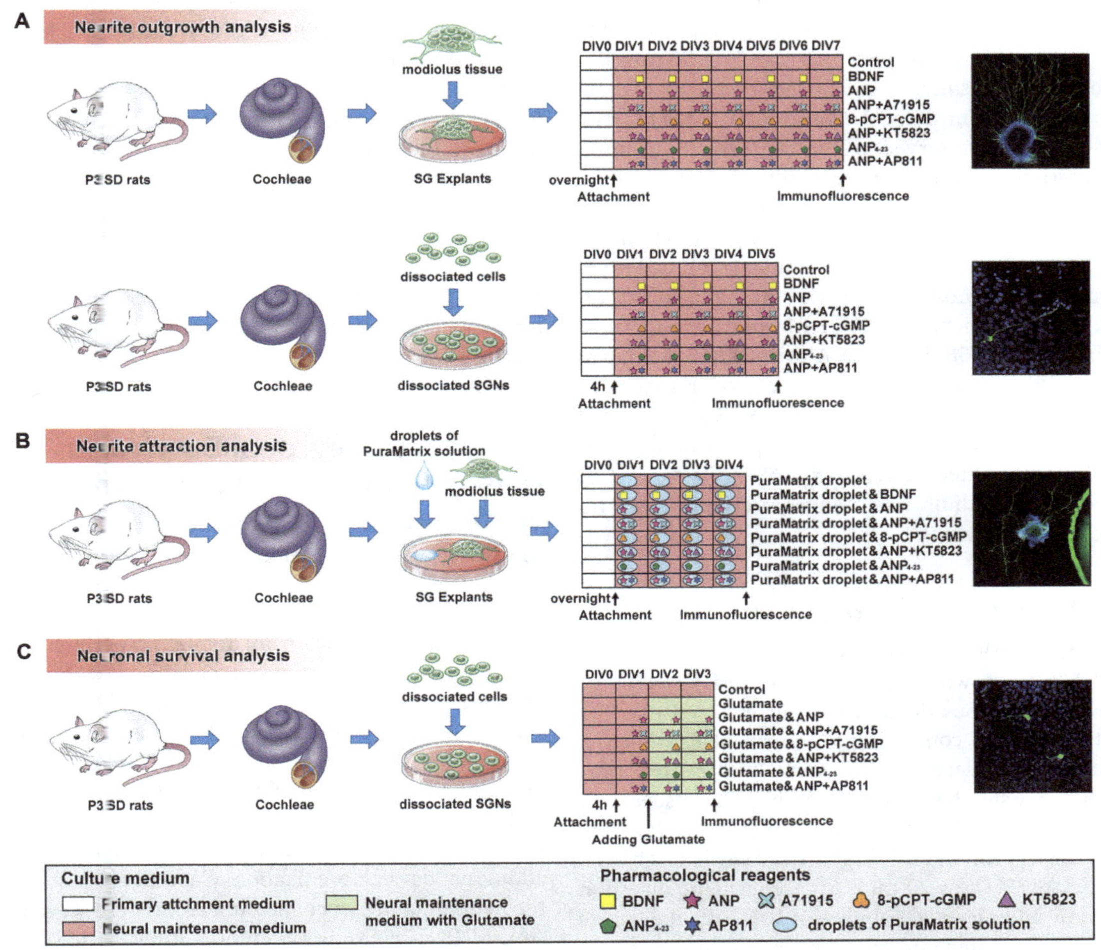

FIGURE 1 | Schematic summary of the protocol and timeline for SG explant or dissociated SGN cultures used for analysis of neurite outgrowth **(A)**, neurite attraction **(B)** and neuronal survival **(C)**.

diluted in an antibody solution at a concentration of 1:500 for 2 h at RT. Cochlear specimens randomly processed for staining in parallel without incubation with primary antibodies were served as a negative control. After counterstaining with Hoechst 33342 at 1:1,000 (Thermo Fisher Scientific) for 15 min at RT, all samples were subsequently mounted with the Prolong Gold anti-fade mounting medium (Thermo Fisher Scientific). All confocal images acquired under a confocal microscope system (FV1000; Olympus) were converted to TIFF format using a confocal software (FV10-ASW 4.2; Olympus) and processed for optimal brightness and contrast with the Adobe Photoshop software (CC 2020; Adobe Systems).

Analysis of Neurite Outgrowth in SG Explant Cultures

The experimental protocol for cochlear SG explant culture was performed according to a previous study (Sun et al., 2016) with a minor modification. Briefly, the membranous labyrinth was revealed after removal of the cochlear capsule from P3 rat cochleae under the dissecting microscope. After the spiral ligament, stria vascularis, and basilar membrane were separated from the modiolus, the remaining spiral lamina containing SG was cautiously dissected into equal pieces of approximately 500 μm. Subsequently, each dissected tissue was adhered to a single 15-mm glass-bottom culture dish (Advance BioScience), previously coated with Cell-Tak (BD Biosciences, #354240), and filled with 100 μl of primary attachment medium consisting of Dulbecco's modified Eagle medium (DMEM), 10% fetal bovine serum (FBS), 25 mM HEPES, and 1% penicillin–streptomycin (all Thermo Fisher Scientific). Samples were kept overnight in an atmosphere of 5% CO_2 and 95% humidity at 37°C. After attachment of explants, the culture medium was aspirated, and 100 μl of 20% Matrigel (BD Biosciences, #356234) mixture diluted with the attachment medium was directly dropped onto each explant culture. Immediately, the culture dish was transferred to the incubator to initiate gelation of the Matrigel for 10 min.

For neurite outgrowth assay, SG explants were cultured in neural maintenance medium consisting of DMEM/Ham's F12 medium (DMEM/F12) supplemented with 1x B27 and 1x N2 (all Thermo Fisher Scientific) and 1% penicillin–streptomycin and simultaneously treated with distinct pharmacological reagents. Explants incubated in medium supplemented with or without 20 ng/ml recombinant brain-derived neurotrophic factor (BDNF; PeproTech, #450-02) were served as control cultures. Cultures from other experimental groups were maintained in medium supplemented with 1 μM of ANP (Caymanchem, #24276), 1 μM of ANP plus 1 μM of NPR-A antagonist A71915 (Bachem, #4030385), 1 μM of the cell-permeable analog of cGMP 8-(4-chlorophenylthio) guanosine-3',5'-cyclic monophosphate (8-pCPT-cGMP; Sigma-Aldrich, #C5438), 1 μM of ANP plus 1 μM of the PKG inhibitor KT5823 (Sigma-Aldrich, #K1388), 1 μM of the specific NPR-C agonist ANP_{4-23} (Echelon Biosciences, #155-40), or 1 μM of ANP plus 1 μM of the NPR-C antagonist AP811 (Tocris Bioscience, #5498). In each experimental group, five explants were incubated at 37°C with 5% CO_2 for 7 days prior to fixation. The medium was changed every other day for the duration of the experiment.

Analysis of Neurite Outgrowth in Dissociated SGN Cultures

Dissociated SGN cultures were conducted in accordance with the procedures from a previous document (Tuft et al., 2013). The cochlear ducts of P3 rats containing the organ of Corti, spiral ligament, and stria vascularis were sequentially dissected away to collect modiolus tissues harboring the SGNs. The tissues were then applied to enzymatic dissociation by using 0.1% collagenase type IV and 0.25% trypsin in Ca^{2+}/Mg^{2+}-free HBSS (all Thermo Fisher Scientific) at 37°C for 20 min. After enzymatic digestion was inactivated by adding equal volumes of 10% FBS, the tissues were mechanically triturated into cell suspensions through a fire-polished glass Pasteur pipette. The dissociated SG cells were resuspended in neural maintenance medium and seeded at a density of 2.0×10^5 cells/poly-L-lysine-coated (Thermo Fisher Scientific) dish for 4 h.

For neurite outgrowth assay, the attached SGNs were maintained in culture medium supplemented with or without the following reagents consistent with those in SG explant cultures: 20 ng/ml BDNF, 1 μM ANP, 1 μM ANP plus 1 μM A71915, 1 μM 8-pCPT-cGMP, 1 μM ANP plus 1 μM KT5823, 1 μM ANP_{4-23}, or 1 μM ANP plus 1 μM AP811. In each group, five culture dishes containing dissociated cells were replenished with a fresh medium every other day and transferred to a 5% CO_2 incubator at 37°C for 5 days before fixation.

Analysis of Neurite Attraction in SG Explant Cultures

The procedures for evaluating the neurite attraction of SG explants cultures were adopted from procedures described previously with several modifications (Frick et al., 2017). Briefly, 1% PuraMatrix solution (BD Biosciences, #354250) was diluted to 0.25% solution with sterile ultrapure water (Milli-Q, Merck) alone or diluted with ultrapure water containing the following reagents to obtain a 0.25% PuraMatrix mixture: 20 ng/ml BDNF, 1 μM ANP, 1 μM ANP plus 1 μM A71915, 1 μM 8-pCPT-cGMP, 1 μM ANP plus 1 μM KT5823, 1 μM ANP_{4-23}, or 1 μM ANP plus 1 μM AP811. Each resulting PuraMatrix hydrogel (diluted solution or mixture) was briefly sonicated for 30 min for homogenization. Subsequently, 5-μl droplets of 0.25% PuraMatrix hydrogel were transferred into Cell-Tak-coated culture dishes, and dishes were maintained by incubation at 37°C for 30 min before settling of SG explants. Each dissected SG explant was plated at approximately 0.5 mm next to a hydrogel droplet in a culture dish and settled to attach as described above. After attachment, all explants were cultured in the neural maintenance medium for 4 days prior to fixation, and the culture medium was refreshed every other day. For each condition, five explants were maintained for neurite attraction study.

Analysis of Neuronal Survival in Dissociated SGN Cultures With Glutamate Excitotoxicity

The dissociated cells from modiolus tissues obtained as described above were incubated in neural maintenance medium at the same density of 2.0×10^5 cells per dish. On the first day *in vitro* (DIV1), dissociated cells from different experimental groups were maintained in a medium supplemented with or without the reagents as follows: 1 μM ANP, 1 μM ANP plus 1 μM A71915, 1 μM 8-pCPT-cGMP, 1 μM ANP plus 1 μM KT5823, 1 μM ANP_{4-23}, or 1 μM ANP plus 1 μM AP811. At DIV2, 100 μM of L-glutamic acid (glutamate, Glu; Sigma-Aldrich, #G5889) was added to the culture medium of different experimental cultures to induce excitotoxicity, and all cultures were maintained for two additional days before fixation. Concurrently, cells incubated in the neural maintenance medium alone were served as a baseline control. In each group, five culture dishes seeded with dissociated SGNs were maintained for neuronal survival study.

Immunofluorescence and Statistical Analysis

Following the culture period, all SG explants and dissociated SGNs were firstly fixed with paraformaldehyde for immunofluorescent analysis. All specimens were then permeabilized and blocked with a PBS solution containing 5% BSA and 0.1% Triton X-100, followed by incubation with the mouse primary antibody against TUJ1 (diluted 1:500) and Alexa Fluor 488-conjugated donkey anti-mouse IgG (diluted 1:500) to visualize the neural components. After nuclear counterstaining with Hoechst 33342 (diluted 1:1,000), all samples in the culture dishes were mounted with the Prolong Gold medium. Images of explant and cell cultures were photographed on the confocal microscope and analyzed for neurite tracing by using the "Neurite Tracer" function in the ImageJ software (version 1.46r; National Institute of Health) according to a previous study (Kempfle et al., 2018). The number and lengths of neurite outgrowth from the SG explants, together with the neuronal number and neurite length of dissociated SGNs, were measured and analyzed. Besides, the capacity of the PuraMatrix hydrogel to attract neurites was evaluated according to the previous research (Frick et al., 2017), by quantifying the probability of neurite attachment to hydrogel surfaces (estimated by the ratio of the number of explants with extended neurites that attached to hydrogel surfaces to the number of explants with extended neurites that contacted hydrogel droplets).

Furthermore, all experimental data are shown as the means ± standard error of the mean (means ± SEM) and analyzed by using the Statistical Program for Social Science software (SPSS, version 22.0; IBM Inc.). One-way analysis of variance (ANOVA) followed by Bonferroni's *post hoc* test was used to assess the statistical significance. *P*-values less than 0.05 ($P < 0.05$) was accepted as statistically significant.

RESULTS

Expression of ANP and Its Receptors in Cochlear SGNs of Postnatal Rats

To confirm the distribution patterns of ANP and its receptors within the cochlear SG of postnatal rats in our previous publications, anti-ANP, NPR-A, and NPR-C immunolabeling were performed on cochlear cryosections from P7 rats co-immunostained with antibodies against neuron-specific β-III tubulin. As shown in **Figure 2**, ANP (**Figure 2A**) and its receptors' (**Figures 2B,C**) immunoreactivities were observed in the SG regions along the length of the cochlear tonotopic axis without any noticeable apical-to-basal gradients. The representative images of cryosectioned tissues from the mid-cochlear turn revealed that the immunoreactivities of ANP (**Figure 2A$_2$**), NPR-A (**Figure 2B$_2$**), or NPR-C (**Figure 2C$_2$**) were colocalized with TUJ1-positive neuronal somata of SGNs, which was consistent with our previous results (Sun et al., 2013, 2014, 2020). The similar distribution patterns of ANP (**Figure 2A$_{2'}$**), NPR-A (**Figure 2B$_{2'}$**), and NPR-C (**Figure 2C$_{2'}$**) were observed in the cochlear SGNs, and they were predominantly immunoreactive in the neuronal perikarya, including the cytoplasm and plasma membrane of SGNs. The fluorescence intensity of NPR-A and NPR-C were more evident than that of our previous results, as we employed a different group of primary and secondary antibodies for labeling of ANP, NPR-A, and NPR-C. No specific immunoreactivity was seen in the negative controls for which the primary antibodies were omitted.

ANP Promotes Neurite Outgrowth of SG Explants and Dissociated SGNs by Activating the NPR-A/cGMP/PKG Pathway

To explore the possible effects of two distinct downstream signaling pathways of ANP receptors on the neurite outgrowth of SGNs, we initially counted the average number of regenerated neurites and the mean length of neurites extended from SG explants of P3 rats in each different distinct experimental group maintained in the culture medium containing specific reagents *in vitro* for 7 days (at DIV7). The explants treated with the culture medium alone were served as a negative control, while the explants that received the BDNF-containing medium for trophic support of neurite extension were used as a positive control. As shown in **Figure 3**, a small number of spontaneous neurite outgrowth with short length were observed in explants from negative controls (**Figure 3A**). As expected, robustly sprouting and elongating neurites were induced from explants treated with 20 ng/ml BDNF (**Figure 3B**). Interestingly, treatment of samples with 1 μM ANP elicited pronounced neurite outgrowth from SG explants (**Figure 3C**). For better understanding the possible mechanism of ANP in promoting the neurite outgrowth of SGNs, we discovered whether this polypeptide hormone acts via its GC-coupled receptor NPR-A or its clearance receptor NPR-C. In the presence of 1 μM NPR-A antagonist A71915, ANP (1 μM) failed to develop neurite elongation, suggesting that ANP-induced cGMP formation was abolished (**Figure 3D**), with respect to significantly less number and length of neurite than those in BDNF-positive control cultures. Treatment with 1 μM of the cell-permeable cGMP analog 8-pCPT-cGMP mimicked the effect of ANP-mediated neurite outgrowth, which would involve stimulation of PKG (**Figure 3E**). Conversely, application of 1 μM KT5823, a selective inhibitor of PKG, appeared to abrogate ANP-induced neurite outgrowth and sprouting (**Figure 3F**). Furthermore, incubation with 1 μM ANP_{4-23}, a specific NPR-C agonist, did not significantly stimulate neurite outgrowth from SG tissues (**Figure 3G**). Despite blockade of NPR-C with its antagonist AP811, ANP considerably elevated the number and the length of elongating neurites (**Figure 3H**) in comparison to the negative controls.

Subsequently, we counted the mean neuronal number and the average neuritic process length of dissociated SGNs from P3 rats incubated in the culture medium with the assigned additives *in vitro* for 5 days (at DIV5). To provide a positive or negative control, the neuronal cultures were maintained in medium with or without the addition of BDNF, respectively. Representative images of neuronal cultures from various experimental groups are illustrated in **Figure 4**. The average number of neurons per culture dish was 47.7 ± 2.3, and the average neurite length per neuron was 227.2 ± 21.4 μm in negative control samples (**Figure 4A**). A significantly increased number of neurons and elongating neurite outgrowth were seen in cell cultures treated with 20 ng/ml BDNF (**Figure 4B**). As expected, the number of neurons and neurite length of ANP-treated (**Figure 4C**) and 8-pCPT-cGMP-treated (**Figure 4E**) neurons were significantly increased compared to the negative control samples. Conversely, 1 μM ANP failed to elevate the neuronal number and neurite elongation of SGNs in the presence of 1 μM A71915 (**Figure 4D**) or 1 μM KT5823 (**Figure 4F**). Furthermore, 1 μM ANP_{4-23} did not elicit the same effect as ANP (**Figure 4G**), while 1 μM AP811 did not suppress the effect of ANP on neuronal maintenance and neurite outgrowth (**Figure 4H**). Significantly, incubation with ANP (**Figure 4C**) and the cGMP analog 8-pCPT-cGMP (**Figure 4E**) inspired branch formation of neurites in cultured SGNs, and a similar phenomenon could be seen in BDNF-treated neurons (**Figure 4B**) and is previously described in our report (Sun et al., 2020), indicating the cascade in which neurotrophins and ANP/NPR-A/cGMP/PKG activation lead to a trophic support for neurite growth and branching. Accordingly, the mechanism of

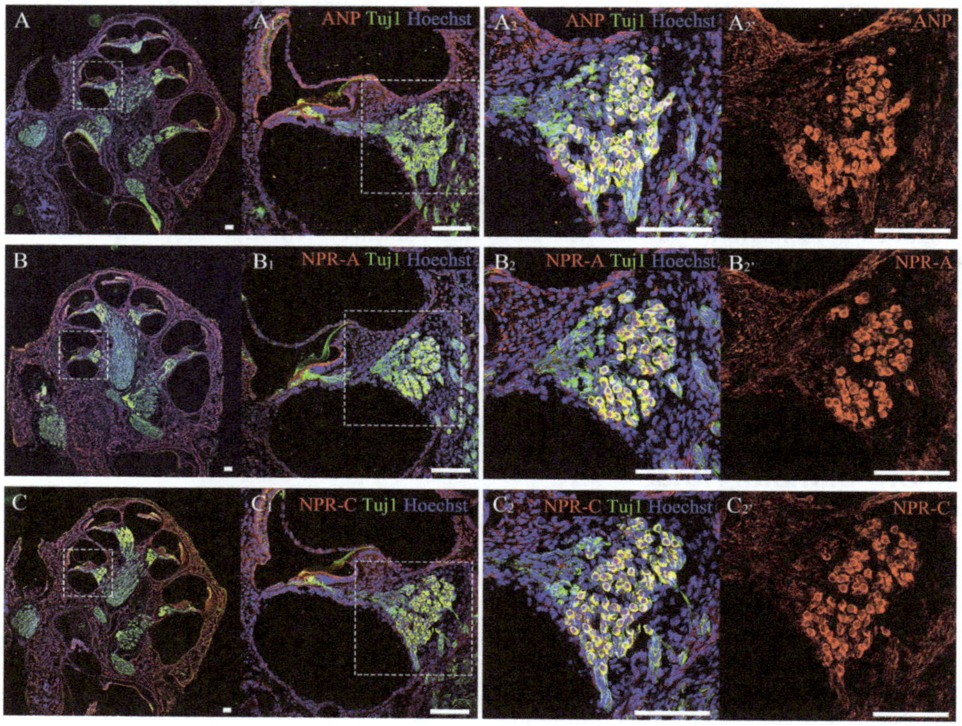

FIGURE 2 | Immunolocalization of ANP, NPR-A and NPR-C in SGNs within cochlear SG from rats at P7. **(A–C)** Gross view of cryosectioned cochlear tissues triple-labeled with antibodies against neural marker β-III Tubulin (TUJ1, green), ANP/NPR-A/NPR-C (red) and Hoechst (blue). **(A_1,B_1,C_1)** High-magnification views of the boxed region of **(A–C)**. **(A_2,B_2,C_2)** Higher-magnification images of the boxed region of **(A_1,B_1,C_1)** reveal that ANP/NPR-A/NPR-C is colocalized with TUJ1-positive SGNs, respectively. **($A_{2'}$,$B_{2'}$,$C_{2'}$)** Immunoreactivities of ANP, NPR-A, and NPR-C are present in the SGNs. Scale bars = 100 μm.

ANP/NPR-A/cGMP/PKG signaling in the regulation of axonal branching or pathfinding requires further exploration during cochlear development to comprehensively elucidate the principle underlying the assembly of auditory circuits.

Collectively, these observations indicate that ANP may promote outgrowth and regeneration of neurites from SGNs by activating the NPR-A/cGMP/PKG pathway. In addition, the variation tendency associated with the number of neurites from SG explants (**Figure 3I**) and cell number of dissociated SGNs (**Figure 4I**) suggested that the ANP/NPR-A/cGMP/PKG pathway may improve neuronal survival *in vitro*, to a certain extent.

ANP Attracts Neurite Outgrowth of SG Explants by Activating the NPR-A/cGMP/PKG Pathway

To evaluate the capacity to attract SGN neurites of downstream signaling pathways mediated by ANP and its receptors, we determined the probability of neurite attaching to surfaces of PuraMatrix hydrogel incorporated with given additives after SG explants of P3 rats were maintained *in vitro* for 4 days (at DIV4). As illustrated in **Figure 5**, a few neurites sprouting from explants contacted the edge of the PuraMatrix droplets but rarely grew onto the hydrogel surface (attachment) and thus yielded a low probability (20%) of neurite attachment to native PuraMatrix (**Figure 5A**). To attract extending neurites from explants, 20 ng/ml of BDNF was incorporated into 0.25% PuraMatrix, which gave rise to increased probability (100%) of neurite attachment (**Figure 5B**). Likewise, a substantial number of neurites were attracted and attached to surfaces of hydrogel incorporated with 1 μM ANP (**Figure 5C**). Similar patterns of neurite attachment could also be noticed on explants settled in proximity to hydrogel incorporated with 1 μM 8-pCPT-cGMP (**Figure 5E**). In contrast, incorporation of 1 μM NPR-A blocker A71915 (**Figure 5D**) or KT5823 (**Figure 5F**) into ANP-supplemented PuraMatrix resulted in drastically reduced probability of neurite attachment. Besides, activation of NPR-C with 1 μM ANP_{4-23} failed to support neurite attachment to hydrogel (**Figure 5G**), whereas blockade of NPR-C with 1 μM AP811 did not compromise the capacity of ANP-incorporated hydrogel to attract neurites (**Figure 5H**). These findings indicate a high capacity of ANP to attract neurites of SG explants by activating the NPR-A/cGMP/PKG pathway.

ANP Promotes Neuronal Survival of Dissociated SGNs Against Glutamate Excitotoxicity by Activating the NPR-A/cGMP/PKG Pathway

To verify the possible neuroprotective effects of ANP receptor-associated downstream signaling pathways on SGNs against glutamate-induced excitotoxicity, we calculated the neuronal

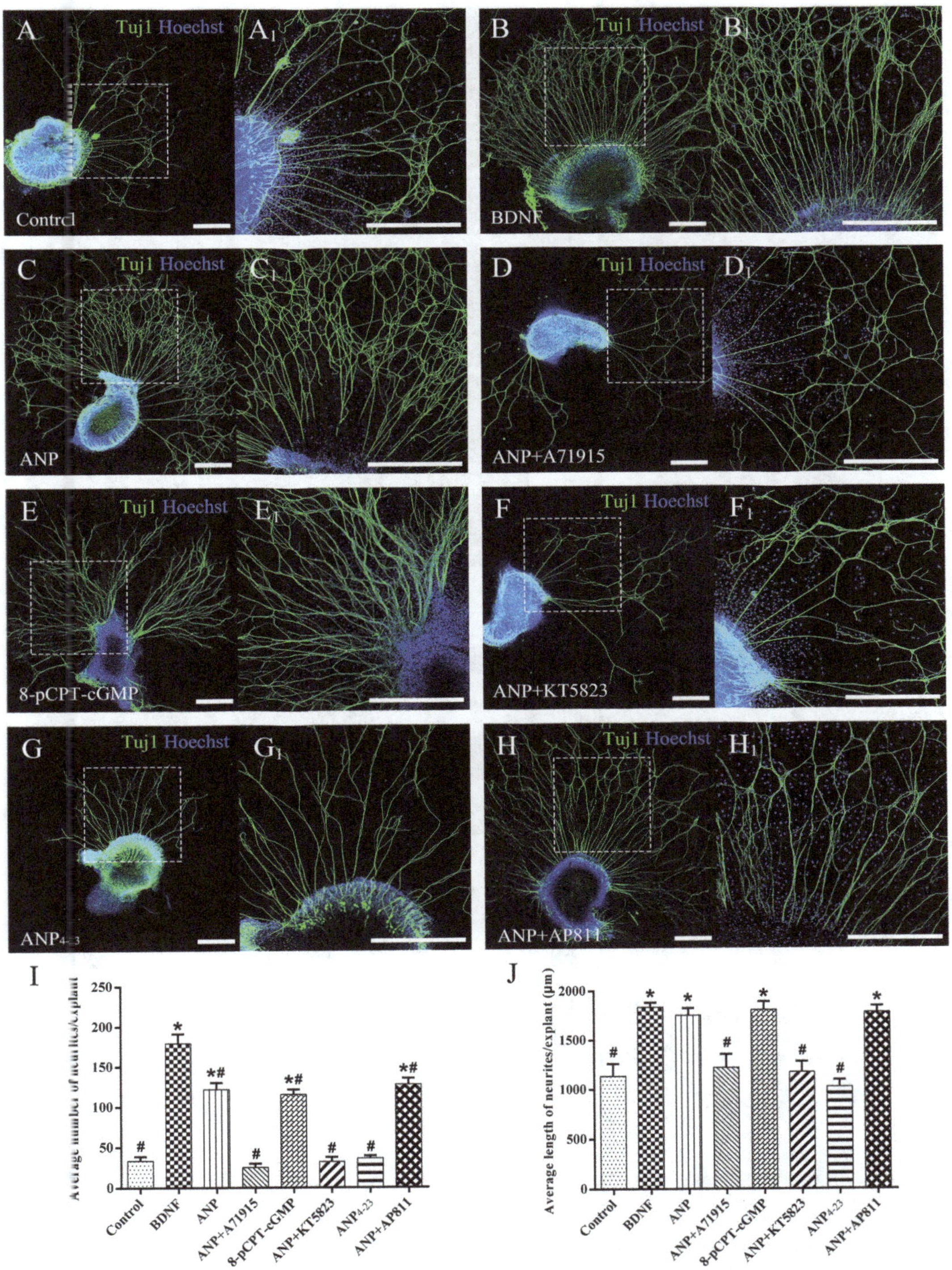

FIGURE 3 | ANP promotes neurite outgrowth of SG explants by activating NPR-A/cGMP/PKG pathway. Cochlear SG explants were maintained in culture medium alone **(A)**, or medium supplemented with 20 ng/mL BDNF **(B)**, 1 μM ANP **(C)**, 1 μM ANP plus 1 μM A71915 **(D)**, 1 μM 8-pCPT-cGMP **(E)**, 1 μM ANP plus 1 μM KT5823 **(F)**, 1 μM ANP_{4-23} **(G)**, or 1 μM ANP plus 1 μM AP811 **(H)** for 7 days. Neurons were double-labeled with TuJ1 antibody (green) and Hoechst (blue). **(A_1–H_1)** High-magnification views of the boxed region of **(A–H)**. Scale bars = 500 μm. The number of neurites **(I)** and average neurite length **(J)** of explants were quantified (N = 5 explants for each group). Results are expressed as mean ± SEM ($^*P < 0.05$, versus negative control samples; $^{\#}P < 0.05$, versus positive control samples/BDNF).

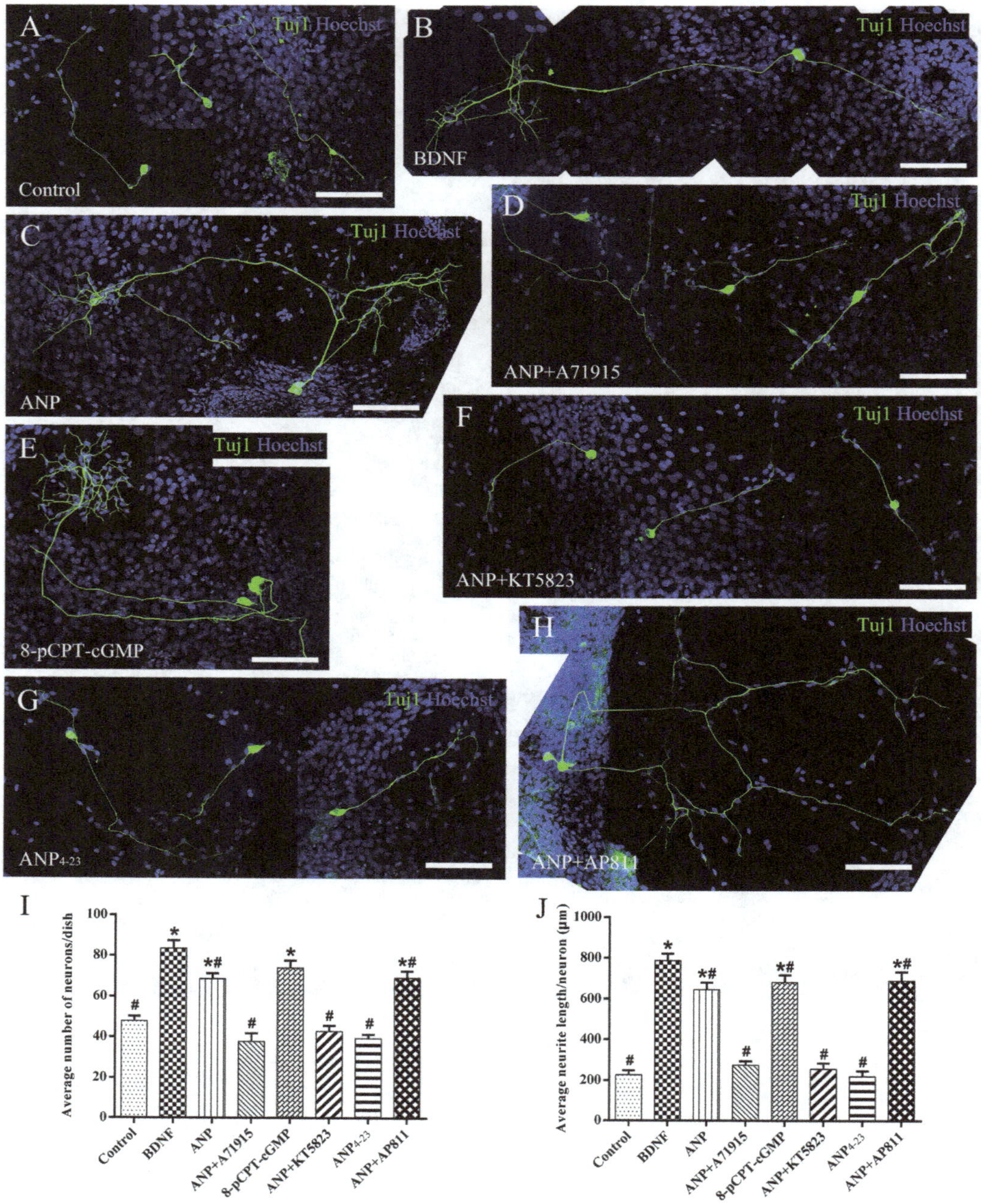

FIGURE 4 | ANP promotes neurite outgrowth of dissociated SGNs by activating NPR-A/cGMP/PKG pathway. Dissociated SGNs were maintained in culture medium alone **(A)**, or medium supplemented with 20 ng/mL BDNF **(B)**, 1 μM ANP **(C)**, 1 μM ANP plus 1 μM A71915 **(D)**, 1 μM 8-pCPT-cGMP **(E)**, 1 μM ANP plus 1 μM KT5823 **(F)**, 1 μM ANP_{4-23} **(G)**, or 1 μM ANP plus 1 μM AP811 **(H)** for 5 days. Neurons were double-labeled with TuJ1 antibody (green) and Hoechst (blue). Scale bars = 100 μm. The cell number **(I)** and average neurite length **(J)** of dissociated SGNs were counted (*N* = 5 culture dishes for each group). Results are expressed as mean ± SEM ($^{*}P < 0.05$, versus negative control samples; $^{\#}P < 0.05$, versus positive control samples/BDNF).

number and neurite length of dissociated SGNs from P3 rats cultured in medium containing the additives for 3 days (at DIV3). Representative images from cultures in different experimental groups are illustrated in **Figure 6**. The average number of neurons per dish was 38.6 ± 4.1, and the average neurite length per neuron was 234.0 ± 13.8 μm in control samples (**Figure 6A**). A drastic decrease in the number and neurite length of adhering neurons was observed in cultures subjected to excitotoxicity elicited by 100 μM glutamate for 48 h (**Figure 6B**), indicating that glutamate excitotoxicity would influence neuronal viability and neurite integrity, contributing directly to neurodegeneration (neuronal loss and neurite retraction) of SGNs. Pretreatment of

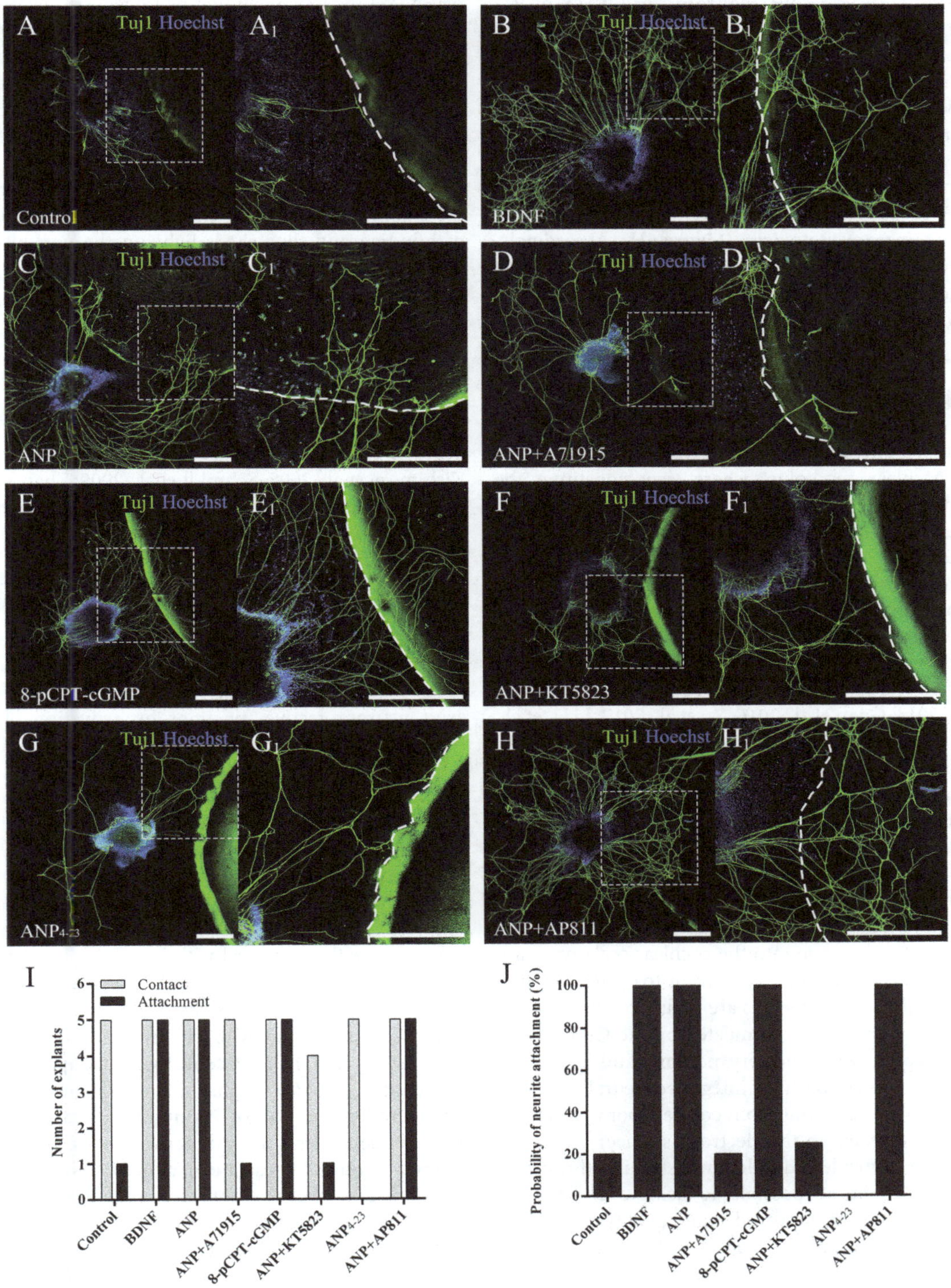

FIGURE 5 | ANP attracts neurite outgrowth of SG explants by activating NPR-A/cGMP/PKG pathway. SG explants were settled in close proximity to droplets of 0.25% native PuraMatrix solution **(A)**, or 0.25% PuraMatrix mixture incorporated with 20 ng/mL BDNF **(B)**, 1 μM ANP **(C)**, 1 μM ANP plus 1 μM A71915 **(D)**, 1 μM 8-pCPT-cGMP **(E)**, 1 μM ANP plus 1 μM KT5823 **(F)**, 1 μM ANP_{4-23} **(G)**, or 1 μM ANP plus 1 μM AP811 **(H)** and maintained in culture medium for 4 d. Neurons were double-labeled with TuJ1 antibody (green) and Hoechst (blue). **(A_1–H_1)** High-magnification views of the boxed region of **(A–H)**. The dashed white line marks the border of the PuraMatrix droplet. Scale bars = 500 μm. The number of explants extended neurites to contact or attach to the droplet surface **(I)** and the probability of neurite attachment to PuraMatrix hydrogel **(J)** were determined (N = 5 explants for each group).

dissociated SGNs with 1 μM ANP (**Figure 6C**) or 1 μM 8-pCPT-cGMP (**Figure 6E**) was able to substantially prevent neuronal loss and neurite retraction induced by glutamate exposure, whereas pre-incubation with 1 μM NPR-A inhibitor A71915 (**Figure 6D**) or 1 μM KT5823 (**Figure 6F**) abolished ANP-mediated neuronal survival and neurite outgrowth. Furthermore, 1 μM NPR-C agonist ANP_{4-23} failed to mimic the effect of ANP on neuronal viability and neurite integrity (**Figure 6G**), while 1 μM NPR-C blocker AP811 did not suppress the protective effect of ANP against glutamate excitotoxicity (**Figure 6H**). Accordingly, these results demonstrate that the neuroprotective effect of ANP on promoting survival of SGNs against glutamate-induced excitotoxicity is mediated by the NPR-A/cGMP/PKG pathway.

DISCUSSION

SGNs are auditory afferent neurons located in the Rosenthal canal in the cochlear modiolus, where they constitute the initial segment of auditory circuit to transmit neural impulse encoding acoustic information from the cochlea to the brain. The peripheral dendrites of SGNs extending from their somata within the modiolus form synaptic contacts with mechanosensory HCs in the organ of Corti, while their central axons connect to the cochlear nuclei within the brainstem (Nayagam et al., 2011). Many stress stimulators like ototoxic drugs and noise exposure had been testified to produce vast ROS in HCs and damage the HCs (Sun et al., 2014; Guan et al., 2016; Yu et al., 2017; Li H. et al., 2018; Zhang Y. et al., 2019; Gao et al., 2020; Zhong et al., 2020). Once the sensory epithelium of the cochlea or contacts with HCs are damaged due to auditory insults, SGNs may retract peripheral neurites and progressively degenerate due to lack of neurotrophic support (Stankovic et al., 2004; Vink et al., 2021). For individuals suffering from profound to severe SNHL, the treatment of choice at present is the implantation of a cochlear electrode array (CIs) by which the function of the missing HCs can be replaced. After insertion of the electrode into the cochlear scala tympani, auditory neurons can be stimulated electrically to create a hearing neural impulse. Benefits from the CIs are influenced by not only the amount of functional SGNs stimulated by the CIs but also the anatomical gap between auditory neurons and implanted cochlear electrodes. To establish an integrated neural-electrode interface, SGN neurites sprouting from cochlear bony structures must grow and be directed to the electrode surface. If neurites extend closer to the electrode and yield lower stimulus thresholds in a CI array, it might be possible to achieve controllable neural stimulation as well as improved sound quality and speech perception (Kwiatkowska et al., 2016; Li et al., 2017). To facilitate regeneration and guidance of peripheral processes from residual auditory neurons toward an implanted electrode, promising neurotrophic molecules (e.g., neurotrophins) are under research, due to their profound impact on neuronal survival, neurite outgrowth, and subsequent performance of CIs (Pfingst et al., 2017; Ma et al., 2019).

The cGMP signaling cascade has a versatile role in a broad spectrum of biological processes and maintains, in both the central and peripheral nervous systems, all aspects of neuronal functions including neurogenesis, synaptic formation, neuroprotection, neuronal excitability, and sensory transduction associated with olfaction, vision, and nociception (Zhao et al., 2009; Zhang et al., 2010). ANP and other members of the NP family, along with their receptors, are widely distributed in the mammalian nervous system and may participate in the regulation of neuroprotection, neural development, synaptic transmission, and information processing. Circumstantial evidence indicates the significance of cGMP signaling for neurite outgrowth and pathfinding and thus sheds light on the possible involvement of NPs in neuronal development and neurite regeneration. Particularly, cGMP signaling that is activated through binding of the ligand CNP to its transmembrane GC-coupled NPR-B (also known as NPR2 or GC-B) controls axonal bifurcation of cranial sensory ganglia neurons including cochlear SGNs entering the hindbrain (Lu et al., 2011, 2014; Ter-Avetisyan et al., 2014, 2018; Wolter et al., 2018; Schmidt and Fritzsch, 2019) and DRG neurons entering the spinal cord (Schmidt et al., 2002, 2007; Kishimoto et al., 2008; Schmidt et al., 2009; Zhao et al., 2009; Xia et al., 2013; Schmidt et al., 2016, 2018; Dumoulin et al., 2018a,b; Tröster et al., 2018). Likewise, knocking out PKGIα (also termed cGKIα) or NPR-B leads to defective central axonal projection of SGNs or DRG neurons in mouse models. Consequently, these studies suggested that the CNP/NPR-B/cGMP/PKG pathway might be implicated in the major events related to neurite outgrowth or pathfinding during neuronal development.

Additionally, increasing evidence indicates that NPs can exert neuroprotective functions by activation of GC-coupled NPRs. It has been reported that the ANP/NPR-A pathway might possess neuroprotective effects on rat retinal neurons against excitotoxicity caused by *N*-methyl-D-aspartate, probably by the activation of D1 dopamine receptors (Kuribayashi et al., 2006). CNP could serve a neuroprotective role which rescued rat retinal ganglion cells from apoptotic impairment *in vitro* or *in vivo* (Ma et al., 2010). ANP and BNP could inhibit apoptosis of cultured PC12 cells induced by serum deprivation and improve their survival with increasing cGMP levels (Fiscus et al., 2001). Pretreatment with ANP alleviated nitric oxide-induced neuronal apoptosis of a cholinergic-neuron-like cell line NG108-15, associated with elevation of cGMP levels (Cheng Chew et al., 2003). ANP could protect dopaminergic neuron-like models *in vitro* against neurotoxic insult for mimicking the neurodegeneration of Parkinson's disease, which might be strongly dependent on the activation of the Wnt/β-catenin pathway (Colini Baldeschi et al., 2018). CNP was also shown to function as an innate neuroprotectant which improved neuronal survival of neonatal brain in mice from hypoxia–ischemia insult through its receptor NPR-B (Ma and Zhang, 2018).

Circumstantial evidence shows that ANP and receptors, i.e., its cognate receptor NPR-A and its clearance receptor NPR-C, are broadly distributed in mammalian CNS and peripheral sensory tissues, suggesting their involvement in regulation of various neuronal functions (Cao and Yang, 2008; Mahinrad et al., 2016). Taking together the results from previous findings and those of our works that demonstrate the colocalization of ANP and its receptors in cochlear SG, we proposed that ANP may also participate in the regulation of certain auditory neuronal

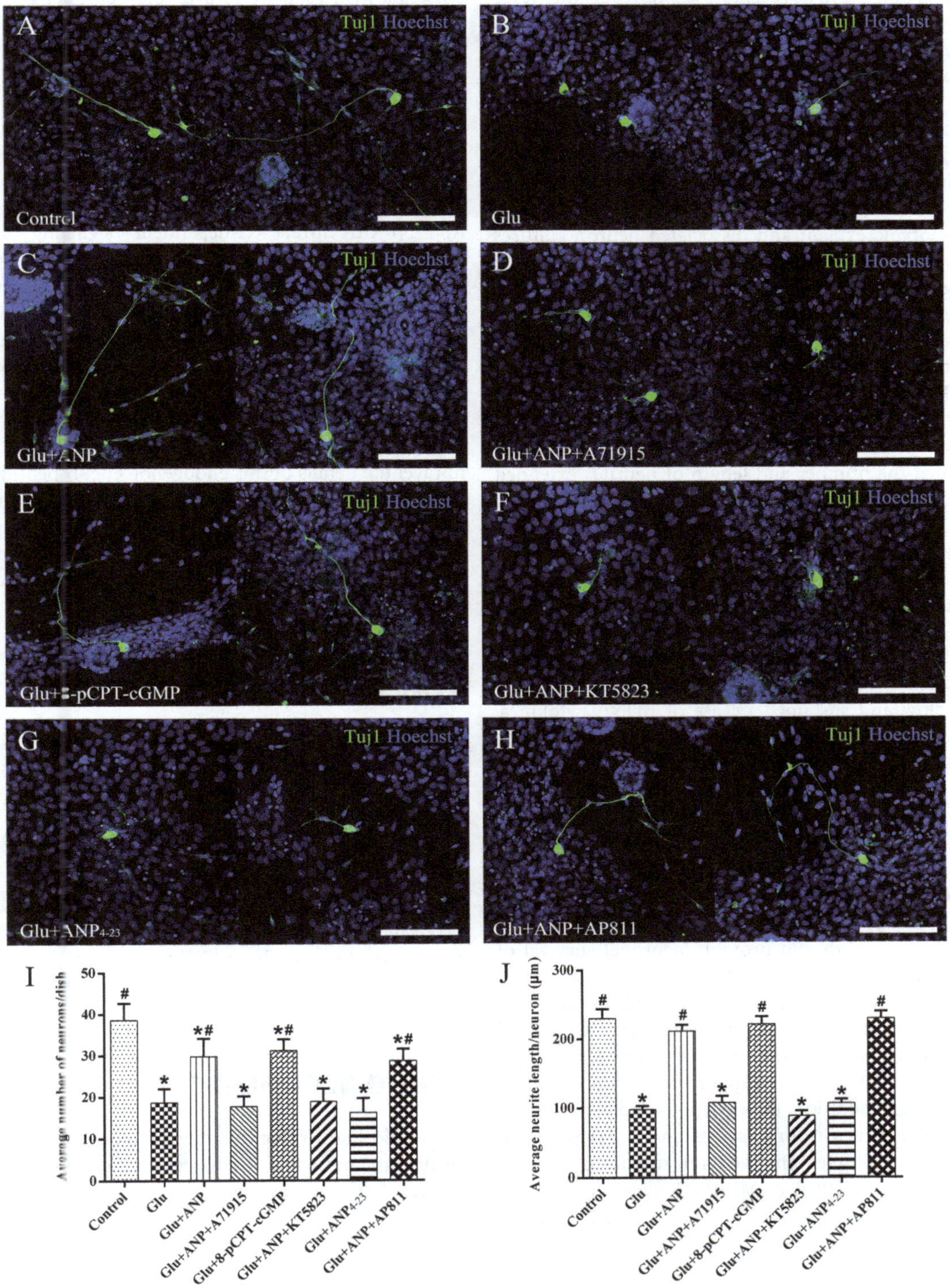

FIGURE 6 | ANP promotes neuronal survival of dissociated SGNs against glutamate induced-excitotoxicity by activating NPR-A/cGMP/PKG pathway. Dissociated SGNs were incubated in culture medium alone **(A,B)**, or medium supplemented with 1 μM ANP **(C)**, 1 μM A71915 **(D)**, 1 μM 8-pCPT-cGMP **(E)**, 1 μM ANP plus 1 μM KT5823 **(F)**, 1 μM ANP$_{4-23}$ **(G)**, or 1 μM ANP plus 1 μM AP811 **(H)** for 24 h. Then, 100 μM glutamate was added to the culture medium of all experimental cultures **(B–G)** and maintained for 48 h. Neurons were double-labeled with TuJ1 antibody (green) and Hoechst (blue). Glu: glutamate. Scale bars = 100 μm. The neuronal number **(I)** and average neurite length **(J)** of dissociated SGNs were calculated (N = 5 culture dishes for each group). Results are expressed as mean ± SEM ($^{*}P < 0.05$, versus control samples; $^{\#}P < 0.05$, versus glutamate treated samples/Glu).

functions through binding to its receptors (Lamprecht and Meyer zum Gottesberge, 1988; Furuta et al., 1995; Sun et al., 2013, 2014). Although our recent study suggests that ANP would stimulate neurite outgrowth of cochlear SGNs by triggering the NPR-A/cGMP/PKG pathway (Sun et al., 2020), the possible influence of NPR-C signaling within this process still needs to be examined, since NPR-C can interact with other second messenger signaling through the inhibition of adenylyl cyclase and activation of phospholipase C (Rose and Giles, 2008). In the present study, we employed organotypic explant and dissociated neuron cultures from SG of postnatal rats *in vitro* to evaluate the influence of ANP on neurite outgrowth, neurite attraction, and neuronal survival of SGNs. To determine which receptor is predominantly involved in the modulatory effects on neuronal functions of SGNs, we used the selective NPR-A antagonist A71915, cGMP analog 8-pCPT-cGMP, PKG inhibitor KT5823, selective NPR-C agonist ANP_{4-23}, and NPR-C antagonist AP811. To explore the effect of ANP receptor pathways on neurite outgrowth of SGNs, we initially calculated the number and length of neurites extended from SG explants and dissociated neurons. Furthermore, the capacity of ANP receptor pathways to attract neurites was assessed by determining the probability of neurite attachment to the hydrogel surface by employing an *in vitro* SG explant model cultured next to PuraMatrix droplets (Frick et al., 2017). In these procedures, BDNF served as positive controls since it acts as a soluble neurotrophin to enhance neurite elongation, as well as a guidance cue to attract the growing neurites toward the hydrogel. The slow and sustained release of BDNF, cytokines, and small molecules from similar hydrogels suggests favorable release kinetics of the PuraMatrix hydrogel that might be utilized to establish a concentration gradient attracting attachment of neurites (Gelain et al., 2010; Frick et al., 2017). At last, the possible neuroprotective effect of ANP receptor pathways on SGNs was explored by calculating the neuron number and neurite length of dissociated SGNs exposed to glutamate excitotoxicity. As illustrated above, our data indicate that ANP would effectively stimulate neurite outgrowth and promote neuronal survival of SGNs by activating the NPR-A/cGMP/PKG cascade, since this activity can be mimicked by 8-pCPT-cGMP and abolished by KT-5823. Specifically, a cGMP signaling pathway composed of the ligand ANP, GC-coupled receptor NPR-A, and the downstream effector PKG could support and attract neurite outgrowth of SGNs. In addition, the variation tendency relevant to the number of neurites from explants and cell number of dissociated SGNs in samples analyzed for neurite outgrowth implied that the ANP/NPR-A/cGMP/PKG signaling cascade may improve neuronal survival. Furthermore, ANP might possess a high capacity to promote neuronal survival of SGNs against glutamate-induced excitotoxicity by activating the NPR-A/cGMP/PKG pathway.

Taken together, our study provides valuable information regarding the distribution of ANP and its receptors as well as their potential modulatory effects on neuronal functions of primary auditory neurons in the inner ear of postnatal rat. The neuroregenerative and neuroprotective nature of ANP/NPRA/cGMP/PKG-dependent signaling also strongly intimates that ANP could perform a vital role in normal neuritogenesis (sprouting, elongation, and branching) of SGN during development of the inner ear. Manipulation of cGMP levels and activation of PKG by activating ANP and receptors signals represent a potential therapeutic strategy to enhance regrowth of SGN neurites and support SGN survival, which promises to be a fruitful area for developing new and effective therapies for SNHL. Future investigations are necessary to unravel the details of this endogenous neuropeptide modulating the physiological functions of cochlear neurons, which will enhance our understanding of the mechanisms underlying normal and pathological states of hearing and provide future clinical applications on effective prophylactic and therapeutic treatment for hearing impairment.

ETHICS STATEMENT

The animal study was reviewed and approved by the Animal Ethics Committee of the Fourth Military Medical University.

AUTHOR CONTRIBUTIONS

FS, KZ, and D-jZ conceived and designed the study. FS, K-yT, X-yZ, and WL performed the experiments. K-yT, JW, and C-pZ interpreted the data. FS and KZ wrote the manuscript. J-hQ and D-jZ reviewed and edited the manuscript. All authors have read and approved the final manuscript.

ACKNOWLEDGMENTS

We would like to thank Guangzhou Sagene Biotech Co., Ltd., for the preparation of the diagrammatic drawing for the culture protocol in the manuscript.

REFERENCES

Abdelalim, E. M., Bellier, J.-P., and Tooyama, I. (2013). Expression of NPR-B in neurons of the dorsal root ganglia of the rat. *Peptides* 43, 56–61. doi: 10.1016/j.peptides.2013.02.013

Abdelalim, E. M., and Tooyama, I. (2010). NPR-C is expressed in the cholinergic and dopaminergic amacrine cells in the rat retina. *Peptides* 31, 180–183. doi: 10.1016/j.peptides.2009.10.014

Cao, L.-H., and Yang, X.-L. (2008). Natriuretic peptides and their receptors in the central nervous system. *Prog. Neurobiol.* 84, 234–248. doi: 10.1016/j.pneurobio.2007.12.003

Chen, Y., Lu, X., Guo, L., Ni, W., Zhang, Y., Zhao, L., et al. (2017). Hedgehog signaling promotes the proliferation and subsequent hair cell formation of progenitor cells in the neonatal mouse cochlea. *Front. Mol. Neurosci.* 10:426. doi: 10.3389/fnmol.2017.00426

Cheng, C., Guo, L., Lu, L., Xu, X., Zhang, S., Gao, J., et al. (2017). Characterization of the Transcriptomes of Lgr5+ Hair cell progenitors and lgr5- supporting cells in the mouse cochlea. *Front. Mol. Neurosci.* 10:122. doi: 10.3389/fnmol.2017.00122

Cheng, C., Wang, Y., Guo, L., Lu, X., Zhu, W., Muhammad, W., et al. (2019). Age-related transcriptome changes in Sox2+ supporting cells in the mouse cochlea. *Stem Cell Res. Ther.* 10:365. doi: 10.1186/s13287-019-1437-0

Cheng Chew, S. B., Leung, P. Y., and Fiscus, R. R. (2003). Preincubation with atrial natriuretic peptide protects NG108-15 cells against the toxic/proapoptotic effects of the nitric oxide donor S-nitroso-N-acetylpenicillamine. *Histochem. Cell Biol.* 120, 163–171. doi: 10.1007/s00418-003-0568-6

Colini Baldeschi, A., Pittaluga, E., Andreola, F., Rossi, S., Cozzolino, M., Nicotera, G., et al. (2018). Atrial natriuretic peptide acts as a neuroprotective agent in in vitro models of parkinson's disease via up-regulation of the Wnt/β-Catenin Pathway. *Front. Aging Neurosci.* 10:20. doi: 10.3389/fnagi.2018.00020

Cox, B. C., Chai, R., Lenoir, A., Liu, Z., Zhang, L., Nguyen, D.-H., et al. (2014). Spontaneous hair cell regeneration in the neonatal mouse cochlea in vivo. *Development* 141, 816–829. doi: 10.1242/dev.103036

Ding, Y., Meng, W., Kong, W., He, Z., and Chai, R. (2020). The role of FoxG1 in the inner ear. *Front. Cell Dev. Biol.* 8:614954. doi: 10.3389/fcell.2020.614954

Dumoulin, A., Dagane, A., Dittmar, G., and Rathjen, F. G. (2018a). S-palmitoylation is required for the control of growth cone morphology of DRG neurons by CNP-Induced cGMP signaling. *Front. Mol. Neurosci.* 11:345. doi: 10.3389/fnmol.2018.00345

Dumoulin, A., Ter-Avetisyan, G., Schmidt, H., and Rathjen, F. G. (2018b). Molecular analysis of sensory axon branching unraveled a cGMP-Dependent signaling cascade. *Int. J. Mol. Sci.* 19:1266. doi: 10.3390/ijms19051266

Fang, Q., Zhang, Y., Chen, X., Li, H., Cheng, L., Zhu, W., et al. (2020). Three-dimensional graphene enhances neural stem cell proliferation through metabolic regulation. *Front. Bioeng. Biotechnol.* 7:436. doi: 10.3389/fbioe.2019.00436

Fang, Q., Zhang, Y., Da, P., Shao, B., Pan, H., He, Z., et al. (2019). Deletion of Limk1 and Limk2 in mice does not alter cochlear development or auditory function. *Sci. Rep.* 9:3357. doi: 10.1038/s41598-019-39769-z

Fiscus, R. R., Tu, A. W. K., and Chew, S. B. C. (2001). Natriuretic peptides inhibit apoptosis and prolong the survival of serum-deprived PC12 cells. *Neuroreport* 12, 185–189. doi: 10.1097/00001756-200102120-00003

Fitzakerley, J. L., and Trachte, G. J. (2018). Genetics of guanylyl cyclase pathways in the cochlea and their influence on hearing. *Physiol. Genomics* 50, 780–806. doi: 10.1152/physiolgenomics.00056.2018

Frick, C., Müller, M., Wank, U., Tropitzsch, A., Kramer, B., Senn, P., et al. (2017). Biofunctionalized peptide-based hydrogels provide permissive scaffolds to attract neurite outgrowth from spiral ganglion neurons. *Colloids Surf. B Biointerfaces* 149, 105–114. doi: 10.1016/j.colsurfb.2016.10.003

Furuta, H., Mori, N., Luo, L., and Ryan, A. F. (1995). Detection of mRNA encoding guanylate cyclase A/atrial natriuretic peptide receptor in the rat cochlea by competitive polymerase chain reaction and in situ hybridization. *Hear. Res.* 92, 78–84. doi: 10.1016/0378-5955(95)00203-0

Gao, S., Cheng, C., Wang, M., Jiang, P., Zhang, L., Wang, Y., et al. (2020). Blebbistatin inhibits neomycin-induced apoptosis in hair Cell-Like HEI-OC-1 cells and in cochlear hair cells. *Front. Cell Neurosci.* 13:590. doi: 10.3389/fncel.2019.00590

Gelain, F., Unsworth, L. D., and Zhang, S. (2010). Slow and sustained release of active cytokines from self-assembling peptide scaffolds. *J. Control Release* 145, 231–239. doi: 10.1016/j.jconrel.2010.04.026

Gottesberge, A. M. M. Z., Gagelmann, M., and Forssmann, W. G. (1991). Atrial natriuretic peptide-like immunoreactive cells in the guinea pig inner ear. *Hear. Res.* 56, 86–92. doi: 10.1016/0378-5955(91)90157-5

Guan, M., Fang, Q., He, Z., Li, Y., Qian, F., Qian, X., et al. (2016). Inhibition of ARC decreases the survival of HEI-OC-1 cells after neomycin damage in vitro. *Oncotarget* 7, 66647–66659. doi: 10.18632/oncotarget.11336

Guo, R., Li, J., Chen, C., Xiao, M., Liao, M., Hu, Y., et al. (2021). Biomimetic 3D bacterial cellulose-graphene foam hybrid scaffold regulates neural stem cell proliferation and differentiation. *Colloids Surf. B Biointerfaces* 200:111590. doi: 10.1016/j.colsurfb.2021.111590

Guo, R., Ma, X., Liao, M., Liu, Y., Hu, Y., Qian, X., et al. (2019). Development and application of cochlear implant-based electric-acoustic stimulation of spiral ganglion neurons. *ACS Biomater. Sci. Eng.* 5, 6735–6741. doi: 10.1021/acsbiomaterials.9b01265

Guo, R., Zhang, S., Xiao, M., Qian, F., He, Z., Li, D., et al. (2016). Accelerating bioelectric functional development of neural stem cells by graphene coupling: implications for neural interfacing with conductive materials. *Biomaterials* 106, 193–204. doi: 10.1016/j.biomaterials.2016.08.019

Guo, R., Xiao, M., Zhao, W., Zhou, S., Hu, Y., Liao, M., et al. (2020). 2D Ti3C2TxMXene couples electrical stimulation to promote proliferation and neural differentiation of neural stem cells. *Acta Biomater.* (in press). doi: 10.1016/j.actbio.2020.12.035

He, Z., Fang, Q., Li, H., Shao, B., Zhang, Y., Zhang, Y., et al. (2019). The role of FOXG1 in the postnatal development and survival of mouse cochlear hair cells. *Neuropharmacology* 144, 43–57. doi: 10.1016/j.neuropharm.2018.10.021

He, Z., Guo, L., Shu, Y., Fang, Q., Zhou, H., Liu, Y., et al. (2017). Autophagy protects auditory hair cells against neomycin-induced damage. *Autophagy* 13, 1884–1904. doi: 10.1080/15548627.2017.1359449

He, Z., Sun, S., Waqas, M., Zhang, X., Qian, F., Cheng, C., et al. (2016). Reduced TRMU expression increases the sensitivity of hair-cell-like HEI-OC-1 cells to neomycin damage in vitro. *Sci. Rep.* 6:29621. doi: 10.1038/srep29621

He, Z.-H., Zou, S.-Y., Li, M., Liao, F.-L., Wu, X., Sun, H.-Y., et al. (2020). The nuclear transcription factor FoxG1 affects the sensitivity of mimetic aging hair cells to inflammation by regulating autophagy pathways. *Redox Biol.* 28:101364. doi: 10.1016/j.redox.2019.101364

Jiang, P., Zhang, S., Cheng, C., Gao, S., Tang, M., Lu, L., et al. (2020). The roles of exosomes in visual and auditory systems. *Front. Bioeng. Biotechnol.* 8:525. doi: 10.3389/fbioe.2020.00525

Kempfle, J. S., Nguyen, K., Hamadani, C., Koen, N., Edge, A. S., Kashemirov, B. A., et al. (2018). Bisphosphonate-Linked TrkB agonist: cochlea-targeted delivery of a neurotrophic agent as a strategy for the treatment of hearing loss. *Bioconjug. Chem.* 29, 1240–1250. doi: 10.1021/acs.bioconjchem.8b00022

Kishimoto, I., Tokudome, T., Horio, T., Soeki, T., Chusho, H., Nakao, K., et al. (2008). C-type natriuretic peptide is a schwann cell-derived factor for development and function of sensory neurones. *J. Neuroendocrinol.* 20, 1213–1223. doi: 10.1111/j.1365-2826.2008.01778.x

Koch, T., Gloddek, B., and Gutzke, S. (1992). Binding sites of atrial natriuretic peptide (ANP) in the mammalian cochlea and stimulation of cyclic GMP synthesis. *Hear. Res.* 63, 197–202. doi: 10.1016/0378-5955(92)90085-2

Krause, G., Meyer Zum Gottesberge, A. M., Wolfram, G., and Gerzer, R. (1997). Transcripts encoding three types of guanylyl-cyclase-coupled trans-membrane receptors in inner ear tissues of guinea pigs. *Hear. Res.* 110, 95–106. doi: 10.1016/S0378-5955(97)00064-6

Kuribayashi, K., Kitaoka, Y., Kumai, T., Munemasa, Y., Kitaoka, Y., Isenoumi, K., et al. (2006). Neuroprotective effect of atrial natriuretic peptide against NMDA-induced neurotoxicity in the rat retina. *Brain Res.* 1071, 34–41. doi: 10.1016/j.brainres.2005.11.068

Kwiatkowska, M., Reinhard, J., Roll, L., Kraft, N., Dazert, S., Faissner, A., et al. (2016). The expression pattern and inhibitory influence of Tenascin-C on the growth of spiral ganglion neurons suggest a regulatory role as boundary formation molecule in the postnatal mouse inner ear. *Neuroscience* 319, 46–58. doi: 10.1016/j.neuroscience.2016.01.039

Lamprecht, J., and Meyer zum Gottesberge, A. M. (1988). The presence and localization of receptors for atrial natriuretic peptide in the inner ear of the guinea pig. *Arch. Otorhinolaryngol.* 245, 300–301. doi: 10.1007/BF00464636

Li, A., You, D., Li, W., Cui, Y., He, Y., Li, W., et al. (2018). Novel compounds protect auditory hair cells against gentamycin-induced apoptosis by maintaining the expression level of H3K4me2. *Drug Delivery* 25, 1033–1043. doi: 10.1080/10717544.2018.1461277

Li, D., Yan, X., Hu, Y., Liu, Y., Guo, R., Liao, M., et al. (2019). Two-photon image tracking of neural stem cells via iridium complexes encapsulated in polymeric nanospheres. *ACS Biomater. Sci. Eng.* 5, 1561–1568. doi: 10.1021/acsbiomaterials.8b01231

Li, G., Chen, K., You, D., Xia, M., Li, W., Fan, S., et al. (2019). Laminin-coated electrospun regenerated silk fibroin mats promote neural progenitor cell proliferation, differentiation, and survival in vitro. *Front. Bioeng. Biotechnol.* 7:190. doi: 10.3389/fbioe.2019.00190

Li, H., Edin, F., Hayashi, H., Gudjonsson, O., Danckwardt-Lillieström, N., Engqvist, H., et al. (2017). Guided growth of auditory neurons: bioactive particles towards gapless neural – electrode interface. *Biomaterials* 122, 1–9. doi: 10.1016/j.biomaterials.2016.12.020

Li, H., Song, Y., He, Z., Chen, X., Wu, X., Li, X., et al. (2018). Meclofenamic acid reduces reactive oxygen species accumulation and apoptosis, inhibits excessive autophagy, and protects hair cell-Like HEI-OC1 cells from cisplatin-induced damage. *Front. Cell Neurosci.* 12:139. doi: 10.3389/fncel.2018.00139

Li, X., Bi, Z., Sun, Y., Li, C., Li, Y., and Liu, Z. (2020). In vivo ectopic Ngn1 and Neurod1 convert neonatal cochlear glial cells into spiral ganglion neurons. *FASEB J.* 34, 4764–4782. doi: 10.1096/fj.201902118R

Liu, L., Chen, Y., Qi, J., Zhang, Y., He, Y., Ni, W., et al. (2016). Wnt activation protects against neomycin-induced hair cell damage in the mouse cochlea. *Cell Death Dis.* 7:e2136. doi: 10.1038/cddis.2016.35

Liu, W., Xu, X., Fan, Z., Sun, G., Han, Y., Zhang, D., et al. (2019). Wnt signaling activates TP53-Induced glycolysis and apoptosis regulator and protects against cisplatin-induced spiral ganglion neuron damage in the mouse cochlea. *Antioxid Redox Signal.* 30, 1389–1410. doi: 10.1089/ars.2017.7288

Liu, Y., Qi, J., Chen, X., Tang, M., Chu, C., Zhu, W., et al. (2019). Critical role of spectrin in hearing development and deafness. *Sci. Adv.* 5:eaav7803. doi: 10.1126/sciadv.aav7803

Loo, L., Shepherd, A. J., Mickle, A. D., Lorca, R. A., Shutov, L. P., Usachev, Y. M., et al. (2012). The C-Type natriuretic peptide induces thermal hyperalgesia through a noncanonical Gβγ-dependent modulation of TRPV1 channel. *J. Neurosci.* 32, 11942–11955. doi: 10.1523/jneurosci.1330-12.2012

Lu, C. C., Appler, J. M., Houseman, E. A., and Goodrich, L. V. (2011). Developmental profiling of spiral ganglion neurons reveals insights into auditory circuit assembly. *J. Neurosci.* 31, 10903–10918. doi: 10.1523/jneurosci.2358-11.2011

Lu, C. C., Cao, X.-J., Wright, S., Ma, L., Oertel, D., and Goodrich, L. V. (2014). Mutation of Npr2 Leads to blurred tonotopic organization of central auditory circuits in mice. *PLoS Genet.* 10:e1004823. doi: 10.1371/journal.pgen.1004823

Lu, X., Sun, S., Qi, J., Li, W., Liu, L., Zhang, Y., et al. (2017). Bmi1 regulates the proliferation of cochlear supporting cells via the canonical wnt signaling pathway. *Mol. Neurobiol.* 54, 1326–1339. doi: 10.1007/s12035-016-9686-8

Lv, J., Fu, X., Li, Y., Hong, G., Li, P., Lin, J., et al. (2021). Deletion of Kcnj16 in mice does not alter auditory function. *Front. Cell Dev. Biol.* 9:630361. doi: 10.3389/fcell.2021.630361

Ma, J., Yu, W., Wang, Y., Cao, G., Cai, S., Chen, X., et al. (2010). Neuroprotective effects of C-Type natriuretic peptide on rat retinal ganglion cells. *Invest. Ophthalmol. Vis. Sci.* 51, 3544–3553. doi: 10.1167/iovs.09-5049

Ma, Q., and Zhang, L. (2018). C-type natriuretic peptide functions as an innate neuroprotectant in neonatal hypoxic-ischemic brain injury in mouse via natriuretic peptide receptor 2. *Exp. Neurol.* 304, 58–66. doi: 10.1016/j.expneurol.2018.02.016

Ma, Y., Wise, A. K., Shepherd, R. K., and Richardson, R. T. (2019). New molecular therapies for the treatment of hearing loss. *Pharmacol. Ther.* 200, 190–209. doi: 10.1016/j.pharmthera.2019.05.003

Mahinrad, S., De Craen, A. J. M., Yasar, S., Van Heemst, D., and Sabayan, B. (2016). Natriuretic peptides in the central nervous system: novel targets for cognitive impairment. *Neurosci. Biobehav. Rev.* 68, 148–156. doi: 10.1016/j.neubiorev.2016.05.022

McLean, W. J., Yin, X., Lu, L., Lenz, D. R., Mclean, D., Langer, R., et al. (2017). Clonal expansion of Lgr5-positive cells from mammalian cochlea and high-purity generation of sensory hair cells. *Cell Rep.* 18, 1917–1929. doi: 10.1016/j.celrep.2017.01.066

Meyer, A. M., and Lamprecht, J. (1989). Localization of the atrial natriuretic peptide binding sites in the inner Ear Tissue—Possibly an additional regulating system. *Acta Otolaryngol.* 108, 53–57. doi: 10.3109/00016488909139021

Meyer Zum Gottesberge, A. M., Schletcher, A., Drummer, C., and Gerzer, R. (1995). The volume protective natriuretic peptide system in the inner ear comparison between vestibular and cochlear compartments. *Acta Otolaryngol.* 115, 170–173. doi: 10.3109/00016489509125219

Nayagam, B. A., Muniak, M. A., and Ryugo, D. K. (2011). The spiral ganglion: connecting the peripheral and central auditory systems. *Hear. Res.* 278, 2–20. doi: 10.1016/j.heares.2011.04.003

Nishimura, K., Nakagawa, T., Sakamoto, T., and Ito, J. (2012). Fates of murine pluripotent stem cell-derived neural progenitors following transplantation into mouse cochleae. *Cell Transplant* 21, 763–771. doi: 10.3727/096368911x623907

Noda, T., Meas, S. J., Nogami, J., Amemiya, Y., Uchi, R., Ohkawa, Y., et al. (2018). Direct reprogramming of spiral ganglion non-neuronal cells into neurons: toward ameliorating sensorineural hearing loss by gene therapy. *Front. Cell Dev. Biol.* 6:16. doi: 10.3389/fcell.2018.00016

Pfingst, B. E., Colesa, D. J., Swiderski, D. L., Hughes, A. P., Strahl, S. B., Sinan, M., et al. (2017). Neurotrophin gene therapy in deafened ears with cochlear implants: long-term effects on nerve survival and functional measures. *J. Assoc. Res. Otolaryngol.* 18, 731–750. doi: 10.1007/s10162-017-0633-9

Potter, L. R., Yoder, A. R., Flora, D. R., Antos, L. K., and Dickey, D. M. (2009). "Natriuretic peptides: their structures, receptors, physiologic functions and therapeutic applications," in *cGMP: Generators, Effectors and Therapeutic Implications*, eds H. H. H. W. Schmidt, F. Hofmann, and J.-P. Stasch (Berlin: Springer Berlin Heidelberg), 341–366. doi: 10.1007/978-3-540-68964-5_15

Qi, J., Liu, Y., Chu, C., Chen, X., Zhu, W., Shu, Y., et al. (2019). A cytoskeleton structure revealed by super-resolution fluorescence imaging in inner ear hair cells. *Cell Discov.* 5:12. doi: 10.1038/s41421-018-0076-4

Qi, J., Zhang, L., Tan, F., Liu, Y., Chu, C., Zhu, W., et al. (2020). Espin distribution as revealed by super-resolution microscopy of stereocilia. *Am. J. Transl. Res.* 12, 130–141.

Qian, F., Wang, X., Yin, Z., Xie, G., Yuan, H., Liu, D., et al. (2020). The slc4a2b gene is required for hair cell development in zebrafish. *Aging* 12, 18804–18821. doi: 10.18632/aging.103840

Roccio, M., Senn, P., and Heller, S. (2020). Novel insights into inner ear development and regeneration for targeted hearing loss therapies. *Hear. Res.* 397:107859. doi: 10.1016/j.heares.2019.107859

Rose, R. A., and Giles, W. R. (2008). Natriuretic peptide C receptor signalling in the heart and vasculature. *J. Physiol.* 586, 353–366. doi: 10.1113/jphysiol.2007.144253

Schmidt, H., Dickey, D. M., Dumoulin, A., Octave, M., Robinson, J. W., Kühn, R., et al. (2018). Regulation of the natriuretic peptide receptor 2 (Npr2) by phosphorylation of juxtamembrane serine and threonine residues is essential for bifurcation of sensory axons. *J. Neurosci.* 38, 9768–9780. doi: 10.1523/jneurosci.0495-18.2018

Schmidt, H., and Fritzsch, B. (2019). Npr2 null mutants show initial overshooting followed by reduction of spiral ganglion axon projections combined with near-normal cochleotopic projection. *Cell Tissue Res.* 378, 15–32. doi: 10.1007/s00441-019-03050-6

Schmidt, H., Peters, S., Frank, K., Wen, L., Feil, R., and Rathjen, F. G. (2016). Dorsal root ganglion axon bifurcation tolerates increased cyclic GMP levels: the role of phosphodiesterase 2A and scavenger receptor Npr3. *Eur. J. Neurosci.* 44, 2991–3000. doi: 10.1111/ejn.13434

Schmidt, H., Stonkute, A., Jüttner, R., Koesling, D., Friebe, A., and Rathjen, F. G. (2009). C-type natriuretic peptide (CNP) is a bifurcation factor for sensory neurons. *Proc. Natl. Acad. Sci. U.S.A.* 106, 16847–16852. doi: 10.1073/pnas.0906571106

Schmidt, H., Stonkute, A., JüTtner, R., SchäFfer, S., Buttgereit, J., Feil, R., et al. (2007). The receptor guanylyl cyclase Npr2 is essential for sensory axon bifurcation within the spinal cord. *J. Cell Biol.* 179, 331–340. doi: 10.1083/jcb.200707176

Schmidt, H., Werner, M., Heppenstall, P. A., Henning, M., Moreì, M. I., and KüHbandner, S. (2002). cGMP-mediated signaling via cGKIα is required for the guidance and connectivity of sensory axons. *J. Cell Biol.* 159, 489–498. doi: 10.1083/jcb.200207058

Seebacher, T., Beitz, E., Kumagami, H., Wild, K., Ruppersberg, J. P., and Schultz, J. E. (1999). Expression of membrane-bound and cytosolic guanylyl cyclases in the rat inner ear. *Hear. Res.* 127, 95–102. doi: 10.1016/S0378-5955(98)00176-2

Solinski, H. J., Dranchak, P., Oliphant, E., Gu, X., Earnest, T. W., Braisted, J., et al. (2019). Inhibition of natriuretic peptide receptor 1 reduces itch in mice. *Sci. Transl. Med.* 11:eaav5464. doi: 10.1126/scitranslmed.aav5464

Stankovic, K., Rio, C., Xia, A., Sugawara, M., Adams, J. C., Liberman, M. C., et al. (2004). Survival of adult spiral ganglion neurons requires erbb receptor signaling in the inner ear. *J. Neurosci.* 24, 8651–8661. doi: 10.1523/jneurosci.0733-04.2004

Sun, F., Zhou, K., Tian, K.-Y., Wang, J., Qiu, J.-H., and Zha, D.-J. (2020). Atrial natriuretic peptide improves neurite outgrowth from spiral ganglion neurons in vitro through a cGMP-Dependent manner. *Neural Plast* 2020, 8831735. doi: 10.1155/2020/8831735

Sun, F., Zhou, K., Wang, S.-J., Liang, P.-F., Wu, Y.-X., Zhu, G.-X., et al. (2013). Expression and localization of atrial natriuretic peptide and its receptors in rat spiral ganglion neurons. *Brain Res. Bull.* 95, 28–32. doi: 10.1016/j.brainresbull.2013.04.001

Sun, F., Zhou, K., Wang, S.-J., Liang, P.-F., Zhu, M.-Z., and Qiu, J.-H. (2014).

Expression patterns of atrial natriuretic peptide and its receptors within the cochlear spiral ganglion of the postnatal rat. *Hear. Res.* 309, 103–112. doi: 10.1016/j.heares.2013.11.010

Sun, G., Liu, W., Fan, Z., Zhang, D., Han, Y., Xu, L., et al. (2016). The three-dimensional culture system with matrigel and neurotrophic factors preserves the structure and function of spiral ganglion neuron in vitro. *Neural Plast* 2016:4280407. doi: 10.1155/2016/4280407

Suzuki, M., Kitano, H., Kitanishi, T., Yazawa, Y., Kitajima, K., Takeda, T., et al. (1998). RT-PCR analysis of mRNA expression of natriuretic peptide family and their receptors in rat inner ear. *Brain Res. Mol. Brain Res.* 55, 165–168. doi: 10.1016/S0169-328X(98)00016-3

Tan, F., Chu, C., Qi, J., Li, W., You, D., Li, K., et al. (2019). AAV-ie enables safe and efficient gene transfer to inner ear cells. *Nat. Commun.* 10:3733. doi: 10.1038/s41467-019-11687-8

Tang, M., Li, J., He, L., Guo, R., Yan, X., Li, D., et al. (2019). Transcriptomic profiling of neural stem cell differentiation on graphene substrates. *Colloids Surf. B Biointerfaces* 182:110324. doi: 10.1016/j.colsurfb.2019.06.054

Ter-Avetisyan, G., Dumoulin, A., Herrel, A., Schmidt, H., Strump, J., Afzal, S., et al. (2018). Loss of axon bifurcation in mesencephalic trigeminal neurons impairs the maximal biting force in npr2-deficient mice. *Front. Cell Neurosci.* 12:153. doi: 10.3389/fncel.2018.00153

Ter-Avetisyan, G., Rathjen, F. G., and Schmidt, H. (2014). Bifurcation of axons from cranial sensory neurons is disabled in the absence of Npr2-Induced cGMP signaling. *J. Neurosci.* 34, 737–747. doi: 10.1523/jneurosci.4183-13.2014

Tröster, P., Haseleu, J., Petersen, J., Drees, O., Schmidtko, A., Schwaller, F., et al. (2018). The absence of sensory axon bifurcation affects nociception and termination fields of afferents in the spinal cord. *Front. Mol. Neurosci.* 11:19. doi: 10.3389/fnmol.2018.00019

Tuft, B. W., Li, S., Xu, L., Clarke, J. C., White, S. P., Guymon, B. A., et al. (2013). Photopolymerized microfeatures for directed spiral ganglion neurite and Schwann cell growth. *Biomaterials* 34, 42–54. doi: 10.1016/j.biomaterials.2012.09.053

Vilotti, S., Marchenkova, A., Ntamati, N., and Nistri, A. (2013). B-Type natriuretic peptide-induced delayed modulation of TRPV1 and P2X3 receptors of mouse trigeminal sensory neurons. *PLoS One* 8:e81138. doi: 10.1371/journal.pone.0081138

Vink, H. A., Versnel, H., Kroon, S., Klis, S. F. L., and Ramekers, D. (2021). BDNF-mediated preservation of spiral ganglion cell peripheral processes and axons in comparison to that of their cell bodies. *Hear. Res.* 400:108114. doi: 10.1016/j.heares.2020.108114

Wang, Y., Li, J., Yao, X., Li, W., Du, H., Tang, M., et al. (2017). Loss of CIB2 causes profound hearing loss and abolishes mechanoelectrical transduction in mice. *Front. Mol. Neurosci.* 10:401. doi: 10.3389/fnmol.2017.00401

Waqas, M., Us-Salam, I., Bibi, Z., Wang, Y., Li, H., Zhu, Z., et al. (2020). Stem cell-based therapeutic approaches to restore sensorineural hearing loss in mammals. *Neural Plast* 2020:8829660. doi: 10.1155/2020/8829660

Wolter, S., Möhrle, D., Schmidt, H., Pfeiffer, S., Zelle, D., Eckert, P., et al. (2018). GC-B deficient mice with axon bifurcation loss exhibit compromised auditory processing. *Front. Neural Circuits* 12:65. doi: 10.3389/fncir.2018.00065

Xia, C., Nguyen, M., Garrison, A. K., Zhao, Z., Wang, Z., Sutherland, C., et al. (2013). CNP/cGMP signaling regulates axon branching and growth by modulating microtubule polymerization. *Dev. Neurobiol.* 73, 673–687. doi: 10.1002/dneu.22078

Xia, L., Shang, Y., Chen, X., Li, H., Xu, X., Liu, W., et al. (2020). Oriented neural spheroid formation and differentiation of neural stem cells guided by anisotropic inverse opals. *Front. Bioeng. Biotechnol.* 8:848. doi: 10.3389/fbioe.2020.00848

Xia, L., Zhu, W., Wang, Y., He, S., and Chai, R. (2019). Regulation of neural stem cell proliferation and differentiation by graphene-based biomaterials. *Neural Plast* 2019:3608386. doi: 10.1155/2019/3608386

Xu, G.-Z., Tian, J., Zhong, Y.-M., and Yang, X.-L. (2010). Natriuretic peptide receptors are expressed in rat retinal ganglion cells. *Brain Res. Bull.* 82, 188–192. doi: 10.1016/j.brainresbull.2010.03.004

Yan, W., Liu, W., Qi, J., Fang, Q., Fan, Z., Sun, G., et al. (2018). A three-dimensional culture system with matrigel promotes purified spiral ganglion neuron survival and function in vitro. *Mol. Neurobiol.* 55, 2070–2084. doi: 10.1007/s12035-017-0471-0

Yang, Y., Zhang, Y., Chai, R., and Gu, Z. (2020). A polydopamine-functionalized carbon microfibrous scaffold accelerates the development of neural stem cells. *Front. Bioeng. Biotechnol.* 8:616. doi: 10.3389/fbioe.2020.00616

Yoon, Y. J., and Anniko, M. (1994). Distribution of Alpha-ANP in the cochlea and the vestibular organs. *ORL* 56, 73–77. doi: 10.1159/000276613

Yoon, Y.-J., and Hellström, S. (1992). Immunohistochemical localization of a-atrial natriuretic polypeptide in the rat cochlea. *Acta Otolaryngol.* 112, 604–610. doi: 10.3109/00016489209137448

Yoon, Y. J., Lee, E. J., Hellstrom, S., and Kim, J. S. (2015). Atrial natriuretic peptide modulates auditory brainstem response of rat. *Acta Otolaryngol.* 135, 1293–1297. doi: 10.3109/00016489.2015.1073354

Yoon, Y. J., Lee, E. J., and Kim, S. H. (2012). Synthesis of atrial natriuretic peptide in the rabbit inner ear. *Laryngoscope* 122, 1605–1608. doi: 10.1002/lary.23235

You, D., Guo, L., Li, W., Sun, S., Chen, Y., Chai, R., et al. (2018). Characterization of Wnt and Notch-Responsive Lgr5+ Hair cell progenitors in the striolar region of the neonatal mouse utricle. *Front. Mol. Neurosci.* 11:137. doi: 10.3389/fnmol.2018.00137

Yu, X., Liu, W., Fan, Z., Qian, F., Zhang, D., Han, Y., et al. (2017). c-Myb knockdown increases the neomycin-induced damage to hair-cell-like HEI-OC1 cells in vitro. *Sci. Rep.* 7:41094. doi: 10.1038/srep41094

Zhang, F.-X., Liu, X.-J., Gong, L.-Q., Yao, J.-R., Li, K.-C., Li, Z.-Y., et al. (2010). Inhibition of inflammatory pain by activating B-Type natriuretic peptide signal pathway in nociceptive sensory neurons. *J. Neurosci.* 30, 10927–10938. doi: 10.1523/jneurosci.0657-10.2010

Zhang, S., Liu, D., Dong, Y., Zhang, Z., Zhang, Y., Zhou, H., et al. (2019). Frizzled-9+ Supporting cells are progenitors for the generation of hair cells in the postnatal mouse cochlea. *Front. Mol. Neurosci.* 12:184. doi: 10.3389/fnmol.2019.00184

Zhang, S., Qiang, R., Dong, Y., Zhang, Y., Chen, Y., Zhou, H., et al. (2020a). Hair cell regeneration from inner ear progenitors in the mammalian cochlea. *Am. J. Stem Cells* 9, 25–35.

Zhang, S., Zhang, Y., Dong, Y., Guo, L., Zhang, Z., Shao, B., et al. (2020b). Knockdown of Foxg1 in supporting cells increases the trans-differentiation of supporting cells into hair cells in the neonatal mouse cochlea. *Cell Mol. Life Sci.* 77, 1401–1419. doi: 10.1007/s00018-019-03291-2

Zhang, Y., Zhang, S., Zhang, Z., Dong, Y., Ma, X., Qiang, R., et al. (2020c). Knockdown of Foxg1 in Sox9+ supporting cells increases the trans-differentiation of supporting cells into hair cells in the neonatal mouse utricle. *Aging* 12, 19834–19851. doi: 10.18632/aging.104009

Zhang, S., Zhang, Y., Yu, P., Hu, Y., Zhou, H., Guo, L., et al. (2017). Characterization of Lgr5+ Progenitor cell transcriptomes after neomycin injury in the neonatal mouse cochlea. *Front. Mol. Neurosci.* 10:213. doi: 10.3389/fnmol.2017.00213

Zhang, Y., Guo, L., Lu, X., Cheng, C., Sun, S., Li, W., et al. (2018). Characterization of Lgr6+ Cells as an enriched population of hair cell progenitors compared to Lgr5+ Cells for hair cell generation in the neonatal mouse cochlea. *Front. Mol. Neurosci.* 11:147. doi: 10.3389/fnmol.2018.00147

Zhang, Y., Li, W., He, Z., Wang, Y., Shao, B., Cheng, C., et al. (2019). Pre-treatment with fasudil prevents neomycin-induced hair cell damage by reducing the accumulation of reactive oxygen species. *Front. Mol. Neurosci.* 12:264. doi: 10.3389/fnmol.2019.00264

Zhao, J., Tang, M., Cao, J., Ye, D., Guo, X., Xi, J., et al. (2019). Structurally tunable reduced graphene oxide substrate maintains mouse embryonic stem cell pluripotency. *Adv. Sci.* 6:1802136. doi: 10.1002/advs.201802136

Zhao, Z., and Ma, L. (2009). Regulation of axonal development by natriuretic peptide hormones. *Proc. Natl. Acad. Sci. U.S.A.* 106, 18016–18021. doi: 10.1073/pnas.0906880106\qr{Citethereference"ZhaoandMa,2009"insidethetext.}

Zhao, Z., Wang, Z., Gu, Y., Feil, R., Hofmann, F., and Ma, L. (2009). Regulate axon branching by the cyclic GMP pathway via inhibition of glycogen synthase kinase 3 in dorsal root ganglion sensory neurons. *J. Neurosci.* 29, 1350–1360. doi: 10.1523/jneurosci.3770-08.2009

Zhong, Z., Fu, X., Li, H., Chen, J., Wang, M., Gao, S., et al. (2020). Citicoline protects auditory hair cells against neomycin-induced damage. *Front. Cell Dev. Biol.* 8:712. doi: 10.3389/fcell.2020.00712

Zhou, H., Qian, X., Xu, N., Zhang, S., Zhu, G., Zhang, Y., et al. (2020). Disruption of Atg7-dependent autophagy causes electromotility disturbances, outer hair cell loss, and deafness in mice. *Cell Death Dis.* 11:913. doi: 10.1038/s41419-020-03110-8

Zhu, C., Cheng, C., Wang, Y., Muhammad, W., Liu, S., Zhu, W., et al. (2018). Loss of ARHGEF6 causes hair cell stereocilia deficits and hearing loss in mice. *Front. Mol. Neurosci.* 11:362. doi: 10.3389/fnmol.2018.00362

12

Effect of High Jugular Bulb on the Hearing Loss Characteristics in Patients With LVAS

Arthur Benjamin Kwesi[1,2†], Jintao Yu[1†], Chenlu Wang[3], Yonghua Wang[2], Fengyi Chuang[3], Xiaohui Yan[2], Wendi Shi[3*] and Yu Sun[1*]*

[1] Department of Otorhinolaryngology, Union Hospital, Tongji Medical College, Huazhong University of Science and Technology, Wuhan, China, [2] Hearing and Speech Rehabilitation Institute, Zhejiang Chinese Medical University, Hangzhou, China, [3] Hangzhou Ren-ai Hearing Rehabilitation Research Centre, Hangzhou, China

***Correspondence:**
Yonghua Wang
wangyh@vip.sina.com
Wendi Shi
shiwd_huier@sina.cn
Yu Sun
sunyu@hust.edu.cn

† These authors have contributed equally to this work

Objective: Both large vestibular aqueduct syndrome (LVAS) and high jugular bulb (HJB) are regarded as abnormalities commonly seen on the temporal bone CT. High jugular bulb has been found to erode the vestibular aqueduct, and there are several studies on jugular bulb vestibular aqueduct dehiscence. However, there is no study that specifically reports LVAS with concurrent HJB and its hearing loss relatedness. This study presents the pure tone audiometry differences between LVAS with HJB, and LVAS without HJB.

Methods: This was a case control study involving 36 bilateral LVAS with concurrent unilateral HJB patients, total of 72 ears. Intra-person comparison was done, by dividing ears into two groups: the case group, 36 ears (LVAS with HJB); and the control group, 36 ears (LVAS without HJB). Air conduction thresholds (250–4000 Hz), bone conduction thresholds (250–1000 Hz), and air bone gap (250–1000 Hz) were analyzed and compared between groups.

Result: There were statistically significant differences in AC thresholds at 250, 500, 2000, and 4000 Hz between the groups, $p < 0.05$. But there was no statistical significant difference at 1000 Hz, $p > 0.05$. There were statistical significant differences in BC thresholds at 250 and 500 Hz, $p < 0.05$, but there was no statistical difference at 1000 Hz. There were no significant differences in air bone gap at 250, 500, and 1000 Hz between the two groups.

Conclusion: LVAS with concurrent HJB was found to have higher air conduction thresholds, especially at 250, 500, 2000, and 4000 Hz. Bone conduction thresholds were higher at 250 and 500 Hz. Air bone gap at 250, 500, and 1000 Hz, were not significantly higher in LVAS with concurrent HJB.

Keywords: high jugular bulb, large vestibular aqueduct syndrome, hearing loss, hearing characteristics, pilot study

INTRODUCTION

Large vestibular aqueduct syndrome (LVAS) is defined as the enlargement of the narrow bony canals (aqueducts), which extends from the vestibule into the skull. It is known to cause about 5–15% of congenital sensorineural hearing loss in children (Madden et al., 2007; Kupfer et al., 2012; Noguchi et al., 2017). The vestibular aqueduct is determined as enlarged, by temporal bone CT showing the diameter of the aqueduct > 1.5 mm at the midpoint or the operculum, or by MRI showing an enlargement of the endolymphatic duct and sac (Aimoni et al., 2017). Studies have revealed no direct relationship with the size of the enlarged vestibular aqueduct and the level of hearing loss (Yan et al., 2003; Zhang et al., 2006). High jugular bulb (HJB) is known as the elevation of the posterior part of the jugular bulb into any of the following parts in the temporal bone: the hypotympanum portion of the middle ear, the base of the cochlear base, and the internal auditory canal, either with dehiscence or without dehiscence (Tanrivermis Sayit et al., 2017). The cause of high jugular bulb could be linked to the imbalanced venous system, which drains blood from the head, and the effect of the blood flow dynamics (Friedmann et al., 2012). High jugular bulb is one of the most common anatomical variations found in the temporal bone and has been reported to have high occurrence in patients with inner ear anomalies (Singla et al., 2016; Tanrivermis Sayit et al., 2017). High jugular bulb has been found to erode inner ear structures including the vestibular aqueduct (Friedmann et al., 2012). Large vestibular aqueduct syndrome with concurrent high jugular bulb has been observed clinically in patients having hearing loss. However, there are no previous studies in literature about the large vestibular aqueduct syndrome with high jugular bulb and its hearing loss relatedness. Some patients with large vestibular aqueduct syndrome were observed to have worse degree of hearing loss and easily experienced hearing fluctuation. Previous studies on high jugular bulb revealed worse hearing thresholds and progressive hearing in the affected ears of patients with bilateral hearing loss (Tsunoda, 2000; Sasindran et al., 2014). As a novel study, the purpose was to ascertain the audiological characteristics of vestibular aqueduct syndrome with concurrent high jugular bulb by finding out the differences in air conduction thresholds, bone conduction thresholds, and air bone gap between LVAS with HJB and LVAS without HJB. The findings of this study are intended to help ear and hearing health professionals to understand the differences that exist among LVAS patients, in order to guide their diagnosis, counseling, and hearing management, as well as to guide future research on LVAS and HJB.

MATERIALS AND METHODS

This is a case control study conducted at the Zhejiang Chinese Medical University's Affiliated Hearing and Speech Rehabilitation Institute. The study protocol was approved by the Institutional Review Committee.

Subject Recruitment

The study involved EVA patients who visited the hearing and speech rehabilitation center between June 2020 and March 2021 for follow-up. Subjects were recruited based on the following inclusion criteria: (1) diagnosed with bilateral large vestibular aqueduct syndrome with unilateral high jugular bulb using CT; (2) ability to perform behavioral audiometry; (3) stable hearing for at least a 3-month period; (4) patients having outer ear and middle ear abnormalities were excluded by otoscopy, CT, and tympanometry; and (5) an informed consent for participation in the study.

Subjects

Thirty-six bilateral large vestibular aqueduct syndrome with unilateral high jugular bulb patients were recruited (**Figure 1**), comprising 19 males and 17 females; ages ranged from 3 to 27 years, and mean age was 8.08 years. A total of 72 large vestibular aqueduct syndrome ears, were divided into two groups: case group, 36 ears (LVAS with HJB) and control group, 36 ears (LVAS without HJB).

Audiological Testing

All tests were performed in a clinical setting and in accordance with standard procedures. Pure tone audiometry and tympanometry were performed in consideration of the respective ages of patients.

Test Equipment

Pure tone audiometry was performed in a double-walled sound booth, using a Grason-Standler Audiostar ProTM audiometer, TDH-39, and B-71 transducers. Interacoustics Titan/IMP440 tympanometer was used to perform the tympanometry.

Pure Tone Audiometry

Using the Hughson Westlake threshold finding approach, air conduction and bone conduction thresholds were measured at octave frequencies from 250 to 4000 Hz. Masking was performed when necessary.

Tympanometry

Using 226 Hz probe tone at 85 dB SPL, and varying pressure from +200 to −400 daPa, the tympanic membrane mobility and middle ear compliance were assessed. Indications for normal tympanogram were ear canal volume, tympanometric peak pressure, and tympanometric peak compliance within the normative data for tympanometry for children and adults (Margolis and Heller, 1987).

Variable and Comparison

Intra-person comparison was done between ears; 72 ears divided into the case group (36 ears) and the control group (36 ears). AC thresholds from 250 to 4000 Hz; BC thresholds from 250 to 1000 Hz; and air bone gap (ABG) from 250 to 1000 Hz were compared between the two groups.

Statistical Analysis

Statistical analysis was conducted using the IBM SPSS version 25.0; paired-samples t-test was performed to determine the differences between the groups, $p < 0.05$.

RESULTS

Demographic Characteristics and Radiological Findings

Thirty-six patients with bilateral large vestibular aqueduct syndrome with unilateral high jugular bulb constituted 19 males

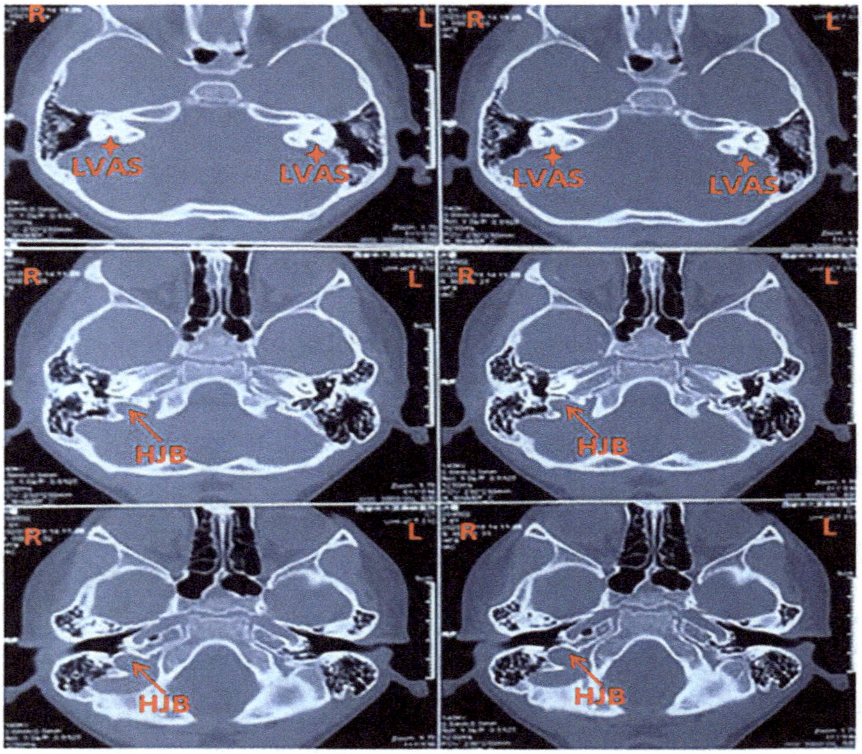

FIGURE 1 | Representative CT (computed tomography) scan images showing bilateral large vestibular aqueduct syndrome with unilateral high jugular bulb (right ear) from a 3-years-old patient.

and 17 females, given a male to female ratio of 1.12:1; ages ranged from 3 to 27 years, and mean age was 8.08 years (**Table 1**).

Seventy-two large vestibular aqueduct syndrome ears were divided in two groups: the case group, 36 ears (LVAS with HJB); and control group, 36 ears (LVAS without HJB). High jugular bulb presented in both left and right ears. The lateralization of high jugular was more in right ears as compared to the left ears. Thirty patients were found to have high jugular bulb in the right ear; 6 patients had high jugular bulb in the left ear, $p < 0.05$.

Pure Tone Audiometry

Air Conduction Thresholds

The statistical analysis of air conduction thresholds from 250 to 4000 Hz showed the following mean thresholds for the case group: 250 Hz (61.94 ± 18.45 dB HL), 500 Hz (66.94 ± 19.50 dB HL), 1000 Hz (73.06 ± 19.10 dB HL), 2000 Hz (82.64 ± 20.96 dB HL), and 4000 Hz (89.44 ± 21.41 dB HL); for the control group: 250 Hz (54.31 ± 17.90 dB HL), 500 Hz (59.58 ± 17.94 dB HL), 1000 Hz (66.67 ± 18.60 dB HL), 2000 Hz (75.00 ± 16.48 dB HL), and 4000 Hz (78.47 ± 22.03 dB HL). The mean differences were 250 Hz (7.63 dB HL), 500 Hz (7.36 dB HL), 1000 Hz (6.39 dB HL), 2000 Hz (7.64 dB HL), and 4000 Hz (10.97 dB HL). Comparison between the two groups showed there were statistical significant differences in AC thresholds at 250, 500, 2000, and 4000 Hz. p Values were <0.05, but there was no statistical significant difference at 1000 Hz, $p > 0.05$ (**Table 2**). The tympanometry results also showed that there was no statistical significant difference in the tympanometric peak compliance between the case group (mean rank = 21.90), and the control group (mean rank = 26.52), $z = -1.313$, $p = 0.189 > 0.05$ (**Supplementary Table 1**).

Bone Conduction Thresholds at Low and Mid Frequencies

The results showed the following mean thresholds for the case group: 250 Hz (20.69 ± 14.70 dB HL), 500 Hz (37.36 ± 15.42 dB HL), and 1000 Hz (51.11 ± 14.50 dB HL); for the control group: 250 Hz (15.56 ± 11.33 dB HL), 500 Hz (32.08 ± 13.91 dB HL), and 1000 Hz (48.75 ± 14.21 dB HL). The mean differences in bone conduction thresholds were 250 Hz (5.14 dB HL), 500 Hz (5.28 dB HL), and 1000 Hz (2.36 dB HL). Comparison between the two groups showed that there were statistically significant differences in BC thresholds at low frequencies: 250 and 500 Hz. p Values were: 250 Hz ($p = 0.008 < 0.05$), 500 Hz ($p = 0.010 < 0.05$), but there was no statistical significant difference at 1000 Hz, $p = 0.245 > 0.05$ (**Table 3**).

Air Bone Gap at Low and Mid Frequencies

Statistical analysis of the air bone gap from 250 to 1000 Hz was performed in 36 patients, 72 ears (36 ears in the case group; 36 ears in the control group). The results showed the following mean ABG for the case group: 250 Hz (41.25 ± 14.46 dB HL), 500 Hz (30.00 ± 13.94 dB HL), and 1000 Hz (21.94 ± 13.11 dB HL); for the control group: 250 Hz (38.75 ± 15.23 dB HL),

TABLE 1 | Gender and age characteristics of subjects.

Gender	<6 years	6–12 years	>12 years	Total
Male	4	10	5	19
Female	4	7	6	17

NB: There was no statistical significance difference, $p > 0.05$.

TABLE 2 | AC thresholds of case group and control group.

Frequency (Hz)	Case group (n = 36)	Control group (n = 36)
250	61.94 ± 18.45*	54.31 ± 17.90
500	66.94 ± 19.50*	59.58 ± 17.94
1000	73.06 ± 19.10	66.67 ± 18.60
2000	82.64 ± 20.96*	75.00 ± 16.48
4000	89.44 ± 21.41*	78.47 ± 22.03

*Paired samples t-test *$p < 0.05$.*

TABLE 3 | BC thresholds of case group and control group.

Frequency (Hz)	Case group (n = 36)	Control group (n = 36)
250	20.69 ± 14.70*	15.56 ± 11.33
500	37.36 ± 15.42*	32.08 ± 13.91
1000	51.11 ± 14.50	48.75 ± 14.21

*Paired samples t-test *$p < 0.05$.*

TABLE 4 | Air bone gap of case group and control group.

Frequency (Hz)	Case group (n = 36)	Control group (n = 36)
250	41.25 ± 14.46	38.75 ± 15.23
500	30.00 ± 13.94	27.50 ± 13.18
1000	21.94 ± 13.11	17.92 ± 11.91

Paired samples t-test $p > 0.05$.

500 Hz (27.50 ± 13.18 dB HL), and 1000 Hz (17.92 ± 11.91 dB HL). The mean differences in air bone gap were 250 Hz (2.50 dB HL), 500 Hz (2.50 dB HL), and 1000 Hz (4.03 dB HL). Comparison between the two groups showed there were no statistically significant differences in air bone gap at low and mid frequencies. p Values were 250 Hz ($p = 0.379 > 0.05$), 500 Hz ($p = 0.320 > 0.05$), and 1000 Hz ($p = 0.078 > 0.05$) (**Table 4**).

DISCUSSION

The laterality of high jugular bulb was found mostly in right ears, the study results showed 30 patients had high jugular bulb in the right ear, and six patients had high jugular bulb in the left ear. Some researches have reported the occurrence of high jugular bulb to be more in the right ears than left ears (Singla et al., 2016; Tanrivermis Sayit et al., 2017). The right side normally has the dominant venous system draining blood from the head, this blood flow dynamics could be linked to the cause of jugular bulb abnormalities. Right sided venous dominance was observed in majority of people with abnormal jugular bulb (Friedmann et al., 2012). The imbalanced system may be linked to the asynchronous development of the embryonic venous sinuses, which may lead to asymmetric blood flow during the early stages of cardiac venous pulsation (Wang et al., 2020). The prevalence of high jugular bulb in males and females and age categories are not significantly different, but the size or area of the jugular bulb may be different with males and females, and with different age categories (Friedmann et al., 2011; Wang et al., 2020).

Air Conduction Thresholds of LVAS With HJB

The study findings revealed that AC thresholds of the case group were higher at all test frequencies, compared to the AC thresholds of the control group. There was a statistically significant difference between the AC thresholds of the two groups at 250, 500, 2000, and 4000 Hz, p values were <0.05; but there was no statistical significant difference at 1000 Hz, $p > 0.05$, although there was an increase of >6 dB HL. Previous studies on jugular bulb abnormalities found that hearing thresholds of the ears with high jugular bulb were higher compared to the ears without jugular bulb abnormalities (Tsunoda, 2000; Sasindran et al., 2014; Tanrivermis Sayit et al., 2017). There was an average increase of 8 dB HL in air conduction thresholds across all the tested frequencies when LVAS with HJB present in single ear.

Low-Frequency AC Thresholds of LVAS With HJB

Findings of this study revealed significant increase in AC thresholds at low frequencies (250 and 500 Hz), an average of >7 dB HL difference was found between the groups. High jugular bulb affects hearing in the low-frequency domain, by interfering with the conductive process hearing. HJB obstructs the tympanic membrane, and the movement of the ossicles, as well as impinges on the round window niche (Weiss et al., 1997; Chennupati et al., 2011; Barr and Singh, 2016; Toman et al., 2016). High jugular bulb presenting in the middle could reduce the middle ear's efficacy to achieve proper impedance matching. In order for a proper impedance matching to be achieved, there needs to be an intact tympanic membrane, a normal ossicular chain, and a conducive middle ear space. There could be a possibility that high jugular bulb changes the normal physiology of the middle ear, hence making it difficult for the middle ear to effectively change the low-pressure high-displacement movements of the eardrum into high-pressure low-displacement movements, required for the cochlear fluid to move. When efficient impedance matching is not achieved, some low-frequency sound energy lost. The obstruction or closure of the round window has been found to cause a threshold shift, a phenomenon known as the cochlear conductive loss, which affects mostly the low-frequency sounds (Weiss et al., 1997). The third window leak out created by the enlarged vestibular aqueduct causes low-frequency sound energy to leak out of the cochlear (Arjmand and Webber, 2004; Merchant et al., 2007; Gopen et al., 2011). Therefore, the interference of the middle ear and obstruction of the round window membrane by HJB, and the third window leakage caused by LVAS, explains the increase in low-frequency thresholds when LVAS with HJB are present in one ear.

High-Frequency AC Thresholds of LVAS With HJB

The findings of our study revealed that there was a significant increase in AC thresholds at high frequencies, 2000 and 4000 Hz;

there was an average difference of >9 dB HL between the groups. Enlarged vestibular aqueduct has been reported to cause endolymphatic reflux, which is the flow back of the endolymph into the cochlear. This causes electrolyte imbalance due to the high volumes of endolymph in the cochlear and affects the ionic pump mechanism of stria vascularis, which could lead to accumulation of toxic metabolites, which may damage the inner ear hair cells (Gopen et al., 2011; Chenlu et al., 2020). The high jugular bulb, which can be found impinging on the cochlear from the base, could add pressure onto the inner ear and disturb the inner ear's homeostasis. The added pressure on cochlear, and electrolyte imbalance in the cochlear, affects the cochlear hair cells, which causes cochlear dead regions mostly at high frequencies. The study results showed 4000 Hz to have the highest increase in thresholds (10.97 dB HL), suggesting having LVAS with HJB in one ear, greatly affecting the hearing at high-frequency hearing thresholds.

There was no statistical significant difference at 1000 Hz, although there was an increase of >6 dB HL in thresholds. LVAS and HJB and the frequencies affect hearing in different frequency spectra. LVAS affects mostly high frequencies, which is seen by a steep sloping audiogram. The hearing loss of HJB is a rising configuration, meaning low frequencies are mostly affected. Now when LVAS and HJB occur in one ear, all frequencies may be affected, but mid-frequency standing waves could not be affected much. Also, the human ear is known to have higher sensitivity to sounds around 1000 Hz; this could explain the statistically insignificant difference between thresholds at 1000 Hz.

Bone Thresholds of LVAS With HJB

The result showed bone conduction thresholds of the case group were higher than bone conduction thresholds of the control group. There were statistically significant differences in bone conduction thresholds at 250 and 500 Hz, $p < 0.05$, but there was no statistically significant difference at 1000 Hz, $p > 0.05$. Round window obstruction has been reported to affect bone conduction thresholds. Normally, vibrations of the osseous cochlear capsule would cause alternating compression and expansion of the labyrinthine fluids. The large volume of the scala vestibuli, relative to the scala tympani, sets a pressure differential across the two partitions of the cochlear duct, and produces a traveling wave in the direction of the scala tympani [16]. When the vibrations of the scala tympani are restricted by the closure of the round window, bone conduction would be affected due to compressed pressure retained in the cochlear. When there are no cochlear outlets, these compressed pressures would spill off forcefully through different outlets (third window), such as the cochlear aqueduct, vestibular aqueduct, semicircular canals, and vascular and neural channels (Weiss et al., 1997; Ho et al., 2017). In the case of LVAS with HJB in one ear, the enlarged vestibular aqueduct becomes the outlet for the compressed pressure to spill off and low-frequency vibrations to leak out. This explains the increased bone conduction thresholds found in LVAS with concurrent HJB. When the round window is immobile but there is an available acoustic outlet, low-frequency vibrations would escape efficiently with minimal bone conduction loss, and with increasing frequencies, the efficiency of the leakage decreases due to a rising impedance and bone thresholds become higher (Weiss et al., 1997). This supports the reason for which the result showed a significantly higher BC threshold at low frequencies, but was not significantly higher at 1000 Hz.

Air Bone Gap of LVAS With HJB

The study results showed there was no statistical significant difference in air bone gap between the two groups, $p > 005$. The mechanism of air bone gap in LVAS patients is caused by the third window created by the enlarged vestibular aqueduct and dehiscence of the semicircular canals. This abnormal opening in the bony labyrinth changes the compliance of the inner ear and results in sound energy being leaked out of the cochlea (Gopen et al., 2011). LVAS increases the impedance difference between scala vestibuli and scala tympani of the cochlear partition by lowering impedance on the vestibuli side, thereby improving cochlear response to bone conduction (Merchant et al., 2007). However, in the case of large vestibular aqueduct syndrome with concurrent high jugular bulb, the mechanism changes. Although LVAS lowers impedance on the vestibuli side to improve the cochlear response to sound vibrations, the obstructed round window membrane would still restrict the formation of the sound traveling wave pressure in the inner ear. This causes the bone conduction thresholds to fall on the audiogram. A study on high jugular bulb reported that both air conduction and bone conduction thresholds would fall simultaneously, by obstruction of the round window membrane with an available leak outlet and the interference with the traveling wave by an additional inner ear pressure (Tsunoda, 2000). This supports our study findings showing increase in both air conduction and bone conduction thresholds in LVAS with HJB. Air bone gap could still be seen on the audiogram of LVAS with HJB, but due to the synchronous decline on air conduction and bone conduction thresholds, the difference would not be high, when compared with LVAS without HJB.

The study findings predict that when LVAS and HJB are together in one ear, it affects low-frequency threshold by the conductive component, caused by the obstruction of the eardrum and ossicles, blocking of the round window niche, and the third window. High = frequency thresholds are affected by increased inner ear pressure and cochlear dead regions. This may account for the significant increase in air conduction thresholds at 250, 500, 2000, and 4000, as well as the increase in bone conduction thresholds at 250 and 500 Hz. Nevertheless, these findings may not be representative of all LVAS with HJB patients, since during the process of this research, some LVAS with HJB still had better thresholds than LVAS without HJB. Therefore, there may be other factors that could contribute to threshold increase in patients with LVAS, but this study presents HJB as a factor that could contribute to higher hearing thresholds in LVAS patients.

CONCLUSION

LVAS with HJB would have higher air conduction thresholds, especially at 250, 500, 2000, and 4000 Hz. Bone conduction thresholds would also be higher at 250 and 500 Hz. LVAS with HJB would have air bone gap at 250, 500, and 1000 Hz, but air bone gap would not be significantly higher than LVAS with HJB.

ETHICS STATEMENT

The studies involving human participants were reviewed and approved by Zhejiang Chinese Medical University's Affiliated Hearing and Speech Rehabilitation Institute. The patients/participants provided their written informed consent to participate in this study. Written informed consent was obtained from the individual(s) for the publication of any potentially identifiable images or data included in this article.

AUTHOR CONTRIBUTIONS

YW, WS, and YS contributed to the conception and design of the study and revised the manuscript. AK, CW, FC, and XY collected the data and performed the statistical analysis. AK and JY drafted and revised the manuscript. All authors have read and approved the submitted version.

REFERENCES

Aimoni, C., Ciorba, A., Cerritelli, L., Ceruti, S., Skarzynski, P. H., and Hatzopoulos, S. (2017). Enlarged vestibular aqueduct: audiological and genetical features in children and adolescents. *Int. J. Pediatr. Otorhinolaryngol.* 101, 254–258. doi: 10.1016/j.ijporl.2017.07.042

Arjmand, E. M., and Webber, A. (2004). Audiometric findings in children with a large vestibular aqueduct. *Arch. Otolaryngol. Head Neck Surg.* 130, 1169–1174. doi: 10.1001/archotol.130.10.1169

Barr, J. G., and Singh, P. K. (2016). A rare cause of conductive hearing loss: high lateralized jugular bulb with bony dehiscence. *Ear Nose Throat J.* 95, 227–229. doi: 10.1177/014556131609500609

Chenlu, W., Wendi, S., Na, Z., and Yonghua, W. (2020). Distribution study of cochlear dead regions in patients with large vestibular aqueduct syndrome. *Chin. Arch. Otolaryngol. Head Neck Surg.* 27, 633–635. doi: 10.16066/j.1672-7002.2020.11.006

Chennupati, S. K., Reddy, N. P., and O'Reilly, R. C. (2011). High-riding jugular bulb presenting as conductive hearing loss. *Int. J. Pediatr. Otorhinolaryngol. Extra* 6, 235–237. doi: 10.1016/j.pedex.2010.10.005

Friedmann, D. R., Eubig, J., McGill, M., Babb, J. S., Pramanik, B. K., and Lalwani, A. K. (2011). Development of the jugular bulb: a radiologic study. *Otol Neurotol.* 32, 1389–1395. doi: 10.1097/MAO.0b013e31822e5b8d

Friedmann, D. R., Eubig, J., Winata, L. S., Pramanik, B. K., Merchant, S. N., and Lalwani, A. K. (2012). A Clinical and Histopathologic Study of Jugular Bulb Abnormalities. *Arch. Otolaryngol. Head Neck Surg.* 138, 66–71. doi: 10.1001/archoto.2011.231

Gopen, Q., Zhou, G., Whittemore, K., and Kenna, M. (2011). Enlarged vestibular aqueduct: review of controversial aspects. *Laryngoscope* 121, 1971–1978. doi: 10.1002/lary.22083

Ho, M. L., Moonis, G., Halpin, C. F., and Curtin, H. D. (2017). Spectrum of Third Window Abnormalities: Semicircular Canal Dehiscence and Beyond. *AJNR Am. J. Neuroradiol.* 38, 2–9. doi: 10.3174/ajnr.a4922

Kupfer, R. A., Hoesli, R. C., Green, G. E., and Thorne, M. C. (2012). The relationship between jugular bulb-vestibular aqueduct dehiscence and hearing loss in pediatric patients. *Otolaryngol. Head Neck Surg.* 146, 473–477. doi: 10.1177/0194599811430045

Madden, C., Halsted, M., Meinzen-Derr, J., Bardo, D., Boston, M., Arjmand, E., et al. (2007). The influence of mutations in the SLC26A4 gene on the temporal bone in a population with enlarged vestibular aqueduct. *Arch. Otolaryngol. Head Neck Surg.* 133, 162–168. doi: 10.1001/archotol.133.2.162

Margolis, R. H., and Heller, J. W. (1987). Screening tympanometry: criteria for medical referral. *Audiology* 26, 197–208. doi: 10.3109/00206098709081549

Merchant, S. N., Nakajima, H. H., Halpin, C., Nadol, J. B., Lee, D. J., Innis, W. P., et al. (2007). Clinical Investigation and Mechanism of Air-Bone Gaps in Large Vestibular Aqueduct Syndrome. *Ann. Otol. Rhinol. Laryngol.* 116, 532–541. doi: 10.1177/000348940711600709

Noguchi, Y., Fukuda, S., Fukushima, K., Gyo, K., Hara, A., Nakashima, T., et al. (2017). A nationwide study on enlargement of the vestibular aqueduct in Japan. *Auris Nasus Larynx* 44, 33–39. doi: 10.1016/j.anl.2016.04.012

Sasindran, V., Abraham, S., Hiremath, S., and Joseph, A. (2014). High-riding jugular bulb: a rare entity. *Indian J. Otol.* 20:129. doi: 10.4103/0971-7749.136863

Singla, A., Gupta, T., Sahni, D., Aggarwal, A., and Gupta, A. (2016). High jugular bulb: different osseous landmarks and their clinical implications. *Surg. Radiol. Anat.* 38, 903–909. doi: 10.1007/s00276-016-1649-2

Tanrivermis Sayit, A., Elmali, M., Kemal, O., and Terzi, Y. (2017). Radiological, clinical and audiological evaluation of jugular bulb-vestibular aqueduct dehiscence. *Acta Otolaryngol.* 137, 1221–1225. doi: 10.1080/00016489.2017.1360516

Toman, J., Wu, X., Malhotra, A., and Michaelides, E. (2016). Conductive Hearing Loss and the Jugular Bulb. *Clin. Neuroradiol.* 26, 235–238. doi: 10.1007/s00062-015-0436-5

Tsunoda, A. (2000). Sensorineural hearing loss caused by a high jugular bulb. *J. Laryngol. Otol.* 114, 867–869. doi: 10.1258/0022215001904194

Wang, J., Feng, Y., Wang, H., Li, C., Wu, Y., Shi, H., et al. (2020). Prevalence of High Jugular Bulb across Different Stages of Adulthood in A Chinese Population. *Aging Dis.* 11, 770–776. doi: 10.14336/AD.2020.0215

Weiss, R. L., Zahtz, G., Goldofsky, E., Parnes, H., and Shikowitz, M. J. (1997). High Jugular Bulb and Conductive Hearing Loss. *Laryngoscope* 107, 321–327. doi: 10.1097/00005537-199703000-00008

Yan, Y. W., Zhen, Z. S., Jun, Z. C., Bo, F., Surgery, N., Pla, C., et al. (2003). Clinical analysis of 95 patients with large vestibular aqueduct syndrome. *Chin. J. Otorhinolaryngol.* 38, 191–194.

Zhang, S. Z., Wei-Yan, Y., and Zi-Ming, W. U. (2006). Relationship between the external aperture and hearing loss in large vestibular aqueduct syndrome. *Chin. Med. J.* 119, 211–216. doi: 10.1097/00029330-200602010-00007

13

Familial Temperature-Sensitive Auditory Neuropathy: Distinctive Clinical Courses Caused by Variants of the *OTOF* Gene

Yi-Ming Zhu[1,2†], *Qi Li*[1†], *Xue Gao*[3], *Yan-Fei Li*[1], *You-Li Liu*[1], *Pu Dai*[1,4*] *and Xiang-Ping Li*[1*]

[1] Department of Otolaryngology-Head and Neck Surgery, Nanfang Hospital, Southern Medical University, Guangzhou, China, [2] Department of Otolaryngology-Head and Neck Surgery, Lanzhou University Second Hospital, Lanzhou, China, [3] Department of Otolaryngology, PLA Rocket Force Characteristic Medical Center, Beijing, China, [4] Department of Otolaryngology-Head and Neck Surgery, Chinese PLA General Hospital, Beijing, China

***Correspondence:**
Xiang-Ping Li
li321162@qq.com
Pu Dai
daipu301@vip.sina.com

† These authors have contributed equally to this work and share first authorship

Objective: To investigate the clinical course and genetic etiology of familial temperature-sensitive auditory neuropathy (TSAN), which is a very rare subtype of auditory neuropathy (AN) that involves an elevation of hearing thresholds due to an increase in the core body temperature, and to evaluate the genotype–phenotype correlations in a family with TSAN.

Methods: Six members of a non-consanguineous Chinese family, including four siblings complaining of communication difficulties when febrile, were enrolled in this study. The clinical and audiological profiles of the four siblings were fully evaluated during both febrile and afebrile episodes, and the genetic etiology of hearing loss (HL) was explored using next-generation sequencing (NGS) technology. Their parents, who had no complaints of fluctuating HL due to body temperature variation, were enrolled for the genetics portion only.

Results: Audiological tests during the patients' febrile episodes met the classical diagnostic criteria for AN, including mild HL, poor speech discrimination, preserved cochlear microphonics (CMs), and absent auditory brainstem responses (ABRs). Importantly, unlike the pattern observed in previously reported cases of TSAN, the ABRs and electrocochleography (ECochG) signals of our patients improved to normal during afebrile periods. Genetic analysis identified a compound heterozygous variant of the *OTOF* gene (which encodes the otoferlin protein), including one previously reported pathogenic variant, c.5098G > C (p.Glu1700Gln), and one novel variant, c.4882C > A (p.Pro1628Thr). Neither of the identified variants affected the C2 domains related to the main function of otoferlin. Both variants faithfully cosegregated with TSAN within the pedigree, suggesting that *OTOF* is the causative gene of the autosomal recessive trait segregation in this family.

Conclusion: The presence of CMs with absent (or markedly abnormal) ABRs is a reliable criterion for diagnosing AN. The severity of the phenotype caused by dysfunctional neurotransmitter release in TSAN may reflect variants that alter the C2 domains of otoferlin. The observations from this study enrich the current understanding of the phenotype and genotype of TSAN and may lay a foundation for further research on its pathogenesis.

Keywords: temperature sensitive, auditory neuropathy, variant, *OTOF*, otoferlin, genotype phenotype correlation, hearing loss

INTRODUCTION

Auditory neuropathy (AN), which is a clinical disorder featuring auditory processing dysfunction, is characterized by normal outer hair cell (OHC) function in the cochlea and abnormal neural function at the level of the inner hair cells (IHCs), the cochlear nerve, or their junction. Patients with AN commonly have normal otoacoustic emissions (OAEs) and cochlear microphonics (CMs) but absent or severely abnormal auditory brainstem responses (ABRs). Pure-tone audiometry can vary widely from normal hearing thresholds to profound hearing loss (HL). Acoustic reflexes (ARs) are often absent, and speech recognition is worse than would be predicted from the pure-tone thresholds, particularly in ambient noise (Starr et al., 1996). Although individuals with AN retain OHC function, they usually have impaired neural coding of sound stimuli as a result of lesions involving the auditory nerve itself, the IHCs and/or their synapses or auditory cortex abnormalities (Kaga et al., 1996). Accordingly, the terms "auditory synaptopathy" and "auditory neuropathy" are applied to this disease when it is due to synaptic and neural deficits, respectively (Moser and Starr, 2016).

Among patients with sensorineural HL, AN accounts for 0.5–15% of cases (Madden et al., 2002; Sanyelbhaa Talaat et al., 2009; Gohari et al., 2019), with a prevalence of approximately 0.23% in at-risk children (Rance et al., 1999); however, the diverse etiologies of AN are only beginning to be characterized. Genetic factors and the effects of a wide range of other etiologies (anoxia, certain infectious diseases, and hyperbilirubinemia) are estimated to account for 42 and 10% of all cases of AN, respectively, and the remaining 48% of cases lack a defined etiology (Starr et al., 2000, 2008). All forms of AN may be present in isolation (non-syndromic AN) or with multisystem involvement, including peripheral and/or optic neuropathies as well as various central nervous system (CNS) disorders (syndromic AN) (Santarelli, 2010).

Due to the distinct clinical and pathological features of non-syndromic AN (NSAN), its diagnosis mainly relies on audiological measures and electrophysiological tests along with ancillary methods, such as OAEs, acoustic immittance, temporal bone high-resolution computed tomography (HRCT) and magnetic resonance imaging (MRI). Pure-tone audiometry enables the degree, type, and configuration of HL to be identified. In addition to revealing impaired speech perception that is out of proportion to HL, electrophysiological tests [including ABRs and electrocochleography (ECochG)] and OAEs can assist in identifying the sites of the lesions along the auditory pathway since dysfunction of the auditory nerve, IHCs and/or IHC ribbon synapses [absent/abnormal ARs, ABRs, and action potential (AP) on ECochG] is accompanied by preserved OHC measurements (OAEs and/or CMs) (Santarelli, 2010). Furthermore, HRCT and MRI approaches have become effective methods for identifying possible structural or inflammatory abnormalities of the auditory nerve and auditory pathway that cause HL (Sharma et al., 2018). Therefore, when diagnosing AN, both imaging modalities are powerful methods for ruling out any organic lesions.

Temperature-sensitive auditory neuropathy (TSAN) is a very rare form of NSAN with distinct phenotypes. The most striking feature of TSAN is that patients present with transient HL after a rise in the core body temperature. This disorder was first described by Gorga et al. (1995) in a child with recurrent but completely reversible HL during febrile conditions. Clinical examinations showed that poor speech understanding emerged earlier than pure-tone HL and resolved more slowly than the loss of auditory function. Tests of cochlear function, including OAEs and ECochG, were normal; however, all the tests related to central connections within the brainstem, such as ARs, ABRs, and mechanically evoked trigeminofacial reflexes, were abnormal regardless of whether auditory function was normal or impaired at the time. Moreover, the middle-latency responses and auditory late potentials appeared normal. The authors predicted that the site of the lesion was the brainstem, rather than the peripheral nervous system or higher levels in the auditory pathway. Three years later, Starr et al. (1998) identified three children—two siblings and an unrelated child—who carried similar phenotypes, as confirmed by tests performed in both febrile and afebrile states. Two of the three children may have had a summating potential (SP), the existence of which was not examined in the first reported patient. Furthermore, all three patients had mild HL either at all frequencies or specifically at low frequencies when afebrile. In addition, one patient showed abnormal median sensory nerve conduction. The authors proposed that the patients' transient deafness resulted from a demyelinating disorder of the auditory nerve and concluded that the reported cases represented an atypical form of AN, which was termed TSAN. Examples of both sporadic and familial TSAN have been described (Cianfrone et al., 2006; Varga et al., 2006; Madanoglu and Derinsu, 2007; Marlin et al., 2010; Dimitrijevic et al., 2011; Matsunaga et al., 2012; Wynne et al., 2013; Kaga, 2016; Zhang et al., 2016). Although fever-associated HL is reversible and OAEs are always normal, all reported cases have two abnormal auditory findings in common: ABRs and ARs are abnormal during both febrile and afebrile episodes. Further research revealed that variants of the *OTOF* gene are the main cause of this disease (Varga et al., 2006; Romanos et al., 2009; Marlin et al., 2010; Wang et al., 2010; Matsunaga et al., 2012; Zhang et al., 2016).

The pathogenic mechanism of TSAN is only beginning to be understood. To date, only one study performed by Strenzke et al. (2016) successfully built an $Otof^{I515T/I515T}$ mutant mouse model, which exhibited a similar severity of HL to that in humans. Further research revealed that impaired exocytosis at hair cell ribbon synapses due to abnormal synaptic vesicles caused by Ile515Thr-otoferlin was the main pathogenic mechanism of TSAN. Notably, the mutant mice failed to show more severe hearing loss at high body temperatures, unlike the patients. The authors concluded that the lack of a human RXR motif (20 amino acids), which is thermally sensitive in mice, was the cause of inconsistent phenotypes between mutant mice and TSAN patients. However, TSAN patients are rare, the relationship between the severity of phenotypes and variants of the *OTOF* gene is still unclear, and clinical tests have never detected any demonstrable structural lesion or underlying mechanism to explain this uncommon type of HL.

Herein, we describe a TSAN-afflicted family with a distinctive pattern of phenotypic and genetic features. Four siblings, including a pair of identical twins, were examined in our clinic, and diagnosed with TSAN. Using next-generation sequencing (NGS) technology, we identified two compound heterozygous variants of the *OTOF* gene that are associated with TSAN. These data reveal genotype–phenotype correlations in TSAN, providing an improved understanding of the diagnostic features and natural history of this disease.

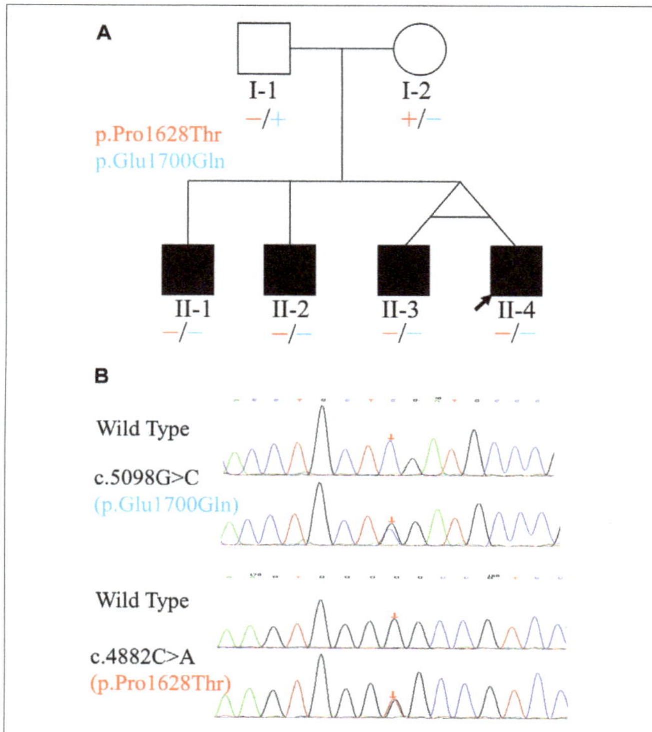

FIGURE 1 | Pedigree and variants of the *OTOF* gene found in the family. **(A)** Pedigree and distribution of *OTOF* variants. Filled symbols represent affected individuals. Circle indicates female and squares indicate males. The two variants are shown in different colors. "−" and "+" represent variant and wild-type *OTOF*, respectively. **(B)** Electropherograms showing the two heterozygous *OTOF* variants (in the reverse direction). The positions of variants are indicated by red arrows.

MATERIALS AND METHODS

Subjects

In 2016, a 13-year-old boy with normal-hearing parents visited our clinic. The boy complained of hearing difficulty and poor speech discrimination only when his body temperature was high due to influenza or other causes. His family history revealed that his three brothers (including a twin brother) had similar complaints. Six individuals from this family were enrolled in the study (**Figure 1**). Detailed medical histories of the four siblings were obtained, and otologic and hearing evaluations of the four patients were performed during both afebrile and febrile states. Their parents were enrolled for the genetics portion only because neither parent complained of fluctuating HL when their body temperature varied. Vestibular function was not evaluated. Body temperature was measured at the axilla using a clinical mercury thermometer (Yuwell, Nanjing, China). Two hundred unrelated, ethnicity- and age-matched individuals (100 males and 100 females) with normal hearing were recruited as normal controls to rule out genetic polymorphisms.

The study was approved by the institutional ethics review board, including committees of medical ethics at the Nanfang Hospital, the Chinese PLA General Hospital, and the Lanzhou University Second Hospital. After written informed consent was obtained from all subjects included in the study or their guardians, genomic DNA (gDNA) was collected from the peripheral blood of all participants using standard procedures.

Auditory Function Examination

All hearing evaluations, including pure-tone and speech audiometry, acoustic immittance, ABRs, ECochG, and distortion product otoacoustic emissions (DPOAEs), were performed according to standard clinical methods in a magnetically shielded and sound-attenuated room in the Department of Otolaryngology, Head and Neck Surgery, Nanfang Hospital, Southern Medical University, Guangzhou, China. Furthermore, imaging examinations, including thin-slice temporal bone HRCT scans and MRIs, were performed when the patients were febrile and afebrile.

Audiometric and Acoustic Immittance Tests

Air- and bone-conduction pure-tone audiometry was performed at octave frequency intervals in the range of 0.125–8 kHz for both ears using a GSI AudioStar Pro audiometer (Grason-Stadler Inc., Eden Prairie, MN, United States). The pure-tone average over four frequencies (0.5, 1, 2, and 4 kHz) from the better-hearing ear was used for data analysis. The severity of HL was graded as normal (0–25 dB HL), mild (26–40 dB HL), moderate (41–55 dB HL), moderately severe (56–70 dB HL), severe (71–90 dB HL), or profound (>90 dB HL) (Schlauch and Nelson, 2015). Speech audiometry measures included the speech reception threshold (SRT) and monosyllabic speech discrimination score (SDS) at 40 dB SL or less above the SRT or at the maximum level (100 dB HL) of the audiometer, depending on the patient's hearing threshold and the highest comfortable level, especially during periods of elevated thresholds. Mandarin speech test materials (MSTM) were used to evaluate speech recognition under quiet conditions. Speech recognition tests were conducted in noise using a 10 dB signal-to-noise ratio at the baseline test. Speech testing in noise was not evaluated upon follow-up testing due to patient reports of discomfort from the noise levels used. Acoustic immittance measurements (including tympanometry and AR) were performed using an Interacoustics AT235h Impedance Audiometer (Middelfart, Denmark). The outcomes of a tympanogram with a 226 Hz probe tone were categorized as either type A, B, or C and accompanied by a cutoff negative pressure for type C at -100 daPa, as defined in the Jerger classification system (Jerger, 1970). ARs were measured ipsilaterally and contralaterally to the stimulated ear at frequencies of 0.5, 1, 2, and 4 kHz.

Electrophysiological Measures

Auditory brainstem responses and ECochG signals were recorded using the IHS SmartEP system (Intelligent Hearing Systems, Miami, FL, United States) with ER-3A insert earphones (Etymotic Research, Elk Grove Village, IL, United States). Click stimuli with a duration of 0.1 ms, which were separated into condensation (C) and rarefaction (R) clicks, were monaurally presented at a repetition rate of 19.3 clicks/s for ABRs and 7.1 clicks/s for ECochG. Furthermore, CMs were measured during the ABRs by examining responses to opposite-polarity stimuli, whereas ECochG was used to examine SP and AP.

Auditory brainstem responses were differentially recorded using alternating polarities, and 1,024 sweeps were averaged and analyzed using a 12-ms epoch (time window) with filtering at 100–1,000 Hz. To better evaluate and monitor the processes of auditory function recovery, stimuli were presented at the maximum level (100 dB nHL) and reduced in 10-dB steps until there was no response. For every condition, at least two replication trials were performed. ABRs were interpreted as having a CM when (1) there was a short latency (approximately 0.8 ms) or no latency shift was observed with variations in the stimulus level (Shi et al., 2012), (2) the response appeared before the normal ABR waveform, (3) the phases were inverted upon the reversal of stimulus polarities (rarefaction and condensation), and (4) clamping of the acoustic conduction tube eliminated the responses. When these criteria for CMs were met, the CM amplitude was enhanced by subtracting the average separate responses to C and R stimuli (C - R) instead of adding the traces (C + R), which resulted in the elimination of CMs.

Tympanic ECochG was performed with a wick electrode (Lilly, Miami, FL, United States) placed against the unanesthetized tympanic membrane (TM) under direct microscopic visualization. To obtain better performance, the clicks used as acoustic stimuli were also delivered at different intensity levels decreasing in 10-dB steps from a maximum intensity of 100 dB nHL to allow visual detection of the AP and SP. For the AP and SP recordings, 512 sweeps with separate opposite click polarities (C and R) as well as alternating polarities (within a single test run) were averaged using an epoch of 5 ms (including 1 ms prestimulus time) and a filter setting of 100–1,500 Hz. The AP and SP amplitudes and the SP/AP amplitude ratio were analyzed accordingly regarding the amplitude recorded. The SP/AP amplitude ratio was defined as enhanced when it was $\geq$0.4, in accordance with a proposed classification (Ohashi et al., 2009).

Distortion Product Otoacoustic Emission Test

Distortion product otoacoustic emissions were tested using a GSI Audera system (Grason-Stadler Inc., Eden Prairie, MN, United States). DPOAEs were evaluated in quarter-octave bands from 500–8,000 Hz using a frequency (F) ratio F2/F1 = 1.22 with levels (L2 and L1) of 65- and 55-dB SPL. When emissions were present at 60% or more of the test frequencies, DPOAE was defined as present; otherwise, it was defined as absent.

Test Frequency

Patients enrolled in this study were followed up for 3 years at the local hospital. Hearing tests were performed daily during febrile episodes and then repeated every day within the first week (when possible) after each febrile event as well as one month later and every 6 months thereafter (**Figure 2**). Otitis and other causes of HL were first excluded during these febrile episodes by physical and imaging examinations.

Analysis of Clinical Features

To better interpret clinical presentations and diagnostic evaluations, we divided the course of each febrile event into three separate periods, i.e., the febrile episode, the recovery episode and the afebrile episode, referring to the day(s) when the patient had a fever, the first 6 days after body temperature recovery, and the period beginning 1 week after body temperature recovery, respectively (**Figure 2**). The results were calculated and plotted using the Origin 8.5 package (OriginLab Corp., Northampton, MA, United States). Data are presented as the mean ± SEM (standard error of the mean).

Genetic Analysis

Determination of Twin Zygosity

To confirm whether the twin brothers were identical or fraternal, the AGCU 17 + 1 STR Kit (AGCU ScienTech Inc., Wuxi, China), which is composed of 17 autosomal unlinked loci and the sex-determining marker amelogenin, was used to determine the twin zygosity. The autosomal loci included D3S1358, D13S317, D7S820, D16S539, Penta E, TPOX, TH01, D2S1338, CSF1PO, D19S433, vWA, D5S818, FGA, D6S1043, D8S1179, D21S11, and D18S51. Polymerase chain reaction (PCR) amplification, sample preparation, and electrophoresis were performed in accordance with the manufacturers' instructions (Fan et al., 2012). Briefly, gDNA (0.5–2.0 ng) from the two twin brothers was added to the reaction mix along with HotStart C-Taq DNA polymerase and

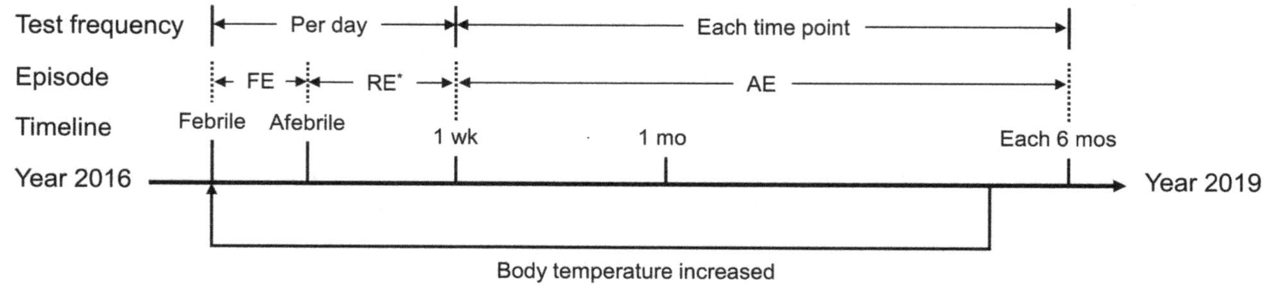

FIGURE 2 | Timeline of the episodes and tests described in the present study. FE, febrile episode; RE, recovery episode; AE, afebrile episode; wk, week; mo, month. *Not available in some days during this period. The axis indicates the timeline from the year 2016 to the year 2019. The phrase "body temperature increased" indicates a round of hearing fluctuation due to a febrile episode. During the follow-up period, the proband experienced three febrile episodes, whereas each of the other three patients experienced only one. Tests were completed at each time point during each febrile episode.

17 + 1 fluorescently labeled primers to give a final volume of 10 μL for PCR (conditions not shown). The targeted products were analyzed using an ABI 3130XL Genetic Analyzer (Applied Biosystems, Foster City, CA, United States). Genotypes were validated by comparing the sizes of the unknown fragments to the allelic ladders provided by the kit.

Targeted Next-Generation Sequencing

After the common deafness genes (*GJB2*, *SLC26A4*, and *MT-RNR1*) had been excluded by direct sequencing (Du et al., 2014), NGS technology was applied to identify the causative gene in this family.

For targeted capture and massively parallel sequencing (MPS), the qualified gDNA of the proband (II-4) was randomly sheared using the Covaris S2 Focused Ultrasonicator (Covaris, Massachusetts, MA, United States) to an average fragment size of 350–400 bp. The fragments were then end-repaired, ligated to adapters, and analyzed using an Agilent 2100 Bioanalyzer. All exons and flanking intronic regions of 159 deafness-related nuclear genes, 6 deafness-related mitochondrial regions, and 3 miRNAs (**Supplementary Tables 1–3**) were captured using a GenCap kit (MyGenostics, Beijing, China). The captured sequences were analyzed by high-throughput sequencing using a NextSeq 500 next-generation sequencer (Illumina Inc., San Diego, CA, United States).

To identify modifier genes for the phenotypic manifestation of TSAN-associated *OTOF* variants, we performed whole-exome sequencing (WES) of DNA from the proband (II-4). For WES confirmation, fragment libraries were prepared using the Nextera Rapid Capture kit (Illumina). The gDNA fragments were end-repaired and purified in accordance with the manufacturer's protocol. The Nimblegen SeqCap EZ Exome v3.0 (64 Mb) Kit (Roche, Madison, WI, United States) was used to capture exons after the manufacturer's protocols, and these exons were then sequenced on the HiSeq XTen PE150 platform (Illumina).

Bioinformatics Analysis

Next-generation sequencing data from the two procedures were analyzed using an in-house bioinformatics pipeline, as we previously described (Yuan et al., 2020). Briefly, qualified reads were obtained after low-quality data were filtered out from the raw data using the Cutadapt program (Martin, 2011) and were then mapped to the human reference genome (GRCh37/hg19) using the program Burrows-Wheeler Aligner (BWA).[1] Subsequently, the Genome Analysis Toolkit (GATK) program was used to call single-nucleotide variants (SNVs) and insertions or deletions (indels). The SNVs and indels were annotated using public databases (including the 1000 Genomes, gnomAD/ExAC, ClinVar, HGMD, and ClinGen databases and the Deafness Variation Database) and in-house databases according to the ACMG/AMP guidelines for genetic HL (Oza et al., 2018).

Variant Confirmation and Screening

The suspected candidate variants were confirmed by Sanger sequencing, and the responsible variants were identified based on co-segregation analysis with the TSAN phenotype among the family members. The primer sequences and PCR conditions are available upon request. Finally, the detected variants were screened in the control group to discard polymorphisms and explore the allele frequencies according to recessive inheritance patterns.

Evolutionary Conservation and Molecular Model Analyses

Evolutionary conservation was evaluated across 11 organisms using Clustal X 2.1 (Larkin et al., 2007). To analyze the effects of the two identified *OTOF* variants, the three-dimensional (3D) structures of otoferlin and its p.Pro1628Thr and p.Glu1700Gln mutants were modeled using AlphaFold (Jumper et al., 2021). The molecular data obtained by homology modeling were represented using the PyMOL 2.5 molecular graphics system.[2]

RESULTS

Clinical Data and Audiological Findings

Four siblings were clinically diagnosed with non-syndromic TSAN based on auditory evaluations, medical histories, and

[1] http://bio-bwa.sourceforge.net/
[2] https://pymol.org/2/

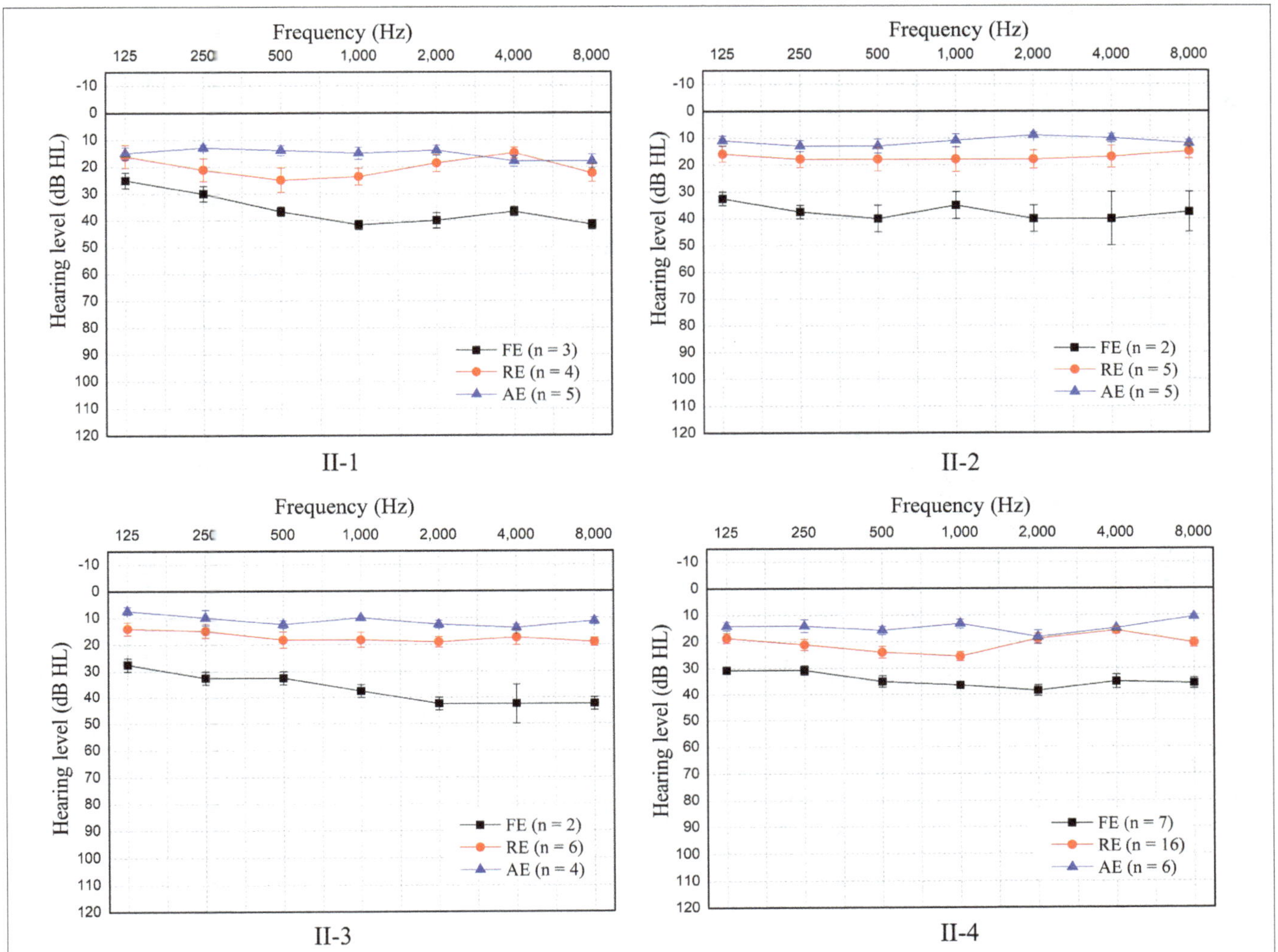

FIGURE 3 | Pure-tone audiometry of the four patients during the three episodes. Since no air-bone gap was found, only pure-tone air-conducted thresholds for the better ear for each patient are shown. Patients experienced mild sensorineural hearing loss during each febrile episode (FE), but hearing returned to normal in the recovery episode (RE) and remained normal in the afebrile episode (AE). The hearing threshold at each frequency is shown as the mean ± SEM of the air-conduction threshold. N: number of test events.

physical examinations. The relationship among the siblings is shown in **Figure 1**. They complained of hearing impairment and a poor ability to discriminate speech during each febrile episode. This phenotype of TSAN was associated with communication difficulties secondary to poor auditory function during febrile episodes, and speech recognition abilities recovered immediately when the core body temperature returned to normal. Although general physical examinations identified no structural or developmental abnormality in any of the four siblings, audiometry results showed that their SDSs improved more rapidly than other test results, such as those for ECochG signals and ABRs. Interestingly, pure-tone thresholds improved from mild HL during the febrile condition to normal levels during the afebrile periods (**Figure 3** and **Table 1**), while CMs were present during all test conditions (**Table 1**). Moreover, the follow-up audiometry assessments, except for the continued absence of ARs, showed improvement to normal levels during afebrile episodes. Importantly, HRCT and MRI scans failed to show any structural or inflammatory abnormalities or abnormal contrast enhancement of the ear (including the outer, middle, and inner ear), auditory nerve or brain, such as tympanitis, acoustic neuromas or brainstem tumors, in febrile or afebrile episodes. Notably, their unaffected parents without similar complaints had clinically normal hearing ability and were able to recognize speech.

During the 3-year follow-up period, the proband suffered from three episodes of "poor hearing," while his three brothers experienced one episode each. Audiological tests revealed that all four brothers had the same pattern of hearing fluctuation. Because of the different auditory phenotypes and test results for the different periods, the results from the febrile, recovery and afebrile periods are shown separately (**Table 2**).

TABLE 1 | Overview of genotype–phenotype correlations of *OTOF* variants in the TSAN patients identified in the present study or previous studies.

	Family 1	Family 2	Family 3	Family 4	Family 5	Family 6	Family 7	Family 8
Genotype								
OTOF variants	c.1544T > C/ c.3346C > T	c.1841G > A/ c.3239G > C	c.5410_ 5412del GAG Hom	c.1621G > A Hom	c.2975_2978delAG/ c.4189C > T	c.4189C > T Hom	c.2382_2383delC/ c.1621G > A	c.5098G > C/ c.4882C > A
Otoferlin changes	p.Ile515Thr/ p.Arg1116Ter	p.Gly614Glu/ p.Arg1080Pro	p.Glu1804del Hom	p.Gly541Ser Hom	p.Gln994Valfs*7/ p.Arg1607Trp	p.Arg1607Trp Hom	p.Leu795Serfs*5/ p.Gly541Ser	p.Glu1700Gln/ p.Pro1628Thr
No. of CAV	2	1	2	2	2	2	2	0
Phenotype								
No. of patient(s)	2	1	3	1	1	1	1	4
Origin	United States	Brazil	Scotland	Japan	China	China	China	China
Sex	Male (1), Female (1)	Female	Male (1), Female (2)	Male	Male	Male	Male	Male
Age at onset (diagnosis)	2 (3, 2) years	–	2 (7–10) years	10 (25) years	13 months	6 years	30 months	Childhood (8–15 years)
Febrile episode								
Body temperature (°C)	38.1/37.8	–	>38	37.2	36.64[†]/36.5	36.9	–	38–40.2
Hearing level	Profound-mild	Severe	Profound/severe	Profound	Severe[†]/moderate	Mild	–	Mild
SDS (%)	0	–	<100	≤15	–[†]/(16–20)	88–80	–	0–20
Tympanometry	A	–	–	–	A	A	A	A × 3/C ×1
AR	Absent	–	–	–	Absent	Absent	Absent	Absent
OAEs	Present	–	Present	Present	Present	Present	Present	Present × 3/Absent × 1
ABR	Absent	–	Abnormal	Absent	Absent	Absent	Absent	Absent
CM	Present	–	–	Present	Present	Present	Present	Present
ECochG	Absent	–	–	Abnormal	–	–	–	Absent
Afebrile episode								
Body temperature (°C)	Normal	–	–	36.8	(36.13–36.32)[†]/36.3	36.6	–	36.3–37.3
Hearing level	Mild in low frequencies	Mild	Normal/mild	Mild	Moderately severe[†]/mild	Moderate[†]/normal	Moderate	Normal
SDS (%)	88–100	–	≤80	≤80	–[†]/16	96	93–98 (after CI)	88–100
Tympanometry	A	–	–	–	A	A	A	A
AR	Absent	–	–	–	Absent	Absent	Absent	Absent
OAEs	Present	Present	Present	Present	Present	Present	Present	Present
ABR	Abnormal	Abnormal	Abnormal	Absent	Absent	Absent	Absent	Normal
CM	Present	–	–	Present	Present	Present	Present	Present
ECochG	SP (possible)	–	–	SP (definite)	Abnormal	–	–	Normal
Auditory rehabilitation	–	–	Hearing aids	–	Improved with age	Improved with age	Cochlear implantation (CI)	No[‡]
References	Starr et al., 1998; Varga et al., 2006; Strenzke et al., 2016	Romanos et al., 2009	Marlin et al., 2010	Matsunaga et al., 2012; Kaga, 2016	Wang et al., 2010; Zhang et al., 2016	Zhang et al., 2016	Zhang et al., 2016	Present study

–, undefined/untested; †, before hearing improvement; ‡, automatically recovered. ABR, auditory brainstem response; AR, acoustic reflex; CAV, C2 domain-affecting variant of otoferlin; CM, cochlear microphonic; ECochG, electrocochleography; Hom, homozygote; OAE, otoacoustic emission; SDS, speech discrimination score.

TABLE 2 | Clinical features of four brothers with temperature-sensitive auditory neuropathy.

	II-1	II-2	II-3	II-4
Sex	Male	Male	Male	Male
Age† (years)	16	14	13	13
Febrile episode				
N	3	2	2	7
Temperature	37.9 ± 0.1	37.7 ± 0.2	38 ± 0.2	38.4 ± 0.3
Hearing level	Mild	Mild	Mild	Mild
Average SDS (%, L/R)	4/12	10/15	13/5	5/4
Tympanogram	A	A	A	C
AR	Abs	Abs	Abs	Abs
ABR	Abs	Abs	Abs	Abs
CM	Pres	Pres	Pres	Pres
ECochG	Abs	Abs	Abs	Abs
DPOAE	Pres	Pres	Pres	Abs‡
Recovery episode				
N	4	5	6	16
Temperature	36.6 ± 0.1	36.2 ± 0.1	36.5 ± 0.1	36.5 ± 0.1
Hearing level	Normal	Normal	Normal	Normal
Average SDS (%, L/R)	98/97	97/96	98/99	97/97
Tympanogram	A	A	A	C × 6/A × 10
AR	Abs	Abs	Abs	Abs
ABR	Abs × 2/Abn × 2	Abs × 3/Abn × 2	Abs × 4/Abn × 2	Abs × 6/Abn × 10
CM	Pres	Pres	Pres	Pres
ECochG	Abs × 2/Abn × 2	Abs × 3/Abn × 2	Abs × 4/Abn × 2	Abs × 6/Abn × 10
DPOAE	Pres	Pres	Pres	Abs‡ × 6/Pres × 10
Afebrile episode				
N	5	5	4	6
Temperature	36.3 ± 0.1	36.2 ± 0.1	36.4 ± 0.1	36.5 ± 0.1
Hearing level	Normal	Normal	Normal	Normal
Average SDS (%, L/R)	99/98	98/97	98/99	98/99
Tympanogram	A	A	A	A
AR	Abs	Abs	Abs	Abs
ABR	Normal	Normal	Normal	Normal
CM	Pres	Pres	Pres	Pres
ECochG	Normal	Normal	Normal	Normal
DPOAE	Pres	Pres	Pres	Pres

†At the time of enrollment in the study.
‡Absent DPOAEs may have been due to abnormal middle ear function.
N, number of test events (results are not available for several days during recovery episodes); ABR, auditory brainstem response; AR, acoustic reflex; CM, cochlear microphonic; DPOAE, distortion product otoacoustic emission; ECochG, electrocochleography; SDS, speech discrimination score; L/R, left/right ear; Abn, abnormal (detectable with an elevated threshold and/or prolonged latency for ABRs or an enlarged SP/AP amplitude ratio for ECochG); Abs, absent (no detectable wave or response); Pres, present.

Febrile Manifestations

The pure-tone thresholds were not consistent with those of SDSs or the electrophysiological examinations of the cochlea. During febrile episodes, the pure-tone thresholds of the four patients indicated bilateral sensorineural mild HL (**Figure 3**), but the average SDSs were very low, varying from 4 to 15% under quiet conditions (**Table 2**) The tympanograms were type C for the proband but type A for the other patients, and ARs (both the ipsilateral and contralateral sides) were consistently absent for both ears from 500 to 4,000 Hz (**Table 2**). Bilateral DPOAEs were absent in the proband but present in the other three brothers (**Table 2**). The neural components of the ABR and the ECochG (AP) were unanimously absent during febrile episodes (**Figure 4**). In contrast, CMs were observed bilaterally in response to a stimulus presented at 100 dB nHL (**Table 2** and **Figure 4**).

Recovery Manifestations

During the recovery period, auditory function improved, but it did so at variable rates. Pure-tone audiometry and SDS returned to normal quickly, whereas the ABRs and ECochG signals progressed from absent to abnormal before recovering to normal (**Table 2** and **Figure 4**). The SDSs exhibited faster recovery than the metrics of the other audiological tests. Although the DPOAEs and tympanograms of the proband transitioned to present and

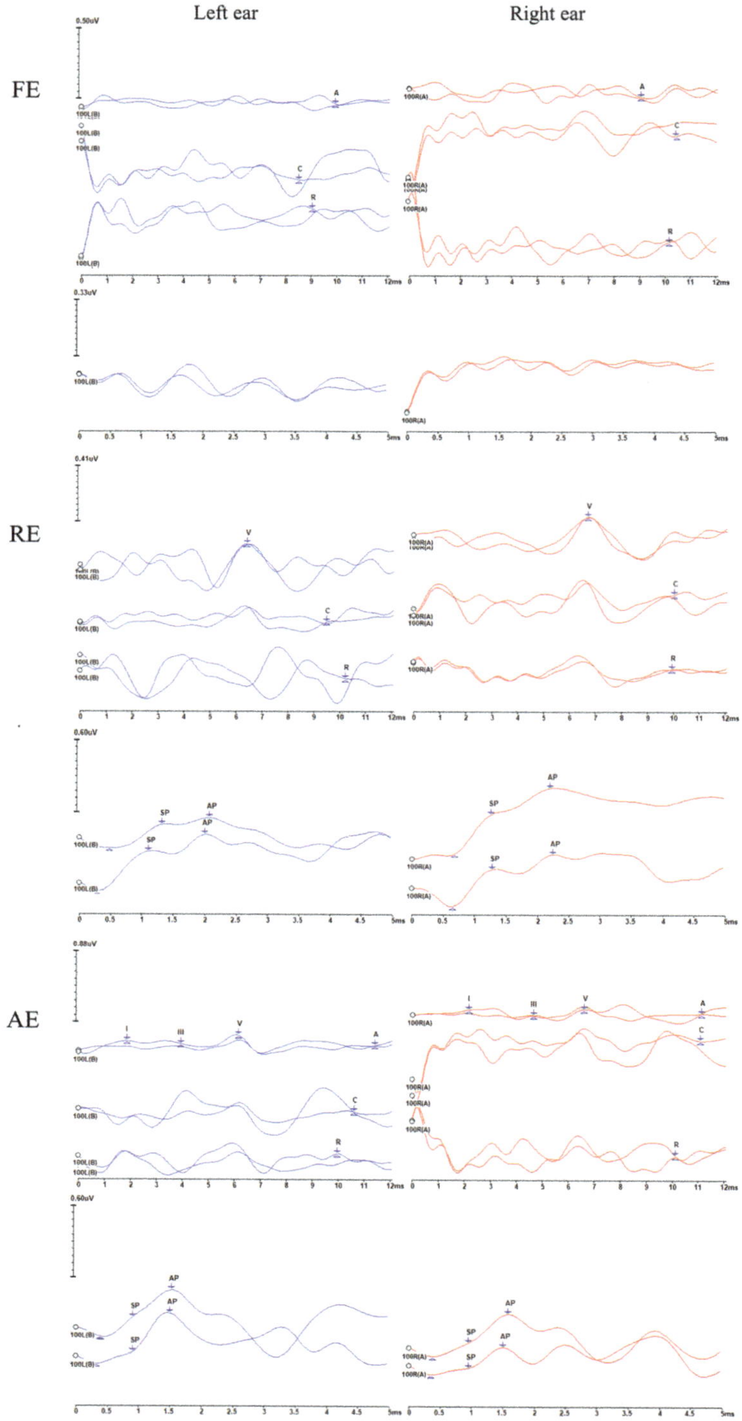

FIGURE 4 | Recordings of the auditory brainstem responses (ABRs), cochlear microphonics (CMs), and electrocochleography (ECochG) waveforms of the proband (II-4) during the three episodes. FE, febrile episode; RE, recovery episode; AE, afebrile episode. For each episode, the upper and lower panels represent the ABRs and CMs and ECochG signals, respectively. The number 100 indicates the click stimulus level. "A" indicates ABRs, and "C" and "R" represent the condensation and rarefaction polarity click responses, respectively. CMs can be identified according to the inverted phases of C and R responses. Waves I, III, and V are marked. The changes in ABRs and CMs differ. ABRs were gradually restored, i.e., absent (FE), then abnormal (with an elevated threshold and prolonged latency) (RE), and finally, almost normal (AE). However, CMs were persistently present, although some were of low amplitude. AP and SP represent the action potential and summating potential, respectively. ECochG signals were absent under febrile conditions (FE). Notably, the results appear show neuroelectric activity and possibly the CMs rather than ECochG. During the RE, the SP/AP amplitude ratios were >0.4. During the AE, the SP/AP amplitude ratios were <0.4, indicating a recovery of auditory function.

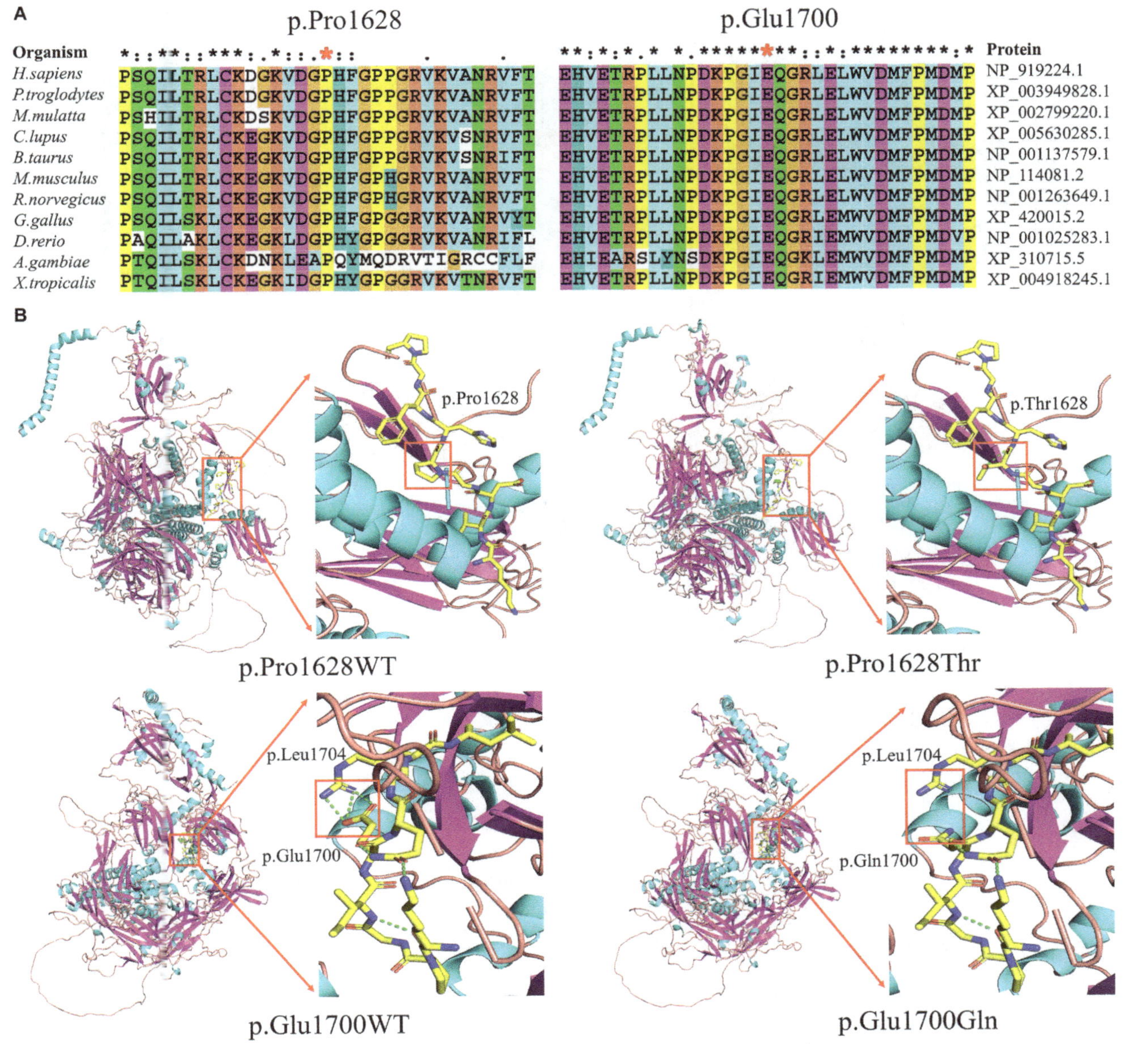

FIGURE 5 | Results of evolutionary conservation and molecular model analyses. **(A)** Amino acid conservation analysis. Protein alignment shows that the Pro1628 **(left)** and Glu1700 **(right)** residues of otoferlin are highly conserved across 11 organisms. The two positions of Pro1628 and Glu1700 are indicated by red stars. **(B)** Molecular models of wild-type (WT) **(left column)** and missense variants **(right column)** in otoferlin. The variant p.Pro1628Thr was found to perturb an amino acid chain and generate an extra hydrogen bond within the mutant p.Thr1628 **(upper row)**. The variant p.Glu1700Gln likely perturbs an amino acid side chain and has lost the hydrogen bonds between p.Glu1700 and p.Leu1704 **(lower row)**.

type A, respectively, those of his brothers remained normal (present DPOAEs and type A tympanograms) (**Table 2**). The ARs and CMs of all four patients were absent and present, respectively.

Afebrile Manifestations

During afebrile episodes, audiological tests showed consistent normal results in pure-tone audiometry, SDSs, DPOAEs, ABR, and ECochG along with absent ARs (**Table 2** and **Figures 3**, **4**). These results indicated that the auditory function of all patients recovered despite the continued absence of ARs.

Genetics Analysis

Determination of Twin Zygosity

All 18 loci investigated with the AGCU 17 + 1 STR Kit showed a consistent allelic pattern; therefore, the twin boys were concluded to be monozygotic (identical) (**Supplementary Table 4**). The 18 investigated loci provided a matching probability high

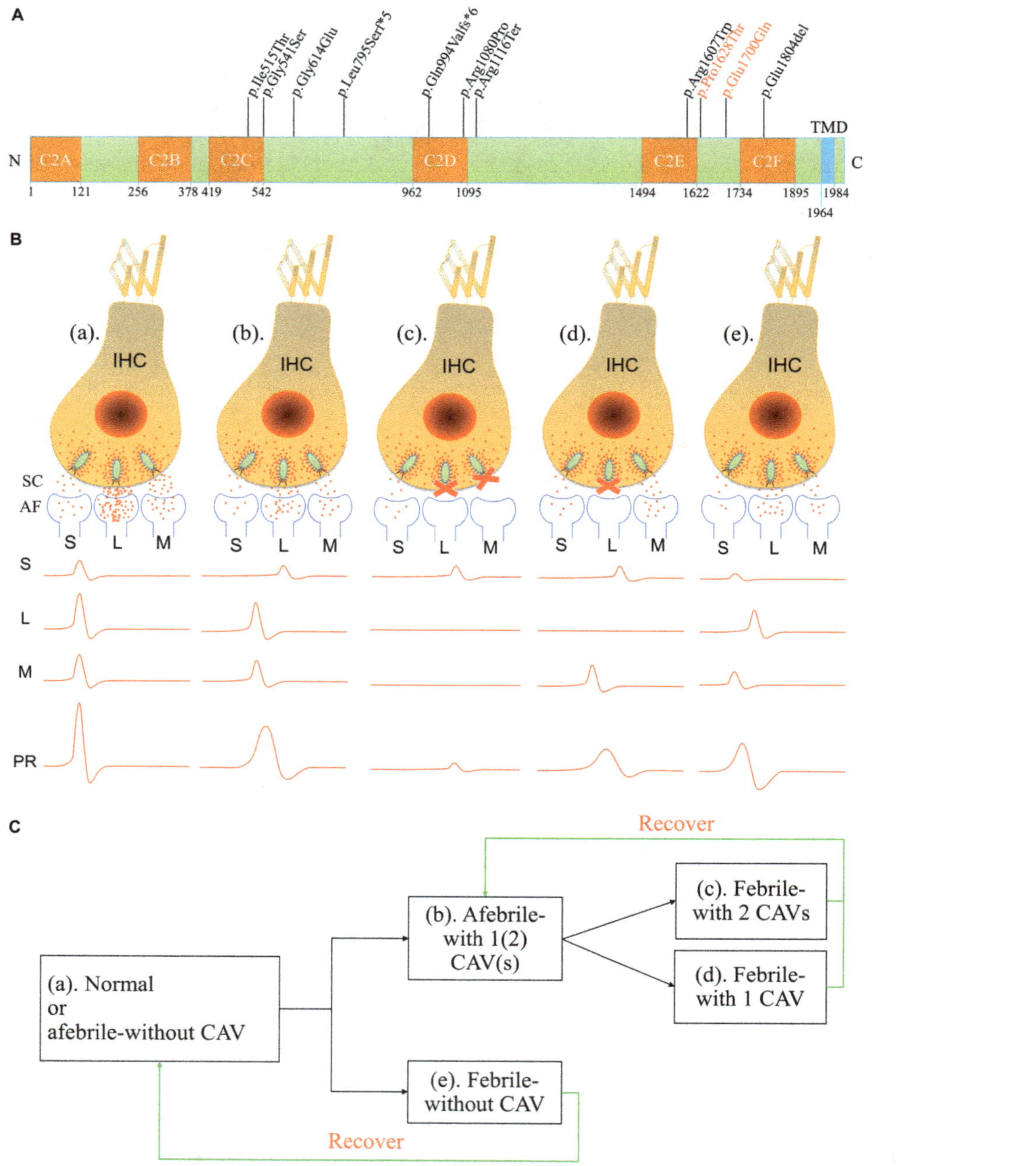

FIGURE 6 | Amino acid variants in otoferlin and possible mechanisms of otoferlin-dependent exocytosis in the inner hair cell (IHC) ribbon synapses of different temperature-sensitive auditory neuropathy (TSAN) patients. **(A)** Locations of otoferlin protein variants identified in TSAN patients. The numbers indicate the domain boundaries of otoferlin. The orange boxes indicate calcium-binding domains C2A through C2F, whereas the light-blue box indicates the transmembrane domain (TMD). Eleven variants have been found to be associated with TSAN, of which three variants (p.Gly614Glu, p.Glu1700Gln and p.Pro1628Thr) do not affect any otoferlin C2 domain. Two variants identified in this study (p.Glu1700Gln and p.Pro1628Thr) are shown in red. **(B)** Abnormal neural representation of sounds due to the dysfunction of synaptic transmission caused by *OTOF* variants in normal-hearing and TSAN patients. **(a)** Normal auditory function with normal synaptic transmission between IHCs and spiral ganglion neurons (SGNs). **(b)** TSAN patients with one or two C2 domain-affecting variants (CAVs) showed persistent partial dysfunction of all IHC–SGN synapses even when afebrile. **(c)** TSAN patients with two CAVs in a febrile state. Synaptic transmitter release was transiently blocked in almost all IHC–SGN synapses in addition to the more seriously affected remaining impaired synapses than those in panel **(b)**. **(d)** TSAN patients with only one CAV in a febrile state. A large number of IHC–SGN synapses temporarily failed to function. In addition, the remaining impaired synapses were more heavily affected in this state than in panel **(b)**. **(e)** TSAN patients with no CAVs in a febrile state. The IHC–SGN synapses were slightly affected but less severely affected than those of patients with one or two CAVs. The red dots represent glutamate (neurotransmitter), and the letters "S," "L," and "M" indicate small, large, and medium numbers, respectively, of IHC–SGN synapses. SC, synaptic cleft; AF, afferent fiber; PR, potential recording. **(C)** The genotype–phenotype relationships between *OTOF* variants and TSAN in patients with variable auditory function in this study and previous studies.

enough to assume that the results were accurate and reliable (Fan et al., 2012).

Targeted Next-Generation Sequencing and Data Analysis

To identify the cause of HL in the family, we first performed targeted NGS analysis to identify the possible variant(s) present in the proband. For MPS, the coverage and average read depth of the targeted regions were 98.26% and 350-fold, respectively. Of the 496 identified variants (**Supplementary Table 5**), seven candidate variants remained after filtering (**Supplementary Table 6**). For WES, the data mapped to the targeted region had a mean depth of 194.57-fold, and the coverage of the targeted bases was 99.19% at a depth of 4×, 98.11% at a depth of 10×, and 96.15% at a depth of 20×. A total of 64,940 variants remained after we filtered out those with allele frequencies greater than 5% in the 1000 Genomes, gnomAD/ExAC and in-house databases. For further analysis, we focused only on variants in splicing and coding regions. After completing this filtering process, we identified 1,381 variants (**Supplementary Table 7**). Finally, seven variants remained after referring to the variation databases [ClinVar, HGMD and Online Mendelian Inheritance in Man (OMIM)] and literature (**Supplementary Table 8**). Under the autosomal recessive mode of inheritance, two variants in two genes (*MHN14* and *OTOF*) from both sequencing processes were selected for further analysis. Notably, we failed to identify any known gene carrying a compound heterozygous or homozygous variant using WES.

Variant Validation and Analysis

Using PCR-Sanger sequencing technology, variants in both *MYH14* (c.1153C > T and c.1301A > G, RefSeq: NM_001145809.1) and *OTOF* (c.5098G > C and c.4882C > A, RefSeq: NM_194248.2) genes were validated. The results revealed that only the two variants of the *OTOF* gene completely co-segregated with deafness in this family. In the three cases (with the identical twin brothers regarded as representing one case) involving subjects who were TSAN patients, the subjects were compound heterozygotes for the two variants, and both parents were unaffected and heterozygous (**Figure 1**). The c.5098G > C variant, which occurred in exon 40 and was inherited from the unaffected mother (I-2), resulted in a glutamic acid-to-glutamine substitution at position 1,700 and has been previously reported as a pathogenic allele (Chiu et al., 2010; Chen et al., 2018; Qiu et al., 2019; Wu et al., 2019). The other variant, c.4882C > A, which was located in exon 39 and passed on from the clinically normal father (I-1), resulted in a single amino acid change from a proline to a threonine at position 1,628 in otoferlin. This variant was first identified in this study and has a high Rare Exome Variant Ensemble Learner (REVEL) score (0.742) and a very low allele frequency in the public database ExAC (8.67×10^{-6}). Furthermore, both variants were located at conserved amino acid positions of the otoferlin protein (**Figure 5A**). Based on these results, the phenotypes of the family, and the ACMG/AMP rules for recessive HL, the novel variant (c.4882C > A) was classified as pathogenic according to the standards of PS4, PM2, PM3, PP1_Strong, PP3 and PP4 (Oza et al., 2018). The patient's phenotypes and the detected variants have been deposited into ClinVar under accession numbers SCV001787151 and SCV001787152.

Variant Screening

Both variants identified in this study were absent in 200 normal-hearing controls matched for Chinese ethnicity, suggesting that *OTOF* was the causative gene of the autosomal recessive trait in this family.

Results of Evolutionary Conservation and Molecular Modeling

The positions of both Proline1628 and Glutamic acid1700 in otoferlin are conserved across 11 organisms (**Figure 5A**). 3D structural analysis revealed that both variants were likely to perturb amino acid (side) chains (**Figure 5B**).

DISCUSSION

In the mammalian inner ear, hair cells (HCs) transform mechanical vibrations into electrical signals (Wang et al., 2017; He et al., 2019; Liu Y. et al., 2019; Qi et al., 2019, 2020; Jiang et al., 2020; Zhou et al., 2020), and spiral ganglion neurons (SGNs) function as electric signal-transduction cells (Sun et al., 2016; Liu et al., 2018, 2021; Guo et al., 2019, 2020, 2021; Zhao et al., 2019). While supporting cells function as potential resources to regenerate HCs after damage (Lu et al., 2017; Zhang et al., 2017; Tan et al., 2019; Zhang S. et al., 2019, 2020; Zhang Y. et al., 2020; Chen et al., 2021). Sensorineural hearing loss has many etiologies, varying from genetic defects (Zhu et al., 2018; Fang et al., 2019; Yang et al., 2019; Qian et al., 2020; Cheng et al., 2021; Fu et al., 2021a; Lv et al., 2021; Zhang et al., 2021) to environmental factors, including aging (Zhang et al., 2017; Fu et al., 2018; Li H. et al., 2018; He et al., 2020, 2021), noise and ototoxic drugs (Liu et al., 2016; He et al., 2017; Li A. et al., 2018; Zhang Y. et al., 2019; Gao et al., 2020; Zhong et al., 2020; Fu et al., 2021b). TSAN is a rare phenotype with high clinical heterogeneity, manifesting as transient bilateral HL due to an increase in the core body temperature. The transient, conditional nature of this HL makes diagnosis challenging. In the present study, the diagnosis of AN was based on normal CM responses and abnormal ABRs during febrile episodes, although the tympanometry and AR measurement results were abnormal in one of four cases at the beginning of febrile episodes. However, further audiometric evaluations showed that the patients' behavioral thresholds, ABRs, and ECochG signals recovered to normal during afebrile episodes. Unlike other patients with TSAN or other forms of AN, the ECochG pattern in our patients during afebrile episodes was reversible, suggesting that auditory function almost completely recovered, although ARs continued to be absent. Therefore, certain exceptions to the usual features of AN often need to be considered when making a diagnosis, as 40% of affected individuals have abnormal rather than absent ABRs, ARs are sometimes present at elevated thresholds rather than being absent, and OAEs are absent in approximately 30% of AN patients upon retesting (Starr et al., 2001, 2008). In the present study, the proband's abnormal DPOAEs with a type C tympanogram and absent ARs during the febrile state were very likely attributable to dysfunction of the middle ear rather than OHC and not related to TSAN, although no abnormality was detected in physical or neuroimaging examinations. More notably, however, negative middle ear pressure should result in a retracted TM, which may or may not be observable upon physical examination, depending on the experience of the person conducting the examination, the amount of negative pressure, and the use of a standard otoscope versus microscopic examination of the TM. Furthermore, imaging studies will not show a retracted TM as an isolated finding. In contrast, his twin brother (II-3) showed consistent normal DPOAEs and a type A tympanogram, regardless of the body temperature, although they shared the same genotype. However, the changes in CMs and ABRs during each febrile event in the twins were the same, indicating that both tests are more reliable than others when diagnosing AN, especially when DPOAEs and tympanograms differ among patients in the same family. Consequently, present CMs with absent ABRs are recommended to diagnose AN (Mittal et al., 2012). Therefore, patients in this study were diagnosed with AN when febrile despite the recovery of their auditory function after fever.

Although several genes are involved in AN, only mutations of the *OTOF* gene are responsible for TSAN (Del Castillo and Del Castillo, 2012). To date, five loci (including four identified genes) and six genes are known to be associated with NSAN: DFNB9 (*OTOF* gene), DFNB59 (*PJVK* gene), and *GJB2* for autosomal recessive AN; AUNA1 (*DIAPH3* gene), AUNA2 (undefined gene), *SLC17A8*, *PCDH9*, *DIAPH1*, and *TMEM43* for autosomal dominant AN; DFNX5 (*AIFM1* gene) for X-linked recessive AN; and mitochondrial 12S rRNA (T1095C) (Varga et al., 2003; Cheng et al., 2005; Wang et al., 2005; Delmaghani et al., 2006; Ruel et al., 2008; Santarelli et al., 2008; Grati et al., 2009; Schoen et al., 2010; Zong et al., 2015; Lang-Roth et al., 2017; Wu et al., 2020; Jang et al., 2021). However, variants of the *OTOF* gene have been shown to be major contributors to NSAN (Varga et al., 2006; Rodríguez-Ballesteros et al., 2008; Romanos et al., 2009; Chiu et al., 2010; Wang et al., 2010). Moreover, DNA variations in *OTOF* differ among regions and ethnic populations (Rodríguez-Ballesteros et al., 2008; Del Castillo and Del Castillo, 2012; Matsunaga et al., 2012; Almontashiri et al., 2018). Two families with familial TSAN have been shown to carry *OTOF* variants. The first family was reported by Starr et al. in 1998 (Starr et al., 1998). Varga et al. (2006) showed that in this family, the two siblings with TSAN carried a heterozygous c.1544T > C (p.Ile515Thr) variant in the *OTOF* gene (Varga et al., 2006). This variant was inherited from their unaffected father and was absent in their mother and maternal siblings, and it is known to contribute to profound prelingual HL in humans and TSAN or NSAN in mouse models (Mirghomizadeh et al., 2002; Strenzke et al., 2016; Michalski et al., 2017). Further study revealed that the other mutant allele containing c.3346C > T (p.Arg1116Ter) in the *OTOF* gene (Strenzke et al., 2016). The second familial TSAN cluster was found in a consanguineous family with three members carrying a homozygous p.Glu1804del variant (Marlin et al., 2010). Furthermore, several sporadic cases of TSAN have been reported to be caused by variants in the *OTOF* gene (Romanos et al., 2009; Matsunaga et al., 2012; Zhang et al., 2016). To date, a total of nine variants of the *OTOF* gene have been identified as associated with TSAN (**Table 1** and **Figure 6A**). In this study, we reported a third cluster of familial TSAN, which includes three cases with two variants of the *OTOF* gene (which encodes otoferlin protein), c.5098G > C (p.Glu1700Gln) and c.4882C > A (p.Pro1628Thr). The reasons why both variants were considered part of the cause of TSAN in this family are as follows: (1) both are missense variants affecting residues that are completely preserved among different species; (2) p.Glu1700Gln has been shown to be pathogenic (Chiu et al., 2010; Chen et al., 2018; Qiu et al., 2019; Wu et al., 2019); (3) p.Pro1628Thr, which is reported here for the first time, was absent in 200 normal controls and has a very low allele frequency in a public database (8.67×10^{-6} in ExAC); and (4) both variants strongly co-segregated with the TSAN phenotype.

Most patients with NSAN caused by *OTOF* variants present with severe prelingual or profound deafness; however, the phenotypes of TSAN patients reported in this and previous studies did not follow this pattern. In previous studies, most TSAN patients had variable HL (normal to mild) when afebrile, and their hearing thresholds dropped to a greater degree of HL, with associated communication difficulties only during febrile episodes. In addition, patients with AN caused by *OTOF* variants tended to have more frequently affected and more severely affected DPOAEs than those with no *OTOF* variants (Kitao et al., 2019). Otoferlin, which is encoded by the *OTOF* gene, is a six-C2 domain (C2A–F) protein that also has a transmembrane domain (TMD), and its function is auditory neurotransmission at the hair cell ribbon synapse in the inner ear (Roux et al., 2006; Vogl et al., 2016; Michalski et al., 2017). C2 domains have been implicated in Ca^{2+} binding, and they play a crucial role in the function of otoferlin, which may contribute to the location specificity of most pathogenic variants of the *OTOF* gene (Del Castillo and Del Castillo, 2012). Notably, at least one of the alleles observed in these cases carries a missense variant affecting a C2 domain of otoferlin (**Figure 6A**). Moreover, subjects with two C2 domain-affecting variants presented with more severe phenotypes than did those with only one (**Table 1**). Relative to subjects in earlier studies, the three subjects in this study showed mild phenotypes, with the improvement in pure-tone thresholds from mild HL during the febrile condition to normal levels during the afebrile periods and the recovery of auditory function (except for ARs) during afebrile periods. Neither of the variants identified in this study is located in a C2 domain (both are between domains C2E and C2F); in addition, the p.Glu1700Gln variant has been shown to cause progressive mild to moderate prelingual HL, and OAEs in patients with AN carrying homozygous or compound heterozygous p.Glu1700Gln may be consistently present, consistently absent, or even present in the first test and absent later (Chiu et al., 2010; Wu et al., 2018). However, in the present study, the causes of the proband's absent DPOAEs only when febrile are still unknown, although he has the same genetic background as his twin brother. Remarkably, we did not identify modifiers using WES technology, suggesting that the variable phenotypes associated with these genotypes may result from environmental and/or genetic factors that have not yet been identified. In addition, the temperature-sensitive phenotype of HL may also be a direct consequence of defects in normal otoferlin-mediated synaptic vesicle trafficking in the inner ear. This issue may be addressed using temperature-sensitive variants that have been reported in several human diseases, including albinism and cystic fibrosis (King et al., 1991; Sharma et al., 2001; Wang et al., 2008), and decreased activity of otoferlin due to structural changes with rising temperatures may have an additive effect on the phenotype, as verified in previous reports (Strenzke et al., 2016).

Although the precise synaptic mechanism of the action of otoferlin at hair cell ribbon synapses remains unclear, the impairment of otoferlin in temperature-sensitive synaptic neurotransmitter release has been suggested to contribute to the phenotype of TSAN (Kaga, 2016; Kindt and Sheets, 2018). Normal auditory function depends on faithful information transfer, which requires otoferlin-dependent IHC exocytosis to be indefatigable, highly efficient, and accurately synchronized (Johnson, 1980; Griesinger et al., 2005; Roux et al., 2006; Kitcher et al., 2021). Reliable and temporally precise cochlear potentials are characterized by fast rise times, short onsets, and short peak latencies (Liu W. et al., 2019; Rutherford et al., 2021). Based on the findings from the present and other studies (**Table 1**), the severity of the phenotype associated with TSAN due to dysfunctional neurotransmitter release appears to reflect variants that alter the C2 domains of otoferlin. Therefore, the patients in previous studies had more severe HL in the febrile and afebrile states than the patients in the present study. We suggest that the possible pathogenesis and phenotype-genotype relations of TSAN caused by the dysfunction of otoferlin-dependent exocytosis in the IHC ribbon synapses are shown in **Figures 6B,C**. According to this hypothesis, three different clinical phenotypes may be interpreted. First, in TSAN patients with two C2 domain-affecting variants (CAVs) who became febrile, synaptic transmitter release was transiently blocked in almost all IHC–SGN synapses, especially the more seriously affected remaining synapses. The recorded cochlear current waves were low and prolonged or, in some cases, were hardly detectable. Second, when febrile, TSAN patients with only one CAV had better hearing thresholds than those with two CAVs. Large numbers of IHC–SGN synapses temporarily failed to release vesicles, with the remaining synapses being more heavily affected than those during afebrile states. Moreover, the initiation and propagation of spikes along the SGNs tended to vary in time and intensity. The measurements revealed the occurrence of cochlear potentials of variable size and shape in this type of TSAN patient under febrile conditions. Third, as in TSAN patients with one or two CAVs, mutant otoferlin in TSAN patients with no CAV exhibited impaired neurotransmitter release at IHC–SGN synapses. However, in a febrile state, the impairment caused by mutant otoferlin was less severe in TSAN patients with no CAV than in patients with one or two CAVs. As a result, synaptic transmission was inhibited for a very short period in the febrile state and rapidly increased after the body temperature decreased. The cochlear potentials, i.e., ABRs and ECochG signals, improved from no response to almost normal after the body temperature dropped. Importantly, the small magnitude of the effect on synaptic transmission may be the main reason why fever-related auditory dysfunction is almost completely reversible (with continued absent ARs) in TSAN patients with no CAV. Although the real molecular mechanisms are only beginning to be understood, otoferlin-induced defective synaptic transmission at the IHC ribbon synapse is one of the most important underlying causes of TSAN.

CONCLUSION

In this study, we described the detailed courses of disease in four male siblings from a non-consanguineous Chinese TSAN family who complained of communication difficulties when febrile, and we explored the genetic etiology of their condition using NGS technology. We investigated the detailed clinical progression of autosomal recessive TSAN in four siblings with two *OTOF* variants that did not affect any C2 domain of otoferlin, and we also identified a unique characterization of normal ABRs in afebrile episodes that was different from previously reported cases. Moreover, the presence of CMs with absent (or markedly abnormal) ABRs is a reliable diagnostic criterion for AN. These observations enrich the current knowledge of the phenotypes and genotypes of TSAN and may lay a foundation for further studies of its pathogenesis.

ETHICS STATEMENT

The studies involving human participants were reviewed and approved by Committees of Medical Ethics at the Nanfang Hospital, the Chinese PLA General Hospital, and the Lanzhou University Second Hospital. Written informed consent to participate in this study was provided by the participants' legal guardian/next of kin. Written informed consent was obtained from the individual(s), and minor(s)' legal guardian/next of kin, for the publication of any potentially identifiable images or data included in this article.

AUTHOR CONTRIBUTIONS

Y-MZ collected and analyzed data and drafted the main manuscript. Y-FL and Y-LL collected and processed the data. QL and X-PL supervised and conceptualized the study. XG and PD designed and conceptualized the study, interpreted the data, and revised and finalized the manuscript. All authors read and approved the final manuscript.

ACKNOWLEDGMENTS

We thank the participants of the study for their cooperation. We also thank Yafang Hu, Professor of Neurology at the Department of Neurology, Nanfang Hospital, for providing

SUPPLEMENTARY MATERIAL

Supplementary Table 1 | The 159 deafness-related nuclear genes.

Supplementary Table 2 | Six mitochondrial deafness-related regions.

Supplementary Table 3 | Three deafness-related miRNAs.

Supplementary Table 4 | STR analysis of the affected twin brothers (II-3 and II-4).

Supplementary Table 5 | Filtered variants of targeted NGS.

Supplementary Table 6 | Likely pathogenic variants of targeted NGS.

Supplementary Table 7 | Filtered variants of WES.

Supplementary Table 8 | Likely pathogenic variants of WES.

REFERENCES

Almontashiri, N. A. M., Alswaid, A., Oza, A., Al-Mazrou, K. A., Elrehim, O., Tayoun, A. A., et al. (2018). Recurrent variants in OTOF are significant contributors to prelingual nonsydromic hearing loss in Saudi patients. *Genet. Med.* 20, 536–544. doi: 10.1038/gim.2017.143

Chen, K., Liu, M., Wu, X., Zong, L., and Jiang, H. (2018). Targeted next generation sequencing reveals OTOF mutations in auditory neuropathy spectrum disorder. *Int. J. Pediatr. Otorhinolaryngol.* 115, 19–23. doi: 10.1016/j.ijporl.2018.09.008

Chen, Y., Gu, Y., Li, Y., Li, G.-L., Chai, R., Li, W., et al. (2021). Generation of mature and functional hair cells by co-expression of Gfi1, Pou4f3, and Atoh1 in the postnatal mouse cochlea. *Cell Rep.* 35:109016. doi: 10.1016/j.celrep.2021.109016

Cheng, C., Hou, Y., Zhang, Z., Wang, Y., Lu, L., Zhang, L., et al. (2021). Disruption of the autism-related gene Pak1 causes stereocilia disorganization, hair cell loss, and deafness in mice. *J. Genet. Genomics* 48, 324–332. doi: 10.1016/j.jgg.2021.03.010

Cheng, X., Li, L., Brashears, S., Morlet, T., Ng, S. S., Berlin, C., et al. (2005). Connexin 26 variants and auditory neuropathy/dys-synchrony among children in schools for the deaf. *Am. J. Med. Genet. A* 139A, 13–18. doi: 10.1002/ajmg.a.30929

Chiu, Y. H., Wu, C. C., Lu, Y. C., Chen, P. J., Lee, W. Y., Liu, A. Y. Z., et al. (2010). Mutations in the OTOF gene in Taiwanese patients with auditory neuropathy. *Audiol. Neurotol.* 15, 364–374. doi: 10.1159/000293992

Cianfrone, G., Turchetta, R., Mazzei, F., Bartolo, M., and Parisi, L. (2006). Temperature-dependent auditory neuropathy: is it an acoustic Uhthoff-like phenomenon? A case report. *Ann. Otol. Rhinol. Laryngol.* 115, 518–527. doi: 10.1177/000348940611500706

Del Castillo, F. J., and Del Castillo, I. (2012). Genetics of isolated auditory neuropathies. *Front. Biosci. (Landmark Ed.)* 17, 1251–1265. doi: 10.2741/3984

Delmaghani, S., del Castillo, F. J., Michel, V., Leibovici, M., Aghaie, A., Ron, U., et al. (2006). Mutations in the gene encoding pejvakin, a newly identified protein of the afferent auditory pathway, cause DFNB59 auditory neuropathy. *Nat. Genet.* 38, 770–778. doi: 10.1038/ng1829

Dimitrijevic, A., Starr, A., Bhatt, S., Michalewski, H. J., Zeng, F.-G., and Pratt, H. (2011). Auditory cortical N100 in pre- and post-synaptic auditory neuropathy to frequency or intensity changes of continuous tones. *Clin. Neurophysiol.* 122, 594–604. doi: 10.1016/j.clinph.2010.08.005

Du, W., Zhu, Y. M., Guo, Y. F., Wang, Q. J., and Liu, X. W. (2014). Prevalence of GJB2 mutations in the Silk Road region of China and a report of three novel variants. *Acta Otolaryngol.* 134, 373–381. doi: 10.3109/00016489.2013.849817

Fan, S.-L., Shen, C.-M., Wang, F., Ma, J., Wang, H.-D., Yang, G., et al. (2012). Population genetics polymorphisms on 17 autosomal STRs from Chinese Bai ethnic minority group. *Forensic Sci. Int. Genet.* 6, e22–e23. doi: 10.1016/j.fsigen.2010.12.014

Fang, Q., Zhang, Y., Da, P., Shao, B., Pan, H., He, Z., et al. (2019). Deletion of Limk1 and Limk2 in mice does not alter cochlear development or auditory function. *Sci. Rep.* 9:3357. doi: 10.1038/s41598-019-39769-z

Fu, X., An, Y., Wang, H., Li, P., Lin, J., Yuan, J., et al. (2021a). Deficiency of Klc2 induces low-frequency sensorineural hearing loss in C57BL/6 J mice and human. *Mol. Neurobiol.* doi: 10.1007/s12035-021-02422-w [Epub ahead of print].

Fu, X., Sun, X., Zhang, L., Jin, Y., Chai, R., Yang, L., et al. (2018). Tuberous sclerosis complex-mediated mTORC1 overactivation promotes age-related hearing loss. *J. Clin. Invest.* 128, 4938–4955. doi: 10.1172/JCI98058

Fu, X., Wan, P., Li, P., Wang, J., Guo, S., Zhang, Y., et al. (2021b). Mechanism and prevention of ototoxicity induced by aminoglycosides. *Front. Cell. Neurosci.* 15:692762. doi: 10.3389/fncel.2021.692762

Gao, S., Cheng, C., Wang, M., Jiang, P., Zhang, L., Wang, Y., et al. (2020). Blebbistatin inhibits neomycin-induced apoptosis in hair cell-Like HEI-OC-1 cells and in cochlear hair cells. *Front. Cell. Neurosci.* 13:590. doi: 10.3389/fncel.2019.00590

Gohari, N., Emami, S. F., Mirbagheri, S. S., Valizadeh, A., Abdollahi, N., and Borzuei, M. (2019). The prevalence and causes of auditory neuropathy/dys-synchrony (AN/AD) in children with hearing impairment. *Indian J. Otolaryngol. Head Neck Surg.* 71, 71–75. doi: 10.1007/s12070-018-1494-1

Gorga, M. P., Stelmachowicz, P. G., Barlow, S. M., and Brookhouser, P. E. (1995). Case of recurrent, reversible, sudden sensorineural hearing loss in a child. *J. Am. Acad. Audiol.* 6, 163–172.

Grati, F. R., Lesperance, M. M., De Toffol, S., Chinetti, S., Selicorni, A., Emery, S., et al. (2009). Pure monosomy and pure trisomy of 13q21.2–31.1 consequent to a familial insertional translocation: exclusion of PCDH9 as the responsible gene for autosomal dominant auditory neuropathy (AUNA1). *Am. J. Med. Genet. A* 149A, 906–913. doi: 10.1002/ajmg.a.32754

Griesinger, C. B., Richards, C. D., and Ashmore, J. F. (2005). Fast vesicle replenishment allows indefatigable signalling at the first auditory synapse. *Nature* 435, 212–215. doi: 10.1038/nature03567

Guo, R., Li, J., Chen, C., Xiao, M., Liao, M., Hu, Y., et al. (2021). Biomimetic 3D bacterial cellulose-graphene foam hybrid scaffold regulates neural stem cell proliferation and differentiation. *Colloids Surf. B Biointerfaces* 200:111590. doi: 10.1016/j.colsurfb.2021.111590

Guo, R., Ma, X., Liao, M., Liu, Y., Hu, Y., Qian, X., et al. (2019). Development and application of cochlear implant-based electric-acoustic stimulation of spiral ganglion neurons. *ACS Biomater. Sci. Eng.* 5, 6735–6741. doi: 10.1021/acsbiomaterials.9b01265

Guo, R., Xiao, M., Zhao, W., Zhou, S., Hu, Y., Liao, M., et al. (2020). 2D $Ti_3C_2T_x$MXene couples electrical stimulation to promote proliferation and neural differentiation of neural stem cells. *Acta Biomater.* doi: 10.1016/j.actbio.2020.12.035 [Epub ahead of print].

He, Z., Fang, Q., Li, H., Shao, B., Zhang, Y., Zhang, Y., et al. (2019). The role of FOXG1 in the postnatal development and survival of mouse cochlear hair cells. *Neuropharmacology* 144, 43–57. doi: 10.1016/j.neuropharm.2018.10.021

He, Z., Guo, L., Shu, Y., Fang, Q., Zhou, H., Liu, Y., et al. (2017). Autophagy protects auditory hair cells against neomycin-induced damage. *Autophagy* 13, 1884–1904. doi: 10.1080/15548627.2017.1359449

He, Z.-H., Li, M., Fang, Q.-J., Liao, F.-L., Zou, S.-Y., Wu, X., et al. (2021). FOXG1 promotes aging inner ear hair cell survival through activation of the autophagy pathway. *Autophagy.* doi: 10.1080/15548627.2021.1916194 [Epub ahead of print].

He, Z.-H., Zou, S.-Y., Li, M., Liao, F.-L., Wu, X., Sun, H.-Y., et al. (2020). The nuclear transcription factor FoxG1 affects the sensitivity of mimetic aging hair cells to inflammation by regulating autophagy pathways. *Redox Biol.* 28:101364. doi: 10.1016/j.redox.2019.101364

Jang, M. W., Oh, D.-Y., Yi, E., Liu, X., Ling, J., Kim, N., et al. (2021). A nonsense TMEM43 variant leads to disruption of connexin-linked function and autosomal dominant auditory neuropathy spectrum disorder. *Proc. Natl. Acad. Sci. U.S.A.* 118:e2019681118. doi: 10.1073/pnas.2019681118

Jerger, J. (1970). Clinical experience with impedance audiometry. *Arch. Otolaryngol.* 92, 311–324. doi: 10.1001/archotol.1970.04310040005002

Jiang, P., Zhang, S., Cheng, C., Gao, S., Tang, M., Lu, L., et al. (2020). The roles of exosomes in visual and auditory systems. *Front. Bioeng. Biotechnol.* 8:525. doi: 10.3389/fbioe.2020.00525

Johnson, D. H. (1980). The relationship between spike rate and synchrony in responses of auditory-nerve fibers to single tones. *J. Acoust. Soc. Am.* 68, 1115–1122. doi: 10.1121/1.384982

Jumper, J., Evans, R., Pritzel, A., Green, T., Figurnov, M., Ronneberger, O., et al. (2021). Highly accurate protein structure prediction with AlphaFold. *Nature* 596, 583–589. doi: 10.1038/s41586-021-03819-2

Kaga, K. (2016). Auditory nerve disease and auditory neuropathy spectrum disorders. *Auris Nasus Larynx* 43, 10–20. doi: 10.1016/j.anl.2015.06.008

Kaga, K., Nakamura, M., Shinogami, M., Tsuzuku, T., Yamada, K., and Shindo, M. (1996). Auditory nerve disease of both ears revealed by auditory brainstem responses, electrocochleography and otoacoustic emissions. *Scand. Audiol.* 25, 233–238. doi: 10.3109/01050399609074960

Kindt, K. S., and Sheets, L. (2018). Transmission disrupted: modeling auditory synaptopathy in zebrafish. *Front. Cell Dev. Biol.* 6:114. doi: 10.3389/fcell.2018.00114

King, R. A., Townsend, D., Oetting, W., Summers, C. G., Olds, D. P., White, J. G., et al. (1991). Temperature-sensitive tyrosinase associated with peripheral pigmentation in oculocutaneous albinism. *J. Clin. Invest.* 87, 1046–1053. doi: 10.1172/JCI115064

Kitao, K., Mutai, H., Namba, K., Morimoto, N., Nakano, A., Arimoto, Y., et al. (2019). Deterioration in distortion product otoacoustic emissions in auditory neuropathy patients with distinct clinical and genetic backgrounds. *Ear Hear.* 40, 184–191. doi: 10.1097/AUD.0000000000000586

Kitcher, S. R., Pederson, A. M., and Weisz, C. J. C. (2021). Diverse identities and sites of action of cochlear neurotransmitters. *Hear. Res.* 108278. doi: 10.1016/j.heares.2021.108278 [Epub ahead of print].

Lang-Roth, R., Fischer-Krall, E., Kornblum, C., Nürnberg, G., Meschede, D., Goebel, I., et al. (2017). AUNA2: a novel type of non-syndromic slowly progressive auditory synaptopathy/auditory neuropathy with autosomal-dominant inheritance. *Audiol. Neurotol.* 22, 30–40. doi: 10.1159/000474929

Larkin, M. A., Blackshields, G., Brown, N. P., Chenna, R., McGettigan, P. A., McWilliam, H., et al. (2007). Clustal W and Clustal X version 2.0. *Bioinformatics* 23, 2947–2948. doi: 10.1093/bioinformatics/btm404

Li, A., You, D., Li, W., Cui, Y., He, Y., Li, W., et al. (2018). Novel compounds protect auditory hair cells against gentamycin-induced apoptosis by maintaining the expression level of H3K4me2. *Drug Deliv.* 25, 1033–1043. doi: 10.1080/10717544.2018.1461277

Li, H., Song, Y., He, Z., Chen, X., Wu, X., Li, X., et al. (2018). Meclofenamic acid reduces reactive oxygen species accumulation and apoptosis, inhibits excessive autophagy, and protects hair cell-like HEI-OC1 cells from cisplatin-induced damage. *Front. Cell. Neurosci.* 12:139. doi: 10.3389/fncel.2018.00139

Liu, L., Chen, Y., Qi, J., Zhang, Y., He, Y., Ni, W., et al. (2016). Wnt activation protects against neomycin-induced hair cell damage in the mouse cochlea. *Cell Death Dis.* 7:e2136. doi: 10.1038/cddis.2016.35

Liu, W., Wang, X., Wang, M., and Wang, H. (2019). "Protection of spiral ganglion neurons and prevention of auditory neuropathy," in *Hearing Loss Mechanisms Prevention and Cure*, 1st Edn, eds H. Li and R. Chai (Singapore: Springer), 93–107.

Liu, W., Xu, L., Wang, X., Zhang, D., Sun, G., Wang, M., et al. (2021). PRDX1 activates autophagy via the PTEN-AKT signaling pathway to protect against cisplatin-induced spiral ganglion neuron damage. *Autophagy.* doi: 10.1080/15548627.2021.1905466 [Epub ahead of print].

Liu, W., Xu, X., Fan, Z., Sun, G., Han, Y., Zhang, D., et al. (2018). Wnt signaling activates TP53-induced glycolysis and apoptosis regulator and protects against cisplatin-induced spiral ganglion neuron damage in the mouse cochlea. *Antioxid. Redox Signal.* 30, 1389–1410. doi: 10.1089/ars.2017.7288

Liu, Y., Qi, J., Chen, X., Tang, M., Chu, C., Zhu, W., et al. (2019). Critical role of spectrin in hearing development and deafness. *Sci. Adv.* 5:eaav7803. doi: 10.1126/sciadv.aav7803

Lu, X., Sun, S., Qi, J., Li, W., Liu, L., Zhang, Y., et al. (2017). Bmi1 regulates the proliferation of cochlear supporting cells via the canonical Wnt signaling pathway. *Mol. Neurobiol.* 54, 1326–1339. doi: 10.1007/s12035-016-9686-8

Lv, J., Fu, X., Li, Y., Hong, G., Li, P., Lin, J., et al. (2021). Deletion of Kcnj16 in mice does not alter auditory function. *Front. Cell Dev. Biol.* 9:630361. doi: 10.3389/fcell.2021.630361

Madanoglu, N., and Derinsu, U. (2007). Familial temperature-sensitive auditory neuropathy/auditory dyssynchrony. *J. Int. Adv. Otol.* 3, 69–74.

Madden, C., Rutter, M., Hilbert, L., Greinwald, J. H. Jr., and Choo, D. I. (2002). Clinical and audiological features in auditory neuropathy. *Arch. Otolaryngol. Head Neck Surg.* 128, 1026–1030. doi: 10.1001/archotol.128.9.1026

Marlin, S., Feldmann, D., Nguyen, Y., Rouillon, I., Loundon, N., Jonard, L., et al. (2010). Temperature-sensitive auditory neuropathy associated with an otoferlin mutation: deafening fever! *Biochem. Biophys. Res. Commun.* 394, 737–742. doi: 10.1016/j.bbrc.2010.03.062

Martin, M. (2011). Cutadapt removes adapter sequences from high-throughput sequencing reads. *EMBnet J.* 17, 10–12. doi: 10.14806/ej.17.1.200

Matsunaga, T., Mutai, H., Kunishima, S., Namba, K., Morimoto, N., Shinjo, Y., et al. (2012). A prevalent founder mutation and genotype–phenotype correlations of OTOF in Japanese patients with auditory neuropathy. *Clin. Genet.* 82, 425–432. doi: 10.1111/j.1399-0004.2012.01897.x

Michalski, N., Goutman, J. D., Auclair, S. M., Boutet, de Monvel, J., Tertrais, M., et al. (2017). Otoferlin acts as a Ca^{2+} sensor for vesicle fusion and vesicle pool replenishment at auditory hair cell ribbon synapses. *eLife* 6:e31013. doi: 10.7554/eLife.31013

Mirghomizadeh, F., Pfister, M., Apaydin, F., Petit, C., Kupka, S., Pusch, C. M., et al. (2002). Substitutions in the conserved C2C domain of otoferlin cause DFNB9, a form of nonsyndromic autosomal recessive deafness. *Neurobiol. Dis.* 10, 157–164. doi: 10.1006/nbdi.2002.0488

Mittal, R., Ramesh, A. V., Panwar, S. S., Nilkanthan, A., Nair, S., and Mehra, P. R. (2012). Auditory neuropathy spectrum disorder: its prevalence and audiological characteristics in an Indian tertiary care hospital. *Int. J. Pediatr. Otorhinolaryngol.* 76, 1351–1354. doi: 10.1016/j.ijporl.2012.06.005

Moser, T., and Starr, A. (2016). Auditory neuropathy — neural and synaptic mechanisms. *Nat. Rev. Neurol.* 12, 135–149. doi: 10.1038/nrneurol.2016.10

Ohashi, T., Nishino, H., Arai, Y., Hyodo, M., and Takatsu, M. (2009). Clinical significance of the summating potential–action potential ratio and the action potential latency difference for condensation and rarefaction clicks in Meniere's disease. *Ann. Otol. Rhinol. Laryngol.* 118, 307–312. doi: 10.1177/000348940911800412

Oza, A. M., DiStefano, M. T., Hemphill, S. E., Cushman, B. J., Grant, A. R., Siegert, R. K., et al. (2018). Expert specification of the ACMG/AMP variant interpretation guidelines for genetic hearing loss. *Hum. Mutat.* 39, 1593–1613. doi: 10.1002/humu.23630

Qi, J., Liu, Y., Chu, C., Chen, X., Zhu, W., Shu, Y., et al. (2019). A cytoskeleton structure revealed by super-resolution fluorescence imaging in inner ear hair cells. *Cell Discov.* 5:12. doi: 10.1038/s41421-018-0076-4

Qi, J., Zhang, L., Tan, F., Liu, Y., Chu, C., Zhu, W., et al. (2020). Espin distribution as revealed by super-resolution microscopy of stereocilia. *Am. J. Transl. Res.* 12, 130–141.

Qian, F., Wang, X., Yin, Z., Xie, G., Yuan, H., Liu, D., et al. (2020). The slc4a2b gene is required for hair cell development in zebrafish. *Aging* 12, 18804–18821. doi: 10.18632/aging.103840

Qiu, Y., Chen, S., Xie, L., Xu, K., Lin, Y., Bai, X., et al. (2019). Auditory neuropathy spectrum disorder due to two novel compound heterozygous OTOF mutations in two Chinese families. *Neural Plast.* 2019:9765276. doi: 10.1155/2019/9765276

Rance, G., Beer, D. E., Cone-Wesson, B., Shepherd, R. K., Dowell, R. C., King, A. M., et al. (1999). Clinical findings for a group of infants and young children with auditory neuropathy. *Ear Hear.* 20, 238–252. doi: 10.1097/00003446-199906000-00006

Rodríguez-Ballesteros, M., Reynoso, R., Olarte, M., Villamar, M., Morera, C., Santarelli, R., et al. (2008). A multicenter study on the prevalence and spectrum of mutations in the otoferlin gene (OTOF) in subjects with nonsyndromic hearing impairment and auditory neuropathy. *Hum. Mutat.* 29, 823–831. doi: 10.1002/humu.20708

Romanos, J., Kimura, L., Favero, M. L., Izarra, F. A. R., de Mello Auricchio, M. T. B., Batissoco, A. C., et al. (2009). Novel OTOF mutations in Brazilian patients with auditory neuropathy. *J. Hum. Genet.* 54, 382–385. doi: 10.1038/jhg.2009.45

Roux, I., Safieddine, S., Nouvian, R., Grati, M. H., Simmler, M.-C., Bahloul, A., et al. (2006). Otoferlin, defective in a human deafness form, is essential for exocytosis at the auditory ribbon synapse. *Cell* 127, 277–289. doi: 10.1016/j.cell.2006.08.040

Ruel, J., Emery, S., Nouvian, R., Bersot, T., Amilhon, B., Van Rybroek, J. M., et al. (2008). Impairment of SLC17A8 encoding vesicular glutamate transporter-3, VGLUT3, underlies nonsyndromic deafness DFNA25 and inner hair cell dysfunction in null mice. *Am. J. Hum. Genet.* 83, 278–292. doi: 10.1016/j.ajhg.2008.07.008

Rutherford, M. A., von Gersdorff, H., and Goutman, J. D. (2021). Encoding sound in the cochlea: from receptor potential to afferent discharge. *J. Physiol.* 599, 2527–2557. doi: 10.1113/JP279189

Santarelli, R. (2010). Information from cochlear potentials and genetic mutations helps localize the lesion site in auditory neuropathy. *Genome Med.* 2:91. doi: 10.1186/gm212

Santarelli, R., Cama, E., Scimemi, P., Dal Monte, E., Genovese, E., and Arslan, E. (2008). Audiological and electrocochleography findings in hearing-impaired children with connexin 26 mutations and otoacoustic emissions. *Eur. Arch. Otorhinolaryngol.* 265, 43–51. doi: 10.1007/s00405-007-0412-z

Sanyelbhaa Talaat, H., Kabel, A. H., Samy, H., and Elbadry, M. (2009). Prevalence of auditory neuropathy (AN) among infants and young children with severe to profound hearing loss. *Int. J. Pediatr. Otorhinolaryngol.* 73, 937–939. doi: 10.1016/j.ijporl.2009.03.009

Schlauch, R. S., and Nelson, P. (2015). "Puretone evaluation," in *Handbook of Clinical Audiology*, 7th Edn, eds J. Katz, M. Chasin, K. English, L. J. Hood, and K. L. Tillery (Philadelphia, PA: Wolters Kluwer Health), 29–47.

Schoen, C. J., Emery, S. B., Thorne, M. C., Ammana, H. R., Śliwerska, E., Arnett, J., et al. (2010). Increased activity of Diaphanous homolog 3 (DIAPH3)/diaphanous causes hearing defects in humans with auditory neuropathy and in Drosophila. *Proc. Natl. Acad. Sci. U.S.A.* 107, 13396–13401. doi: 10.1073/pnas.1003027107

Sharma, A., Kirsch, C. F. E., Aulino, J. M., Chakraborty, S., Choudhri, A. F., Germano, I. M., et al. (2018). ACR appropriateness criteria® hearing loss and/or vertigo. *J. Am. Coll. Radiol.* 15, S321–S331. doi: 10.1016/j.jacr.2018.09.020

Sharma, M., Benharouga, M., Hu, W., and Lukacs, G. L. (2001). Conformational and temperature-sensitive stability defects of the ΔF508 cystic fibrosis transmembrane conductance regulator in post-endoplasmic reticulum compartments. *J. Biol. Chem.* 276, 8942–8950. doi: 10.1074/jbc.M009172200

Shi, W., Ji, F., Lan, L., Liang, S.-C., Ding, H.-N., Wang, H., et al. (2012). Characteristics of cochlear microphonics in infants and young children with auditory neuropathy. *Acta Otolaryngol.* 132, 188–196. doi: 10.3109/00016489.2011.630016

Starr, A., Picton, T. W., Sininger, Y., Hood, L. J., and Berlin, C. I. (1996). Auditory neuropathy. *Brain* 119, 741–753. doi: 10.1093/brain/119.3.741

Starr, A., Sininger, Y., Nguyen, T., Michalewski, H. J., Oba, S., and Abdala, C. (2001). Cochlear receptor (microphonic and summating potentials, otoacoustic emissions) and auditory pathway (auditory brain stem potentials) activity in auditory neuropathy. *Ear Hear.* 22, 91–99. doi: 10.1097/00003446-200104000-00002

Starr, A., Sininger, Y., Winter, M., Derebery, M. J., Oba, S., and Michalewski, H. J. (1998). Transient deafness due to temperature-sensitive auditory neuropathy. *Ear Hear.* 19, 169–179. doi: 10.1097/00003446-199806000-00001

Starr, A., Sininger, Y. S., and Pratt, H. (2000). The varieties of auditory neuropathy. *J. Basic Clin. Physiol. Pharmacol.* 11, 215–230. doi: 10.1515/jbcpp.2000.11.3.215

Starr, A., Zeng, F. G., Michalewski, H. J., and Moser, T. (2008). "3.23 - Perspectives on auditory neuropathy: disorders of inner hair cell, auditory nerve, and their synapse," in *The Senses: A Comprehensive Reference*, 1st Edn, eds R. H. Masland, T. D. Albright, T. D. Albright, R. H. Masland, P. Dallos, D. Oertel, et al. (New York, NY: Academic Press), 397–412.

Strenzke, N., Chakrabarti, R., Al-Moyed, H., Müller, A., Hoch, G., Pangrsic, T., et al. (2016). Hair cell synaptic dysfunction, auditory fatigue and thermal sensitivity in otoferlin Ile515Thr mutants. *EMBO J.* 35, 2519–2535. doi: 10.15252/embj.201694564

Sun, G., Liu, W., Fan, Z., Zhang, D., Han, Y., Xu, L., et al. (2016). The three-dimensional culture system with matrigel and neurotrophic factors preserves the structure and function of spiral ganglion neuron *in vitro*. *Neural Plast.* 2016:4280407. doi: 10.1155/2016/4280407

Tan, F., Chu, C., Qi, J., Li, W., You, D., Li, K., et al. (2019). AAV-ie enables safe and efficient gene transfer to inner ear cells. *Nat. Commun.* 10:3733. doi: 10.1038/s41467-019-11687-8

Varga, R., Avenarius, M. R., Kelley, P. M., Keats, B. J., Berlin, C. I., Hood, L. J., et al. (2006). OTOF mutations revealed by genetic analysis of hearing loss families including a potential temperature sensitive auditory neuropathy allele. *J. Med. Genet.* 43, 576–581. doi: 10.1136/jmg.2005.038612

Varga, R., Kelley, P. M., Keats, B. J., Starr, A., Leal, S. M., Cohn, E., et al. (2003). Non-syndromic recessive auditory neuropathy is the result of mutations in the otoferlin (OTOF) gene. *J. Med. Genet.* 40, 45–50. doi: 10.1136/jmg.40.1.45

Vogl, C., Panou, I., Yamanbaeva, G., Wichmann, C., Mangosing, S. J., Vilardi, F., et al. (2016). Tryptophan-rich basic protein (WRB) mediates insertion of the tail-anchored protein otoferlin and is required for hair cell exocytosis and hearing. *EMBO J.* 35, 2536–2552. doi: 10.15252/embj.201593565

Wang, D.-Y., Wang, Y.-C., Weil, D., Zhao, Y.-L., Rao, S.-Q., Zong, L., et al. (2010). Screening mutations of OTOF gene in Chinese patients with auditory neuropathy, including a familial case of temperature-sensitive auditory neuropathy. *BMC Med. Genet.* 11:79. doi: 10.1186/1471-2350-11-79

Wang, Q., Li, R., Zhao, H., Peters, J. L., Liu, Q., Yang, L., et al. (2005). Clinical and molecular characterization of a Chinese patient with auditory neuropathy associated with mitochondrial 12S rRNA T1095C mutation. *Am. J. Med. Genet. A* 133A, 27–30. doi: 10.1002/ajmg.a.30424

Wang, X., Koulov, A. V., Kellner, W. A., Riordan, J. R., and Balch, W. E. (2008). Chemical and biological folding contribute to temperature-sensitive ΔF508 CFTR trafficking. *Traffic* 9, 1878–1893. doi: 10.1111/j.1600-0854.2008.00806.x

Wang, Y., Li, J., Yao, X., Li, W., Du, H., Tang, M., et al. (2017). Loss of CIB2 causes profound hearing loss and abolishes mechanoelectrical transduction in mice. *Front. Mol. Neurosci.* 10:401. doi: 10.3389/fnmol.2017.00401

Wu, C. C., Hsu, C. J., Huang, F. L., Lin, Y. H., Lin, Y. H., Liu, T. C., et al. (2018). Timing of cochlear implantation in auditory neuropathy patients with OTOF mutations: our experience with 10 patients. *Clin. Otolaryngol.* 43, 352–357. doi: 10.1111/coa.12949

Wu, C.-C., Tsai, C.-Y., Lin, Y.-H., Chen, P.-Y., Lin, P.-H., Cheng, Y.-F., et al. (2019). Genetic epidemiology and clinical features of hereditary hearing impairment in the Taiwanese population. *Genes* 10:772. doi: 10.3390/genes10100772

Wu, K., Wang, H., Guan, J., Lan, L., Zhao, C., Zhang, M., et al. (2020). A novel variant in diaphanous homolog 1 (DIAPH1) as the cause of auditory neuropathy in a Chinese family. *Int. J. Pediatr. Otorhinolaryngol.* 133:109947. doi: 10.1016/j.ijporl.2020.109947

Wynne, D. P., Zeng, F.-G., Bhatt, S., Michalewski, H. J., Dimitrijevic, A., and Starr, A. (2013). Loudness adaptation accompanying ribbon synapse and auditory nerve disorders. *Brain* 136, 1626–1638. doi: 10.1093/brain/awt056

Yang, T., Guo, L., Wang, L., and Yu, X. (2019). "Diagnosis, intervention, and prevention of genetic hearing loss," in *Hearing Loss: Mechanisms, Prevention and Cure*, 1st Edn, eds H. Li and R. Chai (Singapore: Springer), 73–92.

Yuan, Y., Li, Q., Su, Y., Lin, Q., Gao, X., Liu, H., et al. (2020). Comprehensive genetic testing of Chinese SNHL patients and variants interpretation using ACMG guidelines and ethnically matched normal controls. *Eur. J. Hum. Genet.* 28, 231–243. doi: 10.1038/s41431-019-0510-6

Zhang, Q., Lan, L., Shi, W., Yu, L., Xie, L.-Y., Xiong, F., et al. (2016). Temperature sensitive auditory neuropathy. *Hear. Res.* 335, 53–63. doi: 10.1016/j.heares.2016.01.008

Zhang, S., Dong, Y., Qiang, R., Zhang, Y., Zhang, X., Chen, Y., et al. (2021). Characterization of Strip1 expression in mouse cochlear hair cells. *Front. Genet.* 12:625867. doi: 10.3389/fgene.2021.625867

Zhang, S., Liu, D., Dong, Y., Zhang, Z., Zhang, Y., Zhou, H., et al. (2019). Frizzled-9+ supporting cells are progenitors for the generation of hair cells in the postnatal mouse cochlea. *Front. Mol. Neurosci.* 12:184. doi: 10.3389/fnmol.2019.00184

Zhang, S., Zhang, Y., Dong, Y., Guo, L., Zhang, Z., Shao, B., et al. (2020). Knockdown of Foxg1 in supporting cells increases the trans-differentiation of supporting cells into hair cells in the neonatal mouse cochlea. *Cell. Mol. Life Sci.* 77, 1401–1419. doi: 10.1007/s00018-019-03291-2

Zhang, S., Zhang, Y., Yu, P., Hu, Y., Zhou, H., Guo, L., et al. (2017). Characterization of Lgr5+ progenitor cell transcriptomes after neomycin injury in the neonatal mouse cochlea. *Front. Mol. Neurosci.* 10:213. doi: 10.3389/fnmol.2017.00213

Zhang, Y., Li, W., He, Z., Wang, Y., Shao, B., Cheng, C., et al. (2019). Pre-treatment with Fasudil prevents neomycin-induced hair cell damage by reducing the accumulation of reactive oxygen species. *Front. Mol. Neurosci.* 12:264. doi: 10.3389/fnmol.2019.00264

Zhang, Y., Zhang, S., Zhang, Z., Dong, Y., Ma, X., Qiang, R., et al. (2020). Knockdown of Foxg1 in Sox9+ supporting cells increases the trans-differentiation of supporting cells into hair cells in the neonatal mouse utricle. *Aging* 12, 19834–19851. doi: 10.18632/aging.104009

Zhao, J., Tang, M., Cao, J., Ye, D., Guo, X., Xi, J., et al. (2019). Structurally tunable reduced graphene oxide substrate maintains mouse embryonic stem cell Pluripotency. *Adv. Sci.* 6:1802136. doi: 10.1002/advs.201802136

Zhong, Z., Fu, X., Li, H., Chen, J., Wang, M., Gao, S., et al. (2020). Citicoline protects auditory hair cells against neomycin-induced damage. *Front. Cell Dev. Biol.* 8:712. doi: 10.3389/fcell.2020.00712

Zhou, H., Qian, X., Xu, N., Zhang, S., Zhu, G., Zhang, Y., et al. (2020). Disruption of Atg7-dependent autophagy causes electromotility disturbances, outer hair cell loss, and deafness in mice. *Cell Death Dis.* 11:913. doi: 10.1038/s41419-020-03110-8

Zhu, C., Cheng, C., Wang, Y., Muhammad, W., Liu, S., Zhu, W., et al. (2018). Loss of ARHGEF6 causes hair cell stereocilia deficits and hearing loss in mice. *Front. Mol. Neurosci.* 11:362. doi: 10.3389/fnmol.2018.00362

Zong, L., Guan, J., Ealy, M., Zhang, Q., Wang, D., Wang, H., et al. (2015). Mutations in apoptosis-inducing factor cause X-linked recessive auditory neuropathy spectrum disorder. *J. Med. Genet.* 52, 523–531. doi: 10.1136/jmedgenet-2014-102961

14

Phenotypic Heterogeneity of Post-lingual and/or Milder Hearing Loss for the Patients With the GJB2 c.235delC Homozygous Mutation

Hongyang Wang[1*†], *Yun Gao*[1,2,3,4†], *Jing Guan*[1,2,3,4], *Lan Lan*[1,2,3,4], *Ju Yang*[1,2,3,4], *Wenping Xiong*[1,2,3,4], *Cui Zhao*[1,2,3,4], *Linyi Xie*[1,2,3,4], *Lan Yu*[1,2,3,4], *Dayong Wang*[1,2,3,4] and *Qiuju Wang*[1,2,3,4*]

[1] College of Otolaryngology, Head and Neck Surgery, Chinese People's Liberation Army (PLA) Institute of Otolaryngology, Chinese People's Liberation Army (PLA) General Hospital, Beijing, China, [2] National Clinical Research Center for Otolaryngologic Diseases, Beijing, China, [3] Key Lab of Hearing Impairment Science of Ministry of Education, Beijing, China, [4] Key Lab of Hearing Impairment Prevention and Treatment of Beijing, Beijing, China

***Correspondence:**
Hongyang Wang
whyx301@foxmail.com
Qiuju Wang
wqcr301@vip.sina.com

† These authors have contributed equally to this work

Objective: To report the phenotypic heterogeneity of *GJB2* c.235delC homozygotes associated with post-lingual and/or milder hearing loss, and explore the possible mechanism of these unconditional phenotypes.

Methods: Mutation screening of *GJB2* was performed on all ascertained members from Family 1006983 and three sporadic patients by polymerase chain reaction (PCR) amplification and Sanger sequencing. Next generation sequencing (NGS) was successively performed on some of the affected members and normal controls from Family 1006983 to explore additional possible genetic codes. Reverse transcriptase–quantitative PCR was conducted to test the expression of Connexin30.

Results: We identified a Chinese autosomal recessive hearing loss family with the *GJB2* c.235delC homozygous mutation, affected members from which had post-lingual moderate to profound hearing impairment, and three sporadic patients with post-lingual moderate hearing impairment, instead of congenital profound hearing loss. NGS showed no other particular variants. Overexpression of Connexin30 in some of these cases was verified.

Conclusion: Post-lingual and/or moderate hearing impairment phenotypes of *GJB2* c.235delC homozygotes are not the most common phenotype, revealing the heterogeneity of *GJB2* pathogenic mutations. To determine the possible mechanism that rescues part of the hearing or postpones onset age of these cases, more cases are required to confirm both Connexin30 overexpression and the existence of modifier genes.

Keywords: GJB2, Connexin30, modifier, heterogeneity, hearing loss

INTRODUCTION

Hearing loss is one of the major disabilities world-widely, which is often induced by loss of sensory hair cells (HCs) in the inner ear cochlea. HCs mainly function in transducing sound waves into the electric signals (Wang et al., 2017; Liu et al., 2019; Qi et al., 2019; He et al., 2020). Hearing loss could be caused by genetic factors, aging, chronic cochlear infections, infectious diseases, ototoxic drugs, and noise exposure (He et al., 2017; Cheng et al., 2019; Zhou et al., 2020); and genetic factors account for more than 60% of the hearing loss. *GJB2*, which encodes the gap junction protein Connexin 26, is the most common cause of genetic non-syndromic hearing loss (NSHL). Among the approximately 200 hearing loss associated *GJB2* mutations (Stenson et al., 2017), the c.235delC mutation, a founder mutation (Yan et al., 2003; Shinagawa et al., 2020), is the most frequently known mutation in some East Asian groups, with a carrier frequency of approximately 1% (Yan et al., 2003). The mutation has a significant ethnic specificity, with increasing risk of NSHL in the East Asian and Southeast Asian populations (Dai et al., 2015), but no susceptibility in Oceania and European populations (Yao et al., 2012). Most patients with the *GJB2* c.235delC homozygous mutation show pre-lingual severe to profound hearing impairment (Zhao et al., 2011). However, even cases with the *GJB2* c.235delC homozygous mutation may be undetected by newborn hearing screening, suggesting that *GJB2* c.235delC homozygous mutation-related hearing loss may not always be congenital at onset (Minami et al., 2013; Dai et al., 2019; Wang et al., 2019). Clinically, except for late-onset hearing impairment, some *GJB2* c.235delC homozygous patients show post-lingual and/or mild to moderate hearing impairment instead of profound hearing loss with a highly heterogeneous phenotype.

In addition to *GJB2*, *GJB6* is another gene located in DFNB1. *GJB6* encodes the gap junction protein Connexin 30, which is co-assemble with Connexin 26 to form hybrid gap junctions (Ahmad et al., 2003). Connexin26 and Connexin 30 are predominant isoforms in the cochlea (Zhao et al., 2006). Deletions in *GJB6* are also common genetic factors for NSHL in some populations, with ethnic specificity (del Castillo et al., 2002; Marlin et al., 2005; Falah et al., 2020). Cases with digenic heterozygous mutations in *GJB2* and *GJB6* are relatively rare in the NSHL population, with various phenotypes, such as prelingual or post-lingual, ranging from mild or moderate to severe or profound hearing loss (Bolz et al., 2004; Cama et al., 2009; Chan et al., 2010; del Castillo and del Castillo, 2011; Mei et al., 2017). In the *GJB6* homozygous knockout mouse model, overexpression of Connexin26 restored hearing sensitivity and prevented hair cell death, suggesting that upregulation of Connexin might be a therapeutic strategy for patients with *GJB6* mutations (Ahmad et al., 2007). However, there is no animal experiment to verify that the overexpression of Connexin30 can restore the hearing loss caused by *GJB2* mutations, since *Gjb2* knockout mice are embryonically lethal (Gabriel et al., 1998).

Modifier genes are a perspective for the study of hearing loss to interpret phenotypic variation. Linkage analysis (families) and association studies (unrelated patients) are two strategies can be adopted to identify modifier genes for human disorders (Bykhovskaya et al., 2004; Dunckley et al., 2007; Tao et al., 2019). However, association studies are not always effective, and a previous whole genome association (WGA) study on *GJB2* c.35delG homozygous patients showed that phenotypic heterogeneity could not be explained by the effect of a single major modifier gene (Azaiez et al., 2004; Hilgert et al., 2009a).

In this study, we focused on some unconditional cases involving *GJB2* c.235delC homozygotes, whose phenotypes were late-onset and/or moderate hearing loss. First, we found a Chinese family (Family 1006983) with the *GJB2* c.235delC mutation, which was segregated with all of the recruited members. Unlike other patients with the *GJB2* c.235delC homozygous mutation, whose phenotype were pre-lingual severe to profound hearing loss, patients in this family showed post-lingual moderate to profound sensorineural hearing loss. In addition, we further identified three sporadic cases with *GJB2* c.235delC homozygotes, the phenotypes of which were post-lingual moderate hearing impairment. To decipher the mechanism of partial or late-onset hearing loss in *GJB2* c.235delC homozygotes cases, we performed next generation sequencing (NGS), including targeted genes capture and genome sequencing on some of the affected members and controls from 1006983, but no pathogenic variations or modifier genes were identified. Since Connexin26 and Connexin 30 are co-assembled to form hybrid gap junctions and a previous mouse experiment suggested that up-regulation of Connexin or the slowing of its degradation might be a therapeutic strategy to prevent and treat deafness caused by Connexin 30 mutations (Ahmad et al., 2007), we hypothesised that for some of the patients with a more minor phenotype than other patients with the *GJB2* c.235delC mutation, it is the overexpression of Connexin30 that plays a compensatory role. Thus, reverse transcriptase-quantitative polymerase chain reaction (RT-qPCR) was also conducted on some of these patients to test the expression of Connexin30, which is encoded by *GJB6* (**Supplementary Figure 1**).

MATERIALS AND METHODS

Ethics Statement

The study was approved by the Committee of Medical Ethics of the Chinese PLA General Hospital. Written informed consents were obtained from all the participants in the family.

Family Recruitment and Clinical Evaluations

A five-generation family (Family 1006983) with 133 members presenting with autosomal recessive non-syndromic sensorineural hearing loss (ARNSHL) was ascertained from the Institute of Otolaryngology, Chinese PLA General Hospital (**Figures 1, 2**). Three independent sporadic patients with homozygous *GJB2* c.235delC were also recruited in our study, who had late-onset moderate hearing impairment (**Figure 3**). Personal or family medical evidence of hearing loss, tinnitus, vestibular symptoms, and other clinical abnormalities of the participants were identified by a team of experienced physicians

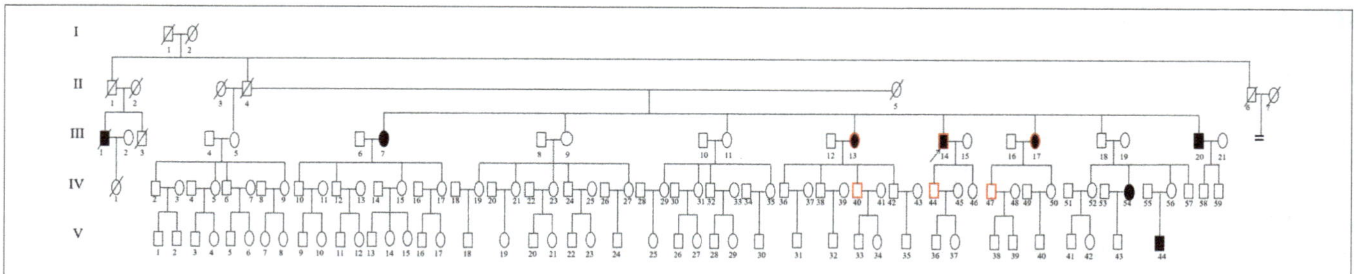

FIGURE 1 | Pedigree of Family 1006983. Filled symbols for males (squares) and females (circles) represent affected individuals, and empty, unaffected individuals. An arrow denotes the proband. The symbols with a red border represent the cases for whom genome sequencing was performed.

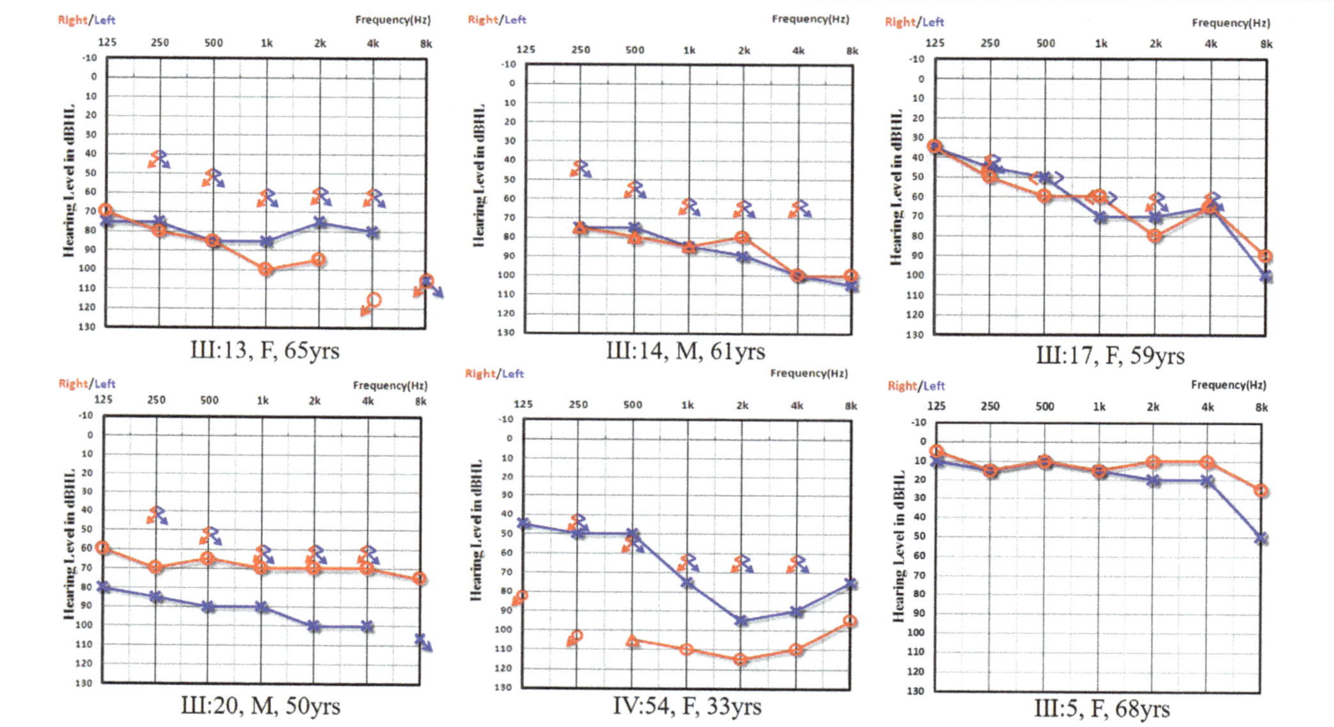

FIGURE 2 | Audiograms of both ears from subjects in Family 1006983. Symbols "o" and "x" denote air conduction pure-tone thresholds at different frequencies in the right and left ear, respectively. dB HL, decibels hearing level; Hz, Hertz. III:13, III:14, III:17, III:20, and IV:54 are the affected cases from Family 1006983 with the *GJB2* c.235delC homozygous mutation. III:5 is a normal control from the family with a *GJB2* c.235delC heterozygous mutation.

and audiologists. Audiometric evaluations included pure tone audiometry (PTA), which was calculated as the average hearing threshold at 0.5, 1, 2, and 4 kHz for the bilateral ears of the ascertained subjects. The severity of hearing impairment was defined as mild (26–40 dB HL), moderate (41–70 dB HL), severe (71–95 dB HL) and profound (>95 dB HL). The speech recognition score was tested and calculated for some patients. Caloric testing was performed on some patients and the normal controls to obtain data on semicircular canal function. Some patients who had tinnitus were estimated by tinnitus assessment. High resolution computed tomography (HRCT) of the temporal bone was conducted for some of the patients.

A cohort of two hundred and ninety-five hearing loss cases who had the homozygous *GJB2* c.235delC mutation in our institute were chosen as the controls to compare phenotypes (Zhao et al., 2011).

Sanger Sequencing

Genomic DNA was extracted from the whole blood samples using a Blood DNA kit according to the standard protocol (TIANGEN BIOTECH, Beijing, China). PCR and Sanger sequencing were performed on all available members from Family 1006983 and the three sporadic patients and their parents to determine whether the potential mutations in causative genes co-segregated with the disease phenotype in these families. Direct PCR products were sequenced using Bigdye Terminator v3.1 Cycle Sequencing Kits (Applied Biosystems, Foster City, CA) and analysed using an ABI 3700XL Genetic Analyser (primers were *GJB2*-Exon2-F:

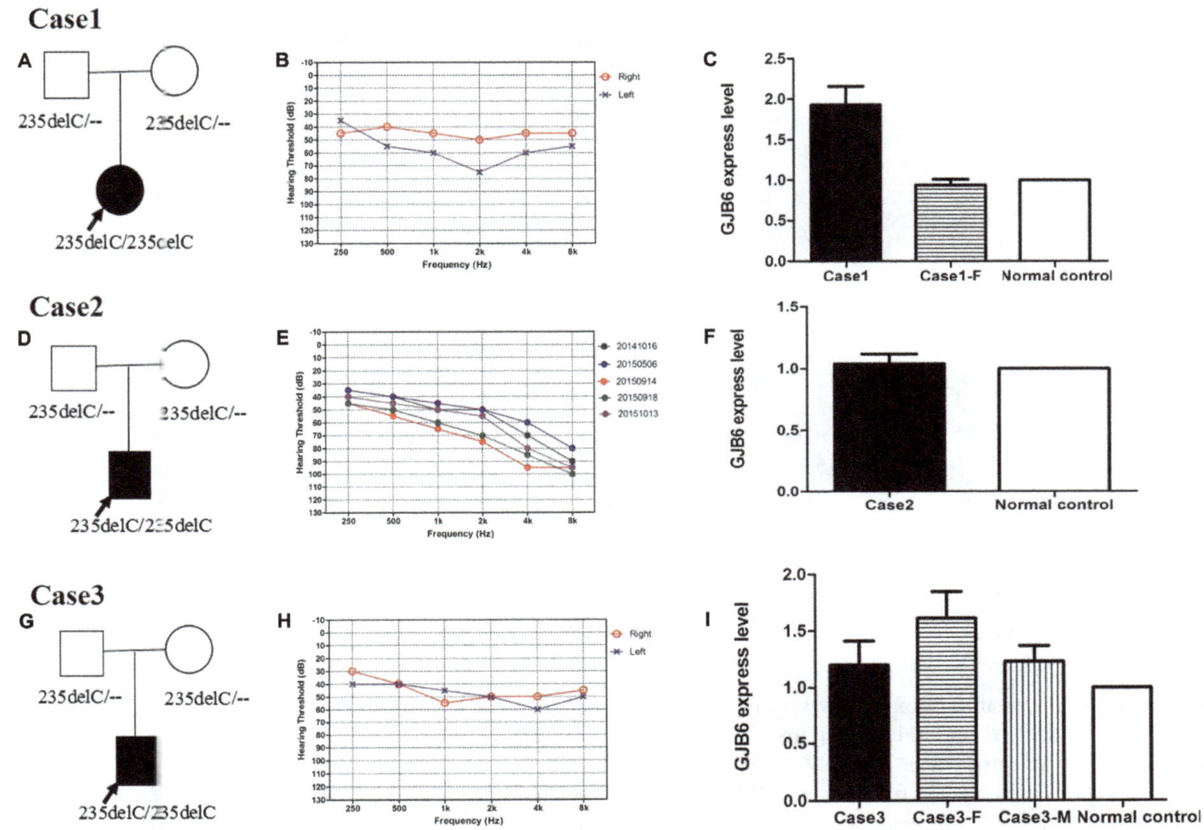

FIGURE 3 | (A,D,G) Pedigree of case 1, case 2, and case 3, respectively. **(B,E,H)** Audiograms of three sporadic cases. **(B)** Audiograms of both ears from case 1. **(E)** Five audiograms of the left ear from case 2 in the last 2 years. Different color audiograms represent audiograms done at different times. **(H)** Audiograms of both ears from case 3. **(B,E,H)** Symbols "o" and "x" denote air conduction pure-tone thresholds at different frequencies in the right and left ear, respectively. dB, decibels; Hz, Hertz. **(C,F,I)** Connexin 30 expression in case 1, case 2, and case 3, respectively. Case 1-F is the father of case 1. Case3-F is the father of case 3, and Case 3-M is the mother of Case 3. Normal control is an independent subject with normal hearing from our institute.

5′-TTGGTGTTTGCTCAGGAAGA-3′ and *GJB2*-Exon2-R: 5′-GGCCTACAGGGGTTTCAAAT-3′).

Next Generation Sequencing

To examine whether other genetic defects or modifier genes were involved, targeted multi-genes capture and NGS were performed on case III:20, who had moderate hearing impairment in the better ear at the age of 50 years when tested. Targeted genes include 307 known and candidate hearing loss associated genes (Wang et al., 2015). And then genome sequencing was further performed on cases III:13, III:14, III:17 and controls IV;40, IV;44, IV:47. Sequencing was carried out on Illumina HiSeq2500 to generate paired end reads. Biologic information analysis was carried out according to a previous process (Wang et al., 2014), and specific analysis strategies to find the modifier genes were conducted on the genome sequencing data.

RT-qPCR of GJB6

Total RNA was extracted from the white cells of the whole blood samples using the cell RAN kit according to the standard protocol (TRIzol Reagent, Life Technologies). Synthesis of cDNA was carried out with a Revert Aid First Strand cDNA Synthesis Kit (Thermo Fisher Scientific). Primers were designed as follows by Primer5: GAPDH-H-F: GGAGCGAGATCCCTCCAAAAT; GAPDH-H-R: GGAGCGAGATCCCTCCAAAAT; GJB6-H-F: CAAGAGGACTTCGTCTGCAAC; GJB6-H-R: GTGGTTTCGTGCCTGTAGTAG. RT-qPCR was conducted according to the protocol of the "Power SYBR Green PCR Master Mix and RT-PCR" by Applied Biosystems. The quantitative analysis conditions were shown in **Supplementary Figure 2.** Expression stability analysis included geNorm analysis, NormFinder analysis and BestKeeper analysis. Statistical analysis was performed using Graphpad Prism version 5.01. All of the quantitative results were duplicated at least twice.

RESULTS

Clinical Description

In Family 1006983, a total of 22 family members, composed of five clinically affected and 17 unaffected individuals were ascertained in this study. In this family, most of the affected

TABLE 1 | Summary of clinical data for hearing impaired members in Family 1006983 and three sporadic cases.

Subject	Gender[a]	Age of test (year)	Age of onset (year)	PTA (dB HL)[b]	Hearing impairment[c]	Audiogram	Tinnitus	Vertigo
III:13 (−3)	F	65	5	L: 81.25	Severe	Flat	+	−
				R: 98.75	Profound	Flat		
III:14 (−4)	M	61	6	L: 87.5	Severe	Flat	+	−
				R: 86.25	Severe	Flat		
III:17 (−7)	F	59	9	L: 63.75	Moderate	Flat	+	−
				R: 66.25	Moderate	Flat		
III:20 (−5)	M	50	7	L: 96.25	Profound	Flat	+	−
				R: 68.75	Moderate	Flat		
IV:54 (−67)	F	33	5	L: 77.5	Severe	Flat	+	−
				R: 110	Profound	Flat		
Case1	F	5	5	L: 45	Moderate	Flat	+	−
				R: 62.5	Moderate	Flat		
Case2	M	37	Not clear	L: 57.5	Moderate	Flat	+	+
				R: 55	Moderate	Flat		
Case3	M	6	6	L: 48.75	Moderate	Flat	+	−
				R: 48.75	Moderate	Flat		

[a]*M, male; F, female.*
[b]*PTA, pure-tone air-conduction averages (0.5, 1, 2, and 4 kHz).*
[c]*Diagnosed at the time of test (case3 showed the last test on 13th October, 2015).*
+, positive finding; −, negative finding.

members showed post-lingual, approximately symmetrical, and bilateral non-syndromic sensorineural hearing loss. The average onset age for all the affected cases was 6.2 years old. The hearing loss was presented at all frequencies (**Table 1** and **Figure 2**). For the other three independent sporadic patients in this study, case 1 was a 5 years old girl who had post-lingual, bilateral symmetrical moderate sensorineural hearing impairment, with an onset age of 5 years old (**Figures 3A,B**); case 2 was a 37-year-old man suffering from sudden hearing loss of left ear accompanied by dizziness and tinnitus when he visited our hospital in 2015, whose hearing threshold had a fluctuation in the last 2 years, and whose onset age was not clear. His hearing threshold was first tested on 16th October, 2014, and the PTAs of the left and right ear were 52.5 and 56.25 dB HL, respectively (**Figures 3D,E**); Case 3 was a 6 year old boy with post-lingual, bilateral symmetrical moderate sensorineural hearing impairment (**Figures 3G,H**). All of these three cases had no family history of hearing loss, no symptoms in other organ systems and no other exposure to risk factors. All of the affected cases had associated tinnitus, but no vestibular symptoms or signs were reported except for case 2. HRCT of the temporal bone in the proband of Family 1006983 (III:14) and three sporadic cases showed normal inner ears structure. No exposure history that may account for the hearing impairment existed in any of the affected members.

Among the 295 cases with the homozygous *GJB2* c.235delC mutation, four patients had late-onset hearing loss, an incidence of 1.36% (4/295) (Zhao et al., 2011). The onset ages of these four cases were 4, 4, 5, and 6 years old, with an average onset age of 4.75 years old. Among these four c.235delC homozygous cases, three children had severe hearing loss, and one had profound hearing impairment. There were also eight patients who had pre-lingual moderate hearing loss, an incidence of 2.71% (8/295).

Mutation Detection and Analysis

The c.235delC is a known pathogenic ARNSHL related mutation. Sanger sequencing confirmed the co-segregation of c.235delC with the disease phenotype in Family 1006983, the three sporadic patients and their parents (**Figures 3A,D,G**). All of the cases with hearing impairment had homozygous c.235delC mutation, and all of the normal controls recruited in this study had either no mutation or heterozygous c.235delC. The genotype frequency in dbSNP137, HapMap, 1,000 Genomes, and local dataset was less than 0.001. This mutation occurred at highly conserved amino acids, and was predicted to be deleterious by the PolyPhen 2, SIFT, and Mutationtaster programs.

A total of 307 hearing loss related genes were captured, and the targeted high-throughput sequencing data were analysed according to the standard process (Wang et al., 2014) and no pathogenic or likely pathogenic variations were identified according to the standards and guidelines for the interpretation of sequence variants (Richards et al., 2015).

To further analyse the modified genes that may exist in the 1006983 family, six samples from the family were selected for genome sequencing analysis. The total amount of data of the whole genome was shown in **Supplementary Table 1**. After screening, a total of 7,132,601 digits of variation were obtained. A total of 6.6% of them were novel variants. Sample sequencing depth and coverage are shown in **Supplementary Table 2**. Variation covers many different types. Four strategies were performed to decipher the possible effective genes. First, assuming that there was a modified gene in this family of patients, all of the heterozygous mutations on chromosome 13 shared by the three patients in Family 1006983, with a frequency of

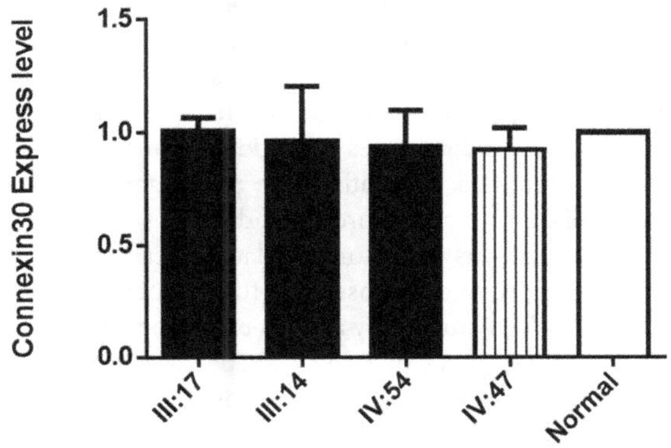

FIGURE 4 | Connexin30 expression of some of the affected members and within-family normal controls from Family 1006983. III:17, III:14, and IV:54 are three hearing loss cases with the *GJB2* 235delC homozygous mutation, IV:47 is a normal control from Family 1006983. Normal represents the Connexin 30 expression of a person who is not a member of the family.

less than 0.0001 and functional mutations were selected (non-coding mutations may also be responsible for the possibility of modification, but due to the huge amount of data, so rare functional mutations were focused on first). Candidate mutation information was shown in **Supplementary Table 3**. Second, genes interacting with *GJB2* were analysed emphatically. Third, copy number variants (CNVs) of genes interacting with *GJB2* gene were analysed[1] by selecting the 20M gene sequence before and after the target genes, with no related CNV were deciphered. Last, related genes located in the *GJB2* signal pathway were determined (**Supplementary Table 4**), and *TJP1* and *TUBA3E* were found to be most likely to be interacting with *GJB2*.

RT-qPCR of GJB6

The expression of Connexin30 in the affected members of Family 1006983 showed no significant difference from that in the control group (**Figure 4**). The expression levels in the three sporadic cases revealed no consistent results, with only case1 having double expression compared to normal control (**Figure 3C**). Case 2 and case 3 showed no significant increase in the expression level from that of the normal controls or the heterozygous controls (**Figures 3F,I**).

DISCUSSION

Phenotype-Genotype Correlation Analysis

There is striking phenotypic heterogeneity in the onset age as well as degree of hearing loss caused by *GJB2* mutations. For most genotypes, however, there is considerable variation. In clinic, cochlea developmental disorders are the mechanism of congenital hearing loss caused by Connexin26 deficiency, whereas the reduction of cochlea active amplification is the cause of late-onset hearing loss induced by Connexin26 deficiency (Mei et al., 2017). A multicenter genotype-phenotype correlation study showed that inactivating mutations cause a more severe phenotype than non-inactivating mutations (Snoeckx et al., 2005). Among c.235delC homozygotes, the majority do have pre-lingual profound hearing loss, while some c.235delC homozygotes have only post-lingual and/or moderate hearing loss. The phenotypic variances found among the cases recruited in this study are as follows.

Late-Onset Phenotype of Homozygous *GJB2* c.235delC

All of the patients from Family 1006983 and the three sporadic cases had late-onset hearing impairment. Previous studies of 295 control cases with homozygous *GJB2* c.235delC by our group reported that post-lingual cases accounted for 1.36% of the cohort, indicating a relatively rare variant (Zhao et al., 2011). Though relatively rare, the *GJB2* c.35delG homozygous mutation, which is the most prevalent mutation in Caucasians, could also contribute to late postnatal onset hearing loss (Pagarkar et al., 2006). There are also some *GJB2* pathogenic mutations associated with post-lingual hearing impairment, such as p.T55N, p.R75Q, p.D179N, and p.C202F (Morle et al., 2000; Primignani et al., 2003; Melchionda et al., 2005; Iossa et al., 2010), which are inherited as autosomal dominant patterns (Wang et al., 2017).

Milder Hearing Impairment Phenotype of Homozygous *GJB2* c.235delC

One affected member from Family 1006983 and three sporadic cases had moderate hearing loss, accounting for 50% of the eight cases recruited in this study, and the other four cases from Family 1006983 had severe to profound hearing loss. In fact, among the four severe to profound cases in Family 1006983, the testing age was 33, 59, 61, and 65 years, showing a progressive hearing impairment tendency according to the complaints of these patients.

GJB2 Mutation and Sudden Hearing Loss

Case 2 complained of sudden hearing loss of the left ear when he came to our clinic on 14th September, 2015. In recent years, some studies have proposed that genetic deafness mutations may be associated with the pathogenesis of sudden hearing loss. Bora et al. once screened the *GJB2*, *GJB3*, and *GJB6* genes in 40 sudden hearing loss patients and 40 normal controls, but the connection between Connexin and sudden hearing loss could not be verified (Bora et al., 2010). In the Chinese population, previous studies showed that the incidence of the *GJB2* c.235delC mutation was low in sudden hearing loss patients (2.1%, 5/234) and had no significant difference from that of normal controls, suggesting that *GJB2* c.235delC has no correlation with sudden hearing loss (Zhan et al., 2014). In our group, we once screened the *GJB2* gene in 93 sudden hearing loss patients and 117 controls with normal hearing. Only two heterozygous c.235delC mutations were identified in the sudden hearing loss group, while five heterozygous c.235delC mutations were identified in the normal control group (data not published).

[1] https://glm.genecards.org/#results

Genetic Counselling and Clinical Management

Genetic diagnosis and counselling is increasingly affecting the clinical practice of genetic hearing loss, especially genotype-phenotype correlation analysis. *GJB2* c.235delC is the most common deafness-related pathogenic variant in the Chinese population, and reporting the phenotypic heterogeneity of *GJB2* c.235delC homozygous cases is helpful throughout the genetic counselling procedure, and would contribute greatly to clinical practice. Except for providing information about incidence, recurrent risk and prevention strategies, phenotype heterogeneity should be accounted both before and after gene testing. For example, information if provided on the possible gene testing results and relevant phenotype prognosis before gene testing, phenotype heterogeneity should be taken into consideration; for the management of an individual with *GJB2* c.235delC homozygous mutation after gene testing, especially for a baby who has passed newborn hearing screening, audiology follow-up seems to be much more critical than performing cochlear implantation directly. Gene therapy as a potential clinical treatment method have been reported to be efficient in inherit hearing loss in animal models (Tan et al., 2019; Delmaghani and El-Amraoui, 2020; Niggemann et al., 2020). However, there are numerous challenges associated with *in vivo* gene therapy targeting the human inner ears to be addressed.

Phenotypic Heterogeneity Mechanisms

Cellular and deafness mechanisms underlying *GJB2* induced hearing impairment are currently unclear, although numerous clinical reports indicate that Connexin26 mutations are associated with hearing impairment. Few studies have been performed on the pathogenesis of Connexin26 mutations. For example, in one clear functional study on a patient who had the Connexin26 c.35delG mutation and a p.E101G missense mutation, microscopic observation revealed nearly complete degeneration of hair cells and agenesis of the SV but no neural degeneration (Jun et al., 2000). In summary, previous studies on Connexin function showed that the cochlear development disorders lead to congenital deafness instead of hair cell degeneration and endocochlear potential reduction, while the reduction of active cochlear amplification leads to late-onset hearing loss, even though cochlear hair cells have no Connexin expression (Wingard and Zhao, 2015).

Most likely, the phenotypic heterogeneity is caused by modifier genes, but none has been identified to date. Modifier genes can be relatively easily identified in mice by crossing parental inbred strains that carry the disease-causing mutation and exhibit a difference in phenotype, such as the modifier gene *Moth1* in the Tubby mouse (Ikeda et al., 2002). However, it is difficult to perform linkage or association analysis to determine the modifier gene in human cases with only one family and a limited number of mild/moderate sporadic patients, such as the situation in this study. In our study, the targeted multi-gene sequence of one of the affected members identified no other variation except for homozygous *GJB2* c.235delC. Their identification could substantially contribute to a more accurate diagnosis and more appropriate genetic counselling (Hilgert et al., 2009b). Exome sequencing or genome sequencing may be better choice to find modifier genes in these unconditional cases. However, although we attempted different strategies, it is difficult to analyse the large amount of data of the genome sequencing, with numerous candidate genes being identified, but no further evidence was obtained to confirm the phenotypic correlation. Another family and many more sporadic cases with the *GJB2* c.235delC homozygous mutation and late-onset milder hearing impairment may provide the possibility to decipher the molecular mechanism. A WGA study may also an effective way to decipher the major modifier genes of *GJB2* c.235delC, as one had been previously performed on a separate set of *GJB2* c.35delG cases (Hilgert et al., 2009a). The WGA study needs a second set of cases to replicate the possible SNPs, however, *GJB2* c.235delC homozygote cases are limited.

From another point of view, we hypothesised that for some of the patients with more minor phenotypes than those with homozygous *GJB2* c.235delC, the overexpression of Connexin30 plays a compensatory role. The mutual pathogenic mechanism of the biallelic *GJB2* and *GJB6* genes is unclear. These two genes have 77% sequence homology. Connexin26 and Connexin30, which are encoded by these two genes, assemble into a complete heterologous gap junction channel together (Liu et al., 2009), playing a key role in inner ear K^+ regulation. *GJB2* overexpression can effectively restore hearing impairment in *GJB6* knockout mice (Ahmad et al., 2007), suggesting that genetic correction by overexpression may restore hearing function effectively. We found some of the cases overexpressed Connexin3, however, we could not find consistency between the family and sporadic patients in this study. In addition, the total RNA extracted from whole blood could not verify the located expression of Connexin30. Furthermore, biopsy of the human cochlear is impossible for now, and measurement of the gene transcription of Connexins by RT-qPCR and of the protein expression of Connexins by western blots analysis cannot be achieved. We will continue focus on the subjects with the same phenotype in this study, to find out the underlying mechanism of the phenotype heterogeneity. In addition, animal experiments are still needed to find out whether increasing the Connexin30 protein level in Gjb2 knock out background could restore hearing. To all knowledge, there is no data to confirm that up-regulation of Connexin6 expression in Gjb2 knockout mice could not rescue the hearing up to date.

CONCLUSION

In conclusion, we reported a family and three sporadic patients with homozygous c.235delC, who had an unconditional phenotype with post-lingual and/or moderate hearing impairment. Multi-genes sequencing showed no other pathogenic mutations or modifier genes. RT-qPCR of Connexin30 expression revealed that some of these cases overexpressed Connexin30, which may play a compensatory role in hearing impairment. However, the mechanism of the phenotypic heterogeneity and the specific mutation-induced pathological changes *in vivo* remain unclear, and there is little information is available for humans. Many more experiments and large series are needed to decipher the genetic code to extend this study in the future.

ETHICS STATEMENT

The studies involving human participants were reviewed and approved by the study was approved by the Committee of Medical Ethics of the Chinese PLA General Hospital. The patients/participants provided their written informed consent to participate in this study. Written informed consent was obtained from the individual(s) for the publication of any potentially identifiable images or data included in this article.

AUTHOR CONTRIBUTIONS

HW and YG conceived and designed the experiments. HW, YG, JG, LL, and JY performed the experiments. HW, JG, WX, LX, and LY analysed the data. JY and CZ contributed reagents, materials, and analysis tools. HW wrote the manuscript. DW and QW performed the critical reading and discussion of manuscript. All authors contributed to the article and approved the submitted version.

SUPPLEMENTARY MATERIAL

Supplementary Figure 1 | Flow chart to state the outline of the manuscript.

Supplementary Figure 2 | Quantitative condition of RT-qPCR.

Supplementary Table 1 | The total amount of the whole genome sequencing data of Family 1006983.

Supplementary Table 2 | The whole genome sequencing depth and coverage of Family 1006983.

Supplementary Table 3 | The candidate gene variants of whole genome sequencing from Family 1006983.

Supplementary Table 4 | related genes located in the *GJB2* signal pathway (Whole genome sequencing data of Family 1006983).

REFERENCES

Ahmad, S., Chen, S., Sun, J., and Lin, X. (2003). Connexins 26 and 30 are co-assembled to form gap junctions in the cochlea of mice. *Biochem. Biophys. Res. Commun.* 307, 362–368. doi: 10.1016/s0006-291x(03)01166-5

Ahmad, S., Tang, W., Chang, Q., Qu, Y., Hibshman, J., Li, Y., et al. (2007). Restoration of connexin26 protein level in the cochlea completely rescues hearing in a mouse model of human connexin30-linked deafness. *Proc. Natl. Acad. Sci. U.S.A.* 104, 1337–1341. doi: 10.1073/pnas.0606855104

Azaiez, H., Chamberlin, G. P., Fischer, S. M., Welp, C. L., Prasad, S. D., Taggart, R. T., et al. (2004). GJB2: the spectrum of deafness-causing allele variants and their phenotype. *Hum. Mutat.* 24, 305–311. doi: 10.1002/humu.20084

Bolz, H., Schade, G., Ehmer, S., Kothe, C., Hess, M., and Gal, A. (2004). Phenotypic variability of non-syndromic hearing loss in patients heterozygous for both c.35delG of GJB2 and the 342-kb deletion involving GJB6. *Hear. Res.* 188, 42–46. doi: 10.1016/s0378-5955(03)00346-0

Bora, A., Altuntas, E. E., Ozdemir, O., Uysal, I. O., and Muderris, S. (2010). [Genetic constitution analysis of idiopathic sudden hearing loss]. *Kulak Burun Bogaz Ihtis. Derg.* 20, 219–225.

Bykhovskaya, Y., Mengesha, E., Wang, D., Yang, H., Estivill, X., Shohat, M., et al. (2004). Phenotype of non-syndromic deafness associated with the mitochondrial A1555G mutation is modulated by mitochondrial RNA modifying enzymes MTO1 and GTPBP3. *Mol. Genet. Metab.* 83, 199–206. doi: 10.1016/j.ymgme.2004.07.009

Cama, E., Melchionda, S., Palladino, T., Carella, M., Santarelli, R., Genovese, E., et al. (2009). Hearing loss features in GJB2 biallelic mutations and GJB2/GJB6 digenic inheritance in a large Italian cohort. *Int. J. Audiol.* 48, 12–17. doi: 10.1080/14992020802400654

Chan, D. K., Schrijver, I., and Chang, K. W. (2010). Connexin-26-associated deafness: phenotypic variability and progression of hearing loss. *Genet. Med.* 12, 174–181. doi: 10.1097/gim.0b013e3181d0d42b

Cheng, C., Wang, Y., Guo, L., Lu, X., Zhu, W., Muhammad, W., et al. (2019). Age-related transcriptome changes in Sox2+ supporting cells in the mouse cochlea. *Stem Cell Res. Ther.* 10:365.

Dai, P., Huang, L. H., Wang, G. J., Gao, X., Qu, C. Y., Chen, X. W., et al. (2019). Concurrent hearing and genetic screening of 180,469 neonates with follow-up in Beijing, China. *Am. J. Hum. Genet.* 105, 803–812.

Dai, Z. Y., Sun, B. C., Huang, S. S., Yuan, Y. Y., Zhu, Y. H., Su, Y., et al. (2015). Correlation analysis of phenotype and genotype of GJB2 in patients with non-syndromic hearing loss in China. *Gene* 570, 272–276. doi: 10.1016/j.gene.2015.06.038

del Castillo, F. J., and del Castillo, I. (2011). The DFNB1 subtype of autosomal recessive non-syndromic hearing impairment. *Front. Biosci.* 16, 3252–3274. doi: 10.2741/3910

del Castillo, I., Villamar, M., Moreno-Pelayo, M. A., del Castillo, F. J., Alvarez, A., Tellería, D., et al. (2002). A deletion involving the connexin 30 gene in nonsyndromic hearing impairment. *N. Engl. J. Med.* 346, 243–249. doi: 10.1056/nejmoa012052

Delmaghani, S., and El-Amraoui, A. (2020). Inner ear gene therapies take off: current promises and future challenges. *J. Clin. Med.* 9:2309. doi: 10.3390/jcm9072309

Dunckley, T., Huentelman, M. J., Craig, D. W., Pearson, J. V., Szelinger, S., Joshipura, K., et al. (2007). Whole-genome analysis of sporadic amyotrophic lateral sclerosis. *N. Engl. J. Med.* 357, 775–788.

Falah, M., Houshmand, M., Balali, M., Asghari, A., Bagher, Z., Alizadeh, R., et al. (2020). Role of GJB2 and GJB6 in Iranian nonsyndromic hearing impairment: from molecular analysis to literature reviews. *Fetal Pediatr. Pathol.* 39, 1–12. doi: 10.1080/15513815.2019.1627625

Gabriel, H. D., Jung, D., Butzler, C., Temme, A., Traub, O., Winterhager, E., et al. (1998). Transplacental uptake of glucose is decreased in embryonic lethal connexin26-deficient mice. *J. Cell Biol.* 140, 1453–1461. doi: 10.1083/jcb.140.6.1453

He, Z., Guo, L., Shu, Y., Fang, Q., Zhou, H., Liu, Y., et al. (2017). Autophagy protects auditory hair cells against neomycin-induced damage. *Autophagy* 13, 1884–1904. doi: 10.1080/15548627.2017.1359449

He, Z. H., Zou, S. Y., Li, M., Liao, F. L., Wu, X., Sun, H. Y., et al. (2020). The nuclear transcription factor FoxG1 affects the sensitivity of mimetic aging hair cells to inflammation by regulating autophagy pathways. *Redox Biol.* 28:101364. doi: 10.1016/j.redox.2019.101364

Hilgert, N., Huentelman, M. J., Thorburn, A. Q., Fransen, E., Dieltjens, N., Mueller-Malesinska, M., et al. (2009a). Phenotypic variability of patients homozygous for the GJB2 mutation 35delG cannot be explained by the influence of one major modifier gene. *Eur. J. H. Genet.* 17, 517–524.

Hilgert, N., Smith, R. J. H., and Van Camp, G. (2009b). Forty-six genes causing nonsyndromic hearing impairment: which ones should be analyzed in DNA diagnostics? *Mutat. Res.* 681, 189–196. doi: 10.1016/j.mrrev.2008.08.002

Ikeda, A., Zheng, Q. Y., Zuberi, A. R., Johnson, K. R., Naggert, J. K., and Nishina, P. M. (2002). Microtubule-associated protein 1A is a modifier of tubby hearing (moth1). *Nat. Genet.* 30, 401–405. doi: 10.1038/ng838

Iossa, S., Chinetti, V., Corvino, V., Marciano, E., and Franze, A. (2010). R75Q dominant mutation in GJB2 gene silenced by the in Cis recessive mutation c.35delG. *Am. J. Med. Genet. A* 152A, 2658–2660. doi: 10.1002/ajmg.a.33630

Jun, A. I., McGuirt, W. T., Hinojosa, R., Green, G. E., Fischel-Ghodsian, N., and Smith, R. J. (2000). Temporal bone histopathology in connexin 26-related hearing loss. *Laryngoscope* 110(Pt 1), 269–275. doi: 10.1097/00005537-200002010-00016

Liu, X. Z., Yuan, Y., Yan, D., Ding, E. H., Ouyang, X. M., Fei, Y., et al. (2009). Digenic inheritance of non-syndromic deafness caused by mutations at the gap junction proteins Cx26 and Cx31. *Hum. Genet.* 125, 53–62. doi: 10.1007/s00439-008-0602-9

Liu, Y., Qi, J., Chen, X., Tang, M., Chu, C., Zhu, W., et al. (2019). Critical role of spectrin in hearing development and deafness. *Sci. Adv.* 5:eaav7803. doi: 10.1126/sciadv.aav7803

Marlin, S., Feldmann, D., Blons, H., Loundon, N., Rouillon, I., Albert, S., et al. (2005). GJB2 and GJB6 mutations: genotypic and phenotypic correlations in a large cohort of hearing-impaired patients. *Arch. Otolaryngol. Head Neck Surg.* 131, 481–487. doi: 10.1001/archotol.131.6.481

Mei, L., Chen, J., Zong, L., Zhu, Y., Liang, C., Jones, R. O., et al. (2017). A deafness mechanism of digenic Cx26 (GJB2) and Cx30 (GJB6) mutations: reduction of endocochlear potential by impairment of heterogeneous gap junctional function in the cochlear lateral wall. *Neurobiol. Dis.* 108, 195–203. doi: 10.1016/j.nbd.2017.08.002

Melchionda, S., Bicego, M., Marciano, E., Franzè, A., Morgutti, M., Bortone, G., et al. (2005). Functional characterization of a novel Cx26 (T55N) mutation associated to non-syndromic hearing loss. *Biochem. Biophys. Res. Commun.* 337, 799–805. doi: 10.1016/j.bbrc.2005.09.116

Minami, S. B., Mutai, H., Nakano, A., Arimoto, Y., Taiji, H., Morimoto, N., et al. (2013). GJB2-associated hearing loss undetected by hearing screening of newborns. *Gene* 532, 41–45. doi: 10.1016/j.gene.2013.08.094

Morle, L., Bozon, M., Alloisio, N., Latour, P., Vandenberghe, A., Plauchu, H., et al. (2000). A novel C202F mutation in the connexin26 gene (GJB2) associated with autosomal dominant isolated hearing loss. *J. Med. Genet.* 37, 368–370. doi: 10.1136/jmg.37.5.368

Niggemann, P., Gyorgy, B., and Chen, Z. Y. (2020). Genome and base editing for genetic hearing loss. *Hear. Res.* 394:107958. doi: 10.1016/j.heares.2020.107958

Pagarkar, W., Bitner-Glindzicz, M., Knight, J., and Sirimanna, T. (2006). Late postnatal onset of hearing loss due to GJB2 mutations. *Int. J. Pediatr. Otorhinolaryngol.* 70, 1119–1124. doi: 10.1016/j.ijporl.2005.10.026

Primignani, P., Castorina, P., Sironi, F., Curcio, C., Ambrosetti, U., and Coviello, D. A. (2003). A novel dominant missense mutation–D179N–in the GJB2 gene (Connexin 26) associated with non-syndromic hearing loss. *Clin. Genet.* 63, 516–521. doi: 10.1034/j.1399-0004.2003.00079.x

Qi, J., Liu, Y., Chu, C., Chen, X., Zhu, W., Shu, Y., et al. (2019). A cytoskeleton structure revealed by super-resolution fluorescence imaging in inner ear hair cells. *Cell Discov.* 5:12.

Richards, S., Aziz, N., Bale, S., Bick, D., Das, S., Gastier-Foster, J., et al. (2015). Standards and guidelines for the interpretation of sequence variants: a joint consensus recommendation of the American college of medical genetics and Genomics and the Association for molecular pathology. *Genet. Med.* 17, 405–424. doi: 10.1038/gim.2015.30

Shinagawa, J., Moteki, H., Nishio, S. Y., Noguchi, Y., and Usami, S. I. (2020). Haplotype analysis of GJB2 mutations: founder effect or mutational hot spot? *Genes* 11:250. doi: 10.3390/genes11030250

Snoeckx, R. L., Huygen, P. L. M., Feldmann, D., Marlin, S., Denoyelle, F., Waligora, J., et al. (2005). GJB2 mutations and degree of hearing loss: a multicenter study. *Am. J. Hum. Genet.* 77, 945–957.

Stenson, P. D., Mort, M., Ball, E. V., Evans, K., Hayden, M., Heywood, S., et al. (2017). The human gene mutation database: towards a comprehensive repository of inherited mutation data for medical research, genetic diagnosis and next-generation sequencing studies. *Hum. Genet.* 136, 665–677. doi: 10.1007/s00439-017-1779-6

Tan, F., Chu, C., Qi, J., Li, W., You, D., Li, K., et al. (2019). AAV-ie enables safe and efficient gene transfer to inner ear cells. *Nat. Commun.* 10:3733.

Tao, F., Beecham, G. W., Rebelo, A. P., Blanton, S. H., Moran, J. J., Lopez-Anido, C., et al. (2019). Modifier gene candidates in Charcot-Marie-Tooth disease type 1a: a case-only genome-wide association study. *J. Neuromuscul. Dis.* 6, 201–211. doi: 10.3233/jnd-190377

Wang, H., Wu, K., Yu, L., Xie, L., Xiong, W., Wang, D., et al. (2017). A novel dominant GJB2 (DFNA3) mutation in a Chinese family. *Sci. Rep.* 7:34425.

Wang, H. Y., Zhao, Y. L., Liu, Q., Yuan, H., Gao, Y., Lan, L., et al. (2015). Identification of two disease-causing genes TJP2 and GJB2 in a Chinese family with unconditional autosomal dominant nonsyndromic hereditary hearing impairment. *Chin. Med. J.* 128, 3345–3351. doi: 10.4103/0366-6999.171440

Wang, H. Y., Zhao, Y. L., Yi, Y. T., Gao, Y., Liu, Q., Wang, D., et al. (2014). Targeted high-throughput sequencing identifies pathogenic mutations in KCNQ4 in two large chinese families with autosomal dominant hearing loss. *PLoS One* 9:e103133. doi: 10.1371/journal.pone.0103133

Wang, Q., Xiang, J., Sun, J., Yang, Y., Guan, J., Wang, D., et al. (2019). Nationwide population genetic screening improves outcomes of newborn screening for hearing loss in China. *Genet. Med.* 21, 2231–2238. doi: 10.1038/s41436-019-0481-6

Wang, Y., Li, J., Yao, X., Li, W., Du, H., Tang, M., et al. (2017). Loss of CIB2 causes profound hearing loss and abolishes mechanoelectrical transduction in mice. *Front. Mol. Neurosci.* 10:401. doi: 10.3389/fnmol.2017.00401

Wingard, J. C., and Zhao, H. B. (2015). Cellular and deafness mechanisms underlying connexin mutation-induced hearing loss – a common hereditary deafness. *Front. Cell. Neurosci.* 9:202. doi: 10.3389/fncel.2015.00202

Yan, D., Park, H. J., Ouyang, X. M., Pandya, A., Doi, K., Erdenetungalag, R., et al. (2003). Evidence of a founder effect for the 235delC mutation of GJB2 (connexin 26) in east Asians. *Hum. Genet.* 114, 44–50. doi: 10.1007/s00439-003-1018-1

Yao, J., Lu, Y., Wei, Q., Cao, X., and Xing, G. (2012). A systematic review and meta-analysis of 235delC mutation of GJB2 gene. *J. Transl. Med.* 10:136. doi: 10.1186/1479-5876-10-136

Zhan, Y., Hu, Y., Huang, X., Chen, H., Guo, C., Xiao, H., et al. (2014). [The study on 235delC mutation of GJB2 gene in patients with idiopathic sudden hearing loss]. *Lin Chuang Er Bi Yan Hou Tou Jing Wai Ke Za Zhi* 28, 621–623, 634.

Zhao, F. F., Ji, Y. B., Wang, D. Y., Lan, L., Han, M. K., Li, Q., et al. (2011). Phenotype-genotype correlation in 295 chinese deaf subjects with biallelic causative mutations in the gjb2 gene. *Genet. Test. Mol. Biomarkers* 15, 619–625. doi: 10.1089/gtmb.2010.0192

Zhao, H. B., Kikuchi, T., Ngezahayo, A., and White, T. W. (2006). Gap junctions and cochlear homeostasis. *J. Membr. Biol.* 209, 177–186. doi: 10.1007/s00232-005-0832-x

Zhou, H., Qian, X., Xu, N., Zhang, S., Zhu, G., Zhang, Y., et al. (2020). Disruption of Atg7-dependent autophagy causes electromotility disturbances, outer hair cell loss, and deafness in mice. *Cell Death Dis.* 11:913.

15

Molecular Behavior of HMGB1 in the Cochlea Following Noise Exposure and *in vitro*

Lili Xiao[1,2,3†], Yan Sun[3†], Chengqi Liu[1,2,3], Zhong Zheng[1,2,3], Ying Shen[1,2,3], Liang Xia[1,2,3], Guang Yang[1,2,3*] and Yanmei Feng[1,2,3*]*

[1] Department of Otolaryngology-Head and Neck Surgery, Shanghai Jiao Tong University Affiliated Sixth People's Hospital, Shanghai, China, [2] Otolaryngology Institute of Shanghai Jiao Tong University, Shanghai, China, [3] Shanghai Key Laboratory of Sleep Disordered Breathing, Shanghai, China, [4] Zhangjiagang TCM Hospital Affiliated to Nanjing University of Chinese Medicine, Zhangjiagang, China

***Correspondence:**
Yanmei Feng
ymfeng@sjtu.edu.cn;
Feng.yanmei@126.com
Guang Yang
77648946@qq.com
Liang Xia
xialiang.sjtu@foxmail.com

† These authors have contributed equally to this work

Noise-induced hearing loss (NIHL) is characterized by cellular damage to the inner ear, which is exacerbated by inflammation. High-mobility group box 1 (HMGB1), a representative damage-associated molecular pattern (DAMP), acts as a mediator of inflammation or an intercellular messenger according to its cellular localization. Blocking or regulating HMGB1 offers an attractive approach in ameliorating NIHL. However, the precise therapeutic intervention must be based on a deeper understanding of its dynamic molecular distribution and function in cochlear pathogenesis after acoustic trauma. Here, we have presented the spatiotemporal dynamics of the expression of HMGB1, exhibiting distribution variability in specific cochlear regions and cells following noise exposure. After gene manipulation, we further investigated the characteristics of cellular HMGB1 in HEI-OC1 cells. The higher cell viability observed in the HMGB1 knocked-down group after stimulation with H_2O_2 indicated the possible negative effect of HMGB1 on cellular lifespan. In conclusion, this study demonstrated that HMGB1 is involved in NIHL pathogenesis and its molecular biology has essential and subtle influences, preserving a translational potential for pharmacological intervention.

Keywords: noise, hearing loss, cochlea, high-mobility group box 1, spatiotemporal distribution

INTRODUCTION

Hearing loss is often induced by loss of sensory hair cells (HCs) in the inner ear cochlea, which functions in the transduction of sound waves into electric signals (Zhu et al., 2018; Liu et al., 2019; Qi et al., 2020). WHO reported that 466 million people suffer from hearing loss worldwide, because of genetic factors, infectious diseases, chronic cochlear infections, aging, exposure to noise, and ototoxic drugs (Gao et al., 2019; Zhang et al., 2019; He et al., 2020). Noise-induced hearing loss (NIHL) is the most common type of sensorineural hearing loss, ranking first among occupational diseases, seriously affecting the lives of patients, and greatly increasing the social burden (Carroll et al., 2017; Murphy et al., 2018). The mechanisms underlying noise-induced damage to critical cochlear cells have been reported to include oxidative damage, mechanical shearing forces, and glutamate excitotoxicity (Zhou et al., 2020), which eventually induce apoptotic cell death in HCs, especially the outer HCs of the basal turn (Sun et al., 2014; Yu et al., 2017; Li et al., 2018a; Zhang et al., 2019).

In recent years, increasing evidence has demonstrated that NIHL could be exacerbated by inflammation of the cochlea (Kalinec et al., 2017; Wood and Zuo, 2017; Hu et al., 2018; Frye et al., 2019). Resident cochlear cells, subsequently infiltrating immune cells, and released cytokines or reactive oxygen species (ROS) have been suggested to all interact toward a positive or negative effect in cochlear pathogenesis (He et al., 2016; Lang et al., 2016; Wood and Zuo, 2017; Hu et al., 2018). Specifically, damage-associated molecular patterns (DAMPs), the cellular byproducts of damage, are known to play an essential role in this inflammation. They could stimulate pattern recognition receptors, leading to the rapid release of proinflammatory cytokines and production of ROS, thus insulting sensorineural cells (Tang et al., 2012; He et al., 2017; Wood and Zuo, 2017). However, the type and function of DAMPs in the cochlea following acoustic trauma is rarely clear.

More specifically, DAMPs include pathogen-associated molecular patterns (PAMPs) and "alarmins," endogenous molecules that signal tissue and cellular damage. The high-mobility group box 1 (HMGB1) protein, a representative alarmin, is known to act as a mediator of inflammation or an intercellular messenger when it reaches the extracellular environment (Bianchi et al., 2017). Extracellular HMGB1 has been shown to be typically involved in various immune responses, such as neuroimmune, chemokine—and cytokine—like activity via recently elucidated signal, and molecular transport mechanisms (Yang et al., 2013; Bianchi et al., 2017). Blocking the release or activation of extracellular HMGB1 has been proposed as a promising therapeutic target for inflammatory diseases. Due to its relatively independent function accompanying its different cellular localization, a deeper understanding of HMGB1 biology in the cochlea is indispensable for guiding future precise therapeutic interventions. However, the spatiotemporal expression of HMGB1 in cochlea with acoustic injury has not been systemically investigated.

Until recently, the molecular biology of HMGB1, especially it signaling and role in inflammation, has been extensively studied and broadly recognized. Of the receptors important for the activity of HMGB1, the toll-like receptor (TLR)-4 and receptor for advanced glycation end products (RAGE) have been reported to be the 2 critical interacting receptors leading to the upregulation of proinflammatory cytokines via the NF-κB and MAP kinase signaling pathways (Andersson and Tracey, 2011; Harris et al., 2012; Ott et al., 2014; Yang et al., 2015a; Paudel et al., 2019). Correspondingly, our recent study demonstrated that the activation of MAPK and NF-κB could facilitate the morphological damage and dysfunction of inner ear tissues during the immune response (Xia et al., 2019). Besides, Shih et al. showed that noise-induced increasing level of HMGB1 in the spiral ligament was significantly reduced in the group given dexamethasone in the middle ear compared with the control group, suggesting that HMGB1 participated in noise-induced cochlear inflammation (Shih et al., 2019). Overall, HMGB1 could be a potentially significant candidate as the initial factor alarming for cochlear damage due to its unique biology and role in immune events. Furthermore, newborn HMGB1-knockout mice were shown to die of hypoglycemia within 24 h, suggesting its important role in gene transcription. However, the effects on transcription were cell-type specific because cell lines lacking HMGB1 have been reported to be able to survive *in vitro* (Calogero et al., 1999). Therefore, gene manipulation could be a possible option for further exploring the function of HMGB1 in specific cochlear cell lines.

In the present study, we investigated the spatiotemporal dynamic expression of HMGB1 in the cochlea following noise exposure (NE), which showed a variable pattern of distribution in specific cochlear regions. The cellular biology of HMGB1 in HEI-OC1 cells was also explored in an oxidative stress model following treatment with H_2O_2, indicating the positive impact of a HMGB1-knockdown on the cellular lifespan. Therefore, selectively targeting HMGB1 at a specific cochlear region with the consideration of temporal factors would offer a novel perspective on the specific intervention for NIHL in the future.

MATERIALS AND METHODS

Animals

A total of 42 male C57BL/6 mice at 4–5 weeks of age were purchased from the Shanghai Songlian Lab Animal Field (Shanghai, China). Animals were maintained in a temperature-controlled room under a 12-h light cycle and were acclimated for at least 1 week before the experiments. All mice were housed in individually ventilated cages (5 per cage) and given access to free water and food. Animals were subjected to auditory brainstem response (ABR) measurements before exposure to ensure they have a normal ABR threshold. Samples from 30 mice (six mice per group) were used for western blotting, while samples from 12 mice (three mice per group) were used for fluorescence immunocytochemical investigations. The cochleae of each side were collected for cryostat sectioning and basilar membrane dissection, respectively. All research protocols involving the use and care of animals were approved by the Ethics Committee of the Shanghai Jiao Tong University Affiliated Sixth People's Hospital (permit number DWLL2017-0295).

Noise Exposure

Awake mice were exposed to white noise high-pass filtered at 4 kHz and 110 dB SPL for 2 h. The noise signal was released from a loudspeaker with an upper-frequency limit of 22 kHz (Pyramid TW67 Super tweeters, Pyramid, Brooklyn, NY, United States). Generally, four mice (one mouse per metal wire cage, 10 cm × 10 cm × 15 cm) were located in the center of the sound chamber, in which animals were left unrestrained.

Electrophysiological Evaluation

The ABR to tone burst (TB) at different frequencies was evaluated for all mice before and 1-, 3-, 7-, and 14-days after NE. Animals were lightly anesthetized with an intraperitoneal injection of 1% sodium pentobarbital (75 mg/kg), and their body temperature was maintained at 37°C with a heating pad. Acoustic stimuli were delivered using an electrostatic speaker (Fostex FT28D Dome Tweeter; Madisound, Middleton, WI, United States), positioned 10 cm in front of the mouse head. The

ABR was recorded with three subdermal electrodes: the recording electrode was inserted at the vertex of the skull, while the reference and grounding electrodes were positioned separately on the mastoid region of the two sides. The biological signals collected by the electrodes were led to a RA4PA preamplifier from Tucker-Davis Technologies (TDT System III; Alachua, FL, United States). Stimulus generation and biosignal acquisition were conducted processed by using the RZ6 BioAMP Processor (TDT System III; Tucker-Davis Technologies, Alachua, FL, United States). Parameters were similar to those used in our previous study (Fan et al., 2020; Zhang et al., 2020). Briefly, the signal of acoustic stimuli is TB for 10 ms at 0.5 ms rise/fall time, and 21.1/s stimulation rate, starting from 90 to 0 dB SPL in decreasing steps of 5 or 10 dB. The ABR threshold was defined as the lowest level of stimulus that yielded a repeatable waveform.

Cell Culture and Hydrogen Peroxide Treatment of HEI-OC1 Cells

HEI-OC1, an inner ear cell line, was purchased from UCLA Technology Development Group (Los Angeles, CA, United States) and cultivated in Dulbecco's modified Eagle's medium (Gibco, United States) supplemented with 10% fetal bovine serum (FBS) (Performance Plus; 16000-044; Gibco) and 10 mg/mL ampicillin sodium solution (sterile) (B540722; Sangon Biotech, Shanghai, China) at 33°C in a humidified 5% CO_2 atmosphere. After 24 h, cells were grown to 70–80% confluency, and the regular medium was exchanged for medium with or without hydrogen peroxide.

Morphology

Mice were anesthetized and decapitated following the ABR recording at the end point. Both the left and right temporal bones were carefully removed, and the bulla was opened to expose the cochlea. The cochleae were perfused locally with a solution of 4% paraformaldehyde in PBS (pH 7.4) and kept in this fixative for 2 h at 4°C, then rinsed with PBS, and decalcified in 10% sodium EDTA solution (adjusted with HCl to pH 7.4) overnight at 4°C. The cochlea of one side was dissected under a microscope, whereas that of the other side was immersed in 15% sucrose solution for 2 h, followed by overnight immersion in sucrose (30%) at 4°C. Cochleae were embedded in optimal cutting temperature compound (OCT), frozen at −80°C, and cryosectioned at a thickness of 12 μm using a cryostat microtome (Leica CM1860, Leica Biosystems Nussloch GmbH, Nussloch, Germany). Sections were processed at the same time for all staining procedures. All slides and the basilar membrane were washed with PBS, incubated in 1% TritonX-100 for 1 h, and immersed in 5% goat serum for 1 h at 25°C and then in primary antibodies at 4°C overnight. Primary antibodies used included: monoclonal rabbit anti-HMGB1 Ig-G (1:200; ab79823, Abcam) and monoclonal mouse anti-beta III tubulin Ig-G (1:200; ab78078, Abcam). Subsequently, they were incubated with either Alexa-Fluor-488 goat anti-rabbit Ig-G (H + L) (1:500; Invitrogen, Carlsbad, CA, United States) or Alexa-Fluor-555 goat anti-mouse Ig-G (H + L) (1:500; Invitrogen) at 25°C for 2 h in darkness, followed by incubation with DAPI (ab104139, Abcam) for 5 min, and then their edges were sealed with nail polish.

Cells were cultured in coverslips and subjected to different treatments. After removing the culture medium, cells were rinsed twice with PBS, fixed with 4% paraformaldehyde for 15–20 min, and then permeabilized with 0.5% TritonX-100 for 40 min. Subsequently, cells were blocked with 5% normal goat serum for 1 h at 25°C, followed by incubation with primary HMGB1 rabbit monoclonal antibody (1:200 in PBS; Abcam) overnight at 4°C. After three washes in PBS, cells were incubated in the dark with Alexa Fluor 488-conjugated goat anti-rabbit IgG (H + L) (1:500 in PBS; Invitrogen) for 2 h at 25°C. After four washes with PBS (30 min each), cells were also stained with Phalloidin iFlour 555 reagent (1:5,000 in PBS; Abcam) for 10 min, to mark cell structure. After rinsing in PBS, specimens were immersed for 5 min in fresh DAPI solution in the dark to label the nuclei of cells. Immunocytochemistry images of basal turn in each cochlear sample and HEI-OC1 cells were taken under a 20× and 63× magnification lens respectively with identical Z-stack conditions using a confocal laser-scanning microscope (LSM 710 META; Zeiss, Shanghai, China) and analyzed using the ZEN 2011 software (Zeiss, Oberkochen, Germany).

Cell Vitality Assay

Cultured HEI-OC1 cells were plated in each well of a 96-well plate in five copies. After attachment, cells were treated with a gradient concentration of H_2O_2 (0.1, 0.2, 0.5, and 1.0 mM) for 4, 8, 12, and 24 h. Following treatment, cells were incubated for 2 h with Cell Counting Kit 8 (CCK-8) reagent (100 μL/mL, MCE, Shanghai, China) at 37°C for 2 h, according to the manufacturer's protocol. Absorbance was measured at 450 nm using a microplate reader (Bio-Rad), with results being normalized to untreated blank control cells (100%).

Small Interfering RNA Gene Silencing

The expression of HMGB1 was knocked down by transfection with candidate HMGB1 small interfering RNA (siRNA) (DNABIO; Shanghai, China). Cells were seeded at 2 × 10^5 cells per well in a six-well plate the day before transfection. Cells were transfected in 2 mL of culture medium containing 5 μL of HMGB1 siRNA or non-targeting control siRNA using Lipofectamine 3,000 in Opti-MEM medium (Invitrogen, Carlsbad, CA, United States), following the manufacturer's protocol. After 48 h of transfection, cells were treated as designated. The sequence of siRNA-1 targeting of the mice HMGB1 gene was sense 5′-CCUCAUAUGCAUUCUUUGUTT-3′ and antisense 5′-ACAAAGAAUGCAUAUGAGGAC-3′. The sequence of siRNA-2 was sense 5′-GCUGAAAAGAGCAAGAAAATT-3′ and antisense 5′-UUUUCUUGCUCUUUUCAGCCT-3′.

Western Blotting

The total protein of cell and cochlea samples was extracted using RIPA lysis buffer (EpiZyme; Shanghai; China). The concentration of each protein sample was quantified using a BCA protein assay kit (EpiZyme). Protein samples (30–40 μg) were subjected to 12.5% polyacrylamide gel electrophoresis and then transferred onto a nitrocellulose membrane (Pierce) and blocked with 5% non-fat milk in EZ Buffer H 1 × TBST Buffer (Sangon Biotech; Shanghai, China) for 1 h. The membranes were washed and then incubated with various primary antibodies (1:30,000 rabbit monoclonal anti-HMGB1, Abcam; 1:1,000 rabbit polyclonal anti-caspase 3, CST) at 4°C overnight. After three washes with TBST (1×), membranes were incubated with appropriate secondary antibodies (1:5,000) for 2 h at 25°C. Following extensive rinsing of membranes, the immunoreactive bands were detected using a chemiluminescence imaging system (Bio-Rad). GAPDH (CST, 1:3,000) was used as a sample loading internal control. Bands were quantified using the ImageJ software (National Institutes of Health, Bethesda, MD, United States).

Statistical Analysis

All data were expressed as the mean ± SD. ANOVAs followed by *post hoc* testing (Holm-Sidak's method) were performed using SigmaPlot (ver. 14; Systat Software Inc., San Jose, CA, United States). In all analyses, a value of $p < 0.05$ was considered statistically significant.

RESULTS

Shift of ABR Threshold and Level of HMGB1

Figure 1 shows the shifts in the ABR threshold and the expression of HMGB1 in the cochlea at different time points after NE. For the ABR result (**Figure 1A**), two-way ANOVA followed by *post hoc* tests were performed for each group. We observed a significant threshold shift as demonstrated by the effect in time points after NE ($F_{3,60} = 21.214$, $p < 0.001$). *Post hoc* pairwise tests showed a significant elevation of the ABR threshold shift at 4 kHz in the 1-day post-noise exposure (1dPNE) group as compared with those in the 3dPNE, 7dPNE, and 14dPNE groups (t = 4.286, 6.231, 9.710, respectively, $p < 0.001$), as well as at 8 kHz with only the 14dPNE group ($t = 3.109$, $p = 0.017$).

Correspondingly, we evaluated the level of total cochlear HMGB1 using western blot analysis and revealed its significance for each group by performing one-way ANOVA ($F_{4,10} = 14.622$, $p < 0.001$). *Post hoc* pairwise tests showed a significant increase in the 7dPNE and 14dPNE groups compared with the control ($t = 5.324$, $p = 0.003$; $t = 3.45$, $p = 0.037$, respectively) and 1dPNE ($t = 6.815$, $p < 0.001$; $t = 4.941$, $p = 0.005$, respectively) groups. We found that the level of HMGB1 increased significantly in the 3dPNE group ($t = 3.706$, $p = 0.028$) but not in the 1dPNE group ($t = 1.874$, $p = 0.315$) compared with the control group. Furthermore, no significance was demonstrated across the 3dPNE, 7dPNE, and 14dPNE groups, suggesting that the level of total cochlear HMGB1 was gradually increased toward a plateau 3 days after NE.

Cellular Expression of HMGB1 in the Basilar Membrane

To investigate the cellular expression of HMGB1 in the cochlea, we performed immunofluorescence experiments. We detected the strong dense optical HMGB1 labeling in the nuclei of all cells examined in this study. **Figure 2** showed distribution of optical density of HMGB1 labeling in the basal turn from the cochlear basilar membrane at different confocal levels in the control, 1dPNE, 3dPNE, and 7dPNE groups. The absence of outer hair cells (OHCs) presented in **Figures 2B′–D′** indicated an irreversible damage caused by NE. Correspondingly, we noted that the arrangement of Deiters cells (DCs) seemed to be disordered in the 7dPNE group because of the increased absence of OHCs. In this study, we mainly focused on several specific confocal levels of immunostaining.

We observed the punctuate labeling of extranuclear HMGB1 in the basilar membrane of all groups, but with a variety of distribution at different confocal levels. We also evaluated the number of punctate labeling in three regions: DCs, OHCs, and inner sulcus (IS) cells. Using one-way ANOVA, we overall detected significant differences in the OHC ($F_{3,12} = 21.26$, $p < 0.001$) and IS cell ($F_{3,12} = 8.314$, $p = 0.003$) regions, but not in the DC region ($F_{3,12} = 1.2$, $p = 0.352$) across groups. We further found that at the OHC level, the number of punctate HMGB1 labeling was significantly increased in the 1dPNE ($t = 4.892$, $p = 0.001$) and 3dPNE ($t = 3.805$, $p = 0.008$) groups compared with the control group. In contrast, it was drastically decreased in the 7dPNE group. When compared with the control group, the number of punctate labeling at the IS level was demonstrated to be significantly elevated following NE at the 1dPNE ($t = 3.358$, $p = 0.02$), 3dPNE ($t = 3.213$, $p = 0.029$), and 7dPNE ($t = 4.389$, $p = 0.002$) groups.

We then investigated the pattern of expression of HMGB1 in the region of OHC and DCs after NE. Interestingly, we observed a specific expression pattern of HMGB1 in both OHC and DCs, as demonstrated in images obtained with the same confocal parameters of samples prepared with the same process (**Figure 3A**). We found that the level of HMGB1 in the OHC region was not evident in the control group, whereas it was shown to subsequently increase to a predominate level at 3dPNE (**Figure 3A**). Regarding DCs, we noted that the dense labeling of HMGB1 was gradually increased toward a plateau at 3dPNE but was then relatively decreased at 7dPNE.

Expression of HMGB1 in the Non-organ of Corti Tissues

Apart from the region of the organ of Corti, we also observed and compared the distinctive expression of HMGB1 in the spiral limbus (**Figure 3B**), spiral ligament (**Figure 3C**), and spiral ganglion cells (SGNs) region (**Figure 4**) at different time points after acoustic trauma. We observed a higher optical labeling density in both the spiral limbus and spiral ligament after NE. Furthermore, we quantitatively measured the average fluorescence density (AFD) of HMGB1 in the spiral ligament region due to its possible essential role in the inflammatory response. Accordingly, using one-way ANOVA we demonstrated a significant difference across groups ($F_{3,8} = 16.966$, $p < 0.001$). A significant elevation of AFD was observed in the 7dPNE group when compared with the AFD of the control ($t = 7.039$, $p < 0.001$), 1dPNE ($t = 4.082$, $p = 0.014$), and 3dPNE ($t = 2.919$, $p = 0.038$), respectively. In addition, the AFD of the 3dPNE group was also shown to be

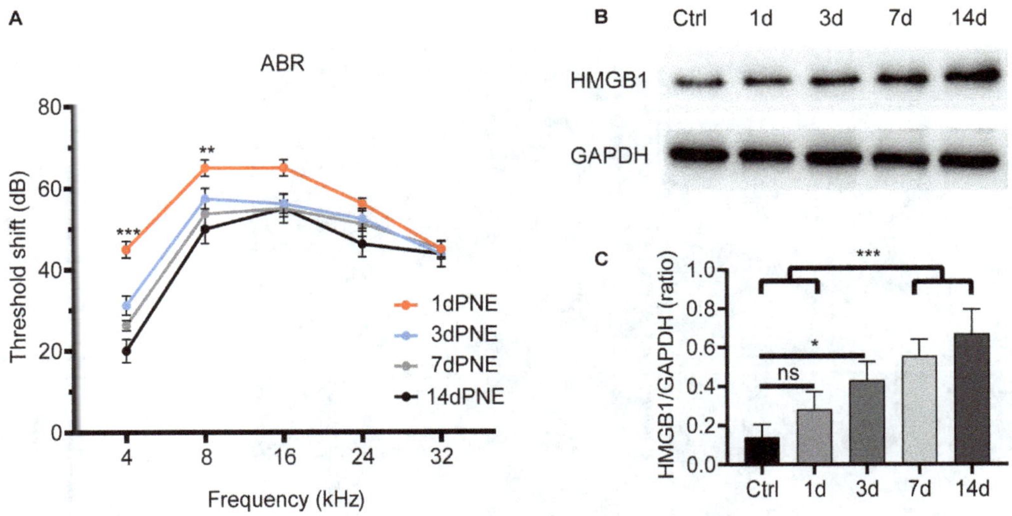

FIGURE 1 | Shift of ABR threshold and total cochlear level of HMGB1 at different time points after noise exposure. **(A)** Threshold shifts (±SD) at 1, 3, 7, and 14 day-PNE (4–22 kHz broadband noise at 110 dB SPL for 2 h). **(B)** Gradual increase in the expression of HMGB1 in the cochlea after noise exposure. **(C)** Densitometry analysis of total HMGB1 band densities normalized to GAPDH confirmed a significant increase in HMGB1 after noise trauma. Data **(C)** is presented as means ± SD, $n = 3$ in each group. PNE, post-noise exposure. $^{*}p < 0.05$, $^{**}p < 0.01$, and $^{***}p < 0.001$ were significant levels of the difference between groups; "ns", no significant.

significantly higher than that of the control group ($t = 4.12$, $p = 0.017$).

We did not observe any evidently increased optical density of HMGB1 in the SGN region, across all groups (**Figure 4**). By specifically labeling the cytoplasm of SGNs for tubulin (red), we could distinguish SGNs and identify their borders from surrounding cells, such as glial cells, as indicated in previous studies (Fang et al., 2018; Liu et al., 2020). The expression of HMGB1 in SGNs was shown to be mainly located in the nucleus and not in the cytoplasm, consistent with two previous reports but contradicting to the results of another study (Ladrech et al., 2017; Fang et al., 2018; Liu et al., 2020). Intriguingly, the proportion of glial cells with a high density of optical HMGB1 was shown to be increased in a time interval-dependent manner post-NE, peaking in the 7dPNE group (white arrows pointed in **Figure 4**). Moreover, the magnified view in the right corner of the merged image shows the possible evolution of the spatial expression of HMGB1 between SGNs and glial cells. We further noted the continuity of HMGB1 immunostaining across SGNs and glial cells in the 3dPNE group, indicating a possible translocation of HMGB1 across them (**Figure 4C‴**).

Impact of HMGB1 Knockdown on the Viability of HEI-OC1 Cells

The HEI-OC1 cell line is known to preserve the specific cell biology of OHCs and it was employed here to explore the underlying molecular mechanisms after acoustic trauma using a gene manipulation method. First, we confirmed the viability of HEI-OC1 cells using the CCK8 test at different time points after stimulation with different concentrations of H_2O_2 (**Figure 5A**). Based on these, 0.5 mM H_2O_2 was identified as the appropriate condition in the following experiments. We accordingly evaluated the level of HMGB1 at 4, 8, and 12 h after treatment with H_2O_2. We performed a one-way ANOVA followed by *post hoc* tests for each group and found that no significant intergroup differences were observed ($F_{3,8} = 1.254$, $p = 0.353$).

As can be observed in the immunostaining image (**Figure 5B**), however, HMGB1 was found to be extensively translocated from the nucleus to the cytoplasm 8 h after stimulation with H_2O_2. The edge of the cell membrane outlined by staining with phalloidin indicated that HMGB1 might be released from the cell before cell disintegration. More importantly, it is worth noting that the overall changes in cell morphology were shown to be quite different at this time. We observed varying degrees of vesicular-like budding that might have been related to the apoptosis or death process in HEI-OC1 cells. Interestingly, at 12 h, most cells were demonstrated to revert to their typical structure, with HMGB1 being redistributed within the nucleus.

Using western blotting, we identified target siRNAs for further knockdown of HMGB1 (**Figure 5D**). Subsequently, we investigated the effect of HMGB1 knockdown on cell viability in the HEI-OC1 oxidative stress model (**Figure 5E**). We found that compared with the control group and the siRNA-HMGB1 group, the cell viability in groups pretreated with H_2O_2 was significantly reduced ($p < 0.001$). However, the group with the HMGB1 knockdown was demonstrated to significantly preserve a higher cell viability compared with the H_2O_2 and the H_2O_2 (siRNA-negative control) groups ($p < 0.001$).

DISCUSSION

Here, we demonstrated the spatiotemporal dynamics of the expression of HMGB1 in the cochlea after NE. We found that the total level of cochlear HMGB1 was gradually increased

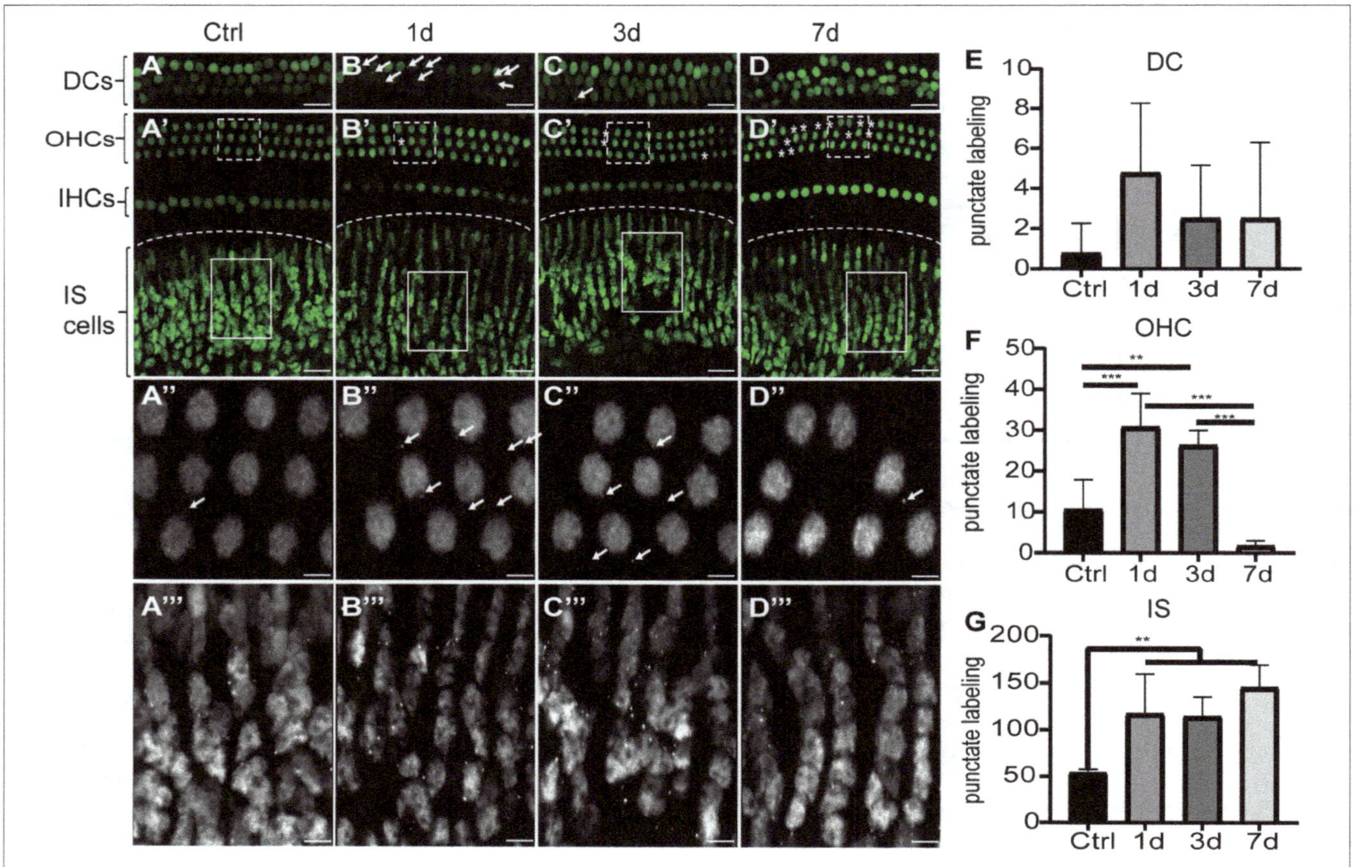

FIGURE 2 | Distribution of optical density of HMGB1 labeling in the basal turn from the cochlear basilar membrane. **(A–D)** Representative images of HMGB1 immunostaining at different confocal levels in the control, 1dPNE, 3dPNE, and 7dPNE groups, respectively. **(E–G)** Quantification of punctate labeling in DCs, OHC, and IS, respectively. White arrows point to the optical HMGB1-immunostained particles. Asterisks represent missed OHCs. Square regions with dash and solid line are magnified below. DCs, Deiters cells; OHCs, outer hair cells; IHCs, inner hair cells; IS cells, inner sulcus cells. All data are presented as means ± SD, $n = 3$ in each group. Scale bars 20 μm **(A–D,A′–D′)**, 5 μm **(A″–D″,A‴–D‴)**. $^{**}p < 0.01$, $^{***}p < 0.001$.

following NE, exhibiting however a distribution variability in specific cochlear regions and cells. Specifically, noise induced a robust accumulation of HMGB1 in the spiral ligament, but not in the region of SGNs, which coincided with the cochlear level as tested by western blotting. In contrast, despite the extranuclear punctate labeling for HMGB1 revealing a varying distribution, we observed that HMGB1 was primarily located in the nuclei of cochlear cells. In addition, we noted the occurrence of a temporary translocation of HMGB1 from the nucleus to the cytoplasm as well as the extracellular space, in HEI-OC1 cells 8 h after treatment with H_2O_2. However, nuclear retention of HMGB1 was shown to recur at 12 h after treatment with H_2O_2, following the completion of apoptotic processes.

Accompanying the activation of the innate immune system in noise-induced cochlear pathologies, HMGB1 might play an essential role as a mediator of inflammation by alarming of the induced cell damage (Tang et al., 2012; Yang et al., 2013; Wood and Zuo, 2017; Frye et al., 2019; He et al., 2020). As a representative DAMP, the biological activity of HMGB1 is known to depend on its location and its interaction with cytokines or other exogenous and endogenous molecules (Andersson and Tracey, 2011). Its dynamic translocation from the nucleus with a state binding DNA to the cytoplasm or extracellular context has been reported to depend on cell activation, injury, or death (Ueda and Yoshida, 2010). In the present study, we investigated the rare high dense extracellular distribution of HMGB1 following NE, even at the local point of absent scattered OHCs. The main reason behind this finding could be the characteristic deposition of HMGB1, which might vary among necrotic and apoptotic cells. Breaking-down cell permeability could facilitate the passive release of HMGB1 from necrotic cells; however, under apoptotic conditions, maintaining nuclear retention of HMGB1 would be necessary for chromatin binding through posttranslational modifications (Scaffidi et al., 2002; Rovere-Querini et al., 2004; Bell et al., 2006; Kazama et al., 2008). Importantly, OHCs are known to be vulnerable to damage induced by excessive noise, with apoptosis appearing to be the most common mechanism of OHC loss (Morrill and He, 2017). Therefore, the release of HMGB1 from the nucleus of OHCs was shown to be highly restricted after acoustic injury. Alternately, a possibility exists that the translocation behavior of HMGB1 could be a temporary process, indicating that more

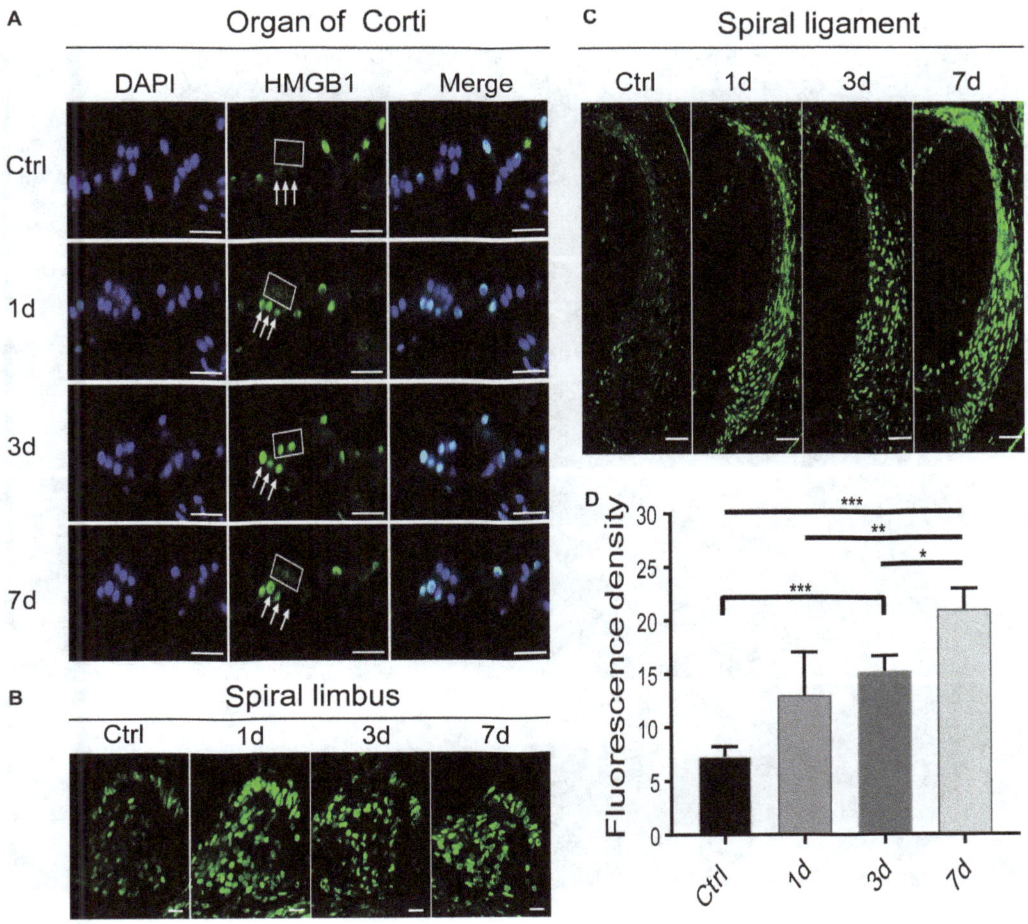

FIGURE 3 | Spatiotemporal dynamics of HMGB1 at the organ of Corti **(A)**, spiral limbus **(B)**, and spiral ligament **(C)** in the basal turn of cochlea after acoustic trauma. The square and arrows in panel **(A)** identify the region of outer hair cells and Deiters cells, respectively. **(D)** Quantitative measurement of average fluorescence density (AFD) in the spiral ligament of panel **(C)**. Data is presented as means ± SD, $n = 3$ in each group. Scale bars 50 μm **(C)**, 20 μm **(A,B)**. $^{*}p < 0.05$, $^{**}p < 0.01$, and $^{***}p < 0.001$.

sensitive and intensive detection methodology might be required for the observation of its dynamic distribution (Gaillard et al., 2008). This was consistent with our results here revealing the presence of a high density of HMGB1 in the cytoplasm of HEI-OC1 cells at 8 h that disappeared at 12 h after treatment with H_2O_2. Furthermore, we evaluated the changes in the expression level of caspase-3 by western blotting. There was a sharp elevation at 12 h after treatment with H_2O_2, indicating an extensive activation of apoptosis, potentially explaining the molecular event of the retention of HMGB1 in the nucleus (Bell et al., 2006).

Maintaining the structural and functional integrity of the basilar membrane in the cochlea, is known to require a highly orchestrated process for the elimination of damaged OHCs (Hu et al., 2018; Li et al., 2018b; Zhou et al., 2020). This process has been shown to always involve the activation of neighbor cells or professional scavengers, such as macrophages. Although the organ of Corti lacks immune cells, the cochlear resident cells, particularly DCs, are known to preserve their phagocytic activity responding to damaged OHCs (Abrashkin et al., 2006; Du et al., 2011; Yang et al., 2015b). This was supported by strong piece of evidence showing that prestin immunopositive fragments of OHCs were located inside the cytoplasm of DCs (Abrashkin et al., 2006). However, the mechanism by which DCs detect the injury of OHCs remains unclear. Ladrech et al. proposed that DCs might regulate the remodeling of the aminoglycoside-injured organ of Corti by releasing HMGB1 (Ladrech et al., 2013). This hypothesis was strongly supported in immunoelectron microscopy experiments, by the detection of HMGB1 particles encapsulated within cytoplasmic membrane-bound vesicles inside DCs. More importantly, these vesicles were labeled as specific markers of processing secretion, indicating the function of DCs to initiatively secrete HMGB1 (Ladrech et al., 2013). In our present study, we found that the density of optical HMGB1 labeling was drastically increased in DCs after acoustic trauma, especially in the 1dPNE group. Overall, the spatiotemporal dynamics of the distribution of HMGB1 in the organ of Corti suggested a specific pattern of immune

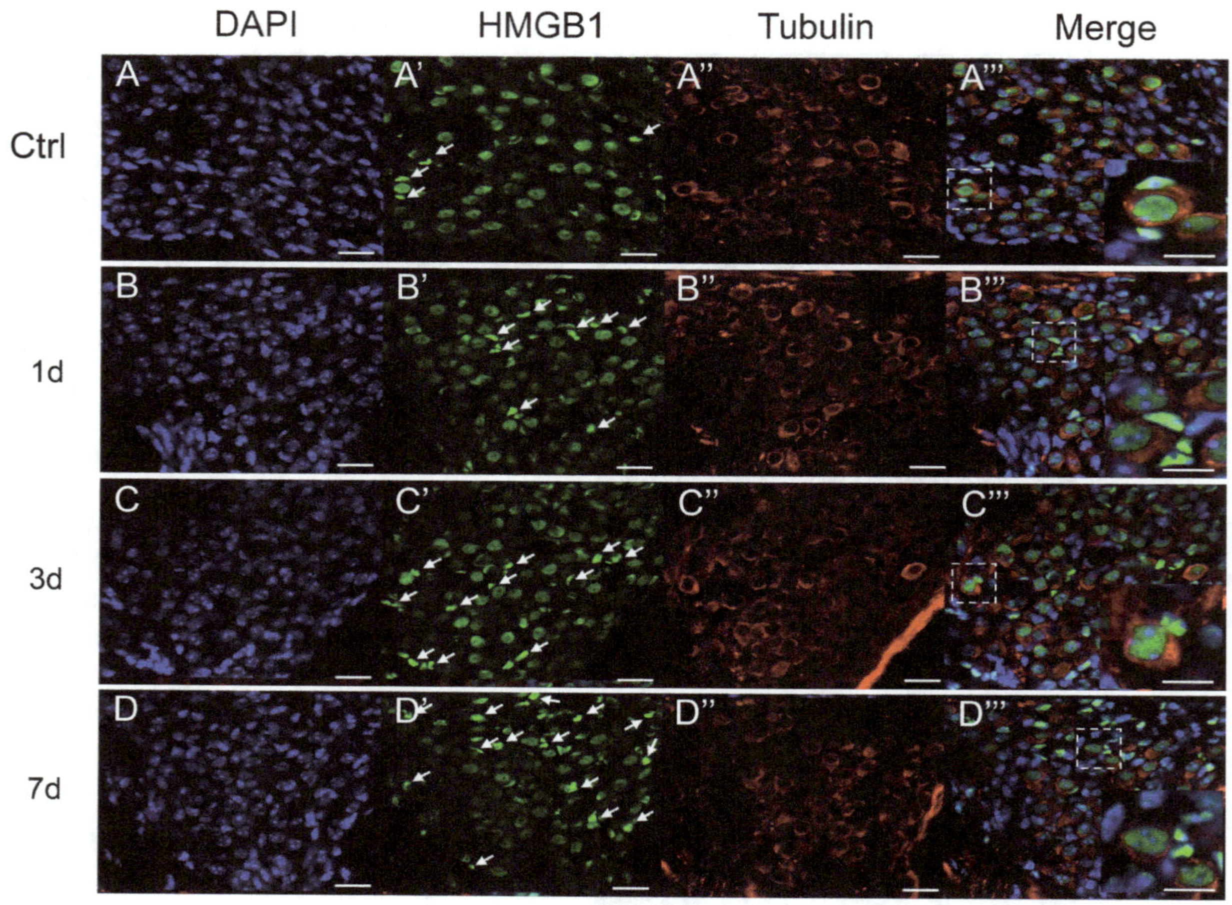

FIGURE 4 | Representative images of immunostaining against HMGB1 (Green) in the SGN region. All images were taken from the cochlear basal turn. White arrows point to glial cells surrounding SGNs with evidently higher density of optical HMGB1. The square region in the merged picture depicts the distribution of HMGB1 in SGNs and glial cells, and is magnified at the right corner. The cytoplasm of SGNs was specifically labeled for tubulin (red), and nuclei were labeled with DAPI (blue). Scale bars 20 μm **(A–D,A′–D′,A′′–D′′)**, 10 μm **(A′′′–D′′′)**.

activity involving DCs, which might exert a direct impact on the pathogenesis of OHCs after acoustic trauma.

Apart from the organ of Corti, the level of HMGB1 was also tested in non-organ of Corti tissues including spiral limbus, spiral ligament, and SGNs. The density of optical labeling of HMGB1 was found to be greatly increased in the spiral ligament, but not SGNs. In the SGN region, the number of glial cells with high level of HMGB1 was demonstrated to be increased in the 3dPNE group, indicating a possible intercellular event between SGN and glial cells. In the spiral ligament, we found that the tendency of AFD elevated (**Figures 3C,D**), which was consistent with the change in the total cochlear level of HMGB1 (**Figure 1B**). Necroptosis-, ferroptosis-, apoptosis- and pyroptosis-mediated mechanism have all been implicated in HMGB1 release from cells (Scaffidi et al., 2002; Bell et al., 2006; Murai et al., 2018; Wen et al., 2019; Volchuk et al., 2020). Specifically, as a marker of cellular damage, the increasing HMGB1 level or the release of HMGB1 in the spiral ligament indicated the activation of cell death pathways. In previous studies, noise-induced apoptosis and necroptosis in the spiral ligament cells have been elucidated, but the pyroptosis and ferroptosis have not been verified and might cause the HMGB1 release here (Wang et al., 2019; Wu et al., 2020). Therefore, our future work will focus on defining HMGB1 sources and secretion pathways in this region during noise-induced inflammation.

In the present study, our *in vitro* experiments showed that knocking down the HMGB1 gene could protect HEI-OC1 cells against hydrogen peroxide stress damage (**Figure 5**), indicating potential therapeutic approaches to prevent NIHL. However, it might not be an optimal approach to manipulate the expression of HMGB1 due to its intracellular functions, such as acting as a critical pro-autophagic protein that enhances cell survival and limits programmed apoptotic cell death (Tang et al., 2010, 2011; New and Thomas, 2019). Moreover, enhancing the autophagic flux has been shown to prevent the cochlea from acoustic injury and reduce the percentage of absent OHCs (Yuan et al., 2015). Therefore, the critical point of any potential therapeutic strategy of NIHL targeting HMGB1 should avoid affecting its positive intracellular functions. Recently, treatments based on antagonists that specifically inhibit the release of

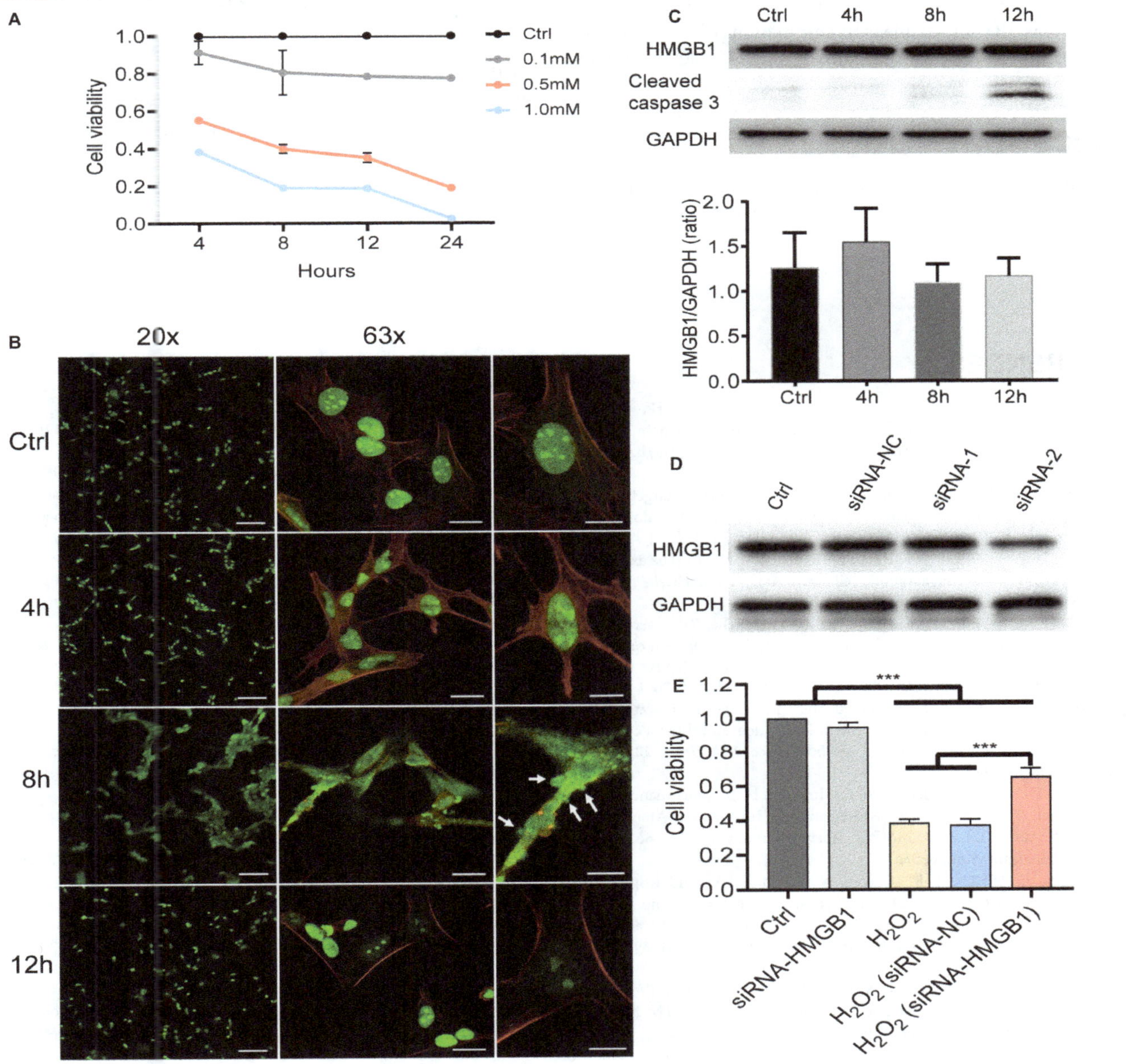

FIGURE 5 | Molecular behavior of HMGB1 and its impact on cell viability *in vitro*. **(A)** Cell viability of HEI-OC1 at 4, 8, 12, and 24 h after stimulation with gradient concentration (0.1, 0.5, and 1 mM) of H_2O_2. Data **(A)** is presented as means ± SD, $n = 3$ in each group. **(B)** Representative images of immunostaining against HMGB1 from low to high field of view of samples pretreated with 0.5 mM H_2O_2 (green: HMGB1; red: phalloidin). **(C)** Level of HMGB1 and caspase-3 at different time points in cells treated with 0.5 mM H_2O_2. Data **(C)** is presented as means ± SD, $n = 3$ in each group. **(D)** Screening result of two candidate siRNAs on knocking down HMGB1. **(E)** Impact of HMGB1 knockdown on the viability of HEI-OC1 cells 8 h after treatment with H_2O_2 (0.5 mM). Data **(E)** is presented as means ± SD, $n = 6$ in each group. Scale bars 100 μm (**B** left panel), 20 μm (**B** middle panel), 10 μm (**B** right panel). $^{***}p < 0.001$.

HMGB1 or extracellular action of HMGB1 have been released. For example, an anti-HMGB1 monoclonal antibody (mAb) has been developed and was shown to be effective in treating many animal models of central nervous system (CNS) diseases, such as Parkinson's disease, Alzheimer's disease, and stroke (Yang et al., 2015b).

Nevertheless, an approach of inhibiting the activities of proinflammatory mediators, such as HMGB1, to treat inflammation-induced diseases might have some considerable challenges: (1) targeting HMGB1 might not be sufficient to obtain significant beneficial results because of homologous molecules playing the same role as HMGB1 in the inflammatory process; (2) triggering a compensatory immune response involving an alternative pathway after inhibiting the extracellular function of HMGB1; (3) risks associated with weakening of a natural defense mechanism in the cochlea (Tabas and Glass, 2013). Furthermore, we still need further *in vivo* experiments to confirm the specific role of HMGB1 in cochlear inflammation in order to fully elucidate the underlying mechanism and be able to intervene to prevent NIHL.

ETHICS STATEMENT

The animal study was reviewed and approved by the Ethics Committee of the Shanghai Jiao Tong University Affiliated Sixth People's Hospital.

AUTHOR CONTRIBUTIONS

LXiao and YSu conducted the experiment, wrote the manuscript, and analyzed the data. LXia, GY, and YF designed the experiment. CL, ZZ, and YSh interpreted the data. All authors have read and approved the final manuscript.

REFERENCES

Abrashkin, K. A., Izumikawa, M., Miyazawa, T., Wang, C. H., Crumling, M. A., Swiderski, D. L., et al. (2006). The fate of outer hair cells after acoustic or ototoxic insults. *Hear Res.* 218, 20–29. doi: 10.1016/j.heares.2006.04.001

Andersson, U., and Tracey, K. J. (2011). HMGB1 is a therapeutic target for sterile inflammation and infection. *Annu. Rev. Immunol.* 29, 139–162. doi: 10.1146/annurev-immunol-030409-101323

Bell, C. W., Jiang, W., Reich, C. F. III, and Pisetsky, D. S. (2006). The extracellular release of HMGB1 during apoptotic cell death. *Am. J. Physiol. Cell Physiol.* 291, C1318–C1325. doi: 10.1152/ajpcell.00616.2005

Bianchi, M. E., Crippa, M. P., Manfredi, A. A., Mezzapelle, R., Rovere Querini, P., and Venereau, E. (2017). High-mobility group box 1 protein orchestrates responses to tissue damage via inflammation, innate and adaptive immunity, and tissue repair. *Immunol. Rev.* 280, 74–82. doi: 10.1111/imr.12601

Calogero, S., Grassi, F., Aguzzi, A., Voigtländer, T., Ferrier, P., Ferrari, S., et al. (1999). The lack of chromosomal protein Hmg1 does not disrupt cell growth but causes lethal hypoglycaemia in newborn mice. *Nat. Genet.* 22, 276–280. doi: 10.1038/10338

Carroll, Y. I., Eichwald, J., Scinicariello, F., Hoffman, H. J., Deitchman, S., Radke, M. S., et al. (2017). Vital Signs: Noise-Induced Hearing Loss Among Adults - United States 2011-2012. *MMWR Morb. Mortal. Wkly Rep.* 66, 139–144. doi: 10.15585/mmwr.mm6605e3

Du, X., Choi, C. H., Chen, K., Cheng, W., Floyd, R. A., and Kopke, R. D. (2011). Reduced formation of oxidative stress biomarkers and migration of mononuclear phagocytes in the cochleae of chinchilla after antioxidant treatment in acute acoustic trauma. *Int. J. Otolaryngol.* 2011:612690. doi: 10.1155/2011/612690

Fan, L., Zhang, Z., Wang, H., Li, C., Xing, Y., Yin, S., et al. (2020). Pre-exposure to Lower-Level Noise Mitigates Cochlear Synaptic Loss Induced by High-Level Noise. *Front. Syst. Neurosci.* 14:25. doi: 10.3389/fnsys.2020.00025

Fang, J., Xing, Y., Chen, H., Yin, S., Shi, H., and Su, K. (2018). Distribution of High Mobility Group Box 1 in Cochlea in C57BL/6J Mice. *Chinese J. Otol.* 16, 888–893.

Frye, M. D., Ryan, A. F., and Kurabi, A. (2019). Inflammation associated with noise-induced hearing loss. *J. Acoustical Soc. Am.* 146, 4020–4032. doi: 10.1121/1.5132545

Gaillard, C., Borde, C., Gozlan, J., Maréchal, V., and Strauss, F. (2008). A high-sensitivity method for detection and measurement of HMGB1 protein concentration by high-affinity binding to DNA hemicatenanes. *PLoS One* 3:e2855. doi: 10.1371/journal.pone.0002855

Gao, S., Cheng, C., Wang, M., Jiang, P., Zhang, L., Wang, Y., et al. (2019). Blebbistatin Inhibits Neomycin-Induced Apoptosis in Hair Cell-Like HEI-OC-1 Cells and in Cochlear Hair Cells. *Front. Cell Neurosci.* 13:590. doi: 10.3389/fncel.2019.00590

Harris, H. E., Andersson, U., and Pisetsky, D. S. (2012). HMGB1: a multifunctional alarmin driving autoimmune and inflammatory disease. *Nat. Rev. Rheumatol.* 8, 195–202. doi: 10.1038/nrrheum.2011.222

He, Z., Guo, L., Shu, Y., Fang, Q., Zhou, H., Liu, Y., et al. (2017). Autophagy protects auditory hair cells against neomycin-induced damage. *Autophagy* 13, 1884–1904. doi: 10.1080/15548627.2017.1359449

He, Z., Sun, S., Waqas, M., Zhang, X., Qian, F., Cheng, C., et al. (2016). Reduced TRMU expression increases the sensitivity of hair-cell-like HEI-OC-1 cells to neomycin damage in vitro. *Sci. Rep.* 6:29621. doi: 10.1038/srep29621

He, Z. H., Zou, S. Y., Li, M., Liao, F. L., Wu, X., Sun, H. Y., et al. (2020). The nuclear transcription factor FoxG1 affects the sensitivity of mimetic aging hair cells to inflammation by regulating autophagy pathways. *Redox Biol.* 28:101364. doi: 10.1016/j.redox.2019.101364

Hu, B. H., Zhang, C., and Frye, M. D. (2018). Immune cells and non-immune cells with immune function in mammalian cochleae. *Hear Res.* 362, 14–24. doi: 10.1016/j.heares.2017.12.009

Kalinec, G. M., Lomberk, G., Urrutia, R. A., and Kalinec, F. (2017). Resolution of Cochlear Inflammation: Novel Target for Preventing or Ameliorating Drug-. Noise Age-related Hearing Loss. *Front. Cell Neurosci.* 11:192. doi: 10.3389/fncel.2017.00192

Kazama, H., Ricci, J. E., Herndon, J. M., Hoppe, G., Green, D. R., and Ferguson, T. A. (2008). Induction of immunological tolerance by apoptotic cells requires caspase-dependent oxidation of high-mobility group box-1 protein. *Immunity* 29, 21–32. doi: 10.1016/j.immuni.2008.05.013

Ladrech, S., Mathieu, M., Puel, J. L., and Lenoir, M. (2013). Supporting cells regulate the remodelling of aminoglycoside-injured organ of Corti, through the release of high mobility group box 1. *Eur. J. Neurosci.* 38, 2962–2972. doi: 10.1111/ejn.12290

Ladrech, S., Wang, J., Mathieu, M., Puel, J. L., and Lenoir, M. (2017). High mobility group box 1 (HMGB1): dual functions in the cochlear auditory neurons in response to stress? *Histochem. Cell Biol.* 147, 307–316. doi: 10.1007/s00418-016-1506-8

Lang, H., Nishimoto, E., Xing, Y., Brown, L. N., Noble, K. V., Barth, J. L., et al. (2016). Contributions of Mouse and Human Hematopoietic Cells to Remodeling of the Adult Auditory Nerve After Neuron Loss. *Mol. Ther.* 24, 2000–2011. doi: 10.1038/mt.2016.174

Li, A., You, D., Li, W., Cui, Y., He, Y., Li, W., et al. (2018a). Novel compounds protect auditory hair cells against gentamycin-induced apoptosis by maintaining the expression level of H3K4me2. *Drug Deliv.* 25, 1033–1043. doi: 10.1080/10717544.2018.1461277

Li, H., Song, Y., He, Z., Chen, X., Wu, X., Li, X., et al. (2018b). Meclofenamic Acid Reduces Reactive Oxygen Species Accumulation and Apoptosis, Inhibits Excessive Autophagy, and Protects Hair Cell-Like HEI-OC1 Cells From Cisplatin-Induced Damage. *Front. Cell Neurosci.* 12:139. doi: 10.3389/fncel.2018.00139

Liu, W., Ding, X., Wang, X., and Yang, J. (2020). Expression and Distribution of High Mobility Group Box 1 (HMGB1) during Cochlear Development in Postnatal Mice. *Chinese J. Otol.* 18, 545–551.

Liu, Y., Qi, J., Chen, X., Tang, M., Chu, C., Zhu, W., et al. (2019). Critical role of spectrin in hearing development and deafness. *Sci. Adv.* 5:eaav7803. doi: 10.1126/sciadv.aav7803

Morrill, S., and He, D. Z. Z. (2017). Apoptosis in inner ear sensory hair cells. *J. Otol.* 12, 151–164. doi: 10.1016/j.joto.2017.08.001

Murai, S., Yamaguchi, Y., Shirasaki, Y., Yamagishi, M., Shindo, R., Hildebrand, J. M., et al. (2018). A FRET biosensor for necroptosis uncovers two different modes of the release of DAMPs. *Nat. Commun.* 9, 4457. doi: 10.1038/s41467-018-06985-6

Murphy, W. J., Eichwald, J., Meinke, D. K., Chadha, S., and Iskander, J. (2018). CDC Grand Rounds: Promoting Hearing Health Across the Lifespan. *MMWR Morb. Mortal. Wkly Rep.* 67, 243–246. doi: 10.15585/mmwr.mm6708a2

New, J., and Thomas, S. M. (2019). Autophagy-dependent secretion: mechanism, factors secreted, and disease implications. *Autophagy* 15, 1682–1693. doi: 10.1080/15548627.2019.1596479

Ott, C., Jacobs, K., Haucke, E., Navarrete Santos, A., Grune, T., and Simm, A. (2014). Role of advanced glycation end products in cellular signaling. *Redox Biol.* 2, 411–429. doi: 10.1016/j.redox.2013.12.016

Paudel, Y. N., Angelopoulou, E., Piperi, C., Balasubramaniam, V., Othman, I., and Shaikh, M. F. (2019). Enlightening the role of high mobility group box 1 (HMGB1) in inflammation: Updates on receptor signalling. *Eur. J. Pharmacol.* 858:172487. doi: 10.1016/j.ejphar.2019.172487

Qi, J., Zhang, L., Tan, F., Liu, Y., Chu, C., Zhu, W., et al. (2020). Espin distribution as revealed by super-resolution microscopy of stereocilia. *Am. J. Transl. Res.* 12, 130–141.

Rovere-Querini, P., Capobianco, A., Scaffidi, P., Valentinis, B., Catalanotti, F., Giazzon, M., et al. (2004). HMGB1 is an endogenous immune adjuvant released by necrotic cells. *EMBO Rep.* 5, 825–830. doi: 10.1038/sj.embor.7400205

Scaffidi, P., Misteli, T., and Bianchi, M. E. (2002). Release of chromatin protein HMGB1 by necrotic cells triggers inflammation. *Nature* 418, 191–195. doi: 10.1038/nature00858

Shih, C.-P., Chen, H.-C., Lin, Y.-C., Chen, H.-K., Wang, H., Kuo, C.-Y., et al. (2019). Middle-ear dexamethasone delivery via ultrasound microbubbles attenuates noise-induced hearing loss. *Laryngoscope* 129, 1907–1914. doi: 10.1002/lary.27713

Sun, S., Sun, M., Zhang, Y., Cheng, C., Waqas, M., Yu, H., et al. (2014). In vivo overexpression of X-linked inhibitor of apoptosis protein protects against neomycin-induced hair cell loss in the apical turn of the cochlea during the ototoxic-sensitive period. *Front. Cell Neurosci.* 8:248. doi: 10.3389/fncel.2014.00248

Tabas, I., and Glass, C. K. (2013). Anti-inflammatory therapy in chronic disease: challenges and opportunities. *Science* 339, 166–172. doi: 10.1126/science.1230720

Tang, D., Kang, R., Coyne, C. B., Zeh, H. J., and Lotze, M. T. (2012). PAMPs and DAMPs: signal 0s that spur autophagy and immunity. *Immunol. Rev.* 249, 158–175. doi: 10.1111/j.1600-065X.2012.01146.x

Tang, D., Kang, R., Livesey, K. M., Cheh, C. W., Farkas, A., Loughran, P., et al. (2010). Endogenous HMGB1 regulates autophagy. *J. Cell Biol.* 190, 881–892. doi: 10.1083/jcb.200911078

Tang, D., Kang, R., Livesey, K. M., Zeh, H. J. III, and Lotze, M. T. (2011). High mobility group box 1 (HMGB1) activates an autophagic response to oxidative stress. *Antioxid Redox Signal* 15, 2185–2195. doi: 10.1089/ars.2010.3666

Ueda, T., and Yoshida, M. (2010). HMGB proteins and transcriptional regulation. *Biochim Biophys Acta* 1799, 114–118. doi: 10.1016/j.bbagrm.2009.11.005

Volchuk, A., Ye, A., Chi, L., Steinberg, B. E., and Goldenberg, N. M. (2020). Indirect regulation of HMGB1 release by gasdermin D. *Nat. Commun.* 11:4561. doi: 10.1038/s41467-020-18443-3

Wang, Y., Qu, Y., Chen, X., Zhang, P., Su, D., Wang, L., et al. (2019). Effects of D-methionine in mice with noise-induced hearing loss mice. *J. Int. Med. Res.* 47, 3874–3885. doi: 10.1177/0300060519860679

Wen, Q., Liu, J., Kang, R., Zhou, B., and Tang, D. (2019). The release and activity of HMGB1 in ferroptosis. *Biochem. Biophys. Res. Commun.* 510, 278–283. doi: 10.1016/j.bbrc.2019.01.090

Wood, M. B., and Zuo, J. (2017). The Contribution of Immune Infiltrates to Ototoxicity and Cochlear Hair Cell Loss. *Front. Cell. Neurosci.* 11:00106. doi: 10.3389/fncel.2017.00106

Wu, J., Ye, J., Kong, W., Zhang, S., and Zheng, Y. (2020). Programmed cell death pathways in hearing loss: A review of apoptosis, autophagy and programmed necrosis. *Cell Prolif.* 53:e12915. doi: 10.1111/cpr.12915

Xia, L., Liu, J., Sun, Y., Shi, H., Yang, G., Feng, Y., et al. (2019). Rosiglitazone Improves Glucocorticoid Resistance in a Sudden Sensorineural Hearing Loss by Promoting MAP Kinase Phosphatase-1 Expression. *Med. Inflamm.* 2019:7915730. doi: 10.1155/2019/7915730

Yang, H., Antoine, D. J., Andersson, U., and Tracey, K. J. (2013). The many faces of HMGB1: molecular structure-functional activity in inflammation, apoptosis, and chemotaxis. *J. Leukoc. Biol.* 93, 865–873. doi: 10.1189/jlb.1212662

Yang, H., Wang, H., Ju, Z., Ragab, A. A., Lundbäck, P., Long, W., et al. (2015a). MD-2 is required for disulfide HMGB1-dependent TLR4 signaling. *J. Exp. Med.* 212, 5–14. doi: 10.1084/jem.20141318

Yang, W., Vethanayagam, R. R., Dong, Y., Cai, Q., and Hu, B. H. (2015b). Activation of the antigen presentation function of mononuclear phagocyte populations associated with the basilar membrane of the cochlea after acoustic overstimulation. *Neuroscience* 303, 1–15. doi: 10.1016/j.neuroscience.2015.05.081

Yu, X., Liu, W., Fan, Z., Qian, F., Zhang, D., Han, Y., et al. (2017). c-Myb knockdown increases the neomycin-induced damage to hair-cell-like HEI-OC1 cells in vitro. *Sci. Rep.* 7:41094. doi: 10.1038/srep41094

Yuan, H., Wang, X., Hill, K., Chen, J., Lemasters, J., Yang, S. M., et al. (2015). Autophagy attenuates noise-induced hearing loss by reducing oxidative stress. *Antioxid Redox Signal* 22, 1308–1324. doi: 10.1089/ars.2014.6004

Zhang, Y., Li, W., He, Z., Wang, Y., Shao, B., Cheng, C., et al. (2019). Pre-treatment With Fasudil Prevents Neomycin-Induced Hair Cell Damage by Reducing the Accumulation of Reactive Oxygen Species. *Front. Mol. Neurosci.* 12:264. doi: 10.3389/fnmol.2019.00264

Zhang, Z., Fan, L., Xing, Y., Wang, J., Aiken, S., Chen, Z., et al. (2020). Temporary Versus Permanent Synaptic Loss from Repeated Noise Exposure in Guinea Pigs and C57 Mice. *Neuroscience* 432, 94–103. doi: 10.1016/j.neuroscience.2020.02.038

Zhou, H., Qian, X., Xu, N., Zhang, S., Zhu, G., Zhang, Y., et al. (2020). Disruption of Atg7-dependent autophagy causes electromotility disturbances, outer hair cell loss, and deafness in mice. *Cell Death Dis.* 11:913. doi: 10.1038/s41419-020-03110-8

Zhu, C., Cheng, C., Wang, Y., Muhammad, W., Liu, S., Zhu, W., et al. (2018). Loss of ARHGEF6 Causes Hair Cell Stereocilia Deficits and Hearing Loss in Mice. *Front. Mol. Neurosci.* 11:362. doi: 10.3389/fnmol.2018.00362

16

Differences in Calcium Clearance at Inner Hair Cell Active Zones May Underlie the Difference in Susceptibility to Noise-Induced Cochlea Synaptopathy of C57BL/6J and CBA/CaJ Mice

Hongchao Liu[1,2,3†], Hu Peng[4†], Longhao Wang[1,2,3], Pengcheng Xu[1,2,3], Zhaoyan Wang[1,2,3], Huihui Liu[1,2,3*] and Hao Wu[1,2,3*]*

[1] Department of Otolaryngology-Head and Neck Surgery, Shanghai Ninth People's Hospital, Shanghai Jiao Tong University School of Medicine, Shanghai, China, [2] Ear Institute, Shanghai Jiao Tong University School of Medicine, Shanghai, China, [3] Shanghai Key Laboratory of Translational Medicine on Ear and Nose Diseases, Shanghai, China, [4] Department of Otolaryngology-Head and Neck Surgery, Changzheng Hospital, Second Military Medical University, Shanghai, China

***Correspondence:**
Zhaoyan Wang
wzyent@126.com
Huihui Liu
liuhent9h@163.com
Hao Wu
haowu@sh-jei.org

[†] These authors have contributed equally to this work

Noise exposure of a short period at a moderate level can produce permanent cochlear synaptopathy without seeing lasting changes in audiometric threshold. However, due to the species differences in inner hair cell (IHC) calcium current that we have recently discovered, the susceptibility to noise exposure may vary, thereby impact outcomes of noise exposure. In this study, we investigate the consequences of noise exposure in the two commonly used animal models in hearing research, CBA/CaJ (CBA) and C57BL/6J (B6) mice, focusing on the functional changes of cochlear IHCs. In the CBA mice, moderate noise exposure resulted in a typical fully recovered audiometric threshold but a reduced wave I amplitude of auditory brainstem responses. In contrast, both auditory brainstem response threshold and wave I amplitude fully recovered in B6 mice at 2 weeks after noise exposure. Confocal microscopy observations found that ribbon synapses of IHCs recovered in B6 mice but not in CBA mice. To further characterize the molecular mechanism underlying these different phenotypes in synaptopathy, we compared the ratio of Bax/Bcl-2 with the expression of cytochrome-C and found increased activity in CBA mice after noise exposure. Under whole-cell patch clamped IHCs, we acquired two-photon calcium imaging around the active zone to evaluate the Ca^{2+} clearance rate and found that CBA mice have a slower calcium clearance rate. Our results indicated that excessive accumulation of calcium due to acoustic overexposure and slow clearance around the presynaptic ribbon might lead to disruption of calcium homeostasis, followed by mitochondrial dysfunction of IHCs that cause susceptibility of noise-induced cochlear synaptopathy in CBA mice.

Keywords: noise-induced cochlear synaptopathy, calcium clearance, mitochondrial, inner hair cell, presynaptic ribbon

INTRODUCTION

Hearing loss is one of the most common health problems that affects communication and impacts life quality (Lin et al., 2011). Hearing loss is often caused by the death of sensory hair cells (HCs) in the inner ear, which function in transducing the sound waves into electric signals (Wang et al., 2017; Zhu et al., 2018; Liu et al., 2019d; Qi et al., 2019, 2020). Damages from a variety of intrinsic and extrinsic sources can impair inner ear function, including mutations in deafness genes, exposure to ototoxic drugs, aging, chronic cochlear infections, and environmental noise overexposure (Kujawa and Liberman, 2009; Gao et al., 2019; Zhang et al., 2019, 2020; He et al., 2020; Qian et al., 2020; Zhong et al., 2020; Zhou et al., 2020), among which, noise-induced hearing loss (NIHL) is the most common form of non-hereditary sensorineural hearing loss, with the incidence increasing annually in our aging society.

Severe noise exposure can damage cells in the inner ear, resulting in HC loss and elevated hearing thresholds. However, recent studies showed that a moderate level of acoustical exposure might not lead to permanent threshold shift but instead cause permanent synapse loss (Kujawa and Liberman, 2009; Liberman et al., 2016; Liberman and Kujawa, 2017). The inner hair cell (IHC) and spiral ganglion neuron (SGN) synapse, both pre- and postsynaptic structures, are vulnerable to noise exposure (Kujawa and Liberman, 2015; Liu et al., 2019b; Michanski et al., 2019). This cochlear synaptopathy is an "auditory processing disorder" that alters auditory information processing and leads to difficulties in speech discrimination in noisy environments (Shi et al., 2016). CBA/CaJ (CBA) and C57BL/6J (B6) mice are two of the most common animal models used in hearing research (Brewton et al., 2016). In our previous study, we compared differences in cellular functions in the cochleae of B6 and CBA mice and concluded that excessive loading of Ca^{2+} over a prolonged period might damage IHCs (Liu et al., 2019a). Cytosolic calcium homeostasis requires efficient Ca^{2+} clearance through a combination of Ca^{2+} pumps, Ca^{2+} buffers, and intracellular Ca^{2+} stores (Tucker and Fettiplace, 1995; Zenisek and Matthews, 2000; Carafoli, 2011). Presynaptic-Ca^{2+} influx through voltage-gated Ca^{2+} channels initiates mitochondrial-Ca^{2+} uptake around the ribbons and subsequent mitochondrial damage (Wong et al., 2019). Based on such a notion, this study further analyzes the functional alterations of IHC ribbon synapses after one episode of noise exposure and explore possible mechanisms in functional differences between B6 and CBA mice.

Noise-induced synaptopathy precedes the more commonly considered form of sensorineural deafness associated with damage to the outer HCs, which leads to the reduction in auditory nerve innervation to the IHCs (Monaghan et al., 2020). This synaptic degeneration may contribute to the generation of tinnitus, hyperacusis, and associated perceptual abnormalities (Kaltenbach and Afman, 2000; Schaette and McAlpine, 2011; Hickox and Liberman, 2014). Gaining understandings of the possible mechanisms underlying damage to the ribbon synapses is an important step in preventing noise-induced cochlear synaptopathy (Vlajkovic et al., 2017; Wang et al., 2019). Our experiments have revealed that excessive accumulation due to slow clearance of calcium around the presynaptic ribbon during acoustic overexposure may lead to disruption of calcium homeostasis, followed by mitochondrial dysfunction of IHCs that cause susceptibility of noise-induced cochlear synaptopathy in CBA mice.

MATERIALS AND METHODS

Animals

Male CBA and B6 mice aged 3–4 weeks old were obtained from SIPPR-BK Laboratory Animals Ltd. (Shanghai, China). Mice were housed for the duration of the experiments in the animal care facility of Ear Institute of Shanghai 9th people's hospital, in affiliation with Shanghai Jiao Tong University School of Medicine. The experimental procedures described were approved by the University Committee of Laboratory Animals of Shanghai 9th people's hospital and followed the guidelines for the Care and Use of Laboratory Animals (8th edition), published by the National Institutes of Health (Bethesda, MD, USA).

Hearing Assessment and Acoustic Exposure

As described previously (El-Hassar et al., 2019; Lin et al., 2019), recordings of the auditory brainstem responses (ABRs) were made on an anesthetized animal (chloral hydrate, 480 mg/kg intraperitoneal), and body temperature was maintained at near 37°C throughout recording with a heating blanket (Harvard Apparatus, Holliston, MA, USA; 55-7020). For the recordings, three needle electrodes were placed subdermally at the vertex (active), left mastoid area (reference), and right shoulder (ground). An MF-1 speaker was placed in front of the animal 10 cm away from the vertex. Short tone burst stimuli (3-ms duration, 1-ms rise/fall times) were delivered free field. Stimulus frequencies rove from 32 to 4 kHz in half-octave steps. For each measured frequency, the sound level starts from 90 to 0 dB of sound pressure level (SPL) with 5 dB decrement or until two levels below visible thresholds. Each waveform was averaged 400 times. The hearing thresholds were determined by the minimal stimulus level that evoked any noticeable ABRs at each frequency. Amplitudes (μV) of ABR wave I were measured and exported offline using BioSigRZ software (Tucker-Davis Technologies, Alachua, FL, USA). Amplitude was measured by averaging the ΔV of both sides of the peak (Tan et al., 2017; Zhao et al., 2020).

Noise exposure was induced by exposing conscious animals in a calibrated reverberating chamber where differences in sound pressure level varied ~1 dB in typical locations. Bandpass noise of 2–20 kHz at 103 dB SPL was delivered for 2 h by an amplifier and loudspeaker (Yamaha). Noise signals were generated by a TDT RZ6 system (Tucker-Davis Technologies) and calibrated to the target sound pressure level immediately before each acoustic overexposure by acoustimeter (type AWA6228+, Hangzhou Aihua). ABR recordings were performed before and repeated at 1 and 14 days after noise exposure.

Two-Photon Ca^{2+} Imaging

Ten mice of each group were used, and the organ of Corti was dissected in the cold extracellular solution containing the following (in millimolar): 115 sodium chloride, 2.8 potassium chloride, 25 tetraethylammonium chloride, 5 calcium chloride, 1 magnesium chloride, 2 sodium pyruvate, 5.6 D-glucose, and 10 4-(2-hydroxyethyl)-1-piperazineethanesulfonic acid (300 mOsm, pH 7.40). For Ca^{2+}-imaging, IHCs were whole-cell patch clamped at the apical turn of the basilar membrane; the selected location corresponds to ~8.0 kHz frequency region. An EPC10 amplifier controlled by Patchmaster 10.0 pulse software (HEKA Elektronik, Harvard Bioscience Inc., Holliston, MA, USA) was used throughout our experiment. Patch pipettes were filled with a cesium-based intracellular solution that contains the following (in millimolar): 115 cesium methanesulfonate, 10 cesium chloride, 10 4-(2-hydroxyethyl)-1-piperazineethanesulfonic acid, 10 tetraethylammonium chloride, 1 ethylene glycol-bis(β-aminoethyl ether)-N,N,N′,N′-tetraacetic acid, 3 adenosine triphosphate magnesium, and 0.5 guanosine 5′-triphosphate sodium salt hydrate, 2.0 mM L-glutathione reduced, 0.375-mM Fluo-4FF (Invitrogen, Carlsbad, USA), and 0.35-mM Cy3-labeled Ribeye-binding peptide (AnaSpec, San Jose, USA), pH 7.20, 290 mOsm. Pipette resistance is 4–6 MΩ range, and cells with a holding current exceeding −40 pA at −80 mV were excluded from the analysis. All patch-clamp experiments were carried out at room temperature, and the liquid junction potential was corrected offline.

Images of IHCs were taken with a two-photon microscope system (Scientifica Ltd., Uckfield, UK) using a 60× water immersion objective (Olympus, Tokyo, Japan). Cells loaded with Ca^{2+}-indicator F4-FF and Cy3-conjugated peptide were excited by ultrafast pulsed titanium–sapphire laser (Coherent Inc., Santa Clara, USA) of 740 nm wavelength. The intracellular Ca^{2+} signal associated with IHC depolarization was acquired by using two-photon line scans (1.0 kHz) across the center of the fluorescent-labeled ribbon. The decay time of Ca^{2+} current transients was measured by fitting the calcium fluorescence decay with the following equation to assess the kinetic properties of Ca^{2+} extrusion.

$$F = F_0 + A1exp\left\{\frac{-(t-x_t)}{\tau 1}\right\} + A2exp\left\{\frac{-(t-t_0)}{\tau 2}\right\}$$

where F_0 is the initial luminescence intensity, $A1$ and $A2$ are pre-exponential factors, and $(t - t_0)$ is the difference between the initial time of measurement after excitation pulse t_0 and time t. $\tau 1$ and $\tau 2$ is the fast and slow decaying component, respectively.

Immunofluorescence Staining and Confocal Imaging

The dissected cochleae were perfused with 4% paraformaldehyde at 4°C overnight. The next day, the organ of Corti was dissected, then permeabilized with 5% Triton X-100 and blocked in 5% bovine serum albumin. Primary antibodies used in this experiment were mouse anti-CtBP2 immunoglobulin (Ig) G1 (BD Biosciences, Franklin Lakes, NJ, USA), mouse anti-GluR2 IgG2a (Merck-Millipore, Darmstadt, Germany), rabbit anti-calretinin (Abcam, Cambridge, UK), and rabbit anti-PNPase (Proteintech, Rosemont, IL, USA). The secondary antibodies used were Alexa Fluor 568-conjugated goat anti-mouse IgG1, Alexa Fluor 647-conjugated IgG2, and Alexa Fluor 488-conjugated goat anti-rabbit IgG (Invitrogen, USA). Confocal

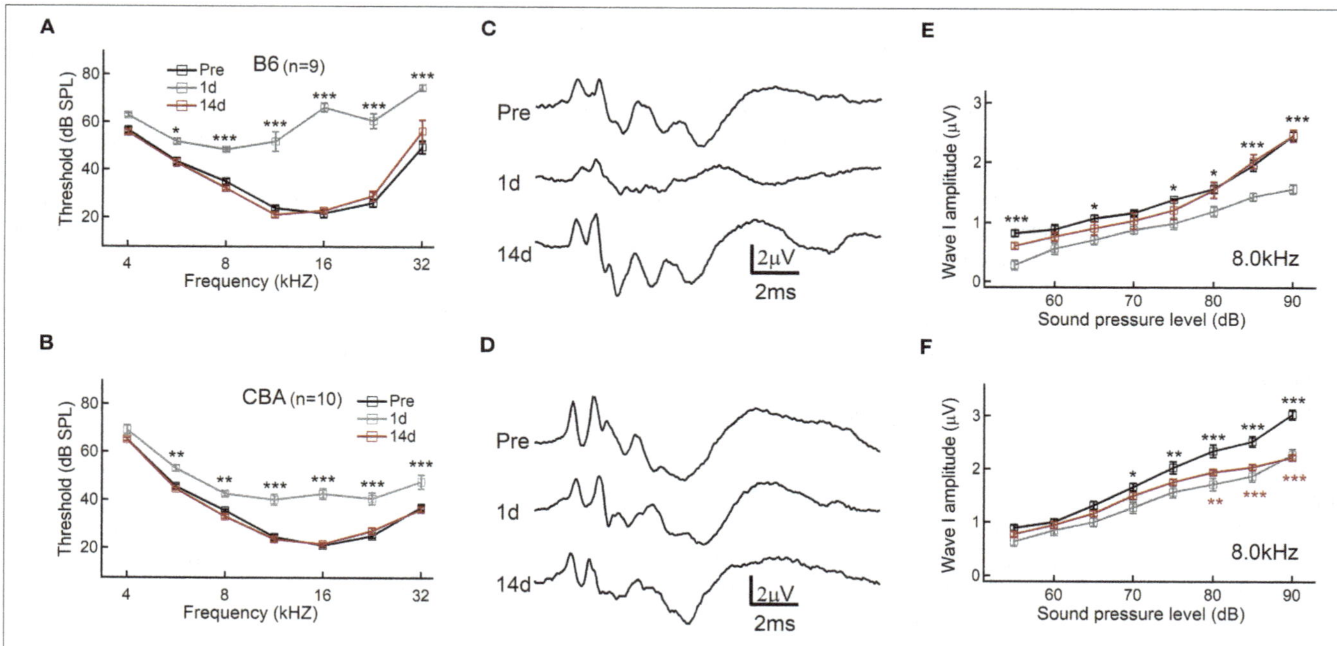

FIGURE 1 | Auditory brainstem response (ABR) threshold and wave I analysis. **(A,B)** Hearing threshold of ABR before and after noise exposure. **(C,D)** Representative traces of ABR response to 80 dB SPL at 8.0 kHz. **(E,F)** ABR wave I amplitudes, evoked by suprathreshold tones at 8.0 kHz. Data are presented as mean ± SEM; statistical significance was assessed by two-way ANOVA followed by the Bonferroni *post-hoc* test, *$P < 0.05$, **$P < 0.01$, and ***$P < 0.001$.

images were acquired on a Zeiss confocal microscope (Carl Zeiss Microscopy GmbH, Jena, Germany). Images were acquired under a Zeiss LSM 880 with a 63×, 1.4 numerical aperture oil objective lens. Pixel size was 0.1 μm in x and y planes and 0.38 μm for the z-axis. For synapse counts, the confocal stacks were created using 3D analysis software (Carl Zeiss Microscopy GmbH, Jena, Germany).

Protein Extraction and Western Blotting

Animals were killed, and cochleae were dissected in ice-cold phosphate-buffered saline. For each sample, tissues from 6 Organs of Corti were collected and pooled, treated with ice-cold radioimmunoprecipitation assay lysis buffer plus protease inhibitor cocktail (Thermo Fisher Scientific, Waltham, MA, USA) and phosphatase inhibitors. The samples were then centrifuged at 10,000 × g at 4°C for 10 min. The supernatants were collected, and the protein concentration was determined by using a BCA Protein Assay Kit (Beyotime Institute of Biotechnology, Jiangsu, China) for protein quantification. Equal amounts of proteins were loaded onto a 10–12% sodium dodecyl sulfate-polyacrylamide gel electrophoresis gel, and after electrophoresis, proteins were transferred onto polyvinylidene difluoride membranes (Merck-Millipore). After blocking with 5% non-fat milk for 1 h at room temperature, the membranes were incubated with anti-cleaved caspase-3, anti-Bcl2, anti-Bax, anti-cytochrome C (Cell Signaling Technology, Danvers, MA, USA), anti-calpain 1/2, anti-calpastatin (Abcam), and anti-GAPDH (Beyotime) overnight at 4°C, with gentle shaking. The next day, the membrane was washed three times (10 min each) with phosphate-buffered saline with Tween 20 buffer and then incubated with an appropriate secondary antibody labeled with horseradish peroxidase (Abcam) for 1 h at 37°C. After extensive washing of the membrane, the protein bands were visualized using an Amersham Imager 600 (G.E. Healthcare, Little Chalfont, UK) using the elevated chemiluminescence procedure. Image J software (National Institutes of Health, Bethesda, MD, USA) was used to calculate the relative densities of the probe protein.

Data Analysis and Statistical Tests

Data analysis was performed by using software Igor Pro (WaveMetrics Inc., Lake Oswego, OR, USA) and GraphPad Prism (GraphPad Software Inc., La Jolla, CA, USA). For

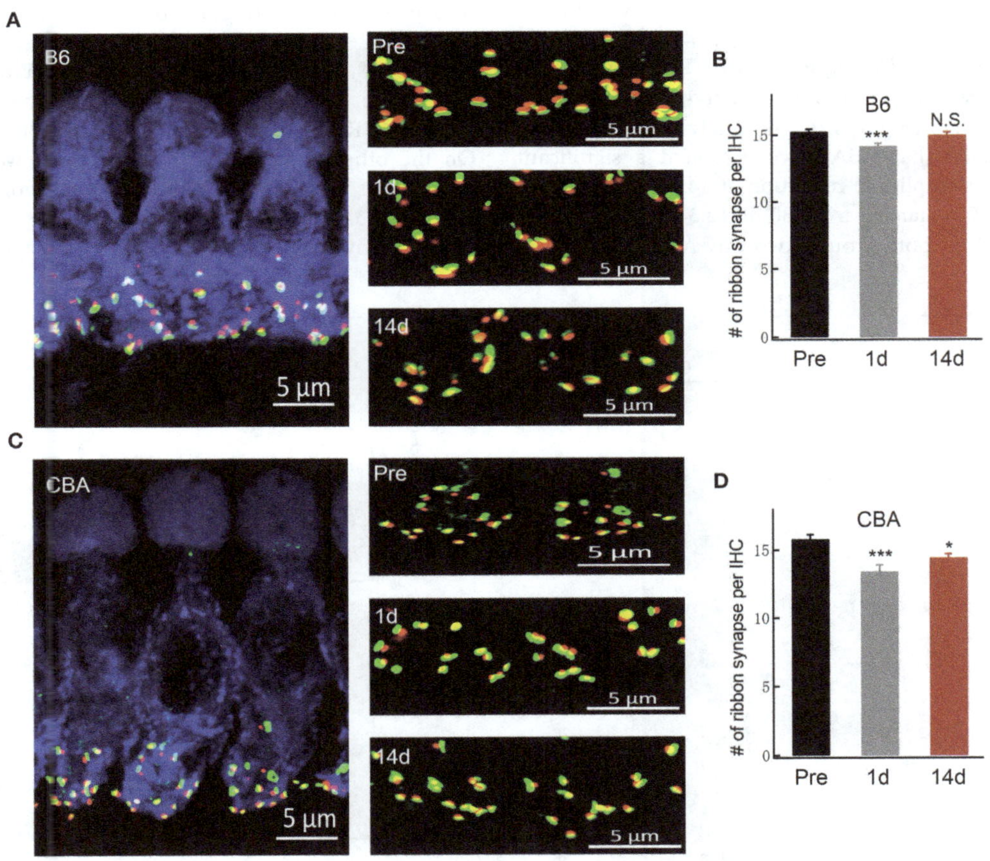

FIGURE 2 | Inner hair cell ribbon synapse counts in B6 and CBA mice before and after noise exposure. **(A,C)** Representative confocal images of IHCs co-labeled for the presynaptic marker CtBP2 (red) and postsynaptic marker GluA2 (green) of B6 and CBA mice at pre, 1 day, and 14 days after noise exposure in the apical turn of the basilar membrane. **(B,D)** Puncta of co-labeling are presumably ribbon synapses, and the numbers of synapses were counted (mean ± SEM) per IHC. Data were analyzed by one-way ANOVA followed by Bonferroni *post-hoc* test. $^{*}P < 0.05$ and $^{***}P < 0.001$. N.S., no significant difference was found.

comparisons between two samples, a two-tailed, unpaired Student's t-test or Mann–Whitney test was used. For multiple group comparison, statistical significance was calculated using one- or two-way ANOVA followed by Bonferroni *post-hoc* test. Cumulative distributions were statistically compared using the Kolmogorov–Smirnov test. Data are presented as mean ± SEM, and values of $P < 0.05$ were considered statistically significant. In figures, N.S. indicates that $P > 0.05$, *indicates that $P < 0.05$, **indicates that $P < 0.01$, and ***indicates that $P < 0.001$.

RESULTS

CBA/CaJ Mice Were More Susceptible to Noise-Induced Synaptopathy

To determine the hearing threshold shift and synaptopathy induced by acoustic exposure, we analyzed ABR recordings before and after noise exposure of B6 and CBA mice. ABR threshold shifts were similar, and temporal threshold shifts were observed in both B6 and CBA mice, which were both significantly elevated at 1 day [$F_{(1,56)} = 574$, $p < 0.0001$; $F_{(1,63)} = 166.9$, $p < 0.0001$, for B6 and CBA mice, respectively, n = 9 and 10, two-way ANOVA] and progressively recovered at 14 days after noise exposure [$F_{(1,56)} = 0.27$, $p = 0.61$; $F_{(1,63)}$, $p = 0.7606$, two-way ANOVA, **Figures 1A,B**]. The first wave of ABR (Wave I) represents the summated activity of responding auditory afferent fibers (**Figures 1C,D**). Analysis of ABR wave I amplitude revealed that CBA mice exhibited a significant reduction of wave I amplitude reduction at 14 days after noise exposure at high SPLs starting from 80 dB (2.34 ± 0.11 vs. 1.93 ± 0.05 μV, n = 10 for both groups, two-way ANOVA followed by Bonferroni *post-hoc* test, $p < 0.01$, **Figure 1F**), whereas B6 wave I amplitude fully recovered (2.46 ± 0.07 vs. 2.45 ± 0.10 μV at 90 dB SPL, n = 9 for both groups, two-way ANOVA followed by Bonferroni *post-hoc* test, $p > 0.05$, **Figure 1E**). Because wave I of ABR is generated by the synchronous firing of auditory nerve fibers, these results indicate that CBA mice's IHC-SGN synaptic functions were more vulnerable to acoustic overexposure. To verify, we then quantify the changes in the synaptic count.

Ribbon Synapse Number Was Incompletely Recovered in CBA/CaJ Mice at 14 Days After Noise Exposure

A functional ribbon synapse consists of a presynaptic ribbon and postsynaptic AMPA receptors (Kim et al., 2019). Excessive noise exposure may lead to excitotoxicity that could damage the synapses. By co-staining the presynaptic ribbons (anti-CtBP2) and postsynaptic AMPA-type glutamate receptors (anti-GluA2) of the organ of Corti before and after noise exposure, we show in B6 mice that the number of ribbon synapses was initially reduced at day 1 after noise exposure but then recovered and indistinguishable from the pre-exposure level at day 14 (15.3 ± 0.16, 14.2 ± 0.19, and 15.0 ± 0.20; n = 31, 28, and 24; respectively, of pre, 1 day, and 14 days) after noise exposure (**Figures 2A,B**), in agreement with the *in vivo* ABR measurement of wave I amplitude measurement. On the other hand, for CBA mice, there was an incomplete recovery of the ribbon synapses after the noise exposure (15.8 ± 0.32, 13.4 ± 0.47, and 14.2 ± 0.47; n = 34, 19, and 26; respectively, of pre, 1 day, and 14 days), which support

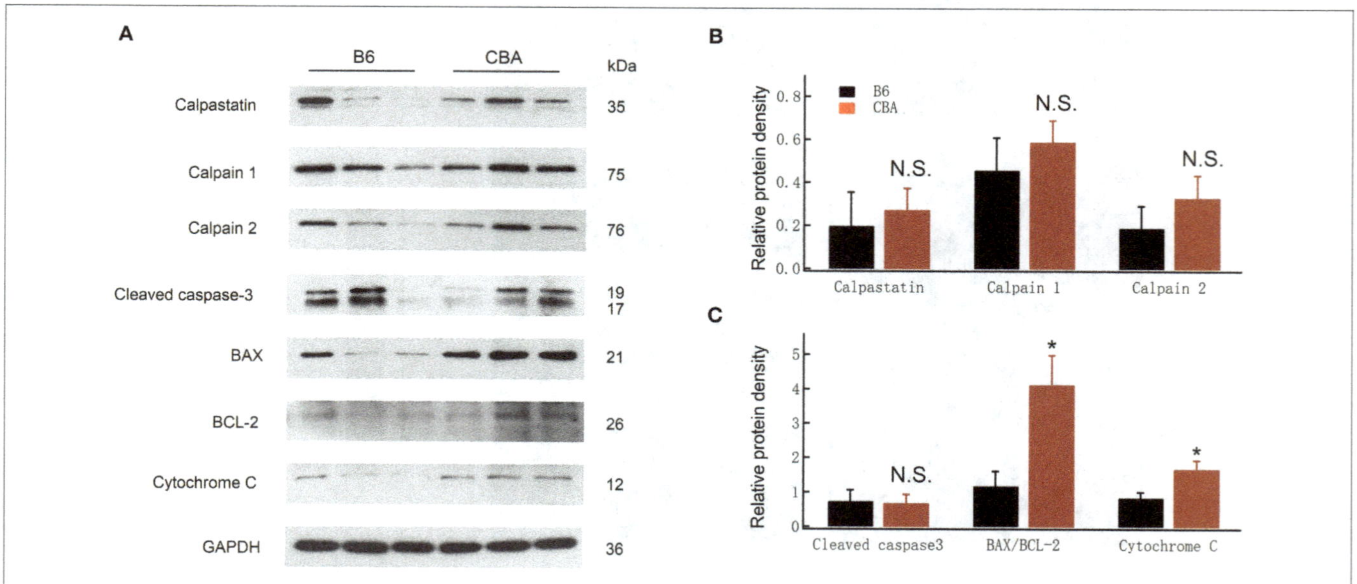

FIGURE 3 | Comparison of protein expression at 1 day after noise exposure between CBA and B6. **(A)** Protein levels of cleaved caspase-3, Bax, Bcl 2, cytochrome-C, calpain 1/2, and calpastatin were detected by Western blotting; GAPDH was used as an internal control. **(B,C)** Relative protein levels are presented as relative ratio of target proteins to GAPDH. Data were analyzed by one-way ANOVA followed by Bonferroni *post-hoc* test. *$P < 0.05$. N.S., no significant difference was found.

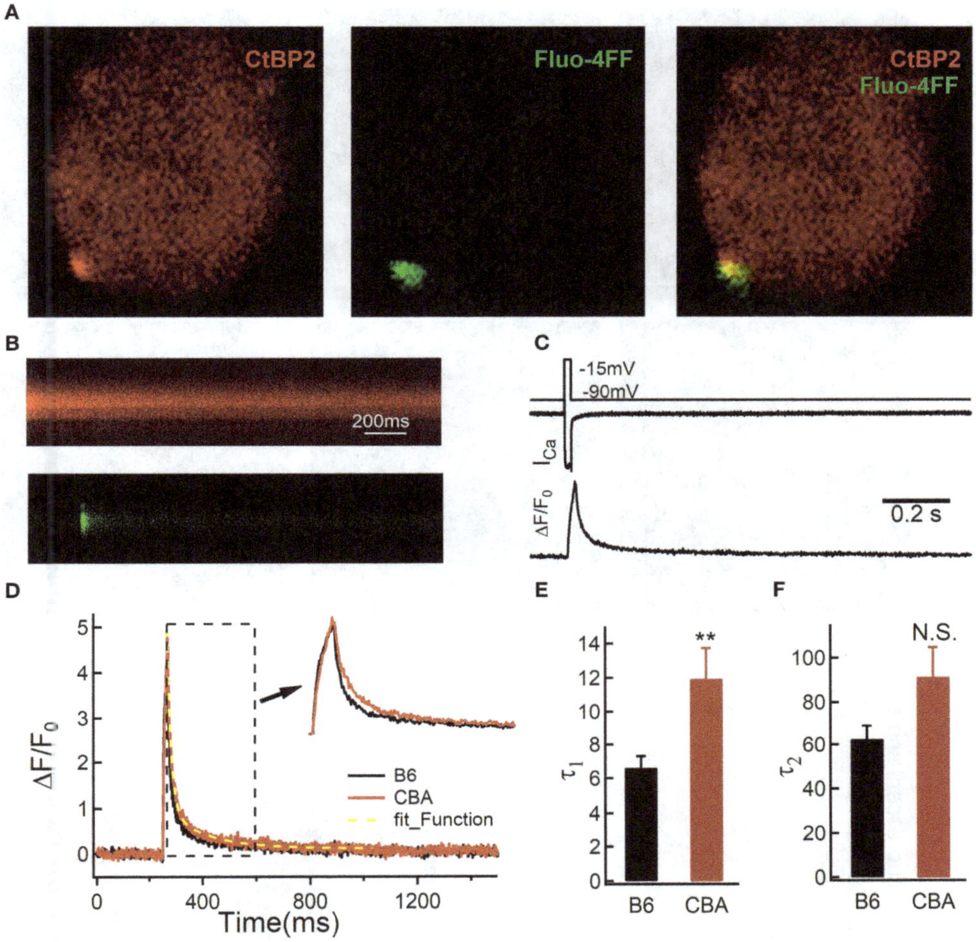

FIGURE 4 | Two-photon calcium imaging in IHCs from the apical turn of the organ of Corti without noise exposure. **(A)** IHCs were loaded with Cy3-conjugated peptide binding to the synaptic ribbon to visualize synaptic ribbons at the active zone, and the hotspots of depolarization-evoked Ca^{2+} influx, visualized by increased fluorescence of the Ca^{2+} indicator Fluo-4FF. **(B)** Example line scan of a fluorescently-labeled ribbon and Fluo-4FF fluorescence change at an individual IHC active zone during 20-ms depolarization. **(C)** Representative recording show the evoked whole-cell Ca^{2+} current and the depolarization-evoked increase in fluorescence at a single active zone; ΔF from line-scans was normalized to their baseline fluorescence F_0 hence $\Delta F/F_0$. **(D–F)** Decay of Ca^{2+} fluorescence intensity was fitted by a double exponential. Statistical significance was assessed by the Mann–Whitney test, $^{**}P < 0.01$. N.S., no significant difference was found.

the finding of significant and lasting ABR wave I reduction (**Figures 2C,D**).

Protein of Bcl-2/Bax Ratio and Cytochrome-C Was Expressed Higher in CBA/CaJ Mice After Noise Exposure

Alterations in calcium homeostasis are widely reported to contribute to synaptic degeneration, and the Ca^{2+}-dependent proteases play a causal role in axonal and synaptic degeneration (Ma et al., 2013). We therefore analyzed the protein levels of calpastatin (0.20 ± 0.16 vs. 0.27 ± 0.10, for B6 and CBA mice, respectively, unpaired *t*-test, $P = 0.71$), calpain 1 (0.46 ± 0.15 vs. 0.59 ± 0.10, for B6 and CBA mice, respectively, unpaired *t*-test, $P = 0.50$), and calpain 2 (0.19 ± 0.10 vs. 0.33 ± 0.10, for B6 and CBA mice, respectively, unpaired *t*-test, $P = 0.39$), but no significant differences were found between the two mouse strains (**Figures 3A,B**).

Free radicals and oxidative stress also play essential roles in the pathogenesis of NIHL (Liu et al., 2016, 2019c; He et al., 2017; Li et al., 2018b; Chen et al., 2020). Cytochrome-c is a biomarker of oxidative stress, which serves as an indicator of oxidative damage (Yamasoba et al., 2005). The activation of caspase-3, known to trigger widespread damage and degeneration, can also modulate synaptic function (Imbriani et al., 2019). Likewise, Bcl-2 expression is reduced, whereas Bax is increased in IHCs after noise exposure (Chen et al., 2020). Therefore, we investigated the expression of mitochondrial-dependent damage markers, such as Bax and cytochrome-c. As shown in **Figure 3C**, an increase in the ratio of Bax/Bcl-2 (1.19 ± 0.42 vs. 4.13 ± 0.85, for B6 and CBA mice, respectively, unpaired *t*-test, $P = 0.036$) and

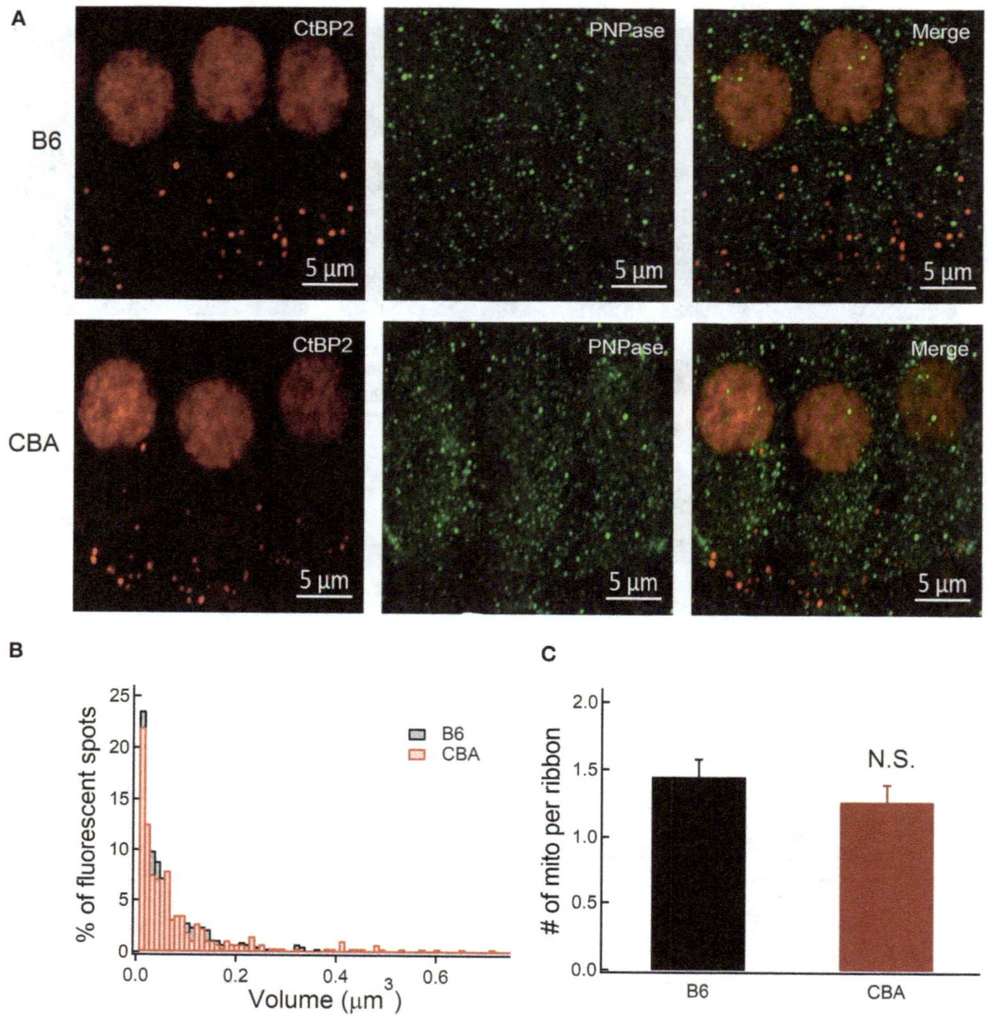

FIGURE 5 | Immunofluorescence analysis of the presynaptic abundance of mitochondria counts between CBA and B6 mice without noise exposure. **(A)** Organ of Corti confocal image stacks of B6 and CBA mice, stained for CtBP2 and PNPase, show similar distribution in IHC at the apical turn of basilar membrane. **(B)** Normalized distributions of volumes of confocal z-sections integrated within a 0.5-μm radius around the center of mass of CtBP2 fluorescence in single confocal sections show near-identical distribution pattern. **(C)** Number of mitochondria within a 0.5-μm radius around the center of mass of CtBP2. Statistical significance was assessed by two-sample Kolmogorov–Smirnov test and unpaired *t*-test. N.S., no significant difference was found.

cytochrome-c release (0.85 ± 0.16 vs. 1.69 ± 0.25, for B6 and CBA mice, respectively, unpaired *t*-test, $P = 0.047$) was found in CBA mice after noise exposure. Meanwhile, the expression of cleaved caspase-3 was similar between the two strains. Taken together, these results revealed that noise-induced mitochondrial damage might be associated with the greater susceptibility to cochlear synaptopathy of CBA mice.

Cytosolic Calcium Clearance at the Active Zone Rate Is Slower in CBA/CaJ mice

During noise exposure, the sustained Ca^{2+} entry could induce mitochondrial dysfunction (Chen et al., 2018). Cytosolic Ca^{2+} homeostasis is maintained through a delicate balance between the influx and efflux of calcium ions. To probe the reasons for the different outcomes after noise exposure, we further analyzed Ca^{2+} dynamics at the single active zone level using two-photon Ca^{2+} imaging (Wong et al., 2014). We loaded IHCs with a Cy3-conjugated Ribeye-binding peptide to locate ribbons (excitation wavelength: 740 nm) and the low-affinity Ca^{2+} indicator Fluo-4FF ($K_d = 9.7$ μM, excitation wavelength: 740 nm; **Figure 4A**). A line scan across the center of fluorescently-labeled ribbons during IHC depolarization (20 ms to −14 mV, 1 kHz) recorded the fluorescence change of Fluo-4FF (**Figures 4B–D**) (Krinner et al., 2017). The time constant fitted by a double exponential function during the decay phase of the Ca^{2+} transient represents the

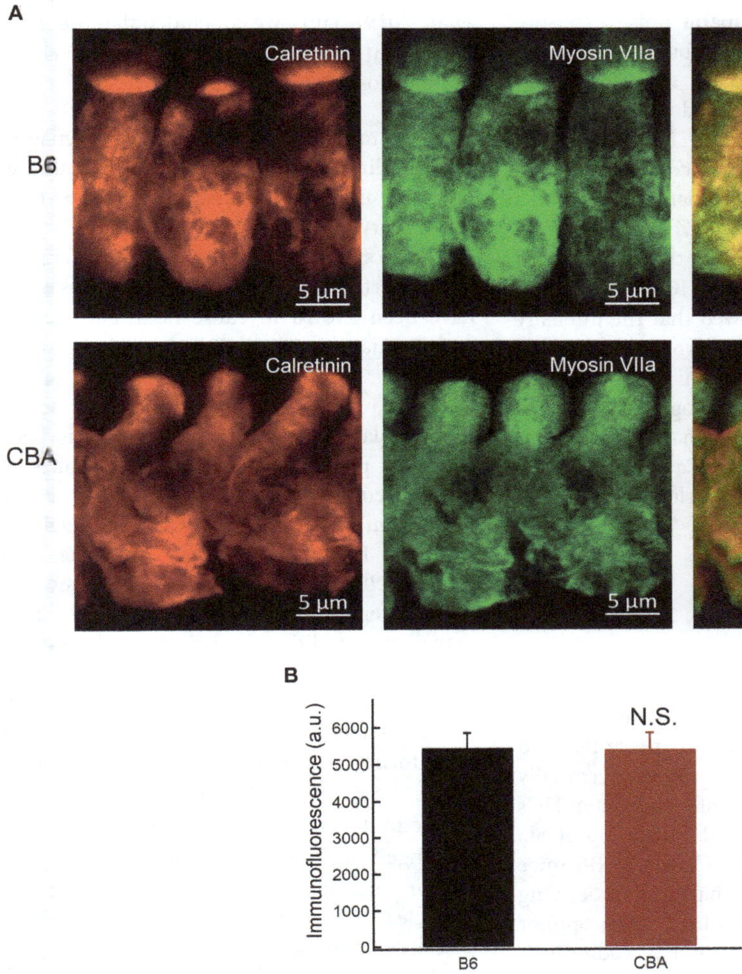

FIGURE 6 | Expression of calretinin in IHCs. **(A)** Whole-mount preparation of organ of Corti double-stained for calretinin and myosin VIIa. **(B)** Quantification of calretinin fluorescence at the base of IHCs in apical region without noise exposure. Statistical significance was assessed by unpaired *t*-test. N.S., no significant difference.

rate of cytosolic Ca^{2+} clearance (Kim et al., 2003; Chamberland et al., 2019). Although the slow-decaying component was similar between the two mouse strains (62.45 ± 26.34 vs. 91.30 ± 49.87 ms, for B6 and CBA mice, respectively, $n = 17$ and 14; Mann–Whitney test, $P = 0.08$; **Figure 4F**), IHCs of B6 mice that had a shorter fast decay time constant (6.62 ± 2.78 vs. 11.93 ± 6.70 ms, for B6 and CBA mice, respectively, $n = 17$ and 14; Mann–Whitney test, $P = 0.001$; **Figure 4E**), suggest that the Ca^{2+} clearance capability of the IHCs was more efficient in B6 mice.

Mitochondria Around a Presynaptic Ribbon and the Expression of Calretinin in Inner Hair Cells Showed No Difference Between C57BL/6J and CBA/CaJ Mice

Mitochondrial calcium overload has been postulated to regulate a wide range of processes involved in NIHL (Wang et al., 2018). The mitochondrial calcium uniporter (MCU) is a major specific calcium channel for calcium uptake, and excessive cellular Ca^{2+} can rapidly enter the mitochondria through the MCU (Rizzuto et al., 2012). Therefore, we compared the volume with the number of mitochondrial around the presynaptic ribbons (**Figure 5**). Presynaptic mitochondrial volumes (integrated within a 0.5-µm radius around the center of mass of CtBP2 fluorescence in single confocal sections) were calculated in a total of 488 and 255 regions of six mice's organ of Corti in each group. There was no difference in the distributions of mitochondrial volumes around the presynaptic ribbon between the two animal strains ($D = 0.05$, two-sample Kolmogorov–Smirnov test, $P = 0.76$; **Figure 5B**). In addition, similar results were observed with regard to the number of mitochondria per ribbon within the region (1.45 ± 0.13 *vs.* 1.26 ± 0.12, for B6 and CBA mice, respectively, unpaired *t*-test, $P = 0.37$; **Figure 5C**).

Neuroprotective Ca^{2+}-buffering proteins have been proposed to be related to protection against traumatic noise exposure (Alvarado et al., 2016). Calretinin is a Ca^{2+}-buffering protein with neuroprotective action (D'Orlando et al., 2002), and the absence of calretinin might be associated with the noise susceptibility of the fibers (Sharma et al., 2018). The expression of calretinin was measured by immunofluorescence quantification. Fluorescence intensity was averaged in Gaussian volumes with standard deviations of 1 μm along the X, Y, and Z axes (Michalski et al., 2017), centered around points selected at the base of IHCs of each confocal stack (for a total of 39 B6 IHCs and 32 CBA IHCs in six mice of each group). We showed that the intensity of calretinin was comparable between the two groups (5.443 ± 412 vs. 5.397 ± 450.4, for B6 and CBA mice, respectively, unpaired t-test, $P = 0.66$; **Figures 6A,B**). Together with the findings mentioned earlier, we hypothesized that mitochondria in IHCs of CBA mice might take up more Ca^{2+} under noise exposure and result in mitochondrial Ca^{2+} overload, resulting in susceptibility to noise-induced synaptopathy.

DISCUSSION

Intense HC stimulation will cause damage to IHC ribbons, as well as to postsynaptic receptors (Kujawa and Liberman, 2009), which has been implicated as a contributor to noise-induced hearing impairment (Henry and Mulroy, 1995), eventually induce apoptotic cell death in HCs, especially the outer HCs of the basal turn (Sun et al., 2014; He et al., 2016; Yu et al., 2017; Li et al., 2018a; Zhang et al., 2019). CBA and B6 mice have been used extensively to explore mechanisms underlying hearing loss for many years (Li and Hultcrantz, 1994; Spongr et al., 1997). B6 mice carry a specific mutation in cadherin23 (Cdh23), which lead to disorganized hair bundles (Noben-Trauth et al., 2003), rendering the mice more susceptible to noise insult (Davis et al., 2001). However, these two animal models exhibited different susceptibilities to noise-induced synaptopathy, in that the ribbon synapse in B6 mice can completely recover (Shi et al., 2015), while not the case in CBA mice. Few studies have been published to focus on this difference and explore the possible mechanisms. Our results identified candidate mechanisms underlying the susceptibility to noise-induced synaptopathy and provide guidance in animal model selection.

As reported in a previous study (Kujawa and Liberman, 2009), we found that CBA mice showed the typical feature of "hidden hearing loss," in which a temporal threshold shift was detected by ABR and a decreased ABR wave I amplitude was observed. Meanwhile, in B6 mice, the ABR wave I was completely recovered, which was consistent with previously published studies (Kim et al., 2019). The repair/regeneration of ribbon synapses, which could present as changes in ABR wave I amplitude (Kujawa and Liberman, 2009), may depend on animal species, experimental conditions, and the actions of neurotrophic factors after acoustic exposure (Shi et al., 2013; Kim et al., 2019). Thus, we concluded that the IHCs of the two strains underwent different cellular/subcellular changes in response to noise exposure.

Calcium channels in the IHC presynaptic active zones are key signaling elements that transform sound-evoked presynaptic potential into neurotransmitter release. Ca^{2+} homeostasis of the sensory HCs is particularly critical for presynaptic electrical activities, synaptic transmission, and efferent modulation (Lenzi and Roberts, 1994). Prolonged alterations of intracellular calcium have been shown to cause neuronal excitotoxicity (Arundine and Tymianski, 2004). During noise exposure, more voltage-gated Ca^{2+} channels continue to open, causing sustained Ca^{2+} entry into IHCs from the extracellular space and elevated the intracellular free Ca^{2+} ions, which has been implicated in a variety of pathological conditions (Brookes et al., 2004). Under these circumstances, the capability of modifying intracellular Ca^{2+} homeostasis appeared to be crucial in maintaining IHC function. Dysfunction of Ca^{2+} extrusion channels can lead to intracellular Ca^{2+} overloading and eventually cell death or neurodegeneration (Hajieva et al., 2018). Thus, Ca^{2+} clearance may play an additional role in neurodegenerative conditions.

The elevation of cytosolic Ca^{2+} alone may not be a major contributing factor to HC death, but the dysfunction of mitochondria is likely the defining event (Esterberg et al., 2014). Low levels of mitochondrial Ca^{2+} uptake can feed energetically active cells through ATP production; however, prolonged uptake can be toxic, leading to an increase in the production of reactive oxygen species production and the release of cytochrome c (Giorgi et al., 2008, 2012). The excessive cytosolic Ca^{2+} uptake by mitochondria through the Ca^{2+} uniporter could lead to mitochondrial dysfunction, which has been implicated in synaptopathy and can contribute to neurodegeneration (Flippo and Strack, 2017). However, the inhibition of MCU activity could attenuate noise-induced loss of sensory HCs, synaptic ribbons, and ABR wave I amplitudes (Wang et al., 2018). Our results found a slower calcium clearance rate and the same levels of Ca^{2+} buffering proteins, which indicated that the mitochondrial might uptake more Ca^{2+}. Taken together, we presented a mechanism that presynaptic- and mito-Ca^{2+} couple to induce the cochlea synaptopathy.

In summary, we demonstrated temporary and persistent alterations of ABR wave I and ribbon synapses in B6 and CBA mice, respectively, and CBA mice showed more susceptibility to noise-induced synaptopathy between the IHCs and SGN. This may be accounted for by the elevated Ca^{2+} around the ribbon and further leads to mitochondrial dysfunction under noise exposure in CBA mice. Further research is required to clarify the possible mechanism between calcium clearance and presynaptic dysfunction in noise-induced synaptopathy.

ETHICS STATEMENT

The animal study was reviewed and approved by University Committee of Laboratory Animals of Shanghai 9th people's hospital.

AUTHOR CONTRIBUTIONS

HuL, ZW, and HW conceived and designed the research. HoL, LW, and PX conducted the experiments. HoL and HP analyzed the generated data and wrote the manuscript. All authors have read and agreed to the published version of the manuscript.

REFERENCES

Alvarado, J. C., Fuentes-Santamaría, V., Gabaldón-Ull, M. C., Jareño-Flores, T., Miller, J. M., and Juiz, J. M. (2016). Noise-induced "toughening" effect in wistar rats: enhanced auditory brainstem responses are related to calretinin and nitric oxide synthase upregulation. *Front. Neuroanat.* 10:19. doi: 10.3389/fnana.2016.00019

Arundine, M., and Tymianski, M. (2004). Molecular mechanisms of glutamate-dependent neurodegeneration in ischemia and traumatic brain injury. *Cell. Mol. Life Sci.* 61, 657–668. doi: 10.1007/s00018-003-3319-x

Brewton, D. H., Kokash, J., Jimenez, O., Pena, E. R., and Razak, K. A. (2016). Age-related deterioration of perineuronal nets in the primary auditory cortex of mice. *Front. Aging Neurosci.* 8:270. doi: 10.3389/fnagi.2016.00270

Brookes, P. S., Yoon, Y., Robotham, J. L., Anders, M. W., and Sheu, S. S. (2004). Calcium, ATP, and ROS: a mitochondrial love-hate triangle. *Am. J. Physiol. Cell Physiol.* 287, C817–C833. doi: 10.1152/ajpcell.00139.2004

Carafoli, E. (2011). The plasma membrane calcium pump in the hearing process: physiology and pathology. *Sci. China Life Sci.* 54, 686–690. doi: 10.1007/s11427-011-4200-z

Chamberland, S., Zamora Moratalla, A., and Topolnik, L. (2019). Calcium extrusion mechanisms in dendrites of mouse hippocampal CA1 inhibitory interneurons. *Cell Calcium* 77, 49–57. doi: 10.1016/j.ceca.2018.12.002

Chen, X. M., Ji, S. F., Liu, Y. H., Xue, X. M., Xu, J., Gu, Z. H., et al. (2020). Ginsenoside Rd ameliorates auditory cortex injury associated with military aviation noise-induced hearing loss by activating SIRT1/PGC-1α signaling pathway. *Front. Physiol.* 11:788. doi: 10.3389/fphys.2020.00788

Chen, Y., Chen, J., Sun, X., Shi, X., Wang, L., Huang, L., et al. (2018). Evaluation of the neuroprotective effect of EGCG: a potential mechanism of mitochondrial dysfunction and mitochondrial dynamics after subarachnoid hemorrhage. *Food Funct.* 9, 6349–6359. doi: 10.1039/c8fo01497c

Davis, R. R., Newlander, J. K., Ling, X., Cortopassi, G. A., Krieg, E. F., and Erway, L. C. (2001). Genetic basis for susceptibility to noise-induced hearing loss in mice. *Hear. Res.* 155, 82–90. doi: 10.1016/s0378-5955(01)00250-7

D'Orlando, C., Celio, M. R., and Schwaller, B. (2002). Calretinin and calbindin D-28k, but not parvalbumin protect against glutamate-induced delayed excitotoxicity in transfected N18-RE 105 neuroblastoma-retina hybrid cells. *Brain Res.* 945, 181–190. doi: 10.1016/s0006-8993(02)02753-1

El-Hassar, L., Song, L., Tan, W. J. T., Large, C. H., Alvaro, G., Santos-Sacchi, J., et al. (2019). Modulators of Kv3 potassium channels rescue the auditory function of fragile X mice. *J. Neurosci.* 39, 4797–4813. doi: 10.1523/jneurosci.0839-18.2019

Esterberg, R., Hailey, D. W., Rubel, E. W., and Raible, D. W. (2014). ER-mitochondrial calcium flow underlies vulnerability of mechanosensory hair cells to damage. *J. Neurosci.* 34, 9703–9719. doi: 10.1523/jneurosci.0281-14.2014

Flippo, K. H., and Strack, S. (2017). Mitochondrial dynamics in neuronal injury, development and plasticity. *J. Cell Sci.* 130, 671–681. doi: 10.1242/jcs.171017

Gao, S., Cheng, C., Wang, M., Jiang, P., Zhang, L., Wang, Y., et al. (2019). Blebbistatin inhibits neomycin-induced apoptosis in hair cell-like HEI-OC-1 cells and in cochlear hair cells. *Front. Cell. Neurosci.* 13:590. doi: 10.3389/fncel.2019.00590

Giorgi, C., Baldassari, F., Bononi, A., Bonora, M., De Marchi, E., Marchi, S., et al. (2012). Mitochondrial Ca(2+) and apoptosis. *Cell Calcium* 52, 36–43. doi: 10.1016/j.ceca.2012.02.008

Giorgi, C., Romagnoli, A., Pinton, P., and Rizzuto, R. (2008). Ca^{2+} signaling, mitochondria and cell death. *Curr. Mol. Med.* 8, 119–130. doi: 10.2174/156652408783769571

Hajieva, P., Baeken, M. W., and Moosmann, B. (2018). The role of Plasma Membrane Calcium ATPases (PMCAs) in neurodegenerative disorders. *Neurosci. Lett.* 663, 29–38. doi: 10.1016/j.neulet.2017.09.033

He, Z., Guo, L., Shu, Y., Fang, Q., Zhou, H., Liu, Y., et al. (2017). Autophagy protects auditory hair cells against neomycin-induced damage. *Autophagy* 13, 1884–1904. doi: 10.1080/15548627.2017.1359449

He, Z., Sun, S., Waqas, M., Zhang, X., Qian, F., Cheng, C., et al. (2016). Reduced TRMU expression increases the sensitivity of hair-cell-like HEI-OC-1 cells to neomycin damage *in vitro*. *Sci. Rep.* 6:29621. doi: 10.1038/srep29621

He, Z. H., Zou, S. Y., Li, M., Liao, F. L., Wu, X., Sun, H. Y., et al. (2020). The nuclear transcription factor FoxG1 affects the sensitivity of mimetic aging hair cells to inflammation by regulating autophagy pathways. *Redox Biol.* 28:101364. doi: 10.1016/j.redox.2019.101364

Henry, W. R., and Mulroy, M. J. (1995). Afferent synaptic changes in auditory hair cells during noise-induced temporary threshold shift. *Hear. Res.* 84, 81–90. doi: 10.1016/0378-5955(95)00014-u

Hickox, A. E., and Liberman, M. C. (2014). Is noise-induced cochlear neuropathy key to the generation of hyperacusis or tinnitus? *J. Neurophysiol.* 111, 552–564. doi: 10.1152/jn.00184.2013

Imbriani, P., Tassone, A., Meringolo, M., Ponterio, G., Madeo, G., Pisani, A., et al. (2019). Loss of Non-apoptotic role of caspase-3 in the PINK1 mouse model of Parkinson's Disease. *Int. J. Mol. Sci* 20:3407. doi: 10.3390/ijms20143407

Kaltenbach, J. A., and Afman, C. E. (2000). Hyperactivity in the dorsal cochlear nucleus after intense sound exposure and its resemblance to tone-evoked activity: a physiological model for tinnitus. *Hear. Res.* 140, 165–172. doi: 10.1016/s0378-5955(99)00197-5

Kim, K. X., Payne, S., Yang-Hood, A., Li, S. Z., Davis, B., Carlquist, J., et al. (2019). Vesicular glutamatergic transmission in noise-induced loss and repair of cochlear ribbon synapses. *J. Neurosci.* 39, 4434–4447. doi: 10.1523/jneurosci.2228-18.2019

Kim, M. H., Lee, S. H., Park, K. H., Ho, W. K., and Lee, S. H. (2003). Distribution of K^+-dependent $Na+/Ca^{2+}$ exchangers in the rat supraoptic magnocellular neuron is polarized to axon terminals. *J. Neurosci.* 23, 11673–11680. doi: 10.1523/jneurosci.23-37-11673.2003

Krinner, S., Butola, T., Jung, S., Wichmann, C., and Moser, T. (2017). RIM-binding protein 2 promotes a large number of Ca(V)1.3 Ca(2+)-channels and contributes to fast synaptic vesicle replenishment at hair cell active zones. *Front. Cell. Neurosci.* 11:334. doi: 10.3389/fncel.2017.00334

Kujawa, S. G., and Liberman, M. C. (2009). Adding insult to injury: cochlear nerve degeneration after "temporary" noise-induced hearing loss. *J. Neurosci.* 29, 14077–14085. doi: 10.1523/jneurosci.2845-09.2009

Kujawa, S. G., and Liberman, M. C. (2015). Synaptopathy in the noise-exposed and aging cochlea: primary neural degeneration in acquired sensorineural hearing loss. *Hear Res.* 330(Pt B), 191–199. doi: 10.1016/j.heares.2015.02.009

Lenzi, D., and Roberts, W. M. (1994). Calcium signalling in hair cells: multiple roles in a compact cell. *Curr. Opin. Neurobiol.* 4, 496–502. doi: 10.1016/0959-4388(94)90049-3

Li, A., You, D., Li, W., Cui, Y., He, Y., Li, W., et al. (2018a). Novel compounds protect auditory hair cells against gentamycin-induced apoptosis by maintaining the expression level of H3K4me2. *Drug Deliv.* 25, 1033–1043. doi: 10.1080/10717544.2018.1461277

Li, H., Song, Y., He, Z., Chen, X., Wu, X., Li, X., et al. (2018b). Meclofenamic acid reduces reactive oxygen species accumulation and apoptosis, inhibits excessive autophagy, and protects hair cell-like HEI-OC1 cells from cisplatin-induced damage. *Front. Cell. Neurosci.* 12:139. doi: 10.3389/fncel.2018.00139

Li, H. S., and Hultcrantz, M. (1994). Age-related degeneration of the organ of Corti in two genotypes of mice. *ORL J. Otorhinolaryngol. Relat. Spec.* 56, 61–67. doi: 10.1159/000276611

Liberman, M. C., Epstein, M. J., Cleveland, S. S., Wang, H., and Maison, S. F.

(2016). Toward a differential diagnosis of hidden hearing loss in humans. *PLoS ONE* 11:e0162726. doi: 10.1371/journal.pone.0162726

Liberman, M. C., and Kujawa, S. G. (2017). Cochlear synaptopathy in acquired sensorineural hearing loss: manifestations and mechanisms. *Hear. Res.* 349, 138–147. doi: 10.1016/j.heares.2017.01.003

Lin, F. R., Niparko, J. K., and Ferrucci, L. (2011). Hearing loss prevalence in the United States. *Arch. Intern. Med.* 171, 1851–1852. doi: 10.1001/archinternmed.2011.506

Lin, X., Li, G., Zhang, Y., Zhao, J., Lu, J., Gao, Y., et al. (2019). Hearing consequences in Gjb2 knock-in mice: implications for human p.V37I mutation. *Aging* 11, 7416–7441. doi: 10.18632/aging.102246

Liu, H., Li, G., Lu, J., Gao, Y. G., Song, L., Li, G. L., et al. (2019a). Cellular differences in the cochlea of CBA and B6 mice may underlie their difference in susceptibility to hearing loss. *Front. Cell. Neurosci* 13:60. doi: 10.3389/fncel.2019.00060

Liu, H., Lu, J., Wang, Z., Song, L., Wang, X., Li, G. L., et al. (2019b). Functional alteration of ribbon synapses in inner hair cells by noise exposure causing hidden hearing loss. *Neurosci. Lett.* 707:134268. doi: 10.1016/j.neulet.2019.05.022

Liu, L., Chen, Y., Qi, J., Zhang, Y., He, Y., Ni, W., et al. (2016). Wnt activation protects against neomycin-induced hair cell damage in the mouse cochlea. *Cell Death Dis.* 7:e2136. doi: 10.1038/cddis.2016.35

Liu, W., Xu, X., Fan, Z., Sun, G., Han, Y., Zhang, D., et al. (2019c). Wnt signaling activates TP53-induced glycolysis and apoptosis regulator and protects against cisplatin-induced spiral ganglion neuron damage in the mouse cochlea. *Antioxid. Redox Signal.* 30, 1389–1410. doi: 10.1089/ars.2017.7288

Liu, Y., Qi, J., Chen, X., Tang, M., Chu, C., Zhu, W., et al. (2019d). Critical role of spectrin in hearing development and deafness. *Sci Adv.* 5:eaav7803. doi: 10.1126/sciadv.aav7803

Ma, M., Ferguson, T. A., Schoch, K. M., Li, J., Qian, Y., Shofer, F. S., et al. (2013). Calpains mediate axonal cytoskeleton disintegration during Wallerian degeneration. *Neurobiol. Dis.* 56, 34–46. doi: 10.1016/j.nbd.2013.03.009

Michalski, N., Goutman, J. D., Auclair, S. M., Boutet de Monvel, J., Tertrais, M., Emptoz, A., et al. (2017). Otoferlin acts as a Ca(2+) sensor for vesicle fusion and vesicle pool replenishment at auditory hair cell ribbon synapses. *Elife* 6:e31013. doi: 10.7554/eLife.31013

Michanski, S., Smaluch, K., Steyer, A. M., Chakrabarti, R., Setz, C., Oestreicher, D., et al. (2019). Mapping developmental maturation of inner hair cell ribbon synapses in the apical mouse cochlea. *Proc. Natl. Acad. Sci. U.S.A.* 116, 6415–6424. doi: 10.1073/pnas.1812029116

Monaghan, J. J. M., Garcia-Lazaro, J. A., McAlpine, D., and Schaette, R. (2020). Hidden hearing loss impacts the neural representation of speech in background noise. *Curr. Biol.* 30, 4710–4721.e4. doi: 10.1016/j.cub.2020.09.046

Noben-Trauth, K., Zheng, Q. Y., and Johnson, K. R. (2003). Association of cadherin 23 with polygenic inheritance and genetic modification of sensorineural hearing loss. *Nat. Genet.* 35, 21–23. doi: 10.1038/ng1226

Qi, J., Liu, Y., Chu, C., Chen, X., Zhu, W., Shu, Y., et al. (2019). A cytoskeleton structure revealed by super-resolution fluorescence imaging in inner ear hair cells. *Cell Discov.* 5:12. doi: 10.1038/s41421-018-0076-4

Qi, J., Zhang, L., Tan, F., Liu, Y., Chu, C., Zhu, W., et al. (2020). Espin distribution as revealed by super-resolution microscopy of stereocilia. *Am. J. Transl. Res.* 12, 130–141.

Qian, F., Wang, X., Yin, Z., Xie, G., Yuan, H., Liu, D., et al. (2020). The slc4a2b gene is required for hair cell development in zebrafish. *Aging* 12, 18804–18821. doi: 10.18632/aging.103840

Rizzuto, R., De Stefani, D., Raffaello, A., and Mammucari, C. (2012). Mitochondria as sensors and regulators of calcium signalling. *Nat. Rev. Mol. Cell Biol.* 13, 566–578. doi: 10.1038/nrm3412

Schaette, R., and McAlpine, D. (2011). Tinnitus with a normal audiogram: physiological evidence for hidden hearing loss and computational model. *J. Neurosci.* 31, 13452–13457. doi: 10.1523/jneurosci.2156-11.2011

Sharma, K., Seo, Y. W., and Yi, E. (2018). Differential expression of Ca(2+)-buffering protein calretinin in cochlear afferent fibers: a possible link to vulnerability to traumatic noise. *Exp. Neurobiol.* 27, 397–407. doi: 10.5607/en.2018.27.5.397

Shi, L., Chang, Y., Li, X., Aiken, S., Liu, L., and Wang, J. (2016). Cochlear synaptopathy and noise-induced hidden hearing loss. *Neural Plast.* 2016:6143164. doi: 10.1155/2016/6143164

Shi, L., Liu, K., Wang, H., Zhang, Y., Hong, Z., Wang, M., et al. (2015). Noise induced reversible changes of cochlear ribbon synapses contribute to temporary hearing loss in mice. *Acta Otolaryngol.* 135, 1093–1102. doi: 10.3109/00016489.2015.1061699

Shi, L., Liu, L., He, T., Guo, X., Yu, Z., Yin, S., et al. (2013). Ribbon synapse plasticity in the cochleae of Guinea pigs after noise-induced silent damage. *PLoS ONE* 8:e81566. doi: 10.1371/journal.pone.0081566

Spongr, V. P., Flood, D. G., Frisina, R. D., and Salvi, R. J. (1997). Quantitative measures of hair cell loss in CBA and C57BL/6 mice throughout their life spans. *J. Acoust. Soc. Am.* 101, 3546–3553. doi: 10.1121/1.418315

Sun, S., Sun, M., Zhang, Y., Cheng, C., Waqas, M., Yu, H., et al. (2014). *In vivo* overexpression of X-linked inhibitor of apoptosis protein protects against neomycin-induced hair cell loss in the apical turn of the cochlea during the ototoxic-sensitive period. *Front. Cell. Neurosci.* 8:248. doi: 10.3389/fncel.2014.00248

Tan, W. J. T., Song, L., Graham, M., Schettino, A., Navaratnam, D., Yarbrough, W. G., et al. (2017). Novel role of the mitochondrial protein Fus1 in protection from premature hearing loss via regulation of oxidative stress and nutrient and energy sensing pathways in the inner ear. *Antioxid. Redox Signal.* 27, 489–509. doi: 10.1089/ars.2016.6851

Tucker, T., and Fettiplace, R. (1995). Confocal imaging of calcium microdomains and calcium extrusion in turtle hair cells. *Neuron* 15, 1323–1335. doi: 10.1016/0896-6273(95)90011-x

Vlajkovic, S. M., Ambepitiya, K., Barclay, M., Boison, D., Housley, G. D., and Thorne, P. R. (2017). Adenosine receptors regulate susceptibility to noise-induced neural injury in the mouse cochlea and hearing loss. *Hear. Res.* 345, 43–51. doi: 10.1016/j.heares.2016.12.015

Wang, J., Yin, S., Chen, H., and Shi, L. (2019). Noise-induced cochlear synaptopathy and ribbon synapse regeneration: repair process and therapeutic target. *Adv. Exp. Med. Biol.* 1130, 37–57. doi: 10.1007/978-981-13-6123-4_3

Wang, X., Zhu, Y., Long, H., Pan, S., Xiong, H., Fang, Q., et al. (2018). Mitochondrial calcium transporters mediate sensitivity to noise-induced losses of hair cells and cochlear synapses. *Front. Mol. Neurosci.* 11:469. doi: 10.3389/fnmol.2018.00469

Wang, Y., Li, J., Yao, X., Li, W., Du, H., Tang, M., et al. (2017). Loss of CIB2 causes profound hearing loss and abolishes mechanoelectrical transduction in mice. *Front. Mol. Neurosci.* 10:401. doi: 10.3389/fnmol.2017.00401

Wong, A. B., Rutherford, M. A., Gabrielaitis, M., Pangrsic, T., Göttfert, F., Frank, T., et al. (2014). Developmental refinement of hair cell synapses tightens the coupling of Ca^{2+} influx to exocytosis. *EMBO J.* 33, 247–264. doi: 10.1002/embj.201387110

Wong, H. C., Zhang, Q., Beirl, A. J., Petralia, R. S., Wang, Y. X., and Kindt, K. (2019). Synaptic mitochondria regulate hair-cell synapse size and function. *Elife* 8:e48914. doi: 10.7554/eLife.48914

Yamasoba, T., Pourbakht, A., Sakamoto, T., and Suzuki, M. (2005). Ebselen prevents noise-induced excitotoxicity and temporary threshold shift. *Neurosci. Lett.* 380, 234–238. doi: 10.1016/j.neulet.2005.0 1.047

Yu, X., Liu, W., Fan, Z., Qian, F., Zhang, D., Han, Y., et al. (2017). c-Myb knockdown increases the neomycin-induced damage to hair-cell-like HEI-OC1 cells *in vitro*. *Sci. Rep.* 7:41094. doi: 10.1038/srep41094

Zenisek, D., and Matthews, G. (2000). The role of mitochondria in presynaptic calcium handling at a ribbon synapse. *Neuron* 25, 229–237. doi: 10.1016/s0896-6273(00)80885-5

Zhang, S., Zhang, Y., Dong, Y., Guo, L., Zhang, Z., Shao, B., et al. (2020). Knockdown of Foxg1 in supporting cells increases the trans-differentiation of supporting cells into hair cells in the neonatal mouse cochlea. *Cell. Mol. Life Sci.* 77, 1401–1419. doi: 10.1007/s00018-019-03291-2

Zhang, Y., Li, W., He, Z., Wang, Y., Shao, B., Cheng, C., et al. (2019). Pre-treatment with fasudil prevents neomycin-induced hair cell damage by reducing the accumulation of reactive oxygen species. *Front. Mol. Neurosci.* 12:264. doi: 10.3389/fnmol.2019.00264

Zhao, J., Li, G., Zhao, X., Lin, X., Gao, Y., Raimundo, N., et al. (2020). Down-regulation of AMPK signaling pathway rescues hearing loss in TFB1 transgenic mice and delays age-related hearing loss. *Aging* 12, 5590–5611. doi: 10.18632/aging.10 2977

Zhong, Z., Fu, X., Li, H., Chen, J., Wang, M., Gao, S., et al. (2020). Citicoline protects auditory hair cells against neomycin-induced damage. *Front. Cell Dev. Biol.* 8:712. doi: 10.3389/fcell.2020.00712

Zhou, H., Qian, X., Xu, N., Zhang, S., Zhu, G., Zhang, Y., et al. (2020). Disruption of Atg7-dependent autophagy causes electromotility disturbances, outer hair cell loss, and deafness in mice. *Cell Death Dis.* 11:913. doi: 10.1038/s41419-020-03110-8

Zhu, C., Cheng, C., Wang, Y., Muhammad, W., Liu, S., Zhu, W., et al. (2018). Loss of ARHGEF6 causes hair cell stereocilia deficits and hearing loss in mice. *Front. Mol. Neurosci.* 11:362. doi: 10.3389/fnmol.2018.00362

17

Claudin h is Essential for Hair Cell Morphogenesis and Auditory Function in Zebrafish

Jie Gong[1†], Peipei Qian[1†], Yuebo Hu[1], Chao Guo[1], Guanyun Wei[1], Cheng Wang[1], Chengyun Cai[1], Haibo Wang[2] and Dong Liu[1*]*

[1] *Nantong Laboratory of Development and Diseases, School of Life Sciences, Co-innovation Center of Neuroregeneration, Key Laboratory of Neuroregeneration of Jiangsu and MOE, Nantong University, Nantong, China,* [2] *Shandong Provincial ENT Hospital, Cheeloo College of Medicine, Shandong University, Jinan, China*

***Correspondence:**
Haibo Wang
whboto11@163.com
Dong Liu
liudongtom@gmail.com;
tom@ntu.edu.cn

† These authors have contributed equally to this work

Hereditary hearing loss caused by defective hair cells is one of the most common congenital diseases, whose nosogenesis is still unclear because many of the causative genes remain unidentified. Claudins are one kind of transmembrane proteins that constitute the most important components of the tight junctions and paracellular barrier and play important roles in neurodevelopment. In this study, we investigated the function of *claudin h* in morphogenesis and auditory function of the hair cell in zebrafish. The results of *in situ* hybridization showed that *claudin h* was specifically localized in the otic vesicle and neuromasts in zebrafish embryos. The deficiency of *claudin h* caused significant reduction of otic vesicle size and loss of utricle otolith. Moreover, the startle response and vestibulo-ocular reflex experiments revealed that loss of *claudin h* led to serious hearing loss and vestibular dysfunction. Importantly, the confocal microscopy observation found that compared to the control zebrafish, the *claudin h* morphants and mutants displayed significantly reduced the number of cristae hair cells and shortened kinocilia. Besides, the deficiency of *claudin h* also caused the loss of hair cells in neuromasts which could be rescued by injecting *claudin h* mRNA into the mutant embryos at one cell stage. Furthermore, the immunohistochemistry experiments demonstrated remarkable apoptosis of hair cells in the neuromasts, which might contribute to the loss of hair cells number. Overall, these data indicated that *claudin h* is indispensable for the development of hair cells, vestibular function, and hearing ability of zebrafish.

Keywords: *claudin h*, otic vesicle, hearing loss, vestibular dysfunction, hair cell, zebrafish

INTRODUCTION

Hair cells are one of the sensory cells in the auditory epithelium of the mammalian inner ear which are necessary for transforming sound vibration and mechanical forces including gravity into neural signals that can be interpreted by the brain (Goutman et al., 2015). In mammals, there are two different hair cells classified as outer hair cells and inner hair cells. Outer hair cells that have three rows of cells can mechanically amplify sound-induced vibrations to increase the responsiveness of sensory epithelium, while inner hair cells have only one row of cells and are functional in transmitting the signals to the spiral ganglion neurons (Ma et al., 2018). Therefore, the number and function of hair cells are crucial for hearing (Liu et al., 2019; Qi et al., 2019; He et al., 2020). Hearing loss could be caused by different reasons including genetic factors, aging, infectious diseases, ototoxic drugs, and noise exposure (Zhu et al., 2018; Gao et al., 2019), among which the genetic factors contribute the most by leading to hereditary and progressive hearing loss. To date, the mechanisms of hair cell damage mainly include mechanical shearing forces and oxidative damage to hair cells, which eventually induce apoptotic cell death in hair cells (Liu et al., 2016; Ding et al., 2020; Zhou et al., 2020). The lower vertebrates have the hair cell regeneration ability though life times; while in mammals, although neonatal mice cochlea have limited hair cell regeneration ability, this regeneration ability is rapidly reduced with age (Wang et al., 2015; Zhang et al., 2020).

A typical characteristic of biological development is to separate the compositionally distinct extracellular fluids by sealing off the paracellular spaces (Madara, 1998). The essential structure of this seal formed with epithelial sheets is the continuous band-like networks of neighboring cells that are known as tight junctions (Nakano et al., 2009). Tight junctions that circumscribe the apical end of the cell can make the membranes of the adjacent cells closely connected and thereby split the cells into the basolateral and apical region, and then form a barrier to restrict paracellular permeability of ions and solutes (Dejana, 2004). In recent years, several integral membrane proteins have been identified to be involved in the function of the tight junctions and the specific expression of these proteins in different tissues may account for various "tightness" of tight junctions (Van Itallie and Anderson, 2004; Li et al., 2018). Nowadays, at least three types of transmembrane proteins, occludin, claudin family, and the junction adhesion molecule family, are reported to compose the tight junctions by interacting with the cytoskeleton and other membrane-associated proteins (Furuse et al., 1993; Martin-Padura et al., 1998; Tsukita and Furuse, 2000).

Claudins have been reported to be the primary components of the tight junctions in many tissues to form the backbone of tight junction strands (Tipsmark et al., 2008). The claudins are conserved in different species for the membrane topology with two extracellular loops, one N-terminal cytoplasmic domain and one C-terminal cytoplasmic domain (Li et al., 2011). The extracellular loops are essential for forming the paracellular barrier structure by polymerizing the intercellular claudins into strands, while the C-terminal cytoplasmic domains of claudins can coordinate with the scaffolding proteins to link the tight junctions to the actin cytoskeleton (Wen et al., 2004; Krause et al., 2008). The epithelia of mammalian nephric tubules utilize abundant tight junctions to transport ions selectively between the intercellular regions (Gong and Hou, 2017). Many different claudins are reported expressing in different segments of nephric tubules and are necessary for kidney function as selective paracellular pores or barriers to regulate the diffusion of different ions and water via tight junctions (Van Itallie et al., 2006; Angelow et al., 2007; Milatz et al., 2010; Li et al., 2011). For example, it has been reported that in the porcine kidney epithelial cell line, Claudin-7 can form a paracellular barrier to Cl-, but serve as a paracellular channel for Na^+ (Alexandre et al., 2005). In addition, there are some claudins which are not merely expressed in tight junctions, but also in some other cellular parts play important roles in embryonic development (Gregory et al., 2001; Kollmar et al., 2001).

The zebrafish has become an excellent model organism in biological research to investigate otic vesicle and neural development which are closely related to the human diseases. The greatest advantage of using zebrafish for research is the convenience for recording and tracking of the developmental process by imaging (Downes and Granato, 2004; Bandmann and Burton, 2010). Moreover, the otic vesicle of zebrafish separates the distinct paracellular fluids compositionally and therefore becomes a great model for investigating the function of claudins and tight junctions on hearing and balance. Recently, loss of both *claudin7b* and *claudin j* was found to lead to the abnormal otolith formation and hair cell function and further cause the inner ear dysfunction in the zebrafish (Hardison et al., 2005; Li et al., 2018). However, the functions of other claudins in the inner ear remain unclear, and thus it promoted us to establish a loss of function model to study the role of claudins in hearing function.

In this study, we found that *claudin h* (*claudin 3* in mammals) were expressed in the otic vesicle and neuromasts of zebrafish embryos by *in situ* hybridization. Loss of function treatments by either morpholino injection or CRISPR-cas9 could both cause hearing loss and vestibular dysfunction. We further found that these dysfunctions might be caused by abnormal otolith formation, hair cell loss, and otic vesicle morphological defects. Moreover, *claudin h* deficiency could induce hair cell apoptosis, which explained the decrease in number of the hair cells. In summary, our study proved that *claudin h* was essential for the formation of hair cell and otoliths and the normal hearing function of the inner ear in zebrafish.

MATERIALS AND METHODS

Zebrafish Husbandry

The zebrafish embryos and adults were maintained in the zebrafish Center of Nantong University under conditions following our previous protocols (Gong et al., 2020). Wild-type (AB) control and *Tg(Brn3c:GFP)* transgenic zebrafish whose hair cells were labeled by GFP were used in this study (Xiao et al., 2005).

Whole Mount *in situ* Hybridization

Whole-mount *in situ* hybridization (WISH) was performed according to our previous procedures (Huang et al., 2013). A 409 bp cDNA fragment of *claudin h* was amplified from zebrafish embryo cDNA library with specific primers (**Table 1**) and inserted into pGEM-T-easy vector. Digoxigenin-labeled antisense probes were synthesized with the linearized pGEM-T inserting with *claudin h* construct by DIG-RNA labeling kit (Roche, Switzerland). Zebrafish embryos without pigment at different developmental stages were collected and fixed with 4% PFA overnight at 4°C. After incubated with the probe overnight, an alkaline phosphatase-conjugated antibody against digoxigenin

TABLE 1 | Summary of primers used.

Primers	Primer sequence (5′-3′)	Purpose
Cldnh-F	CGATGGGACTGGAAATTGGG	Riboprobe amplification for *Cldnh*
Cldnh-R	CCCAGGCTGAAGGAATGAGA	Riboprobe amplification for *Cldnh*
Cldnh-gRNA	GGTGTGATGATCTCCGTCAT	Fragment amplification for gRNA
Cldnh-gRNA F	ATGTGGCGTGTCTCGGCCTT	Fragment amplification for *Cldnh* gRNA
Cldnh-gRNA R	ACAGCATGGCTCCTCCAATG	Fragment amplification for *Cldnh* gRNA

and AP-substrate NBT/BCIP solution (Roche, Switzerland) was used to detect the digoxigenin-labeled RNA probe.

Morpholino and mRNAs Injections

Splicing-blocking Morpholino (5′- ATGAATGTCATTTACCAA GTGTCGA -3′) that was specific for *claudin h* gene was synthesized by Gene Tools. *Tg(Brn3c:GFP)* zebrafish were naturally mated to obtain embryos for microinjection. The Morpholino was diluted to 0.3 mM with RNase-free water and injected into one cell stage embryos and then raised in E3 medium at 28.5°C for imaging.

Immunohistochemistry

The larvae at 96 hpf were fixed with 4% PFA for 2 h at room temperature and then washed with PBST for 30 min followed with antigen retrieval at 98°C for 15 min. After washed three times with PBST, the larvae were incubated in blocking solution for 1 h and then were transferred to the primary antibody solutions (anti-GFP, 1:1000 dilution; Abcam, Cambridge, United Kingdom and anti-cleaved caspase-3, 1:500 dilution; Cell Signaling Technology Inc., Danvers, MA, United States) overnight at 4°C. Then, the Alexa Fluor 488 and Alexa Fluor 647 conjugated secondary antibodies were added to larvae at a dilution of 1:500 in blocking solution and incubated for 1 h at room temperature after washed three times with PBST. Nuclei were labeled with 4,6-diamidino-2-phenylindole (DAPI) (1:1000 dilution; Invitrogen, Carlsbad, CA, United States) for 20 min at room temperature and then mounted for imaging.

sgRNA/Cas9 mRNA Synthesis and Injection

Cas9 mRNA was obtained by *in vitro* transcription with the linearized plasmid pXT7-Cas9 by the mMESSAGE mMACHIN Kit according to the manufacturer's instruction. For the sgRNA synthesis, a forward primer that contained the *claudin h* specific primers and a universal reverse gRNAR primer (**Table 1**) were used for sgDNA amplification with pT7 plasmid as the template, and then transcribed into sgRNA using the MAXIscript® kits according to the manufacturer's instruction. One-cell stage zebrafish embryos were injected with 2–3 nl solution containing 250 ng/μl Cas9 mRNA and 15 ng/μl sgRNA. At 72 and 96 hpf, zebrafish embryos that developed normally were randomly sampled for the confocal imaging and genomic DNA extraction to determine the mutations by DNA sequencing.

mRNA Rescue Experiments

The *claudin h* mRNA was transcribed *in vitro* using linearized artificial PCS2+ vector with the *claudin h* open reading frame cDNAs by the mMESSAGE mMACHIN Kit according to the manufacturer's instruction (Ambion, United States). After purified using RNeasy Mini Kit (Qiagen, Germany), 2 nl capped mRNA was co-injected with *claudin h* Mo into one-cell stage embryos.

Vestibulo-Ocular Reflex (VOR) Testing

The zebrafish larva was gently mounted in the larva-shaped chamber in a dorsal-up position with the tail glued by 5% methylcellulose and covered with a piece of glass coverslip on the chamber. After adding E3 embryo media in the head region, the chamber unit was then mounted on a device for quantifying linear vestibulo-ocular reflex (VOR) from Southern University of Science and Technology (Sun et al., 2018). After aligning the larval eyes to the center of the infrared camera, the platform started to rotate back and forth around a horizontal axis at a speed of 30 rpm, and the VOR was recorded by the camera.

Acoustic Startle Reflex

About 20 larvae were put in a thin layer of culture media in a petri dish attached to mini vibrator. The response of larvae to sound stimulus (a tone burst 9 dB re. m s^{-2}, 600 Hz, for 30 ms) generated by the vibrator was recorded from above by an infrared camera over a 6 s period. The mean moving distance and peak speed were used to quantify the startle response.

Microscopy and Statistical Analysis

After being anesthetized with tricaine, the zebrafish embryos were mounted in 0.8% low melt agarose, and then photographed by Leica TCS-SP5 LSM confocal microscope. For the *in situ* hybridization, photographs were taken using an Olympus stereomicroscope MVX10. Statistical analyses were performed by one-way analysis of variance (ANOVA), student's *t*-test or chi-squared test, and *P* values < 0.05 were considered statistically significant.

RESULTS

Claudin h Gene Is Evolutionarily Conserved and Expressed in the Otic Vesicle and Hair Cells

To determine the relationships of zebrafish *claudin h* with other homologous genes, the multiple alignments of *claudin h* from different species were performed and the phylogenetic tree of the *claudin h* was constructed using the Neighbor-joining method. As shown in **Figure 1A**, the zebrafish *claudin h* gene had significantly high amino acid sequence similarities to other species. The NJ tree of *claudin h* showed that the *claudin h* from osteichthyes

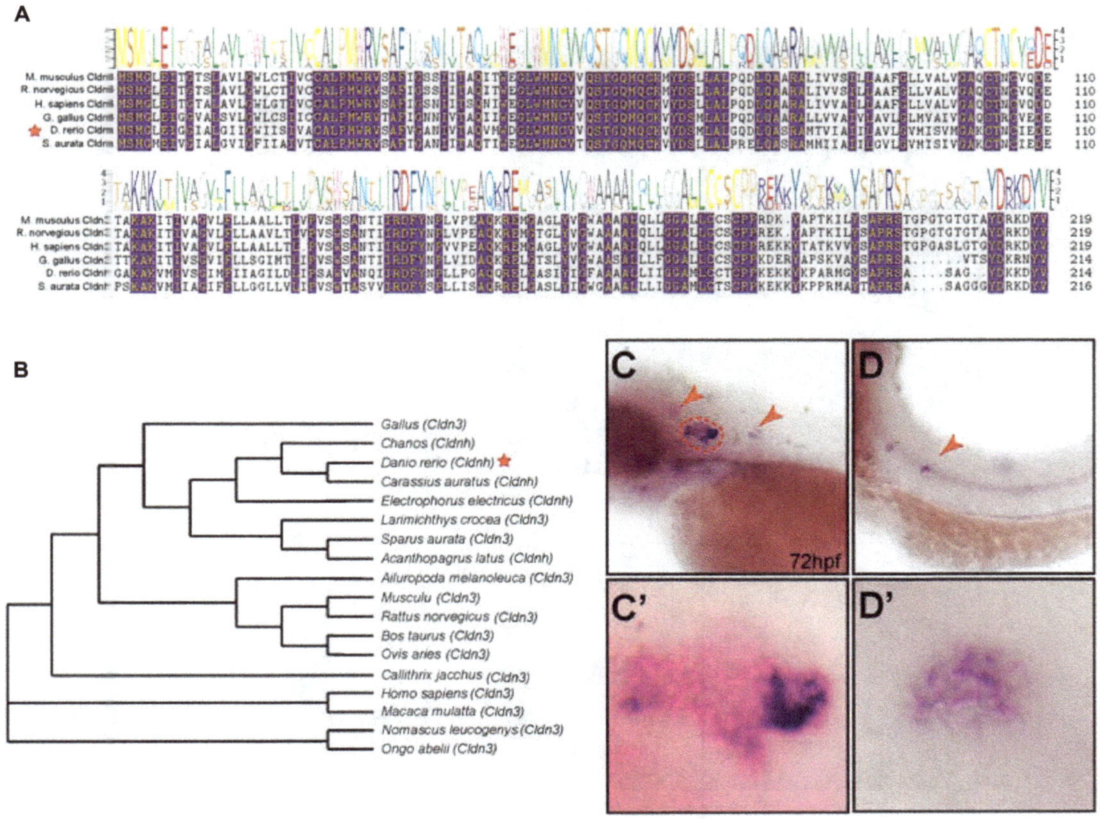

FIGURE 1 | The phylogenetic and expression analysis of zebrafish *claudin h*. **(A)** The alignment of *claudin h* amino acid sequences from different species, and the identical aa residues among all the aligned sequences are labeled with color. **(B)** Phylogenetic analysis of *claudin h*. Neighbor-joining tree was produced with the Mega 5.0 software and the red star marked the zebrafish. **(C,D)** At 72 hpf, the *in situ* hybridization signal of *claudin h* is localized in the otic vesicle and neuromast. The red dotted line marked the boundary of the otic vesicle and the red arrow head marked the neuromast in the head and posterior lateral line. **(C′,D′)** The magnified figure of the positive signals in otic vesicle and neuromast line.

and birds were clustered in a separate clade from rodents and primates *claudin h* (**Figure 1B**).

To investigate the role of *claudin h* during embryonic development, we tested the expression profile of *claudin h* in zebrafish by WISH with a digoxigenin-labeled *claudin h* probe. The results showed that at 24 hpf, *claudin h* was expressed in the otic vesicle, posterior lateral line primordium and pronephros (**Supplementary Figure 1A**), while from 36 hpf, the gene started to be localized in lateral line neuromasts (**Figures 1D,D'** and **Supplementary Figure 1B**). Besides, the *claudin h* was also detected in the neuromasts of the head with continued development (**Figures 1C,C'** and **Supplementary Figure 1**). Together these results suggested that *claudin h* might be vital for the development of otic vesicle and neuromast.

Deficiency of *Claudin h* Caused Developmental Defects of Otic Vesicle and Otoliths

Since a significant expression of *claudin h* was found in the otic vesicle, we examined the morphology of otic vesicle and otolith in the *claudin h* knocking down zebrafish by confocal microscopy at 72 and 96 hpf to investigate whether *claudin h* regulates the formation of otic vesicle. The results showed that although the morphants had no remarkable malformation, the otic vesicle size was significantly smaller compared to that in the control fish at both 72 and 96 hpf (**Figures 2A–C**). Moreover, the *claudin h* morphants also showed obvious defects in both number and shape of the otoliths. Different from the wild type zebrafish who possessed a big otolith (saccular) and a small otolith (utricle), 83% of *claudin h* morphants either lost the utricle otolith or had an abnormal saccular otolith (**Figures 2D–E**).

Deficiency of the *Claudin h* Caused Vestibular Dysfunction and Hearing Defects

To test whether abnormalities of the otic vesicles and otoliths in the *claudin h* morphants caused defects of balance perception or vestibular dysfunction, we tested VOR of AB zebrafish and *claudin h* morphants at 5 dpf using a customized VOR testing system (**Figure 3A**, Sun et al., 2018). The results showed that compared with the AB zebrafish who had robust eye movements,

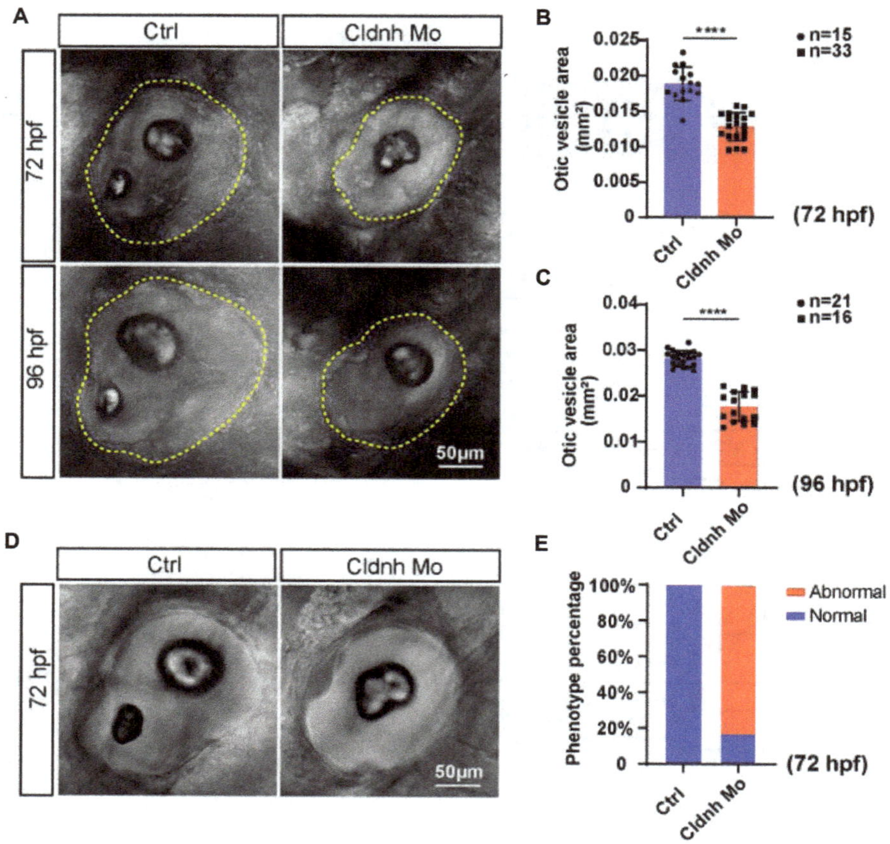

FIGURE 2 | Loss function of *claudin h* caused the defects of otic vesicle and otoliths. **(A,D)** Imaging analysis of otic vesicle and otoliths in control and *claudin h* knocking down groups at 72 and 96 hpf. The yellow dotted line marked the boundary of the otic vesicle. Scale bar = 50 μm. **(B,C)** The statistical analysis of otic vesicle area in the control and *claudin h* morphants at 72 and 96 hpf. **(E)** Quantification of zebrafish embryos with abnormal otolith (defects in both number and shape of otoliths: *claudin h* morphants lost the utricle otolith or had a unnormal saccular otolith). Each bar represents the mean ± SE. Values with **** above the bars are significantly different ($P < 0.0001$).

most of the *claudin h* morphants showed slight eye movements while rotating in the vertical plane in the machine (**Figure 3B**). The statistical analysis also showed that the amplitude of eye movements in *claudin h* morphants was significantly lower than that in AB zebrafish during VOR ($P < 0.0001$, **Figures 3C,D**).

To test whether malformation of the otic vesicles could also result in hearing dysfunction, a startle response experiment was performed. The results showed that the movement trajectory, swimming distance, and velocity of the *claudin h* morphants zebrafish larvae were significantly decreased compared to that of the controls at 5 dpf in startle responses (**Figures 3E–H**). These results indicated that the zebrafish hearing might be impaired by the *claudin h* Mo injection.

Deficiency of the *Claudin h* Led to Decreased Hair Cells and Neuromasts

As we know, the hair cells in the inner ear of zebrafish are involved in balance perception and hearing. Therefore, to further investigate the cellular mechanisms of *claudin h* regulation on the ear function, morpholino-mediated gene knockdown was performed in the transgenic zebrafish line *Tg(Brn3c:mGFP)* where the hair cells are specifically labeled by GFP. The imaging results showed that although the three different cristae hair cell clusters, anterior cristae hair cells, lateral cristae hair cells, and posterior cristae hair cells still existed, the numbers of hair cells in each cluster were significantly decreased after the *claudin h* Mo injection at 72 and 96 hpf (**Figures 4A–D**). In addition, the growth of the cilia in the three different hair cell clusters was also affected by loss of *claudin h* and the statistical analysis demonstrated that the lengths of kinocilia in the *claudin h* morphants were significantly shorter than that in the control zebrafish at 72 and 96 hpf (**Figures 4E,F**).

The WISH results showed that *claudin h* was also localized in the neuromasts of the trunk. As we know the hair cells in the lateral line are crucial for perceiving changes in the surroundings. Therefore, we further detected whether *claudin h* was also involved in the formation of neuromasts in the trunk. Interestingly, the results showed that the number of hair cell clusters in the posterior lateral line of *claudin h* morphants were remarkably reduced (**Figures 5A–C**). Besides, in order to detect whether hair cells in the remaining clusters were affected, we

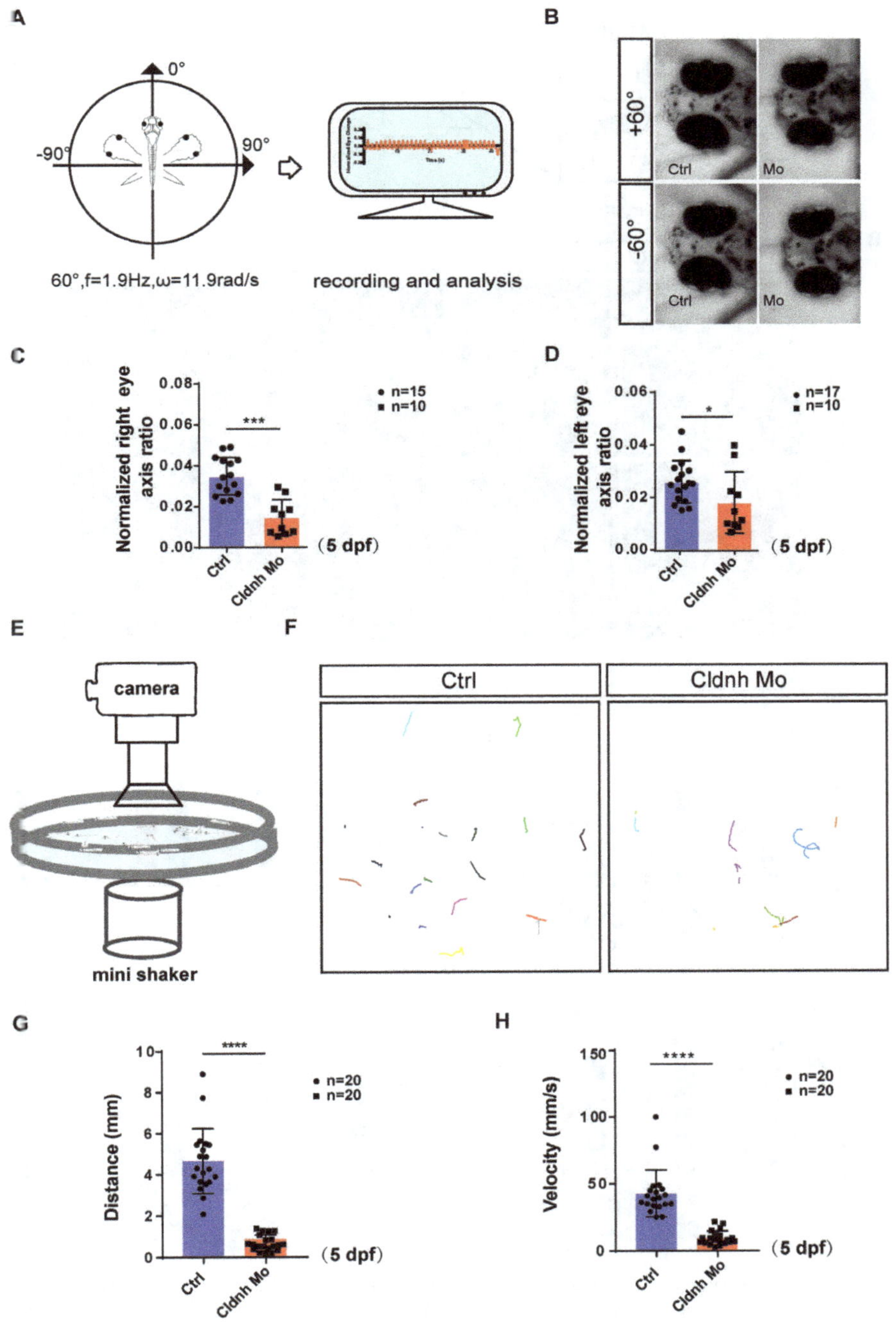

FIGURE 3 | Loss function of the *claudin h* caused the vestibular dysfunction and hearing defects. **(A)** The schematic diagram shows the rotatory trajectory of the larva during VOR. **(B)** The heads and eyes of control and *claudin h* morphants acquired during VOR test at extreme tilting positions. **(C,D)** The vestibular function of zebrafish larvae at 5 dpf is evaluated by vestibular head tilt response measurement (right and left eyes, respectively). **(E)** The schematic diagram shows the startle response testing equipment. **(F)** The swimming trajectory of the control and *claudin h* morphants. **(G,H)** Swimming distance and peak velocity of zebrafish larvae at 5 dpf that reflected the auditory function of zebrafish larvae by examining the startle response. Values with *, ***, and ****above the bars are significantly different ($P < 0.05$, $P < 0.001$, and $P < 0.0001$, respectively).

further imaged and counted the number of L1 hair cells and found that it was significantly decreased after the morpholino injection at 72 and 96 hpf (**Figures 5D–G**). Moreover, we also performed WISH using the probe of eya1 gene, which was reported to be localized in neuromasts of zebrafish (Qian et al., 2020), and the result indicated that the loss of the *claudin h* could also reduce the numbers of neuromasts in the lateral line of zebrafish (**Figure 6I**).

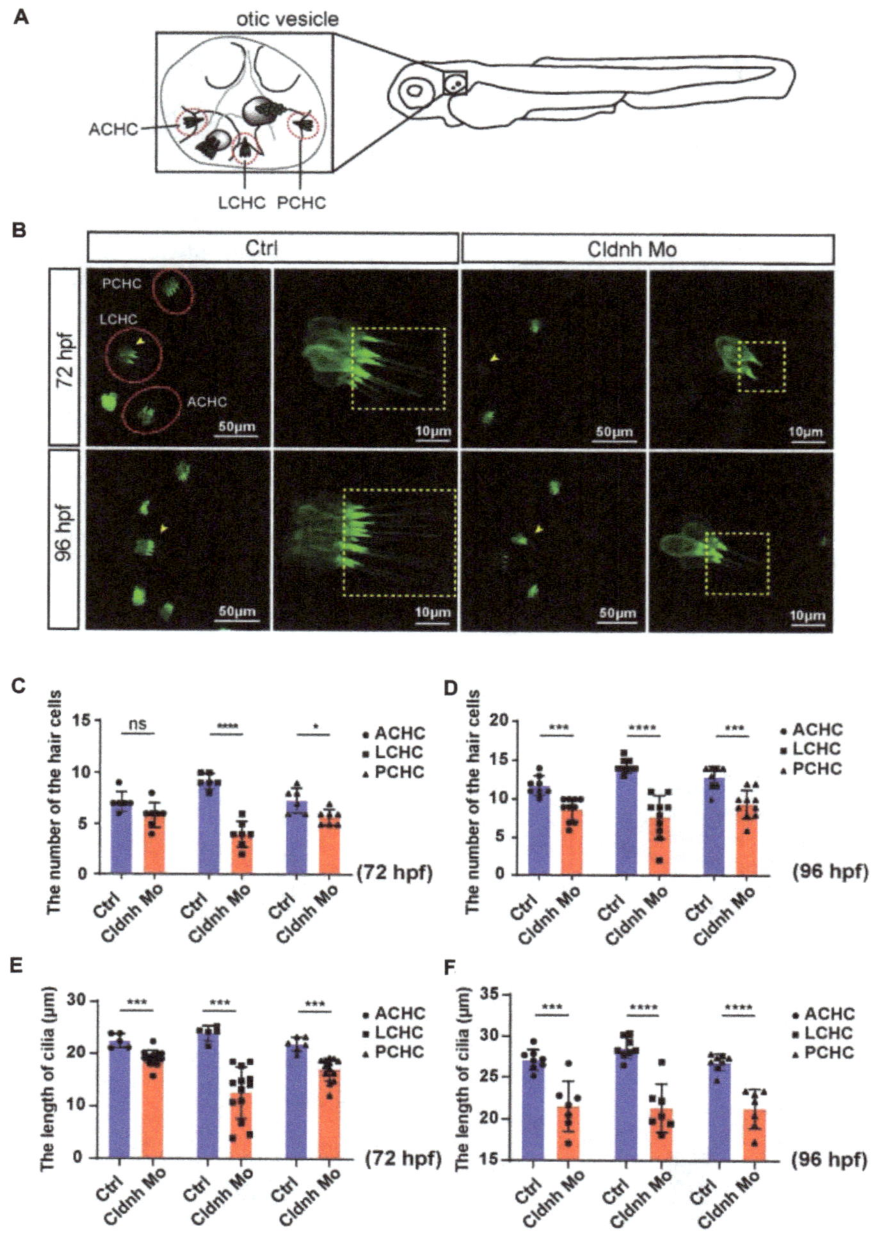

FIGURE 4 | *Claudin h* deficiency suppressed cristae hair cells development. **(A)** The schematic for three different cristae hair cells in the otic vesicle. ACHC, anterior cristae hair cells; LCHC, lateral cristae hair cells; PCHC, posterior cristae hair cells. **(B)** Confocal imaging analysis of cristae hair cells in the otic vesicle of control and *claudin h* deficiency zebrafish at 72 and 96 hpf. The red dotted circle line marked the three different cristae hair cell clusters and magnified lateral cristae hair cell clusters (yellow arrow head) was shown in right and the yellow dotted square line marked the cilia of cristae hair cells. **(C,D)** The statistical analysis of the numbers of different cristae hair cells in the control and *claudin h* morphants at 72 and 96 hpf. **(E,F)** The statistical analysis of the cilia lengths of different cristae hair cells in the control and *claudin h* morphants at 72 and 96 hpf. Values with *, ***, and ****above the bars are significantly different ($P < 0.05$, $P < 0.001$, and $P < 0.0001$, respectively).

The Reduction of Hair Cells in the *Claudin h* Deficient Zebrafish Was Caused by Cell Apoptosis

To investigate cellular mechanism for the loss of the hair cells, immunohistochemistry assay was performed on the *claudin h* deficient and control zebrafish at 72 hpf with the antibody against cleaved caspase-3, one of the apoptosis markers. In the results, though very little signal was detected in controls, much more cleaved caspase-3-positive cells emerged and overlapped with the hair cells in the *claudin h* morphants (**Figure 7**), indicating the lack of hair cells might be caused by the hair cells apoptosis.

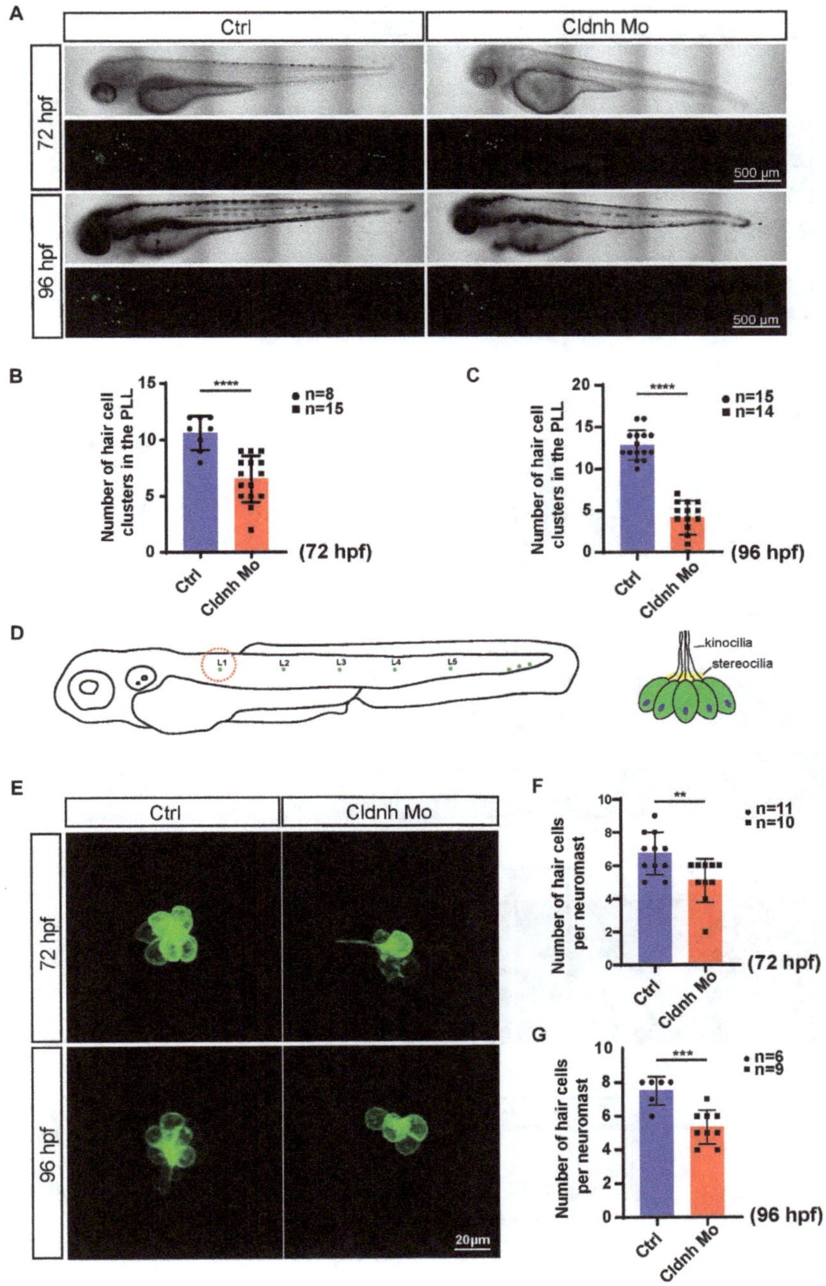

FIGURE 5 | *Claudin h* knockdown decreased hair cell in the posterior lateral line of zebrafish. **(A)** The imaging analysis of control and *claudin h* morphants at 72 and 96 hpf in bright field and fluorescent field. Scale bar = 500 μm. **(B,C)** Quantification of the number of hair cell clusters in the posterior lateral line of control and *claudin h* morphants at 72 and 96 hpf. **(D)** The schematic for different hair cell clusters in the posterior lateral line. Scale bar = 10 μm. **(E)** Confocal imaging analysis of L1 hair cell clusters in the posterior lateral line of control and *claudin h* deficiency zebrafish at 72 and 96 hpf. **(F,G)** Quantification of the number of hair cells per L1 neuromast in the control and *claudin h* morphants at 72 and 96 hpf. Values with **, ***, and ****above the bars are significantly different ($P < 0.01$, $P < 0.001$, and $P < 0.0001$, respectively).

The Defective Phenotype of the *Claudin h* Morphants Could Be Rescued by *Claudin h* mRNA

In order to confirm that the hair cell morphological defects were specifically caused by the *claudin h* deficiency, we co-injected the *in vitro* synthesized *claudin h* mRNA containing an intact open reading frame with *claudin h* Mo into one cell stage zebrafish embryos to test whether exogenous *claudin h* could rescue the phenotype that was found in the *claudin h* morphants. Interestingly, the *claudin h* mRNA co-injection could partially rescue the abnormal phenotypes including the smaller size of

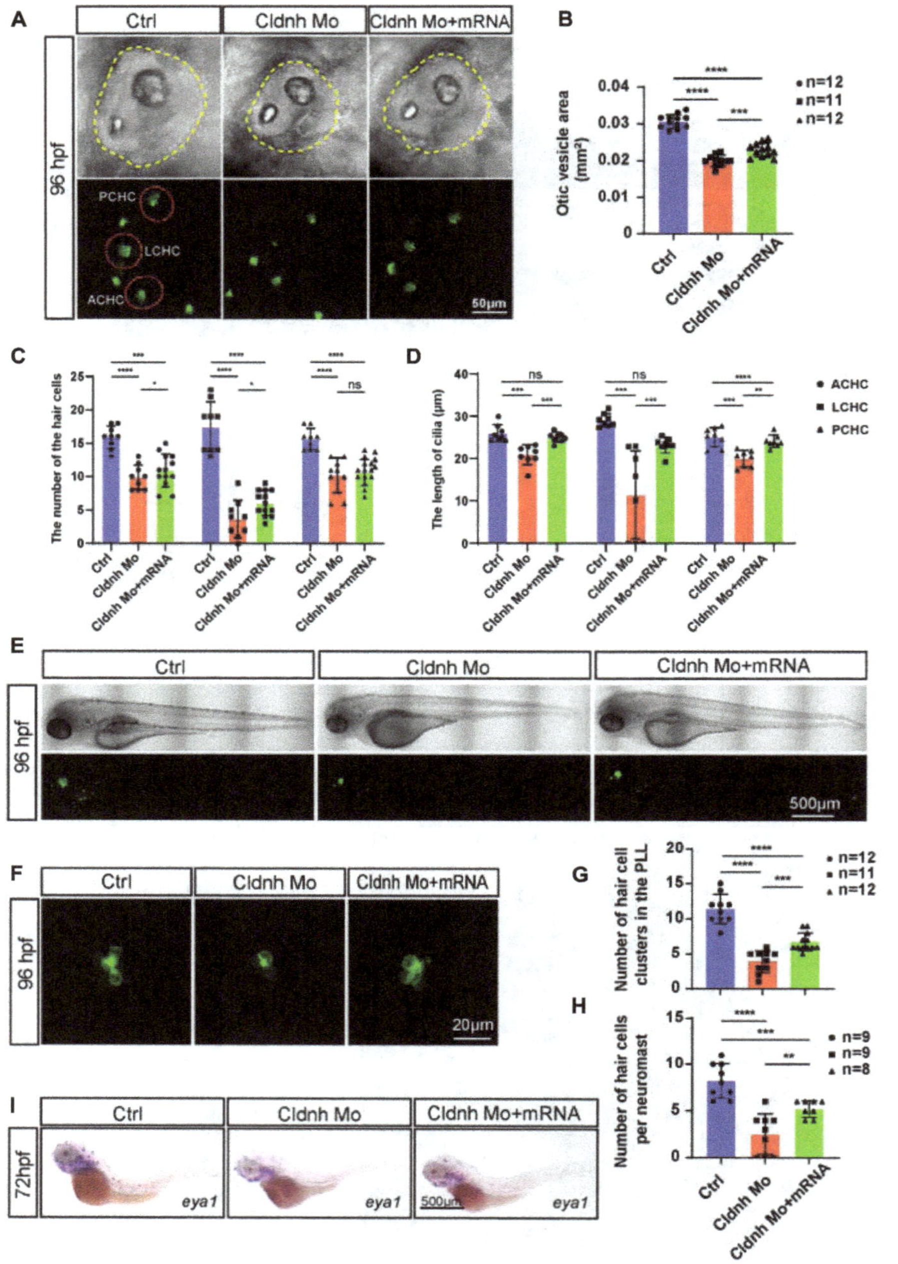

FIGURE 6 | Overexpression of *claudin h* could rescue the development defects of hair cells in claudin morphants. **(A)** Imaging analysis of otic vesicle and cristae hair cells in control, *claudin h* morphants, and rescue group at 96 hpf. The yellow dotted line marked the boundary of the otic vesicle. Scale bar = 50 mm. **(B,C)** The statistical analysis of otic vesicle area in different groups at 96 hpf. **(C,D)** The statistical analysis of the number of different cristae hair cells and the cilia lengths in different groups at 96 hpf. **(E)** WISH results of the eya1 gene and the imaging analysis of control, *claudin h* morphants and rescue zebrafish at 96 hpf in bright field and fluorescent field. Scale bar = 500 μm. **(F)** Quantification of the number of hair cell clusters in the posterior lateral line of different groups at 96 hpf. **(G)** Confocal imaging analysis of L1 hair cell clusters in the posterior lateral line of different groups at 96 hpf. **(H)** Quantification of the number of hair cells per L1 neuromast in the control, *claudin h* morphants, and rescue zebrafish at 96 hpf. Values with *, **, ***, and ****above the bars are significantly different ($P < 0.05$, $P < 0.01$, $P < 0.001$, and $P < 0.0001$, respectively). **(I)** At 72 hpf, the *in situ* hybridization signal of *claudin h* in the control zebrafish, claudin h morphants, and rescue zebrafish.

the otic vesicle and the reducing number of hair cells in the otic vesicle compared to the *claudin h* morphants (**Figures 6A–D**). Similarly, both the number of hair cell clusters in the lateral line and in each L1 cluster were also partially recovered after the *claudin h* mRNA coinjection (**Figures 6E–H**). Taken together, these results indicated that those otic vesicle and hair cell defects found in this study were specifically caused by loss of *claudin h*.

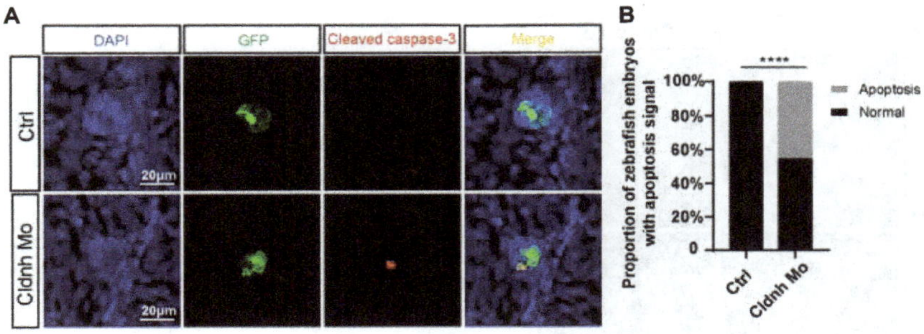

FIGURE 7 | *Claudin h* deficiency caused the hair cells apoptosis. **(A)** DAPI and cleaved caspase-3 staining for the L1 hair cell clusters in the posterior lateral line of the control zebrafish and *claudin h* morphants. Scale bar = 10 μm. **(B)** Quantification of zebrafish embryos with the hair cell apoptosis in the control and *claudin h* morphants. Values with **** above the bars are significantly different ($P < 0.0001$).

CRISPR/Cas9-Mediated *Claudin h* Mutation Disrupts Hair Cell Development

In order to further validate the function of *claudin h* during the hair cell development, the CRISPR/Cas9 system was utilized to knockout *claudin h* in *Tg(Brn3c:mGFP)* transgenic zebrafish. As shown in **Supplementary Figure 3A**, we chose a sgRNA target site near the translation start codon (ATG) in the exon1 of *claudin h* for CRISPR/Cas9-mediated mutation to abolish the protein translation. The mutations were successfully induced into the targeting site which was verified by PCR and sequencing (**Supplementary Figure 3B**).

Similar to the results of the *claudin h* morphants, the otic vesicle size of the *claudin h* mutants was remarkably smaller than that of the control fish at 96 hpf (**Figures 8A,B**). Meanwhile, the number of hair cells in the anterior cristae, lateral cristae, and posterior cristae was significantly decreased and the lengths of the hair cell cilia were shortened as well in the *claudin h* mutant zebrafish at 96 hpf (**Figures 8C,D**). Moreover, we also found that the number of hair cell clusters and the number of hair cells in each neuromast in the lateral line were also decreased significantly after knocking out of *claudin h*, which was consistent with the *claudin h* morphants (**Figures 8E–H**).

DISCUSSION

It is well known that tight junction strands composed of claudins are crucial for the function of permeability barrier of the emunctory like the kidney. However, more and more studies found that many *claudins*, such as *claudin a*, *claudin b*, *claudin j*, *claudin 7b*, *claudin 9*, and *claudin14*, are expressed in the inner ear and necessary for its development, implying that tight junctions in the inner ear might also contain multiple claudins to tightly seal the different regions to regulate the function of the ear including hearing and balance perception during the development (Ben-Yosef et al., 2003; Hardison et al., 2005; Nakano et al., 2009; Li et al., 2018). In this study, the *claudin h* was also found to express in the otic vesicle and the lateral line neuromast, indicating *claudin h* might be also involved in the formation and function of otic vesicle and lateral line.

The development of otic vesicle and formation of otoliths were clearly impaired in the zebrafish lacking *claudin h* in this study. Similarly, it has been reported that though the deficiency of *claudin j* did not directly affect the generation of the calcium carbonate and protein complex, it remarkably prevented these crystallites from efficiently aggregating into the otoliths (Hardison et al., 2005). Moreover, *claudin 7b* was also reported to regulate the formation of otoliths in zebrafish (Li et al., 2018). As we know claudins are necessary for the tight junctions to separate the extracellular fluids by sealing off the paracellular spaces, and many studies have shown that altering or removing the claudins in the tight junctions can alter the ionic permeability barrier (Furuse et al., 2001; Colegio et al., 2003). During the development of zebrafish, the otic vesicle gradually develops into a well-balanced ionic and fluid-filled vesicle with compositional division of the distinct paracellular fluids with tight junctions and thereby to support the normal development of hair cells and otoliths (Li et al., 2018). Therefore, the otolith phenotype might be due to the loss of *claudins* which disrupted the ionic composition in the otic vesicle and further prevented the fusion of crystallites, which was indispensable for normal otolith formation (Hardison et al., 2005).

Otoliths can transmit acoustic vibrations and acceleration forces to the hair cells. The utricular otolith is indispensable for vestibular function, while saccular otoliths are only necessary for hearing (Popper and Fay, 1993; Riley and Moorman, 1999). It has been reported that in zebrafish, *claudin j* expressed in the otic placode and loss of function of *claudin j* caused severe reduction in otoliths size, insensitivity to tapping stimulus, and inability to control balance, which indicated that the hearing and vestibular function were significantly affected by the deficiency of *claudin j* (Hardison et al., 2005). Nowadays, eyes movement detected by VOR have been used to assess the vestibular function. In this study, significant vestibular dysfunction was also detected in the *claudin h* morphants by VOR, which was consistent with the loss of the utricle otolith in *claudin h* morphants. In addition, the startle response of zebrafish that has been used as a reliable evaluation of hearing (Yang et al., 2017) was also performed in this study, and revealed an auditory defect in the *claudin h* morphants (**Figures 3F–H**). Overall, these results clarified that the loss of *claudin h* could lead to the defects of otic vesicle

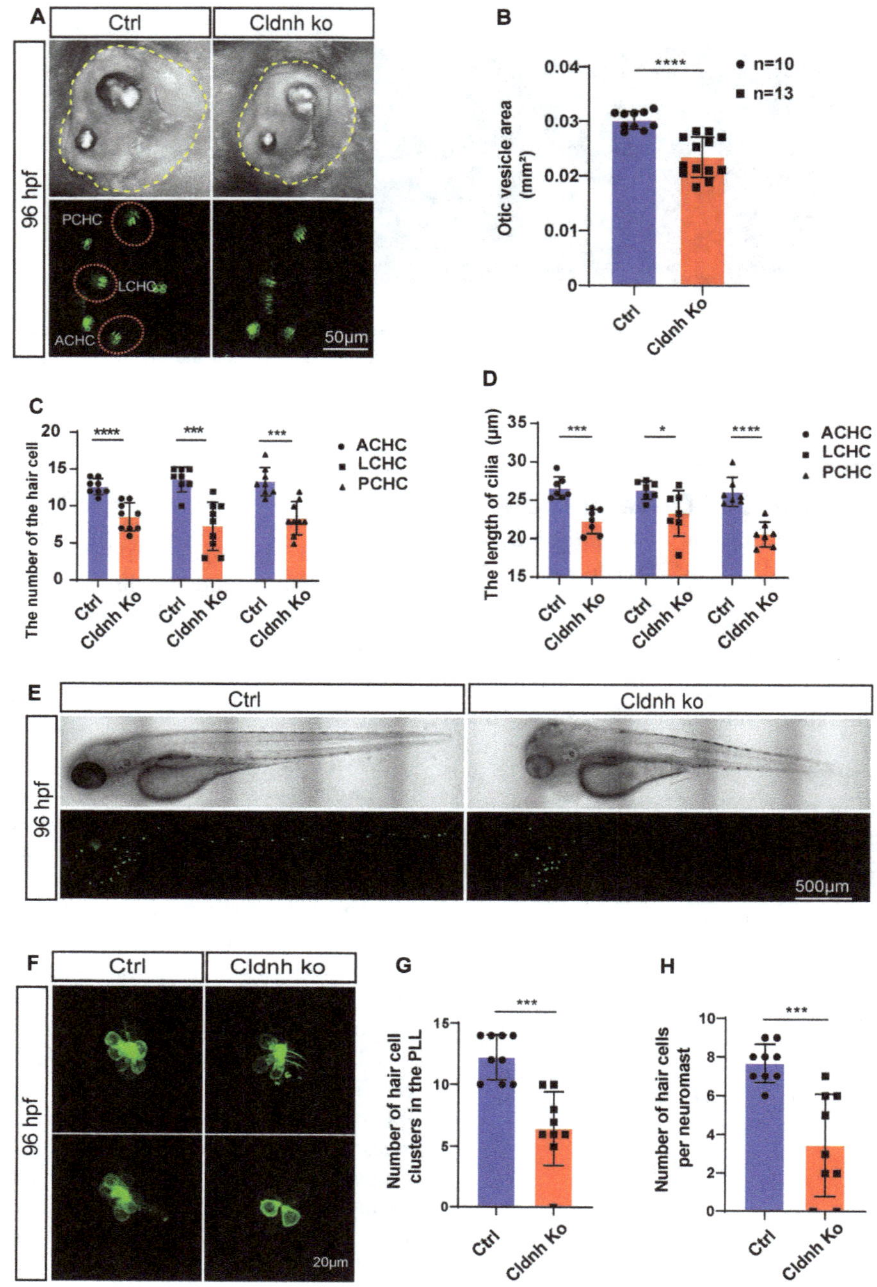

FIGURE 8 | Knocking out of *claudin h* caused the defects of otic vesicle and impaired the development of cristae hair cells and neuromast hair cells. **(A)** Imaging analysis of otic vesicle and cristae hair cells in control and *claudin h* mutants at 96 hpf. The yellow dotted line marked the boundary of the otic vesicle. **(B)** The statistical analysis of otic vesicle area in control and *claudin h* mutants at 96 hpf. **(C,D)** The statistical analysis of the number of different cristae hair cells and the cilia lengths in control and *claudin h* mutants at 96 hpf. **(E)** The imaging analysis of control and *claudin h* mutants at 96 hpf in bright field and fluorescent field.
(F) Confocal imaging analysis of L1 hair cell clusters in the posterior lateral line of control and *claudin h* mutants at 96 hpf. **(G,H)** Quantification of the number of hair cell clusters and the number of hair cells per L1 neuromast in the posterior lateral line of control and *claudin h* mutants at 96 hpf. Values with *, ***, and ****above the bars are significantly different ($P < 0.05$, $P < 0.001$, and $P < 0.0001$, respectively).

and otolith, and further result in vestibular dysfunction and auditory handicap.

Sensory hair cells in the membranous labyrinth of otic vesicle and lateral line neuromasts in zebrafish serve as the receptors for the acoustic signals and pressure acceleration in the surrounding area which then transform these signals or mechanical pressure into chemical or electrical signals to activate auditory or vestibular circuitry (Baxendale and Whitfield, 2016).

A large number of studies have shown that hair cell damage is a leading cause for hearing loss (He et al., 2016; Yu et al., 2017; Zhang et al., 2019). Therefore, investigating whether the development and formation of the hair cells were affected by the *claudin h* deficiency could further illustrate the potential cellular mechanisms of the vestibular and auditory dysfunction found in this study. It has been reported that *claudin14* was expressed in the outer hair cells, cochlear and supporting cells in mice, and the deletion of this gene would lead to significant degeneration of both cochlear outer hair cells and inner hair cells which further cause the congenital hearing deficiency during the first 3 weeks of life (Ben-Yosef et al., 2003). Similarly, we also found the hair cell numbers were remarkably decreased in both otic vesicle and lateral line of *claudin h* morphants and mutants, though most of the hair cell clusters still existed. Moreover, the growth of the hair cell kinocilia was also significantly suppressed by the defects of *claudin h* in this study. These results indicated that the abnormal morphogenesis and formation of hair cells might be a crucial reason for the inner ear dysfunction. Nowadays, many *claudin* genes, such as *claudin a*, *claudin b*, *claudin 7b*, *claudin f*, and *claudin j*, have been reported to be expressed in otic vesicle or lateral line neuromasts during zebrafish larvae development[1] and mutation of them might cause different developmental defects. For example, *claudin 7b* was indispensable for the otic epithelial structure, the otolith formation and sound stimulation sensitiveness by sustaining initial integrity of otic epithelia during embryogenesis; nevertheless, it had no impact on the number and morphology of hair cells (Li et al., 2018). Moreover, although similar otolith phenotype and hearing defects were also found in the *claudin j* mutants, the epithelial structure of the otocyst does not seem to be protruding disrupted (Hardison et al., 2005). Taken together, these results indicated that multiple *claudins* are involved and properly orchestrated to regulate the development and function of the otic vesicle during zebrafish larvae development.

In this study, apoptosis analysis results showed that more cleaved caspase-3-positive cells that were colocalized with the hair cell emerged in the *claudin h* morphants, indicating the lack of hair cells was caused by the hair cell apoptosis. Apoptosis is one of the common pathways for cell death which was characterized by DNA degradation (Morrill and He, 2017). Nowadays, apoptosis is also considered to be one of the mechanisms for the sensory hair cell death induced by acoustic trauma and the caspase-3 activation is a key step during this process (Qian et al., 2020). As the most important components of the tight junctions, claudins play a central role in regulation of paracellular permeability and could create charge-selective channels in the paracellular space with varied combinations or expression levels of claudins (Ben-Yosef et al., 2003). It has been reported that claudin 9 is necessary to form a paracellular ion permeable barrier for Na^+ and K^+. Knocking out of the *claudin 9* in mice would eliminate this ion barrier function and thereby increase the K^+ concentration in the basolateral fluid of the hair cells (Nakano et al., 2009). Similarly, *claudin 14* mutation was also reported to induce the hair cell degeneration by altering ionic permeability of the paracellular barrier for K^+ to further cause human deafness (Ben-Yosef et al., 2003). Besides, longtime exposure in high concentration of K^+ was significantly toxic to hair cells and could suppress hair cell repolarization which eventually led to the hair cells death (Hibino and Kurachi, 2006). Altogether, we hypothesize that the deficiency of *claudin h* in the otic vesicle might have changed the ionic composition through the disruption of paracellular ionic permeability which then induced the hair cell apoptosis and further caused the hearing loss and vestibular dysfunction. However, more details need to be confirmed in future studies. In summary, our characterization of the *claudin h* morphants and mutants not only revealed the biological significance of *claudin h* for the development and function of the hearing organs, but also provided new insights into the pathogenesis of human deafness due to loss of claudin proteins.

ETHICS STATEMENT

The animal study was reviewed and approved by Administration Committee of Experimental Animals, Jiangsu Province, China.

AUTHOR CONTRIBUTIONS

DL conceived the project. JG, PQ, YH, CG, CW, CC, and HW performed most of the experiments. DL, JG, and HW analyzed the data and prepared the manuscript. All authors commented and approved the manuscript.

SUPPLEMENTARY MATERIAL

Supplementary Figure 1 | *Claudin h* expression analyses in the otic vesicle and hair cells. **(A)** At 24 hpf, the *in situ* hybridization signal of *claudin h* is localized in the otic vesicle, posterior lateral line primordium, and pronephros. **(A')** The magnified figure of the region squared in dashed line. **(B–D)** *Claudin h* expressed in the in the otic vesicle and neuromast.

Supplementary Figure 2 | The verification of *fgfbp3* Mo efficiency. **(A)** Schematic diagram for the transcription after fgfbp3 Mo injection. **(B)** The result of RT-PCR of wild type zebrafish and *fgfbp3* morphants.

Supplementary Figure 3 | Generation of zebrafish *claudin h* mutant using CRISPR/Cas9 system. **(A)** Schematic diagram showing the targeting site of the sgRNA on the first exon of *claudin h* gene. **(B)** Mutations occurred in the target site of the *claudin h* gene in mutant zebrafish compared to the wild-type fish.

Supplementary Sequences | The sequencing results for *claudin h* mutant and wildtype zebrafish.

[1] http://ZFIN.org

REFERENCES

Alexandre, M. D., Lu, Q., and Chen, Y. H. (2005). Overexpression of claudin-7 decreases the paracellular Cl- conductance and increases the paracellular Na+ conductance in LLC-PK1 cells. *J. Cell Sci.* 118, 2683–2693. doi: 10.1242/jcs.02406

Angelow, S., El-Husseini, R., Kanzawa, S. A., and Yu, A. S. (2007). Renal localization and function of the tight junction protein, claudin-19. *Am. J. Physiol. Renal. Physiol.* 293, F166–F177.

Bandmann, O., and Burton, E. A. (2010). Genetic zebrafish models of neurodegenerative diseases. *Neurobiol. Dis.* 40, 58–65. doi: 10.1016/j.nbd.2010.05.017

Baxendale, S., and Whitfield, T. T. (2016). Methods to study the development, anatomy, and function of the zebrafish inner ear across the life course. *Zebrafish: Cell. Dev. Biol. Pt B: Dev. Biol.* 134, 165–209. doi: 10.1016/bs.mcb.2016.02.007

Ben-Yosef, T., Belyantseva, I. A., Saunders, T. L., Hughes, E. D., Kawamoto, K., Van Itallie, C. M., et al. (2003). Claudin 14 knockout mice, a model for autosomal recessive deafness DFNB29, are deaf due to cochlear hair cell degeneration. *Hum. Mol. Genet.* 12, 2049–2061. doi: 10.1093/hmg/ddg210

Colegio, O. R., Van Itallie, C., Rahner, C., and Anderson, J. M. (2003). Claudin extracellular domains determine paracellular charge selectivity and resistance but not tight junction fibril architecture. *Am. J. Physiol. Cell Physiol.* 284, C1346–C1354.

Dejana, E. (2004). Endothelial cell-cell junctions: happy together. *Nat. Rev. Mol. Cell Biol.* 5, 261–270. doi: 10.1038/nrm1357

Ding, Y., Meng, W., Kong, W., He, Z., and Chai, R. (2020). The role of FoxG1 in the inner ear. *Front. Cell Dev. Biol.* 8:614954. doi: 10.3389/fcell.2020.614954

Downes, G. B., and Granato, M. (2004). Acetylcholinesterase function is dispensable for sensory neurite growth but is critical for neuromuscular synapse stability. *Dev. Biol.* 270, 232–245. doi: 10.1016/j.ydbio.2004.02.027

Furuse, M., Furuse, K., Sasaki, H., and Tsukita, S. (2001). Conversion of zonulae occludentes from tight to leaky strand type by introducing claudin-2 into Madin-Darby canine kidney I cells. *J. Cell Biol.* 153, 263–272. doi: 10.1083/jcb.153.2.263

Furuse, M., Hirase, T., Itoh, M., Nagafuchi, A., Yonemura, S., Tsukita, S., et al. (1993). Occludin: a novel integral membrane protein localizing at tight junctions. *J. Cell Biol.* 123, 1777–1788. doi: 10.1083/jcb.123.6.1777

Gao, S., Cheng, C., Wang, M., Jiang, P., Zhang, L., Wang, Y., et al. (2019). Blebbistatin inhibits neomycin-induced apoptosis in hair cell-like HEI-OC-1 cells and in cochlear hair cells. *Front. Cell Neurosci.* 13:590. doi: 10.3389/fncel.2019.00590

Gong, J., Hu, S., Huang, Z., Hu, Y., Wang, X., Zhao, J., et al. (2020). The requirement of Sox2 for the spinal cord motor neuron development of Zebrafish. *Front. Mol. Neurosci.* 13:34. doi: 10.3389/fnmol.2020.00034

Gong, Y., and Hou, J. (2017). Claudins in barrier and transport function-the kidney. *Pflugers Arch.* 469, 105–113. doi: 10.1007/s00424-016-1906-6

Goutman, J. D., Elgoyhen, A. B., and Gomez-Casati, M. E. (2015). Cochlear hair cells: the sound-sensing machines. *FEBS Lett.* 589, 3354–3361. doi: 10.1016/j.febslet.2015.08.030

Gregory, M., Dufresne, J., Hermo, L., and Cyr, D. (2001). Claudin-1 is not restricted to tight junctions in the rat epididymis. *Endocrinology* 142, 854–863. doi: 10.1210/endo.142.2.7975

Hardison, A. L., Lichten, L., Banerjee-Basu, S., Becker, T. S., and Burgess, S. M. (2005). The zebrafish gene claudinj is essential for normal ear function and important for the formation of the otoliths. *Mech. Dev.* 122, 949–958. doi: 10.1016/j.mod.2005.03.009

He, Z., Sun, S., Waqas, M., Zhang, X., Qian, F., Cheng, C., et al. (2016). Reduced TRMU expression increases the sensitivity of hair-cell-like HEI-OC-1 cells to neomycin damage in vitro. *Sci. Rep.* 6:29621.

He, Z. H., Zou, S. Y., Li, M., Liao, F. L., Wu, X., Sun, H. Y., et al. (2020). The nuclear transcription factor FoxG1 affects the sensitivity of mimetic aging hair cells to inflammation by regulating autophagy pathways. *Redox Biol.* 28:101364. doi: 10.1016/j.redox.2019.101364

Hibino, H., and Kurachi, Y. (2006). Molecular and physiological bases of the K+ circulation in the mammalian inner ear. *Physiology (Bethesda)* 21, 336–345. doi: 10.1152/physiol.00023.2006

Huang, Y., Wang, X., Wang, X., Xu, M., Liu, M., and Liu, D. (2013). Nonmuscle myosin II-B (myh10) expression analysis during zebrafish embryonic development. *Gene Expr. Patterns* 13, 265–270. doi: 10.1016/j.gep.2013.04.005

Kollmar, R., Nakamura, S. K., Kappler, J. A., and Hudspeth, A. J. (2001). Expression and phylogeny of claudins in vertebrate primordia. *Proc. Natl. Acad. Sci. U.S.A.* 98, 10196–10201. doi: 10.1073/pnas.171325898

Krause, G., Winkler, L., Mueller, S. L., Haseloff, R. F., Piontek, J., and Blasig, I. E. (2008). Structure and function of claudins. *Biochim. Biophys. Acta* 1778, 631–645. doi: 10.1016/j.bbamem.2007.10.018

Li, J., Ananthapanyasut, W., and Yu, A. S. (2011). Claudins in renal physiology and disease. *Pediatr. Nephrol.* 26, 2133–2142. doi: 10.1007/s00467-011-1824-y

Li, X., Song, G., Zhao, Y., Zhao, F., Liu, C., Liu, D., et al. (2018). Claudin7b is required for the formation and function of inner ear in zebrafish. *J. Cell Physiol.* 233, 3195–3206. doi: 10.1002/jcp.26162

Liu, L., Chen, Y., Qi, J., Zhang, Y., He, Y., Ni, W., et al. (2016). Wnt activation protects against neomycin-induced hair cell damage in the mouse cochlea. *Cell Death Dis.* 7:e2136. doi: 10.1038/cddis.2016.35

Liu, Y., Qi, J., Chen, X., Tang, M., Chu, C., Zhu, W., et al. (2019). Critical role of spectrin in hearing development and deafness. *Sci. Adv.* 5:eaav7803. doi: 10.1126/sciadv.aav7803

Ma, J. H., Kim, H. P., Bok, J., and Shin, J. O. (2018). CTCF is required for maintenance of auditory hair cells and hearing function in the mouse cochlea. *Biochem. Biophys. Res. Commun.* 503, 2646–2652. doi: 10.1016/j.bbrc.2018.08.017

Madara, J. L. (1998). Regulation of the movement of solutes across tight junctions. *Annu. Rev. Physiol.* 60, 143–159. doi: 10.1146/annurev.physiol.60.1.143

Martin-Padura, I., Lostaglio, S., Schneemann, M., Williams, L., Romano, M., Fruscella, P., et al. (1998). Junctional adhesion molecule, a novel member of the immunoglobulin superfamily that distributes at intercellular junctions and modulates monocyte transmigration. *J. Cell Biol.* 142, 117–127. doi: 10.1083/jcb.142.1.117

Milatz, S., Krug, S. M., Rosenthal, R., Gunzel, D., Muller, D., Schulzke, J. D., et al. (2010). Claudin-3 acts as a sealing component of the tight junction for ions of either charge and uncharged solutes. *Biochim. Biophys. Acta-Biomembranes* 1798, 2048–2057. doi: 10.1016/j.bbamem.2010.07.014

Morrill, S., and He, D. Z. Z. (2017). Apoptosis in inner ear sensory hair cells. *J. Otol.* 12, 151–164. doi: 10.1016/j.joto.2017.08.001

Nakano, Y., Kim, S. H., Kim, H. M., Sanneman, J. D., Zhang, Y., Smith, R. J., et al. (2009). A claudin-9-based ion permeability barrier is essential for hearing. *PLoS Genet.* 5:e1000610. doi: 10.1371/journal.pgen.1000610

Popper, A. N., and Fay, R. R. (1993). Sound detection and processing by fish: critical review and major research questions. *Brain Behav. Evol.* 41, 14–38. doi: 10.1159/000113821

Qi, J., Liu, Y., Chu, C., Chen, X., Zhu, W., Shu, Y., et al. (2019). A cytoskeleton structure revealed by super-resolution fluorescence imaging in inner ear hair cells. *Cell Discov.* 5:12.

Qian, F., Wand, X., Yin, Z., Xie, G., Yuan, H., Liu, D., et al. (2020). The slc4a2b gene is required for hair cell development in zebrafish. *Aging* 12, 18804–18821. doi: 10.18632/aging.103840

Riley, B. B., and Moorman, S. J. (1999). Development of utricular otoliths, but not saccular otoliths, is necessary for vestibular function and survival in zebrafish. *J. Neurobiol.* 43, 329–337. doi: 10.1002/1097-4695(20000615)43:4<329::aid-neu2>3.0.co;2-h

Sun, P., Zhang, Y., Zhao, F., Wu, J. P., Pun, S. H., Peng, C., et al. (2018). An assay for systematically quantifying the vestibulo-ocular reflex to assess vestibular function in zebrafish larvae. *Front. Cell Neurosci.* 12:257. doi: 10.3389/fncel.2018.00257

Tipsmark, C. K., Kiilerich, P., Nilsen, T. O., Ebbesson, L. O. E., Stefansson, S. O., and Madsen, S. S. (2008). Branchial expression patterns of claudin isoforms in Atlantic salmon during seawater acclimation and smoltification. *Am. J. Phys.-Regulatory Integrative Comparative Physiol.* 294, R1563–R1574.

Tsukita, S., and Furuse, M. (2000). Pores in the wall: claudins constitute tight junction strands containing aqueous pores. *J. Cell Biol.* 149, 13–16.

Van Itallie, C. M., and Anderson, J. M. (2004). The molecular physiology of tight junction pores. *Physiol (Bethesda)* 19, 331–338. doi: 10.1152/physiol.00027.2004

Van Itallie, C. M., Rogan, S., Yu, A., Vidal, L. S., Holmes, J., and Anderson, J. M.

(2006). Two splice variants of claudin-10 in the kidney create paracellular pores with different ion selectivities. *Am. J. Physiol. Renal Physiol.* 291, F1288–F1299.

Wang, T., Chai, R., Kim, G. S., Pham, N., Jansson, L., Nguyen, D. H., et al. (2015). Lgr5+ cells regenerate hair cells via proliferation and direct transdifferentiation in damaged neonatal mouse utricle. *Nat. Commun.* 6:6613.

Wen, H., Watry, D. D., Marcondes, M. C., and Fox, H. S. (2004). Selective decrease in paracellular conductance of tight junctions: role of the first extracellular domain of claudin-5. *Mol. Cell Biol.* 24, 8408–8417. doi: 10.1128/mcb.24.19.8408-8417.2004

Xiao, T., Roeser, T., Staub, W., and Baier, H. (2005). A GFP-based genetic screen reveals mutations that disrupt the architecture of the zebrafish retinotectal projection. *Development* 132, 2955–2967. doi: 10.1242/dev.01861

Yang, Q., Sun, P., Chen, S., Li, H., and Chen, F. (2017). Behavioral methods for the functional assessment of hair cells in zebrafish. *Front. Med.* 11, 178–190. doi: 10.1007/s11684-017-0507-x

Yu, X., Liu, W., Fan, Z., Qian, F., Zhang, D., Han, Y., et al. (2017). c-Myb knockdown increases the neomycin-induced damage to hair-cell-like HEI-OC1 cells in vitro. *Sci. Rep.* 7:41094.

Zhang, S. S., Zhang, Y., Dong, Y., Guo, L. N., Zhang, Z., Shao, B. W., et al. (2020). Knockdown of Foxg1 in supporting cells increases the trans-differentiation of supporting cells into hair cells in the neonatal mouse cochlea. *Cell. Mol. Life Sci.* 77, 1401–1419. doi: 10.1007/s00018-019-03291-2

Zhang, Y., Li, W., He, Z., Wang, Y., Shao, B., Cheng, C., et al. (2019). Pre-treatment with fasudil prevents neomycin-induced hair cell damage by reducing the accumulation of reactive oxygen species. *Front. Mol. Neurosci.* 12:264. doi: 10.3389/fnmol.2019.00264

Zhou, H., Qian, X., Xu, N., Zhang, S., Zhu, G., Zhang, Y., et al. (2020). Disruption of Atg7-dependent autophagy causes electromotility disturbances, outer hair cell loss, and deafness in mice. *Cell Death Dis* 11:913.

Zhu, C., Cheng, C., Wang, Y., Muhammad, W., Liu, S., Zhu, W., et al. (2018). Loss of ARHGEF6 causes hair cell stereocilia deficits and hearing loss in mice. *Front. Mol. Neurosci.* 11:362. doi: 10.3389/fnmol.2018.00362

18

Hearing Loss and Cognition: What We Know and Where We Need to Go

Danielle S. Powell[1,2], Esther S. Oh[2,3], Nicholas S. Reed[2,4,5], Frank R. Lin[2,4,5] and Jennifer A. Deal[2,4,5]*

[1] Department of Health Policy and Management, Johns Hopkins Bloomberg School of Public Health, Baltimore, MD, United States, [2] Cochlear Center for Hearing and Public Health, Johns Hopkins Bloomberg School of Public Health, Baltimore, MD, United States, [3] Division of Geriatric Medicine and Gerontology, Johns Hopkins University School of Medicine, Baltimore, MD, United States, [4] Department of Epidemiology, Johns Hopkins Bloomberg School of Public Health, Baltimore, MD, United States, [5] Department of Otolaryngology, Johns Hopkins University School of Medicine, Baltimore, MD, United States

***Correspondence:**
Danielle S. Powell
dpowel33@jhu.edu

Although a causal association remains to be determined, epidemiologic evidence suggests an association between hearing loss and increased risk of dementia. If we determine the association is causal, opportunity for targeted intervention for hearing loss may play a fundamental role in dementia prevention. In this discussion, we summarize current research on the association between hearing loss and dementia and review potential casual mechanisms behind the association (e.g., sensory-deprivation hypothesis, information-degradation hypothesis, common cause). We emphasize key areas of research which might best inform our investigation of this potential casual association. These selected research priorities include examination of the causal mechanism, measurement of co-existing hearing loss and cognitive impairment and determination of any bias in testing, potential for managing hearing loss for prevention of dementia and cognitive decline, or the potential to reduce dementia-related symptoms through the management of hearing loss. Addressing these research gaps and how results are then translated for clinical use may prove paramount for dementia prevention, management, and overall health of older adults.

Keywords: hearing loss, cognitive decline, dementia, prevention, dementia management, sensory loss, risk factor

INTRODUCTION

Hearing loss is the leading potentially modifiable risk factor for dementia; up to 8% of global dementia cases are estimated as being attributable to hearing loss (Livingston et al., 2017, 2020). Following foundational initial research from over 5 decades ago, recent years have seen a steep rise in scientific investigation of the hearing-dementia association. As far back as 1968, participants demonstrated poorer performance on word-recall cognitive tasks in an experimental condition designed to mimic hearing loss and decreased speech intelligibility compared to normal listening conditions (Rabbitt, 1968). Two decades later, a seminal case-control study (Uhlmann et al., 1989) reported greater odds of dementia in those with hearing loss compared to normal hearing.

Even with our expanding knowledge of the association between hearing loss and dementia, significant gaps in our understanding persist. In this article, we aim to (1) provide a foundational understanding of hearing loss presentation and diagnosis; (2) review current hearing loss epidemiology (3) provide context to the existing research on the relationship between hearing loss and dementia to guide dementia prevention and intervention recommendations or research; (4) discuss the leading theories on the pathways behind the hearing-dementia association; and (5) present four crucial areas for future research. With the demographic changes in the coming decades, we conclude with calls for inter-disciplinary collaboration and posit a unique opportunity to alter the landscape of cognitive aging and dementia care. Understanding the role and presentation of hearing loss in the adult population allows for better appreciation of where the field of auditory science may fit into a broader picture of dementia prevention and interventions.

HEARING MEASUREMENT AND THE PRESENTATION OF HEARING LOSS

Measuring Hearing Ability

The act of hearing involves two inter-related processes and components of the auditory system – the peripheral auditory system and the central auditory system (Musiek and Baran, 2018) and additional non-auditory influences such as cognitive processing, education, situational influences, and self-perception, among others (**Figure 1**). Yet, both parts of the auditory system must work in tandem for an individual to appropriately detect and understand a sound. This process is essential for auditory interaction with the environment and is instrumental for quality communication. Yet most commonly, it is the peripheral auditory system that is considered in discussion of hearing loss. The few epidemiologic studies that include a formalized measure of hearing primarily consider peripheral hearing ability alone. Moreover, many epidemiologic studies rely on the self-reported measures of hearing. While measures of self-report hearing have their utility, self-report hearing is complex and represents perceived functional ability of hearing, incorporating aspects of the peripheral and central auditory system as well as the social environment, psychosocial aspects, and listening demands.

Peripheral Auditory Function

The peripheral auditory system includes the outer ear (pinna), ear drum (tympanic membrane), middle ear bones (malleus, incus, and stapes), and cochlea (Musiek and Baran, 2018). These components work together to transform auditory sound waves or acoustic energy of the surrounding environment captured by the outer ear and ear drum into mechanical energy in the middle ear space, and, eventually, encoding information as an electrical signal in the cochlea to be sent along the central auditory system to the brain (Musiek and Baran, 2018). While a discussion of the complete anatomy and physiology of the peripheral auditory system is beyond the focus of this article, an individual's ability to detect the presence of auditory stimuli initiates within and is dependent upon the peripheral system.

The most common clinical tool for measurement of peripheral hearing acuity in adults is pure tone audiometry (Katz, 2015), with results graphically recorded on an audiogram (**Figure 2**). This gold standard for testing is performed in a sound-proof booth using calibrated headphones. An auditory stimulus (i.e., pure tone) is presented at particular frequencies [measured in Hertz (Hz)] commonly within the range of 250–8000 Hz. The presentation level of each pure tone begins at an audible listening level for each individual and is decreased to ascertain the lowest threshold level [i.e., the volume in decibels hearing level (dB HL)], at which the individual indicates detection of the tone. In the epidemiologic literature, results are often summarized using the World Health Organization criteria as a four-frequency pure tone average (PTA), or the average of responses at 500, 1000, 2000, and 4000 Hz (Katz, 2015). Hearing loss may also be discussed within common clinical categories (i.e., normal [PTA < 20 dB], mild [20 to <35 dB], moderate [35 to <50 dB], moderately severe [50 to <65 dB], severe [65 to < 80 dB], or profound [80 dB or greater]) (World Report on Hearing, 2021) or other categorizations (Clark, 1981) which are not currently adhered to in clinical audiology.

Central Auditory Function

Following passage through the peripheral auditory system, the electrical signal created by the cochlea is sent to the auditory nerve where it is then decoded by the brain (Musiek and Baran, 2018; **Figure 2**). Central hearing ability is therefore dependent upon the integrity of the auditory signal passed from the peripheral auditory system as well as additional cognitive processing (Gates, 2012; Humes et al., 2012). While peripheral hearing ability may be simplified as the ability to detect sound, central hearing ability then is the ability for the brain to understand and make sense of environmental sounds, requiring significant higher-level processing (i.e., identifying signals of interest from ambient noise, giving spatial awareness, adding together several pure tone signals to create complex signals such as speech, etc.).

Measurement of central auditory function is often completed through the presentation of speech within the presence of increasing volume of selected types of background noise (i.e., speech-in-noise testing) or specialized tests of central auditory processing ability that involve specific tasks like listening to degraded or temporally modified speech (Gates, 2012). However, this testing is far less frequently completed in either adult clinical visits or large-scale epidemiologic studies as compared to smaller research studies. Measurement tools for central auditory function transcends the auditory pathway with varied emphasis on how much peripheral auditory function has on performance. Measures might include the presentation of carefully selected single words via tests of word recognition, or presentation of sentences which additionally might provide context clues for word identification either in quiet or increasing levels of background noise. While central hearing ability encompasses more than speech-in-noise ability as noted, current clinical audiologic testing primarily considers basic speech-in-noise ability and not necessarily higher-level auditory cognitive processing tasks [i.e., the differentiation of sound sources within a complex environment (Bregman, 1993)]. However, tests of auditory cognitive ability designed to account for general cognitive ability or specific cognitive domains, in addition to peripheral hearing ability, have been developed (Goll et al., 2010, 2011, 2012; Grube et al., 2016) yet are in limited clinical use. It is conceivable these targeted auditory cognitive tests, with further study and if adopted more widely, may aid in

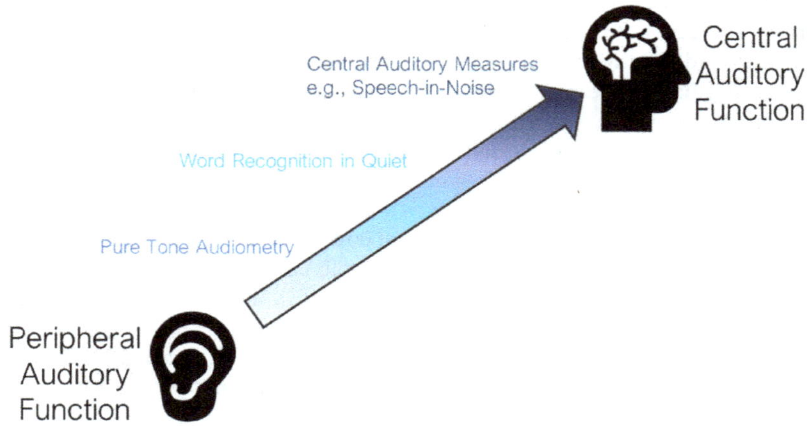

FIGURE 1 | Levels of auditory function. The auditory system spans between peripheral and central auditory function, gaining complexity and higher cognitive processing as you activate more central auditory function. Pure tone audiometry is the most common metric for measurement of peripheral function. Word recognition (i.e., repeating back a single word heard without the use of visual cues) requires additional input of central auditory function. Central auditory measures such as speech-in-noise testing are the most complex and objective measures of central auditory function commonly performed.

understanding of the connection between neurobiological and specific central auditory ability and dementia subtypes and 1 day be included within clinical neurological work-ups as an additional indicator or early-stage dementia. However, until differentiation is feasible, the interdependence between central auditory function and cognitive processing blurs the distinction between the two processing abilities. In addition, heterogeneity in prior study has created significant barriers to pooled evidence and causal inference regarding the role of central hearing ability within cognitive impairment and testing. While more detailed description is beyond the scope of this article, a functional understanding of both aspects of the hearing system is important when considering dementia prevention strategies.

The Presentation of Age-Related Hearing Loss

Age-related hearing loss (ARHL), also known as presbycusis, accounts for the largest percentage of hearing loss cases around the world and presents as a gradual decrease in hearing ability. The outer hair cells and other sensory cells in the cochlea are progressively damaged and unable to regenerate (Pickles, 2013). The result is the impaired encoding of sound, decreased precision, and a distorted auditory signal sent to the brain. This form of hearing loss commonly leads to decreased detection of the higher frequency sounds of speech before lower frequency sounds. The result is reduced ability to hear high-frequency consonants (i.e., /s/, /f/, th/), the parts of speech that provide crispness and clarity. In turn, many with ARHL do not necessarily report difficulty with volume of speech but instead indicate speech sounds muddled or garbled, especially when in the presence of background noise. For everyday function, this may lead to difficulty communicating or interacting with others depending on the listening environment. Those with ARHL may have difficulty hearing or understanding what others are saying in a crowded or noisy setting, such as a restaurant. They may also have difficulty hearing and understanding the television, on the phone, when someone speaks from another room or with their back turned.

The impact of a given pattern of hearing function as represented on the audiogram on communicative performance may vary widely from individual to individual (George et al., 2007; Chang et al., 2009). An individual's functional performance with their hearing depends on not only their peripheral hearing (audiogram) but also their central hearing ability (i.e., central auditory processing, speech-in-noise performance), personal motivation, self-efficacy, listening environments and demands. The availability of cognitive resources to help support interpretation of a degraded auditory signal may also have a significant role in individual experience.

EPIDEMIOLOGY OF HEARING LOSS

The Prevalence and Cost of Hearing Loss

Hearing loss currently impacts an estimated 20% of the global population, or more than 1.5 billion people (World Report on Hearing, 2021). By 2050, estimates now project nearly 2.5 billion people with hearing loss, such that nearly 1 in 4 individuals will have some degree of loss (World Report on Hearing, 2021). The breakdown in hearing loss prevalence by age category varies by country, with Western countries demonstrating greater prevalence at older ages. In the United States, over two-thirds of adults age 70 years and older have a bilateral hearing loss (i.e., hearing loss in both ears) (Lin et al., 2011; Goman and Lin, 2016; **Figure 3**). It was estimated over 44 million older adults would have hearing loss in 2020 with expected increase to over 73 million by 2060 (Goman et al., 2017). However, analysis in a nationally representative sample of older adults suggests that while the overall prevalence of hearing loss is increasing due to greater numbers of older adults, the age-specific prevalence of hearing loss in the United States appears

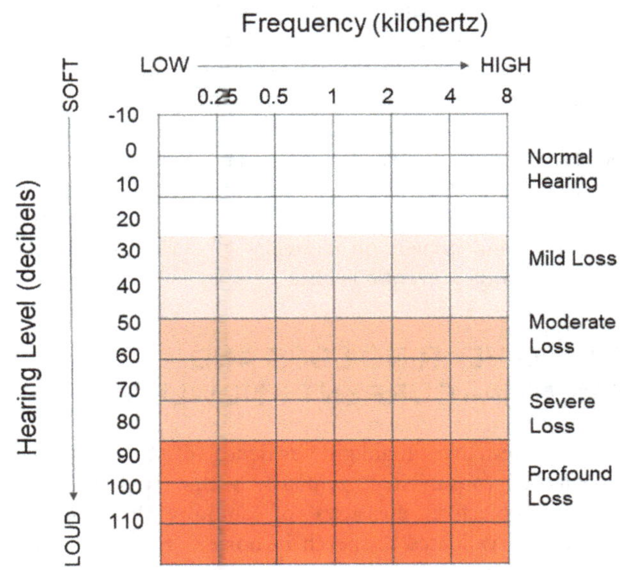

FIGURE 2 | Audiogram. Graphical clinical tool used to depict peripheral hearing ability and record peripheral hearing thresholds as measured via pure tone audiometry. *X* axis represents the frequency (kHz) of sound going from low frequency to high frequency 0.25–8 kHz. *Y* axis represents the volume of the presented pure tone, going from very soft to very loud (–10 to 110 dB). Common clinical categories to describe hearing loss are indicated ranging from normal hearing to a profound hearing loss. The lowest volume at each frequency an individual indicates they can hear the tone is recorded for each ear on the graph.

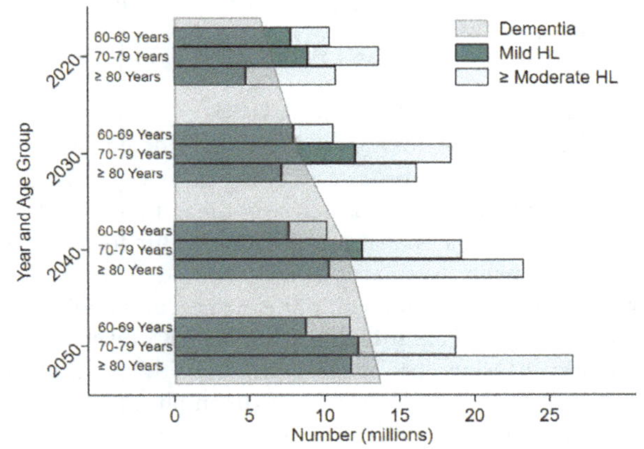

FIGURE 3 | Estimated and projected trends in prevalence of hearing loss (mild hearing loss and moderate or greater hearing loss) and dementia in older adults by age categories in the United States from 2020 to 2050. Data compiled from Goman et al. (2017) and the Alzheimer's Disease Facts and Figures 2020 Report. Adapted from Powell et al. (2021).

to be decreasing over the last decade, by about 2% in adults compared to the prior decade (Hoffman et al., 2017). This age-specific decrease may be related to improvements in health care or access to care and prevention of known risk factors for hearing loss, improved education, environmental noise protections [e.g., workplace hearing protection, time limits for noise exposure, community noise level limits], and management of vascular or disease risk factors.

Globally, the cost of unaddressed hearing loss is estimated at over $980 billion annually (World Report on Hearing, 2021). Economic costs of lost productivity due to hearing loss is estimated widely at $1.8–$194 billion in the United States alone. Excess medical costs due to hearing loss was estimated at $3.3–$12.8 billion (Huddle et al., 2017). Individually, over a span of 10 years, the difference in mean total healthcare costs for someone with hearing loss compared to someone without hearing loss is over $22,000 in the United States (Reed et al., 2019), due in part to increased rate of hospitalizations, higher risk of hospital readmission, and longer hospital stays. This economic cost may take a toll on societies and families managing the social, economic, and healthcare needs of older adults. While hearing loss has its greatest prevalence among older adults, significant hearing loss is not necessarily an inevitable consequence of aging, as everyone has a different hearing trajectory shaped by genetic, environmental, and health related factors from across the life course.

Risk Factors for Hearing Loss

The prevalence of hearing loss varies by non-modifiable factors such as certain identified syndromes and genetic factors (World Report on Hearing, 2021). Additional non-modifiable factors include race/ethnicity and possibly biological sex (Curhan et al., 2017). While a lower prevalence of hearing loss is noted among women compared to men, thought primarily related to behavioral and lifestyle choices (i.e., increased noise exposure), some evidence suggests a biological protective effect of estrogen among women (Hultcrantz et al., 2006; Shuster et al., 2019). Additionally, hearing loss has a lower prevalence in Black adults compared to Hispanic or non-Hispanic White adults (Bainbridge and Wallhagen, 2014; Goman and Lin, 2016), suspected in part due to a protective effect of melanin in the inner ear (Lin et al., 2017).

Additional potential causative risk factors for hearing loss across the life course have also been identified (World Report on Hearing, 2021). While many risk factors for hearing loss stem from prenatal or perinatal causes/determinants (i.e., intrauterine infections, delivery complications), other risk factors for hearing loss in adolescence and adulthood have also been identified (World Report on Hearing, 2021). These include: otitis media (i.e., ear infections), viral infections or pathogens (e.g., measles, mumps, meningitis, HIV, Lassa virus, Ebola), chronic disease (e.g., hypertension, cardiovascular disease, diabetes), smoking, use of ototoxic medications (i.e., cisplatin, carboplatin, gentamicin) head trauma, excessive noise exposure from occupational, recreational, or environmental noise, ear-related conditions such as Meniere's disease, autoimmune disease, or vestibular schwannomas, and nutritional deficiencies from nutrients like Vitamin A, zinc, and iron. As stated, one of the greatest risk factors for hearing loss is increasing age due to age-related sensorineural hearing loss. This is a multifactorial condition thought influenced by genetics, environmental factors, lifestyle, and illnesses. While it is not yet determined if all of these factors are causal, each is correlated with increased risk of hearing loss.

Modifiability of Hearing Loss

Historically, hearing loss has been considered a benign component of the aging process resulting primarily in impaired communication. However, research over the last few decades has highlighted hearing loss as a precipitating factor for additional functional and neuropsychiatric disorders in older adults and has spurred changes in thought within the medical and public health community (Lopez et al., 2011; Lin et al., 2013; Kamil et al., 2014). Importantly, hearing loss is generally considered modifiable through amplification (i.e., hearing aids or amplification devices). The overall goal of amplification is to aid in the restoration of auditory input from impaired peripheral hearing and serve as a tool to help manage the presence of background or competing noise for communication and comfort. Therefore, the scientific and clinical community has begun to recognize the potential protective benefit of hearing loss management, particularly for neuropsychiatric conditions like depression and dementia (Rutherford et al., 2018). Therapeutic opportunity exists, as hearing aids are vastly underutilized: on average only ~30% of eligible adults obtain hearing aids in the United States (Bainbridge and Wallhagen, 2014), with similar uptake reflected in peer countries (World Report on Hearing, 2021). Recent investigation suggests trends in improved uptake of amplification devices in the United States, however disparities and divergences are noted for lower income older adults (Reed et al., 2021). While significant barriers and disparities in hearing health care and accessibility of care and services remain, as will be discussed later, the potential room for intervention growth and public health benefit is substantial. Management of hearing loss through amplification options may not only decrease risk for neuropsychiatric conditions (Rutherford et al., 2018), but may also improve treatment adherence, patient satisfaction, and improve overall health-related quality of life for older adults (Bigelow et al., 2020). Understanding subgroups of older adults who may receive particular benefit from increased amplification use may therefore save health care costs, reduce burden, and improve outcomes – including dementia.

Dementia Prevention Through Hearing Loss

The expected rise in dementia cases around the world requires action on dementia prevention and intervention across innovative and multi-disciplinary channels to meet the pressing societal and health needs. With no known dementia cure, epidemiologic research then seeks to discern risk factors associated with the progression of dementia pathology, progression of dementia symptoms, or with dementia diagnosis to delay or minimize the impact of clinical symptoms (Livingston et al., 2020). If we can identify such risk factors, we may cultivate increased focus and direction for research to possibly delay dementia onset. Delaying the onset of dementia by just 5 years through intervention could lead to a 57% reduction in the number of dementia cases (Sperling et al., 2011) and 40% lower cost for care and services in 30 years (Zissimopoulos, 2014). Epidemiologic research has provided much of the foundational evidence for the association between hearing loss and dementia. This research has allowed for recognition of how the under-utilization of hearing loss treatment strategies presents an opportunity for potential advancement. With potential collaboration across the unique disciplines associated with cognitive aging and auditory science, opportunity for novel intervention and prevention strategies to enrich our evidence base for dementia prevention exists.

LINKING HEARING LOSS AND DEMENTIA– CURRENT KNOWLEDGE

In this review, we highlight evidence of the association and potential causal effect primarily within studies utilizing completed objective measures of auditory function (i.e., audiogram, validated speech-in-noise testing). While consideration of self-reported hearing is important, it integrates aspects of not only peripheral auditory function but also of an individual's perceived hearing and communication ability, incorporating environmental and communication demands, mental health, listening motivation and expectations, and central auditory function.

Heterogeneity in study methodology and design creates challenges to synthesize data from hearing and cognition research. Heterogeneity exists across audiometric and cognitive parameters as well as sample sizes, populations studied, and consideration of confounders, to name a few. Within auditory science, heterogeneity includes aspects such as differing means to define hearing loss, pure tone frequencies used, or how hearing ability is categorized. For cognitive research, variability in the neurocognitive tests used, domains investigated, utilization of cognitive screeners, patient or physician report, and ways of defining cognitive change (i.e., cognitive decline, subjective cognitive impairment, mild cognitive impairment, or diagnosed dementia) all create obstacles for evidence synthesis.

Peripheral Auditory Function

The *Lancet* Commission (Livingston et al., 2017, 2020) reported a pooled relative risk of 1.9 times greater risk of incident dementia among hearing impaired individuals 55 years of age and older compared to those with normal hearing. However, only three longitudinal studies (Lin et al., 2011; Gallacher et al., 2012; Deal et al., 2016) on the association between peripheral hearing impairment and incident dementia met the Commissions specified inclusion criteria of audiometrically (objective) measured hearing, longitudinal evaluation (at least 5 years), and covariate adjustment. While requirement of longitudinal evaluation and covariate adjustment require little justification, audiometrically measured hearing allows for measurement of a more isolated effect of peripheral hearing loss due to cochlear damage rather than the more convoluted measurement of central auditory function or self-report hearing. As audiometry serves as the gold-standard for objective measures of hearing, its validity has been well investigated in a variety of populations. As audiometry is a measure of peripheral function, it is likely not strongly influenced by cortical changes from dementia and can be appropriately completed within populations even with early dementia (Uhlmann et al., 1989; McClannahan et al., 2021). These aspects support minimal concern of the association resulting from reverse causation with dementia leading to impaired audiometry and PTA, although other studies suggest differing conclusions (Brenowitz et al., 2020). Detailed summaries of current evidence have been provided in a handful of other publications (Albers et al., 2015; Fortunato et al., 2016; Thomson et al., 2017 Loughrey et al., 2018; Yuan et al., 2018; Sharma et al., 2021).

A previous meta-analysis (Loughrey et al., 2018) found the odds of cognitive impairment for those with age related hearing loss was 1.22 (95% CI: 1.09, 1.36) and odds of dementia was 1.28 (95% CI: 1.02, 1 59) times higher than those with normal hearing. Prior work has noted an association between hearing loss and declines in global cognitive function, executive function, processing speed, and memory (Lin et al., 2011; Loughrey et al., 2018; Alattar et al., 2020; Gao et al., 2020; Brewster et al., 2021). However, what constitutes hearing ability or cognitive impairment often differs across studies. Some studies have included continuous measures of hearing as decibels hearing level (dB HL) (Armstrong et al., 2019), while others have categorized hearing ability by clinically recognized categories [i.e., mild or greater loss (Lin et al., 2011, 2013; Deal et al., 2016; World Report on Hearing, 2021)] or have only considered specific frequency ranges (Uhlmann et al., 1989; Gates et al., 1996) as compared to the common clinically utilized range of 500–4000 Hz or 500–8000 Hz. The diverse definitions of hearing loss make it challenging to synthesize the current evidence base as the degree of hearing difficulty varies by categorization used and represents different levels of resultant impairment and functional ability. For example, categorization of those with *any* measured hearing loss (i.e., Pure Tone Average [PTA] $\geq$ 25 dB HL) vs. consideration of those with *a moderate or greater* hearing loss (PTA > 40 dB HL) as the hearing-impaired group likely constitutes different comparison groups and underlying idea of what is a hearing "loss" across different studies.

Varied measures of cognition used have also placed challenging demands on synthesis of prior results. A plethora of validated neurocognitive assessments exist both across cognitive domains and as global screeners. Variation in domain, mode of administration, if accommodations for hearing loss were considered, whether cognitive status was determined by provider or proxy report exist across studies, among others. While the importance of evaluating cognitive ability in multiple ways should not be ignored due to the complexity of cognitive processing and complex diagnostic presentation, synthesis of results across studies remains aloof.

Central Auditory Function

While an association between cognitive decline/dementia and peripheral auditory function is well established (Livingston et al., 2020), the relationship between cognitive decline/dementia with central auditory function has been less studied in the epidemiologic literature. Given the interdependence between central auditory function and cognitive processing, it becomes difficult to distinguish between the two processing abilities. For speech to be properly understood, the auditory stimuli must first maintain sufficient integrity to be accurately encoded by the peripheral auditory system and must then be decoded by the central auditory system (Humes, 2021). For the auditory signal to be decoded by the central auditory system, higher level cognitive processing is required. Research over the last few decades has attempted to distinguish the boundaries between central auditory dysfunction (CAD) and cognitive impairment (CHABA, 1988; Humes et al., 2013a). Heterogeneity in defining central auditory function and cognitive processing has led to significant barriers to evidence synthesis and causal inference. As with peripheral hearing loss, a diverse array of definitions, tests, cognitive domains, and sample populations has been utilized for studies across disciplines.

Prior systematic reviews have revealed mixed quality and potential bias in previous work on central auditory function and cognition (Dryden et al., 2017). Dryden et al. (2017) report an overall weak correlation between cognitive performance and speech perception/central auditory function depending on the cognitive domain and speech-in-noise assessment used. The strongest correlation was observed between central auditory function and processing speed. It has yet to be determined what degree un-aided peripheral hearing ability has in the moderating or modifying of the association between central hearing (e.g., decoding of speech stimuli or speech perception ability in noise) and cognitive performance. Overall, results demonstrate an interconnection in cortical resources utilized for both processes (Humes, 2013; Humes et al., 2013b; Humes and Young, 2016; Sardone et al., 2019), presenting challenges for inference but also noteworthy opportunity to identify novel targets for intervention or prevention.

It has been hypothesized CAD may serve as an early marker and therefore a possible prodromal symptom of cognitive decline (Gates et al., 1996). We know AD pathology reaches the auditory cortex. Nearly 30 years ago, Sinha et al. (1993) demonstrated the presence of plaques and neurofibrillary tangles within the medial geniculate body and central nucleus of the inferior colliculus in patients diagnosed with AD compared to those without a diagnosis. Additionally, neurofibrillary plaques and tangles were found in the primary auditory and auditory association cortices of patients diagnosed with AD. While, Braak staging (Braak and Braak, 1991, 1997) suggests these auditory cortices are some of the final brain regions affected by AD pathology. However, evidence indicates functional disconnection effects from the involvement in higher order cortical areas may affect the primary auditory cortex in early Alzheimer's disease (Sardone et al., 2019). Importantly, the cortical areas associated with age related hearing loss and compensatory cortical activation to support language processing like the cingulate cortex are also involved in cognitive function like episodic memory and are affected early in the AD disease process, having specific implications for complex auditory processing (Goll et al., 2010, 2011, 2012; Sardone et al., 2019). These ideas support CAD as a marker of AD, but with unclear indication of CAD as an *early* marker (Sardone et al., 2020). How this presentation of pathology at later stages of progression translates to earlier identification of AD, beyond abilities from currently identified neurological and biological biomarkers is unclear. Yet behavioral testing of central auditory function suggests utility. Gates et al. (2011) demonstrated in a sample of volunteers from a dementia surveillance cohort over nine times greater hazard for incident dementia (95% CI: 3.6, 26.7) among those with severe CAD compared to those with proposed normal function. A pilot study in a well-characterized aging cohort found poor cognitive performance on memory, language, executive function, and global function for those with poor speech-in-noise performance regardless of peripheral hearing status (Mamo et al., 2019). The associations for some domains were attenuated after excluding those with a moderate or greater hearing loss, suggesting peripheral hearing may play a role in performance within certain cognitive domains that are dependent on speech tasks.

Many prior studies have employed the Dichotic Sentence Identification test (DSI) as a measure of central auditory function. The DSI presents a meaningless but grammatically correct sentence to each ear simultaneously and the listener is to then identify the sentences, with designated systematically differing modes of reporting the sentence items (Fifer et al., 1983). This diagnostic tool, primarily used currently in research settings, was designed to be less susceptible to peripheral hearing ability when presented at a conversational level of 50 dB HL. Therefore, some propose poor performance on the DSI test may be more reflective of cognitive ability rather than incorporating influence from peripheral hearing and the simple inability to hear the test (Jerger, 2019). DSI has been used to differentiate memory impairment among those demonstrating mild memory impairment without dementia (Gates et al., 2008). However, the DSI test and many other central auditory function assessments have minimal clinical utility due to complex presentation requirements and time-intensiveness.

Investigation of various means to define and measure central auditory function suggest an association with subjective memory complaints/impairment (Idrizbegovic et al., 2011; Fausto et al., 2018). In a small sample, subjective memory complaints were associated with poor performance on certain central auditory processing evaluations but not with peripheral hearing ability (Jayakody et al., 2020), potentially further supporting speech-in-noise difficulty as a marker of cognitive function. Yet proper implementation of this information for dementia prevention and intervention remains unclarified.

Across measures of central auditory processing, an association has been observed between biomarkers such as CSF tau, cortical thickness and volumetric measures of AD-related brain regions (Tuwaig et al., 2017), although existing supporting evidence remains limited. Given the rapidly expanding identification of dementia related biomarkers, what central auditory processing measures may add to our existing repertoire is an important consideration for future research and identification of pre-clinical dementia, whether considering generic 'dementia' and all subtypes, or considering more targeted research on AD specifically given its epidemiologic importance. Consideration of sensory loss more broadly (i.e., hearing, vision, and olfactory ability) has received more recent attention as indicators of pre-clinical dementia. For example, advances in retinal imaging may shed light on early brain changes associated with Alzheimer's disease (Snyder et al., 2016; Zhang et al., 2021). Yet, like central auditory processing, there is much we still must determine regarding these measures and neurological pathways to understand any potential role of sensory biomarkers in identification of preclinical dementia.

Dementia Prevention Through Management of Hearing Loss

Due to low-risk auditory rehabilitation tools such as hearing aids, hearing loss in older adults is readily considered modifiable and therefore makes it a worthy target of interest among dementia risk factors. The current limited use of hearing aids and challenges with accessibility of hearing devices and services have been a focus of both health research and public policy in recent years (National Academies of Sciences, Engineering, and Medicine, 2016), bringing new force behind the idea of hearing loss management as a means for dementia intervention. Existing data and reports of the use of hearing aids for cognitive decline stem largely from observational and cross-sectional study and present mixed findings (Amieva et al., 2015; Maharani et al., 2018; Ray et al., 2018; Dawes et al., 2019; Amieva and Ouvrard, 2020). In observational studies, we are often not able to completely control for factors which determine or influence if an individual pursues or uses hearing aids or other forms of hearing treatment (e.g., socioeconomic status, education background, social support and engagement, access to healthcare) — many of these factors are also protective against cognitive decline. These challenges present difficulty when trying to isolate the potential protective effect from hearing aids from that of these external factors, potentially influencing estimated effects due to aspects of selection into study of hearing aid use. Well-designed pilot interventions and clinical trials have taken up this challenge in recent years to determine if the use of hearing aids may alter subsequent risk of dementia (Brewster et al., 2020). These clinical trials present unique opportunity inherent within study design by minimizing this potential bias from confounding factors through design tools like randomization and masking (Celentano and Szklo, 2020). One of the largest and longest clinical trials to date on the use of hearing aids for dementia prevention is currently underway in The Aging and Cognitive Health Evaluation in Elders (ACHIEVE) clinical trial (Deal et al., 2018). While not powered to detect a difference for memory scores, the ACHIEVE pilot study demonstrated suggestion of an efficacy signal in memory test performance for participants randomized to hearing treatment, including hearing aid use, compared to a health education control (Deal et al., 2017). The pilot study also indicated positive proximal outcomes of improved participant perception of hearing handicap and improved social network. We have yet to determine how age and rapidity of hearing loss onset and its proximity to hearing aid uptake may modify dementia risk. The influence of other rehabilitation strategies on dementia risk, such as basic communication strategies, cochlear implants, or auditory training, is vastly understudied.

POTENTIAL PATHWAYS LINKING HEARING TO COGNITION

The complexities and interdependence between central auditory function and cognitive processing present challenges for causal inference. Therefore, current hypotheses of mechanistic pathways predominantly view peripheral hearing loss as a potential cause of dementia and consider central auditory function as a marker of cognitive decline. Current hypotheses of the causal mechanistic pathways have been well articulated in other works (Lin and Albert, 2014; Wayne and Johnsrude, 2015; Griffiths et al., 2020; Johnson et al., 2021; Powell et al., 2021). Clarifying this mechanistic pathway has far-reaching implications for research, the design, implementation, and evaluation of dementia prevention strategies, and the translation of the evidence to recommendations for patient care or health policy. A smaller body of evidence currently supports the notion that dementia leads to hearing loss (CHABA, 1988; Baltes and Lindenberger, 1997). A larger collection of evidence supports the notion hearing loss may contribute toward cognitive decline— directly through what is commonly known as the sensory deprivation hypothesis, or indirectly through the information-degradation hypothesis (Wayne and Johnsrude, 2015). Alternatively, hearing loss and dementia may result from an additional external factor through what is considered the common-cause hypothesis (Wayne and Johnsrude, 2015; Powell et al., 2021). In this article, we briefly review evidence to support each hypothesized pathway as depicted in our modified mechanistic framework (**Figure 4**).

Sensory Deprivation

A growing body of evidence indicates prolonged sensory deprivation has an adverse effect on the brain, with enduring changes to brain structure and function. Due to auditory deprivation from ARHL, neural deafferentation, cortical re-allocation for support of other processes, and atrophy in brain regions important for speech perception processing may occur. The resultant reorganization may add to existing brain pathology (e.g., amyloid burden, neuronal loss) at the detriment of general cognitive performance by altering critical brain regions which could otherwise be utilized for higher-level cognitive processing. Reduced gray matter density and reductions in temporal lobe volume are observed in those with peripheral hearing loss (Lin et al., 2014; Wingfield and Peelle, 2015; Armstrong et al., 2019), as prolonged sensory deprivation may lead to changes and decreases in cortical brain volume in conjunction with that seen with expected cognitive aging or neurodegenerative disease (Lin et al., 2014; Eckert et al., 2019). The brain regions most notably affected are pertinent for semantic memory and preclude advancement along the continuum of cognitive decline, including frontal and pre-frontal regions, the superior temporal gyrus and Heschel's gyrus (Husain et al., 2011). Cortical regions enlisted for speech understanding like the frontal cortex and hippocampus are also associated with reductions in whole-brain gray matter volume (Rudner et al., 2019). Even among those older adults considered free of dementia, hearing loss appears to be associated with reduced white matter microstructural integrity in cortical regions crucial for cognitive processing (Rigters et al., 2017; Alfandari et al., 2018; Armstrong et al., 2019; Croll et al., 2020). Research has yet to determine importance of the duration of sensory deprivation or evidence for a sensitive period in age of onset of hearing loss and how this relates to the structural changes observed. While cortical changes and reorganization from hearing loss is evident even among those in the earliest stages of cognitive impairment (Campbell and Sharma, 2014; Sharma and Glick, 2017), the extent of cortical reorganization necessary to evoke brain atrophy and changes to cognitive performance is unclear. Prolonged sensory deprivation, therefore, may result in physical reductions in cortical volume in addition to that experienced from dementia pathology alone. This sensory deprivation may necessitate cortical reorganization resulting in further restriction of cortical capacity available for cognitive processing. How and if these brain volume changes represent specific pathologic changes for types of dementia remains to be clarified. Longitudinal study of the role of peripheral hearing loss and association with AD amyloid pathology on PET imaging did not suggest an association (Parker et al., 2020) but work in this space using specified biomarkers of dementia has been understudied.

Information Degradation

While the sensory deprivation hypothesis suggests physical changes to the brain due to prolonged hearing loss which subsequently impacts cognitive processing, the information degradation hypothesis proposes the association stems from increased demands on cognitive processing in order to compensate for impoverished sensory input. The additional processing required to compensate for degraded auditory perception draws on the same resources needed for other higher-level cognitive processing and semantic encoding (Peelle, 2018). These increased cognitive demands required to appropriately encode auditory stimuli requires extensive listening effort particularly with memory, attention, and executive function (Wingfield et al., 2005; Tun et al., 2009, 2012; Pichora-Fuller et al., 2016; Peelle, 2018). An individual's ability to compensate for subsequent diminished cognitive performance is heterogeneous and may contribute toward the known variability in cognitive performance, presentation, and clinical symptoms among similar existing brain pathology. With hearing loss, this increased cognitive and listening effort may increase cognitive load at any time of day as the auditory system never "turns off," thereby drawing on the cognitive buffer of the individual and their ability to compensate for cognitive changes and resulting in earlier presentation of clinical symptoms and dementia (Whitson et al., 2018). The compensatory mechanisms activated on cognitive tasks between older and younger adults with sensory deficits differ, with older adults demonstrating increased fatigue on dual tasks that rely on both listening and understanding (Schneider et al., 2002). Essentially, the information degradation hypothesis implies acute cognitive impairment. If we are able to restore

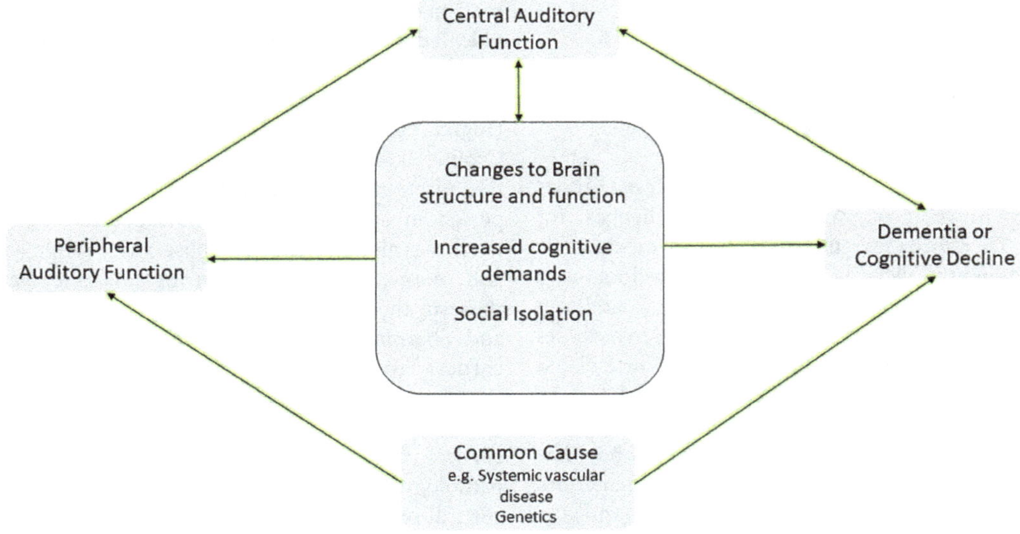

FIGURE 4 | Hypothesized framework for the mechanism of the hearing and dementia association. The center square includes potential causal paths between peripheral hearing loss and cognitive decline or dementia, including changes to brain structure and function (i.e., sensory deprivation hypothesis), increased cognitive demands (i.e., information degradation hypothesis), and other effects such as social isolation. Additionally, a common cause such as systemic vascular disease or genetic factors may lead to both peripheral hearing loss and cognitive decline and dementia. Further inclusion of central auditory function resulting from direct and indirect effects of this causal pathway is depicted and may serve as a marker of cognitive decline or dementia. It is likely more than one of the pathways depicted may explain the link between hearing and dementia. Adapted from Powell et al. (2021).

auditory input, we may therefore see at least some restoration of cognitive performance on higher-level tasks.

A Common Cause of Both Conditions

Alternatively, both hearing loss and cognitive impairment may merely stem from the same underlying mechanism (Baltes and Lindenberger, 1997; Wayne and Johnsrude, 2015). Given the presumed independent effect of peripheral hearing on cognitive processing when measured through audiometry, investigation of a common cause which may be associated with hearing and cognition has largely been evaluated via pure tone audiometry. A potential common mechanism might include the overall neural degeneration common with aging, resulting in both decreased auditory ability and decreased cognitive performance (Surprenant and Neath, 2006; Wayne and Johnsrude, 2015). Additionally, a given dementia pathology (most commonly discussed as AD pathology) may lead to early CAD and impaired hearing prior to more general cognitive decline (Johnson et al., 2021). Decreased processing speed with age may lead to slower cognitive functioning overall as well as slower processing speed for sensory integration and perception (CHABA, 1988; Salthouse, 1996). Dementia pathology from a central cause may therefore produce early dysfunction within the central auditory system resulting in impaired hearing ability (i.e., auditory scene analysis or ability in complex listening environments) prior to the presentation of more general cognitive decline or impairments. As described in the review by Griffiths et al. (2020), it is also possible degraded peripheral signals lead to dysfunctional pattern processing within the central auditory system (particularly the medial temporal lobe) and interacts with existing neurodegenerative or AD pathology, resulting in the observed association. With this hypothesis, whether the increased neuronal activity from degraded auditory input causing or increasing AD pathology, or the degraded auditory input from hearing loss may reduced activity for auditory cognitive processes within the medial temporal lobe remains to be clarified, however, either speculation supports early identification of hearing loss prior to prolonged duration of decreased auditory input and broad hearing-dementia intervention strategies.

It is possible both auditory and neural functioning are altered by systemic vascular pathology impacting the spiral ganglion or stria vascularis of the auditory system and bran vasculature. Therefore, vascular disease in older adults may also subsequently lead to concurrent cognitive and sensory changes (Eckert et al., 2013; Laughlin et al., 2013; Livingston et al., 2017), although this hypothesis is challenging to confirm due to the long prodromal stage of some dementias like AD. Exploration of a common genetic risk between AD and hearing loss using a weighted sum of AD polymorphisms and AD inflammatory pathway suggests a possible genetic link with poorer speech-in-noise performance and self-reported difficulty hearing in background noise (Brenowitz et al., 2020). However, study of Apolipoprotein ε4 (*APOE* ε4) has shown no association with hearing loss (Morita et al., 2019), nor does it modify the association between hearing loss and cognitive decline (Alattar et al., 2020). Other work suggests the presence of one or more *APOE*ε4 alleles may actually be marginally associated with better hearing in older adults as measured via pure tone audiometry, perhaps because *APOE* ε4 is more common in Black adults, but hearing loss is more prevalent in White adults (Mener et al., 2016). While *APOE* ε4 serves as a strong risk factor for dementia, based on current evidence, it does not appear to be a driving factor in the hearing-dementia association. Although the genetic determinants of ARHL are largely unknown, identifying what (if any) genetic determinants exist may provide further insight toward additional avenues of a common cause between hearing loss and dementia (Wells et al., 2019). Overall, few studies have investigated the role of genetic risk on causality in the hearing-dementia link, therefore some question of association with shared genes remains (Mitchell et al., 2020).

Potential Mediators of the Hearing Loss-Dementia Association

Other risk factors for dementia may also mediate the association of hearing and cognition including: loneliness, social isolation, depression, decreased physical activity, or frailty. Studies have demonstrated the presence of hearing loss leads to increased social isolation and/or loneliness for some older adults as individuals with hearing loss may withdraw from previously enjoyed activities or social interactions due to the inability to engage and communicate with others. Links between social isolation or loneliness and dementia are well established (Rutherford et al., 2018; Maharani et al., 2019; Rafnsson et al., 2020; Shukla et al., 2020). The evidence for link between hearing loss and depression, which may serve as a risk factor and/or prodromal sign of dementia, remains mixed (Rutherford et al., 2018). While an increasing body of evidence suggests increased risk of depression with hearing loss, the direction of association remains to be clarified. The heterogeneous course of depression in older adults as it relates to hearing loss has received minimal investigation (Brewster et al., 2018). It is possible hearing loss leads to reduced physical activity and physical functioning, each a known risk factor for dementia, due to decreased auditory awareness with surroundings and anxiety (Chen et al., 2015; Choi et al., 2016; Martinez-Amezcua et al., 2021). Some evidence suggests a greater prevalence of frailty among those with hearing loss, another condition which has been suggested as an independent risk factor or early marker of dementia (Panza et al., 2015; Liljas et al., 2017). Each proposed potential mediator and pathway presents an identified opportunity for targeted intervention, yet how each may fit within a larger dementia framework remains to be clarified.

The Challenges of Multiple Potential Pathways

Multiple potential pathways area likely involved in the association between hearing and dementia, but with unknown understanding of the specific contribution of each pathway and if this contribution varies by the individual. While common risk factors (i.e., age, education, vascular disease) are thought to contribute toward the association (Whalley et al., 2004; Humes, 2013; Wayne and Johnsrude, 2015), these factors likely do not explain the full story. Even in large epidemiologic studies which have attempted to control for these additional factors, the association persists, suggesting additional pathways are likely involved but have yet to be differentiated.

TARGETED FUTURE RESEARCH

Identification of research priorities given the transdisciplinary scope of study on hearing and dementia will aid in achieving foundational dementia research goals: to advance our identification of subgroups of adults who may present greater risk for cognitive decline/dementia or suggest novel options for intervention or prevention. Numerous pressing research questions and additional perspectives on the importance of these questions prevail (Wayne and Johnsrude, 2015; Whitson et al., 2018; Powell et al., 2021). Here we feature four research priorities which, in our opinion, will provide leading advancements in the possible causal role of hearing loss along the dementia continuum: (1) determination of the pathway of association, (2) management of potential bias due to sensory loss in cognitive testing, (3) determining if we can modify dementia risk by treating hearing loss, (4) understanding if biomarkers or indicators of sensory loss are useful for identification of pre-clinical dementia (**Figure 5**).

By What Pathway Does the Hearing-Cognition Association Act?

Given the varied temporal contributions of each proposed mechanistic pathway, determination of which pathway(s) serve as the primary driver behind the association is vital. This determination may allow for improved study design and planning and well as more informed clinical intervention to delay or prevent the onset of cognitive symptoms and delay the progression along or alter the trajectory of the clinical course of dementia. With the current insufficient evidence to declare hearing loss has an independent effect on cognitive impairment for older adults, how we should intervene on hearing loss, when to do so, and if such interventions are effective in decreasing or delaying dementia risk will all largely depend on the underlying mechanism. We know the presentation of dementia symptomatology is heterogeneous across individuals even with the same underlying pathology. We have yet to determine by what manner hearing loss may influence a potential buffer which delays/prevents the presentation of symptoms in some individuals yet fails do so in others, leading to earlier symptomatology.

If the association between hearing loss and dementia is only due to a common cause, the potential for directly delaying or preventing changes in the presentation of dementia symptoms or pathology through hearing would be extremely limited as the underlying cause would remain untreated. The research intervention focus would ultimately turn toward the underlying common confounder, which could then have downstream effects for hearing and cognition. However, the use of hearing management such as hearing aids may support cognition through indirect pathways like improving social engagement and communication yet decreasing cognitive load and strain on central auditory function through improvement of peripheral auditory input, directly preventing dementia would remain elusive.

A direct effect of hearing loss on cognitive function is inferred with the sensory-deprivation and information

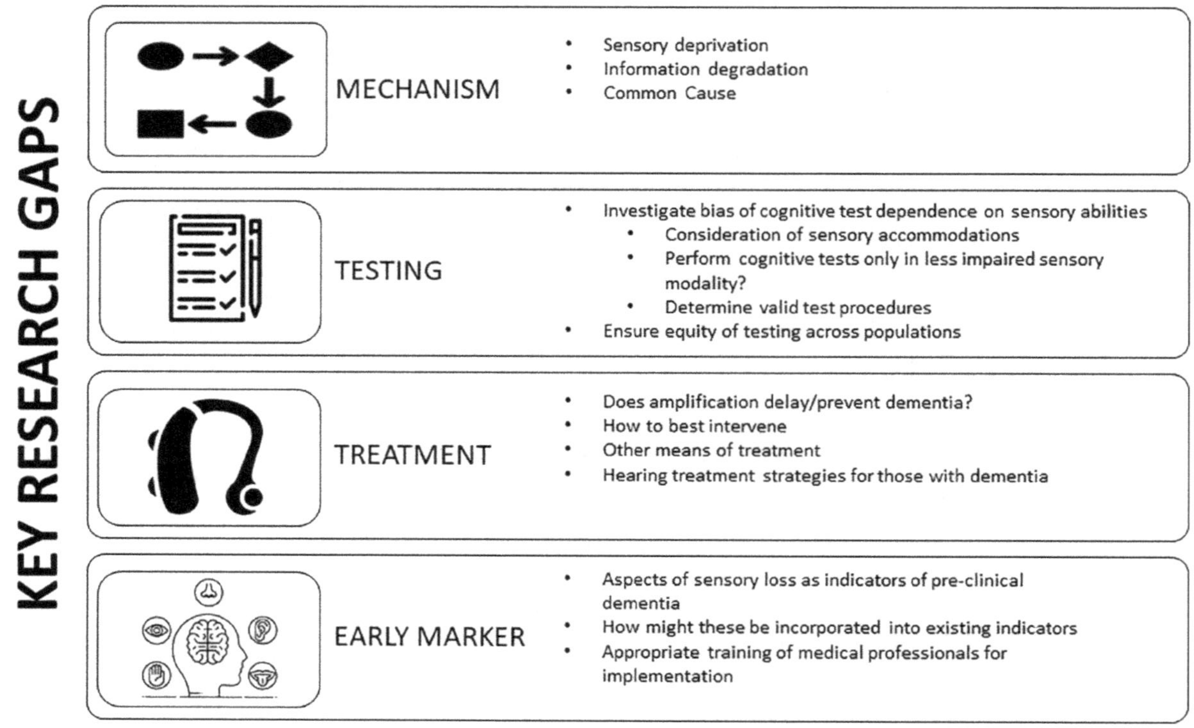

FIGURE 5 | Key research gaps in hearing impairment and cognition. Targeted research on the mechanism behind the association between hearing and cognition will guide intervention and prevention strategies. Additional research gaps include an understanding of potential bias in cognitive testing due to dependence on sensory abilities and how best to study and minimize this bias. Further understanding of if treating hearing loss via amplification or another means influences dementia risk is vital for public health. Determination if markers of sensory impairment may serve as indicators of pre-clinical dementia and how this may be incorporated with existing biomarkers. Adapted from Powell et al. (2021).

degradation hypotheses. A long-term versus short term-effect is implied depending on the proposed pathway, yet both advocate that hearing loss, and notably untreated hearing loss, leads to downstream consequences for cognitive resources with important implications for approaches to intervention. The sensory deprivation hypothesis posits structural and functional changes in the brain due to lack of auditory stimulation. Therefore, preemptive identification of hearing loss and early adoption of treatment strategies which delay or prevent deafferentation or atrophy within the auditory or sensory regions of the brain are essential to prevent lasting structural damage. Importantly, auditory rehabilitation to prevent structural and functional changes in the brain through sensory deprivation may even have benefit at later stages of hearing loss by delaying additional neural reorganization or atrophy. For comparison, the information degradation hypothesis strongly supports hearing intervention at any time in the disease process. With restoration of the integrity of auditory stimuli via rehabilitation or hearing management, the cognitive demands and utilized cognitive resources for speech and environmental awareness would in theory be reduced, allowing for cognitive resources to again be allocated to overall cognitive processing and compensation.

It is imperative we determine how to disentangle CAD and cognitive decline if we are to consider its use in targeting prevention efforts or early identification of subgroups at greater risk for cognitive decline. How to differentiate between changes in cognitive processing and CAD, the temporality between each processing condition, and whether CAD may serve as an early marker for specific subtypes of dementia remains a challenging barrier for characterizing the link between hearing loss and dementia. While the majority of research to date has focused on the association between hearing loss and Alzheimer's disease since the most common form of dementia and pathology observed, distinctions in association with other dementia pathologies is paramount. The dependence and entanglement of both forms of hearing on higher-level cognitive functioning stirs question of how to interpret the role of each process along the auditory pathway. If CAD may serve as an early marker of dementia remains to be determined.

As stated, it is likely multiple mechanistic pathways are involved in the hearing-dementia association. Determining if one pathway serves as the primary driver, or if the pathway is unique to the individual may provide an opportunity for a person-centered approach to dementia prevention and intervention. Furthermore, while not mutually exclusive, determining the role of central vs. peripheral hearing in the hearing-dementia association will further inform research and clinical use of hearing and prevention or as an early marker of dementia.

How Do We Manage Potential Bias Due to Sensory Loss in Cognitive Testing?

A goal of any neurocognitive test battery is to accurately measure cognitive function for all individuals. Yet the validity of cognitive assessments inherently depends on an individual's auditory or visual ability to access test materials. This interdependence has led some to question whether there is a bias or confounding introduced by a sensory impairment during cognitive testing for older adults (Guerreiro and Van Gerven, 2017; Füllgrabe, 2020). An investigation testing this hypothesis used item response theory methods to disentangle the true effect of sensory impairment on test performance (Nichols et al., 2021) in two longitudinal aging cohorts. Results suggest some differences in performance related to sensory loss, particularly among those with the poorest health or greatest cognitive impairment. However, for the vast majority of participants, cognitive performance on testing was not found to be biased due to sensory impairment (Villeneuve et al., 2017; Bott et al., 2019, 2020). Further determination of how best to conduct cognitive testing among those with sensory loss is vital for clinical and research settings.

While exclusion of those with severe sensory loss from testing might ensure completion of evaluations, this exclusion limits our understanding of the role of sensory loss in cognition. One way to assess cognitive function among those with hearing loss may be to utilize cognitive test batteries that are administered via visual modality rather than auditory. However, this strategy does not fully address issues that arise among those with dual sensory impairment (i.e., those with both vision and hearing loss).

An alternative approach to address sensory loss when administering cognitive assessments is to consider accommodations for the sensory loss (Littlejohn et al., 2021). If an individual usually wears a hearing aid or glasses, it would be important to remind the individual to bring these sensory aids for optimal completion of evaluations. Accommodations for sensory loss might include offering test instructions in written (i.e., large print) as well as oral format, ensuring the testing is completed in a quiet and well-lit environment, or provision of a personal amplifier such as a pocket-talker or a visual aid for test takers. Accounting for hearing and vision needs during study conception, design and analysis, as well as during test administration will be important for confidence in study results. Regardless of the different types of cognitive test used, it is imperative that we include individuals with different types and degrees of sensory loss in studies, in order to advance our understanding of the role of sensory loss in cognition (Pye et al., 2017; Littlejohn et al., 2021).

Can We Modify Dementia Risk and Its Associated Behaviors by Treating Hearing Loss?

Recent decades have seen an accumulation of evidence for the impact of treating hearing loss on cognitive decline or dementia. Our observational studies have provided foundational and pivotal insights into the hearing-dementia association, however, evidence of causality for decreased or delayed cognitive decline due to hearing aid use is more challenging. From a neurocognitive perspective on this investigation, challenges include selection effects of older adults into studies. Individuals who pursue and obtain a hearing aid are generally a select group of adults— often with higher education, higher income, and greater health seeking behaviors— all of which are considered protective factors for cognitive decline (National Academies of Sciences, Engineering, and Medicine, 2016; Livingston et al., 2020; Reed et al., 2021).

Many barriers to obtaining hearing aids still exist within the United States and must be considered within the context of existing research on the use of hearing aids as dementia prevention or intervention. Hearing aid and aural rehabilitation services are not covered under Medicare or many private insurances, placing the cost of the device and services (often $1000 or more) on the individual and family. Further, an audiologic evaluation and aural rehabilitation appointments are not currently available through direct-access to patients under some American insurances, but require referral from a primary care physician or specialist (National Academies of Sciences, Engineering, and Medicine, 2016). This added barrier with a need for both patients and providers to understand how to navigate the healthcare system and for patients to attend additional medical appointments currently creates added barriers to hearing treatment which may prevent or deter some individuals from seeking care. While access to hearing devices and services is improved in some countries, global barriers remain as far as availability of trained professionals or cost of devices (World Report on Hearing, 2021). Additional challenges include collection of hearing data and data on hearing aid use, and unmeasured confounding. Data on hearing ability is often not collected or collected only in very limited form in many epidemiologic or non-auditory based studies. Additionally, data on hearing aid use and amount of use is virtually non-existent. Owning a hearing aid is not synonymous with using a hearing aid. Further, individuals vastly over-report their use of the hearing aid (Taubman et al., 1999), yet wearing a device regularly and often is the only means to ensure the brain has had the ability to adapt to increased auditory stimuli. What constitutes "regularly and often" remains to be clarified and may be individualized (Hickson et al., 2014). Without this information, it remains challenging for us to determine how hearing aid use may modify the hearing-dementia association, or any other health outcome for older adults.

Without understanding the mechanism(s) behind the hearing-dementia association, it is challenging to determine how and when is best to intervene on cognitive decline and dementia. Evidence for treatment of hearing loss throughout the dementia continuum is growing, yet many questions remain. Evidence of efficacy, effectiveness and cost efficiency will aid in determining the best aural rehabilitation choices for prevention — all areas with extensive gaps in evidence for hearing loss and dementia.

In addition to potentially serving as a dementia prevention strategy, hearing aids may present opportunity for intervention for neuropsychiatric symptoms (NPS) at all stages of dementia and negative health outcomes associated with NPS (Kales et al., 2014). Breakdowns in communication between those individuals with dementia/cognitive impairment and their caregivers along with decreased awareness of surroundings may contribute to behavioral changes commonly noted with more progressed disease (Littlejohn et al., 2021). The use of a hearing assistive device in older adults with cognitive impairment has been found to result in fewer and less severe NPSs and less severe depressive symptoms (Kim et al., 2020). Therefore, hearing aid use among dementia patients demonstrate improved communication, reduced NPS, decreased perception of hearing handicap, and improved quality of life for both individuals and their caregivers (Dawes et al., 2015, 2019; Mamo et al., 2018; Littlejohn et al., 2021).

Additional work is needed to determine how best to provide auditory rehabilitation for adults with cognitive impairment. A recent study (Hubbard et al., 2018) suggests treating hearing loss in cognitively impaired older adults yields benefits for both the older adult as well as caregiver dyads. A recent internationally gathered task force on identification and management of hearing and vision loss among those living with dementia (Littlejohn et al., 2021) highlighted six key areas of practice recommendations and identified targeted areas for improvement, including: awareness and knowledge, recognition and detection, evaluation, management, support, services and policies. However, the group acknowledged that a dearth of evidence across many of these areas left the basis of broad recommendations to be placed on expert and patient input at times, vowing to revisit recommendations in a few years in the hopes of improved scientific evidence. Even with expert recommendations for management, hearing is not automatically "restored" with the use of a hearing aid. Instead, hearing aids should be considered a tool to improve audibility and access to environmental and speech sounds. For a new hearing aid user, most individuals require an adjustment period as the brain re-habituates to increased access to the auditory environment and stimulation after a potentially prolonged period of sensory deprivation. This aspect of hearing loss management may be unclear or unknown to patients and non-auditory science researchers without the appropriate training and counseling. How to provide this counseling for persons with dementia and their families has, to our knowledge, not been studied.

While hearing aids serve as the most prominent means of hearing intervention, other means of aural rehabilitation are available such as personal amplifiers, general assistive listening devices, or auditory training strategies. Research is limited on the use of these alternative strategies for treatment of hearing loss along the dementia continuum, yet determination of a variety of accessible alternative strategies is fundamental for providing communication ability and social engagement for older adults. Hearing aids may not be feasible for some older adults (e.g., those with severe cognitive impairment) and likely do not meet the listening needs of many adults when used as the only form of rehabilitation. As mentioned, adaptation to increased auditory stimuli requires extensive cortical adjustment which may overwhelm some individuals without proper counseling and consideration. Non-technology driven alternative strategies (e.g., training in communication strategies such as speaking face-to-face, turning off or reducing the presence of competing background noise, talking from the same room, use of additional visual cues/aids, improving self-efficacy advocacy) (Nieman et al., 2017) require further evaluation to determine how these proven strategies might be utilized for older adults with cognitive impairment.

Importantly, the use of hearing aids has a primary role in management of peripheral hearing loss, contributing to the focused effort of public health research on peripheral rather than central hearing ability and the association with cognitive decline/dementia. If the pathway linking hearing to cognition is related (directly or in part) due to central auditory processing and ability, the use of hearing aids as a prevention and intervention option for dementia will have minimal effect given the state of current technology and auditory processing treatments. While hearing aid use may not delay the progression of dementia pathology if the association is due to a common cause, as stated above the use of hearing aids may still indirectly support intervention of progression of the clinical presentation of dementia symptoms through indirect pathways such as decreased cognitive load and improved social stimulation. Future advances in hearing aid technology which may better address cognitive and central auditory demands may provide even greater benefit. Currently, evidence for the role of central auditory processing and central hearing disorders for early identification of dementia will have heightened importance and emphasize the need for consideration of greater use in neuropsychological and medical evaluations.

Can Sensory Loss Be an Additional Tool for Identification of Pre-clinical Dementia?

The high prevalence of not only hearing loss, but also vision loss, among older adults presents opportunity for additional access points for identification of pre-clinical dementia *if* hearing or vision may serve as an early marker of dementia- a point which has yet to be determined and has received minimal study (Brenowitz et al., 2019; Johnson et al., 2021). We do not yet know if sensory loss indicators (i.e., optical coherence tomography, fundus photography, speech-in-noise testing, auditory scene analysis or auditory cognitive testing, electrophysiology, etc.) aid in earlier identification of cognitive change. If sensory loss *does* prove to be a valuable tool for identification of pre-clinical dementia, then we must determine how to use this tool in patient-provider planning and diagnosis as well as within our research models. Additionally, training on discussion with health care professionals for the appropriate referrals and how to convey results within each represented scope of practice is essential for appropriate dementia planning (Littlejohn et al., 2021).

CONCLUSION

Although research on the role of hearing loss on dementia risk initiated over 40 years ago, recent surge in the evidence supporting adverse outcomes across health and care among older adults with hearing loss has come to the attention of patients and their families, clinicians, and policy makers. The human and economic expense of caring for the expected growing number of adults reaching or past retirement age demands interdisciplinary collaboration. While the fields of cognitive science, neuroscience, and gerontology have been at the core of dementia research, allied-health disciplines such as auditory science present untapped opportunity to contribute toward efforts to reduce the burden of dementia across societies. A thorough understanding of the current evidence, identification of leading hypothesis and elucidation of the mechanism(s) driving the association between hearing and dementia, consideration of sensory loss during cognitive testing or in care strategies for those with dementia or dementia prevention, and targeted future directions of research can have a significant impact on prevention and intervention strategies for older adults. The interdependent and synergistic processes of hearing and cognition require careful approach for research and clinical care. The current limitations in dementia treatment necessitate innovative approaches for dementia intervention. Identification of additional early markers of dementia, a potential role of central auditory function with continued research may aid in this process, as well as inform optimal strategies for hearing management itself. Considering the presence of other conditions, like hearing loss, and optimizing our strategies to evaluate and treat hearing loss could diminish the risk of adverse outcomes and enhance health and quality of life for older adults.

AUTHOR CONTRIBUTIONS

DP was responsible for the initial drafting, editing, and formatting. EO, NR, FL, and JD contributed to content and editing. All authors contributed to the article and approved the submitted version.

ACKNOWLEDGMENTS

Parts of this manuscript were adapted from that printed in the Journal of the Association for Research in Otolaryngology. 2021 July; 22(4): 387–403. doi: 10.1007/s10162-021-00799-y. While common ideas are represented across manuscripts for consistency across disciplines related to current knowledge and key gaps in future research, differences in scientific writing and discussions of emphasis are uniquely tailored to the respective journal of publication.

REFERENCES

Alattar, A., Bergstrom, J., Laughlin, G., Kritz-Silberstein, D., Richard, E., Reas, E., et al. (2020). Hearing impairment and cognitive decline in older, community dwelling adults. *J. Gerontol. A Biol. Sci. Med. Sci.* 75, 567–573.

Albers, M. W., Gilmore, G. C., Kaye, J., Murphy, C., Wingfield, A., Bennett, D., et al. (2015). At the interface of sensory and motor dysfunctions and Alzheimer's disease. *Alzheimer's Dementia* 11, 70–98. doi: 10.1016/j.jalz.2014.04.514

Alfandari, D., Criend, C., Heslenfeld, D. J., Versfeld, N. J., Kramer, S. E., and Zekveld, A. D. (2018). Brain volume differences associated with hearing impairment in adults. *Trends Hear.* 22, 1–8.

Amieva, H., and Ouvrard, C. (2020). Does treating hearing loss in older adults improve cognitive outcomes? a review. *J. Clin. Med.* 9:805. doi: 10.3390/jcm9030805

Amieva, H., Ouvrard, C., Giulioli, C., Meillon, C., Rullier, L., and Dartigues, J.-F. (2015). Self-reported hearing loss, hearing aids, and cognitive decline in elderly adults: a 25-year study. *J. Am. Geriatr. Soc.* 63, 2099–2104. doi: 10.1111/jgs.13649

Armstrong, N. M., An, Y., Doshi, J., Erus, G., Ferrucci, L., Davatzikos, C., et al. (2019). Association of midlife hearing impairment with late-life temporal lobe volume loss. *JAMA Otolaryngology-Head Neck Surg.* 145, 794–802. doi: 10.1001/jamaoto.2019.1610

Bainbridge, K. K., and Wallhagen, M. I. (2014). Hearing loss in an aging american population: extent, impact, and management. *Ann. Rev. Public Health* 35, 139–152. doi: 10.1146/annurev-publhealth-032013-182510

Baltes, P. B., and Lindenberger, U. (1997). Emergence of a powerful connection between sensory and cognitive function across the adult lifespan: a new window to the study of cognitive aging? *Psychol. Aging* 12, 12–21. doi: 10.1037//0882-7974.12.1.12

Bigelow, R., Reed, N., Brewster, N., Huang, A., Rebok, G., Rutherford, B. R., et al. (2020). Association of hearing loss with psychological distress and utilization of mental health services among adults in the United States. *JAMA Network Open* 3:e2010986. doi: 10.1001/jamanetworkopen.2020.10986

Bott, A., Hickson, L., Meyer, C., Bardy, F., Van dun, B., Pachana, N., et al. (2020). Is cortical automatic threshold estimation a feasible alternative for hearing threshold estimation with adults with dementia living in aged care? *Int. J. Audiol.* 59, 745–752. doi: 10.1080/14992027.2020.1746976

Bott, A., Meyer, C., Hickson, L., and Pachana, N. A. (2019). Can adults living with dementia complete pure-tone audiometry. *Int. J. Audiol.* 58, 185–192.

Braak, H., and Braak, E. (1991). Neuropathological stageing of Alzheimer-related changes. *Acta Neuropathol.* 82, 239–259.

Braak, H., and Braak, E. (1997). Frequency of stages of Alzheimer-related lesions in different age categories. *Neurobiol. Aging* 18, 551–357.

Bregman, A. S. (1993). "Auditory scene analysis: hearing in complex environments," in *Thinking in Sound: the Cognitive Psychology of Human Audition*, eds S. McAdams and E. Bigand (Oxford: Oxford University Press).

Brenowitz, W., Kaup, A., and Yaffe, K. (2019). Multiple sensory impairment is associated with increased risk of dementia among black and white older adults. *J. Gerontol. Med. Sci.* 74, 890–896. doi: 10.1093/gerona/gly264

Brenowitz, W. D., Filshtein, T. J., Yaffe, K., Walter, S., Ackley, S. F., Hoffman, T. J., et al. (2020). Association of genetic risk score for Alzheimer disease and hearing impairment. *Neurology* 95, e2225–e2234.

Brewster, K. K., Ciarleglio, A., Brown, P. J., Chen, C., and Kim, H. (2018). Age-Related hearing loss and its association with depression in later life. *Am. J. Geriatric Psychiatry* 26, 788–796. doi: 10.1016/j.jagp.2018.04.003

Brewster, K. K., Hu, M., Wall, M., Brown, P., Zilcha-Mano, S., Roose, S. P., et al. (2021). Age-related hearing loss, neuropsychological performance, and incident dementia in older adults. *J. Alzheimer's Dis.* 80, 855–864. doi: 10.3233/jad-200908

Brewster, K. K., Pavlicova, M., Stein, A., Chen, M., Chen, C., Brown, P. J., et al. (2020). A pilot randomized controlled trial of hearing aids to improve mood and cognition in older adults. *Int. J. Geriatr. Psychiatry* 35, 842–850. doi: 10.1002/gps.5311

Campbell, J., and Sharma, A. (2014). Cross-modal re-organization in adults with early stage hearing loss. *PLoS One* 9:e90594. doi: 10.1371/journal.pone.0090594

Celentano, D. D., and Szklo, M. (2020). *Gordis Epidemiology*, 6th Edn. Philadelphia, PA: Elsevier.

CHABA (1988). Speech understanding and aging. working group on speech understanding and aging. committee on hearing, bioacoustics, and biomechanics, commission on behavioral and social sciences and Education, National Research Council. *J. Acoustical Soc. Am.* 83, 859–895. doi: 10.1121/1.395965

Chang, H., Ho, C., and Chou, P. (2009). The factors associated with a self-perceived hearing handicap in elderly people with hearing impairment- results from a community-based study. *Ear. Hear.* 30, 576–583. doi: 10.1097/AUD.0b013e3181ac127a

Chen, D. S., Betz, J., Yaffe, K., Ayonayon, H. N., Kritchevsky, S., Martin, K. R., et al. (2015). Association of hearing impairment with declines in physical functioning and the risk of disability in older adults. *J. Gerontol. Series A Biol. Sci. Med. Sci.* 70, 654–661. doi: 10.1093/gerona/glu207

Choi, J. S., Betz, J., Deal, J., Contrera, K. J., and Genther, D. J. (2016). A comparison of self-report and audiometric measures of hearing and their associations with functional outcomes in older adults. *J. Aging Health* 28, 890–910. doi: 10.1177/0898264315614006

Clark, J. G. (1981). Uses and abuses of hearing loss classification. *ASHA* 23, 493–500.

Croll, P. H., Vernooij, M. W., Reid, R. I., Goedegebure, A., Power, M. C., Rigters, S. C., et al. (2020). Hearing loss and microstructural integrity of the brain in a dementia-free older population. *Alzheimer's Dementia* 16, 1515–1523. doi: 10.1002/alz.12151

Curhan, S. G., Eliassen, A. H., Eavey, R. D., Wang, M., Lin, B. M., and Curhan, G. C. (2017). Menopause and postmenopausal hormone therapy and risk of hearing loss. *Menopause* 24, 1049–1056. doi: 10.1097/gme.0000000000000878

Dawes, P., Emsley, R., Cruickshanks, K. J., Moore, D. R., Fortnum, H., Edmondson-Jones, M., et al. (2015). Hearing loss and cognition: the role of hearing aids, social isolation and depression. *PLoS One* 10:e0119616. doi: 10.1371/journal.pone.0119616

Dawes, P., Wolski, L., Himmelsbach, I., Regan, J., and Leroi, I. (2019). Interventions for hearing and vision impairment to improve outcomes for people with dementia: a scoping review. *Int. Psychogeriatr.* 31, 203–221.

Deal, J. A., Albert, M. S., Arnold, M., Bangdiwala, S. I., Chisolm, T., Davis, S., et al. (2017). A randomized feasibility pilot trial of hearing treatment for reducing cognitive decline: results from the aging and cognitive health evaluation in Elders Pilot Study. *Alzheimer's Dementia: Transl. Res. Clin. Interventions* 3, 410–415. doi: 10.1016/j.trci.2017.06.003

Deal, J. A., Beta, J., Yaffe, K., Harris, T., Purchase-Helzner, E., Satterfield, S., et al. (2016). Hearing impairment and incident dementia and cognitive decline in older adults: the health ABC Study. *J. Gerontol. Ser. A: Biol. Sci. Med. Sci.* 72, 703–709.

Deal, J. A., Goman, A. M., Albert, M. S., Arnold, M. L., Burgard, S., Chisolm, T., et al. (2018). Hearing treatment for reducing cognitive decline: design and methods of the aging and cognitive health evaluation in Elders randomized controlled trial. *Alzheimer's Dementia: Transl. Res. Clin. Interventions* 4, 499–507. doi: 10.1016/j.trci.2018.08.007

Dryden, A., Allen, H. A., Henshaw, H., and Heinrich, A. (2017). The association between cognitive performance and speech-in-noise perception for adult listeners: a systematic literature review and meta-analysis. *Trends Hear.* 21:2331216517744675. doi: 10.1177/2331216517744675

Eckert, M. A., Kuchinsky, S. E., Vaden, K. I., Cute, S. L., Spampinato, M. V., and Dubno, J. (2013). White matter hyperintensities predict low frequency hearing in older adults. *J. Assoc. Res. Otolaryngol.* 14, 425–433. doi: 10.1007/s10162-013-0381-4

Eckert, M. A., Vaden, K. I. Jr., and Dubno, J. R. (2019). Age-related hearing loss associations with changes in brain morphology. *Trends in Hearing* 23:2331216519857267.

Fausto, B., Badana, A., Arnold, M., Lister, J., and Edwards, J. (2018). Comparison of subjective and objective measures of hearing, auditory processing, and cognition among older adults with and without mild cognitive impairment. *J. Speech Lang. Hear Res.* 61, 945–956. doi: 10.1044/2017_JSLHR-H-17-0263

Fifer, R., Berger, J., Berlin, C., Tobey, E. A., and Campbell, J. C. (1983). Development of a dichotic sentence identification test for hearing-impaired adults. *Ear Hear.* 4, 300–305. doi: 10.1097/00003446-198311000-00007

Fortunato, S., Forli, F., Guglielmi, V., De Corso, E., Paludetti, G., Berrettini, S., et al. (2016). A review of new insights on the association between hearing loss and cognitive decline in ageing. *Acta Otorhinolaryngol. Ital.* 36, 155–166.

Füllgrabe, C. (2020). On the possible overestimation of cognitive decline: the impact of age-related hearing loss on cognitive-test performance. *Front. Neurosci.* 14:454. doi: 10.3389/fnins.2020.00454

Gallacher, J., Ilubaera, V., Ben-Shlomo, Y., Bayer, A., Fish, M., Babisch, W., et al. (2012). Auditory threshold, phonologic demand, and incident dementia. *Neurology* 79, 1583–1590. doi: 10.1212/WNL.0b013e31826e263d

Gao, J., Armstrong, N., Deal, J., Lin, F., and He, P. (2020). Hearing loss and cognitive function among Chinese older adults: the role of participation in leisure activities. *BMC Geriatrics* 20:215. doi: 10.1186/s12877-020-01615-7

Gates, G. A. (2012). Central presbycusis: an emerging view. *Otolaryngology-Head Neck Surg.* 141, 1–2. doi: 10.1177/0194599812446282

Gates, G. A., Anderson, M. L., McCurry, S. M., Feeney, M. P., and Larson, E. B. (2008). Central auditory dysfunction in older people with memory impairment or Alzheimer's dementia. *Arch. Otolaryngol. Head Neck Surg.* 134, 771–777. doi: 10.1001/archotol.134.7.771

Gates, G. A., Anderson, M. L., McCurry, S. M., Feeney, M. P., and Larson, E. B. (2011). Central auditory dysfunction as a harbinger of Alzheimer's dementia. *Arch. Otolaryngol. Head Neck Surg.* 137, 390–395. doi: 10.1001/archoto.2011.28

Gates, G. A., Cogg, J. L., Linn, R. T., Rees, T., Wolf, P. A., and D'Agostino, R. B. (1996). Central auditory dysfunction, cognitive dysfunction, and dementia in older people. *Arch. Otolaryngol. Head Neck Surg.* 122, 161–167. doi: 10.1001/archotol.1996.01890140047010

George, E., Zekveld, A., Kramer, S., Goverts, T., Festen, J., and Houtgast, T. (2007). Auditory and nonauditory factors affecting speech reception in noise by older listeners. *J. Acoust. Soc. Am.* 121:2362. doi: 10.1121/1.2642072

Goll, J. C., Crutch, S. J., Loo, J. H. Y., Rohrer, J. D., Frost, C., Bamiou, D. E., et al. (2010). Non-verbal sound processing in the primary progressive aphasia. *Brain* 133, 272–285. doi: 10.1093/brain/awp235

Goll, J. C., Kim, L. G., Hailstone, J. C., Lehman, M., Buckley, A., Crutch, S. J., et al. (2011). Auditory object cognition in dementia. *Neuropsychologia* 49, 2755–2765. doi: 10.1016/j.neuropsychologia.2011.06.004

Goll, J. C., Kim, L. G., Ridgway, G. R., Hailston, J. C., Lehman, M., and Buckley, A. H. (2012). Impairments of auditory scene analysis in Alzheimer's disease. *Brain* 135, 190–200.

Goman, A., and Lin, F. R. (2016). Prevalence of hearing loss by severity in the United States. *Am. J. Public Health* 106, 1820–1822. doi: 10.2105/ajph.2016.303299

Goman, A., Reed, N. S., and Lin, F. R. (2017). Addressing estimated hearing loss in adults in 2060. *JAMA Otolaryngol. Head Neck Surg.* 143, 732–734.

Griffiths, T. D., Lad, M., Kumar, S., Holmes, E., McMurrary, B., Maguire, E., et al. (2020). How can hearing loss cause dementia? *Neuron* 108, 401–412. doi: 10.1016/j.neuron.2020.08.003

Grube, M., Bruffaerts, R., Schaeverbeke, J., Neyens, V., De Weer, A. S., Seghers, A., et al. (2016). Core auditory processing deficits in primary progressive aphasia. *Brain* 139, 1817–1829. doi: 10.1093/brain/aww067

Guerreiro, M. J. S., and Van Gerven, P. W. M. (2017). Disregarding hearing loss leads to overestimation of age-related cognitive decline. *Neurobiol. Aging* 56, 180–189. doi: 10.1016/j.neurobiolaging.2017.05.001

Hickson, L., Meyer, C., Lovelock, K., Lampert, M., and Khan, A. (2014). Factors associated with success with hearing aids in older adults. *Int. J. Audiol.* 53, 18–27.

Hoffman, H. J., Dobie, R. A., Losonczy, K. G., Themann, C. L., and Flamme, G. A. (2017). Declining prevalence of hearing loss in US adults aged 20 to 69 Years. *JAMA Otolaryngol. Head Neck Surg.* 143, 274–285. doi: 10.1001/jamaoto.2016.3527

Hubbard, H. I., Mamo, S. K., and Hopper, T. (2018). Dementia and hearing loss: interrelationships and treatment considerations. *Sem. Speech Lang.* 39, 197–210. doi: 10.1055/s-0038-1660779

Huddle, M. G., Goman, A. M., Kernizan, F. C., Foley, D. M., Price, C., Frick, K. D., et al. (2017). The economic impact of adult hearing loss: a systematic review.

JAMA Otolaryngol. Head Neck Surg. 143, 1040–1048. doi: 10.1001/jamaoto.2017.1243

Hultcrantz, M., Simonoska, R., and Stenberg, A. (2006). Estrogen and hearing: a summary of recent investigations. *Acta Otolaryngol.* 126, 10–14. doi: 10.1080/00016480510038617

Humes, L. E. (2013). Understanding the speech-understanding problems of older adults. *Am. J. Audiol.* 22, 303–305. doi: 10.1044/1059-0889(2013/12-0066)

Humes, L. E. (2021). Factors underlying individual differences in speech-recognition thresholds (SRT) in noise among older adults. *Front. Aging Neurosci.* 13:702739. doi: 10.3389/fnagi.2021.702739

Humes, L. E., Busey, R. A., Craig, J., and Kewley-Port, D. (2013a). Are age-related changes in cognitive function driven by age-related changes in sensory processing? *Atten. Percept. Psychophys.* 75, 508–524. doi: 10.3758/s13414-012-0406-9

Humes, L. E., Kidd, G. R., and Lentz, J. L. (2013b). Auditory and cognitive factors underlying individuals differences in aided-speech-understanding among older adults. *Front. Systems Neurosci.* 7:55. doi: 10.3389/fnsys.2013.00055

Humes, L. E., Dubno, J., Gordon-Salant, S., Lister, J. L., Cacae, A. T., Cruickshanks, K. J., et al. (2012). Central presbycusis: a review and evaluation of the evidence. *J. Am. Acad. Audiol.* 23, 635–666. doi: 10.3766/jaaa.23.8.5

Humes, L. E., and Young, L. A. (2016). Sensory-cognitive interactions in older adults. *Ear Hear.* 37(Suppl. 1), 52S–61S.

Husain, F. T., Medina, R. E., Davis, C. W., Szymko-Bennett, Y., Simonyan, K., Pajor, N. M., et al. (2011). Neuoanatomical changes due to hearing loss and chronic tinnitus: a combined VBM and DTI study. *Brain Res.* 1369, 74–88. doi: 10.1016/j.brainres.2010.10.095

Idrizbegovic, E., Hederstierna, C., Dahlquist, M., Kämpfe Nordström, C., Jelic, V., and Rosenhall, U. (2011). Central auditory function in early Alzheimer's disease and in mild cognitive impairment. *Age. Ageing* 40, 249–254.

Jayakody, D., Menegola, H., Yiannos, J., Goodman-Simpson, J., Fiedland, P., and Taddei, K. (2020). The peripheral hearing and central auditory processing skills of individuals with subjective memory complaints. *Front. Neurosci.* doi: 10.3389/fnins.2020.00888

Jerger, J. (2019). Toward differentiation between SNHL, SNHL with cognitive decline, and SNHL with APD. *Hear. Rev.* 26, 18–22.

Johnson, J. C. S., Marshall, C. R., Weil, R. S., Bamiou, D. E., Hardy, C. J. D., and Warren, J. D. (2021). Hearing and dementia: from ears to brain. *Brain* 144, 391–401.

Kales, H. C., Gitlin, L. N., and Lyketsos, C. G. (2014). Detroit expert panel on the assessment, and management of the neuropsychiatric symptoms of dementia. management of neuropsychiatric symptoms of dementia in clinical settings: recommendations from a multisensory expert panel. *J. Am. Geriatr. Soc.* 62, 762–769. doi: 10.1111/jgs.12730

Kamil, R. J., Li, L., and Lin, F. R. (2014). Association of hearing impairment and frailty in older adults. *J. Am. Geriatric Soc.* 62, 1186–1188. doi: 10.1111/jgs.12860

Katz, J. (ed.) (2015). *Handbook of Clinical Audiology*, 7th Edn. Alphen aan den Rijn: Wolters Kluwer.

Kim, A. S., Garcia Morales, E. E., Amjad, H., Cotter, V. T., Lin, F. R., Lyketsos, C. G., et al. (2020). Association of hearing loss with neuropsychiatric symptoms in older adults with cognitive impairment. *Am. J. Psychiatry* 29, 544–553. doi: 10.1016/j.jagp.2020.10.002

Laughlin, G. A., McEvoy, L. K., Barrett-Connor, E., Daniels, L. B., and Ix, J. H. (2013). Fetuin-A, a new vascular biomarker of cognitive decline in older adults. *Clin. Endocrinol.* 81, 134–140. doi: 10.1111/cen.12382

Liljas, A., Carvalho, L., Papachristou, E., De Oliveira, C., Wannamethee, G., Ramsay, S. E., et al. (2017). Self-reported hearing impairment and incident frailty in English community-dwelling older adults: a 4-year follow-up study. *J. Am. Geriatr. Soc.* 65, 958–965. doi: 10.1111/jgs.14687

Lin, B., Li, W., Curhan, S., Stankovic, K., Qureshi, A. A., and Curhan, G. C. (2017). Skin pigmentation and risk of hearing loss in women. *Am. J. Epidemiol.* 186, 1–10.

Lin, F. L., Metter, J., O'Brien, R. J., Resnick, S. M., Zonderman, A. B., and Ferrucci, L. (2011). Hearing loss and incident dementia. *Arch. Neurol.* 68, 214–220.

Lin, F. R., and Albert, M. (2014). Hearing loss and dementia- who's listening? *Aging Ment. Health* 18, 671–673. doi: 10.1080/13607863.2014.915924

Lin, F. R., Ferrucci, L., An, Y., Goh, J. O., Doshi, J., Metter, E. J., et al. (2014). Association of hearing impairment with brain volume changes in older adults. *Neuorimage* 90, 84–92.

Lin, F. R., Yaffe, K., Xia, J., Xue, Q., Harris, T., Purchase-Helzner, E., et al. (2013). Hearing loss and cognitive decline among older adults. *JAMA Int. Med.* 173:10.1001/jamainternmed.2013.1868

Littlejohn, J., Bowen, M., Constantinidou, F., Dawes, P., Dickinson, C., Heyn, P., et al. (2021). International practice recommendations for the recognition and management of hearing and vision impairment in people with dementia. *Gerontology* doi: 10.1159/000515892

Livingston, G., Huntley, J., Sommerlad, A., Ames, D., Ballad, C., Banerjee, S., et al. (2020). Dementia prevention, intervention, and care. *Lancet* 396, 413–446.

Livingston, G., Sommerlad, A., Orgeta, V., Costafreda, S. G., Huntley, J., Ames, D., et al. (2017). Dementia prevention, intervention, and care. *Lancet* 390, 2673–2734.

Lopez, D., McCaul, K., Hankey, G., Norman, P., Almeida, O., Dobson, A., et al. (2011). Falls, injuries from falls, health related quality of life and mortality in older adults with vision and hearing impairment—is there a gender difference? *Maturitas* 69, 359–364. doi: 10.1016/j.maturitas.2011.05.006

Loughrey, D. G., Kelly, M. E., Kelley, G. A., Brennan, S., and Lawlor, B. A. (2018). Association of age-related hearing loss with cognitive function, cognitive impairment and dementia: a systematic review and meta-analysis. *JAMA Otolaryngology-Head Neck Surg.* 144, 115–126. doi: 10.1001/jamaoto.2017.2513

Maharani, A., Dawes, P., Nazroo, J., Tampubolon, G., and Pendleton, N. (2018). Longitudinal relationship between hearing aid use and cognitive function in older Americans. *J. Am. Geriatr. Soc.* 66, 1130–1136. doi: 10.1111/jgs.15363

Maharani, A., Pendleton, N., and Leroi, I. (2019). Hearing impairment, loneliness, social isolation, and cognitive function: longitudinal analysis using English Longitudinal Study on Ageing. *Am. J. Geriatric Psychiatry* 27, 1348–1356. doi: 10.1016/j.jagp.2019.07.010

Mamo, S., Reed, N., Sharrett, R., Albert, M., Coresh, J., Mosley, T., et al. (2019). Relationship between domain-specific cognitive function and speech-in-noise performance in older adults: the Atherosclerosis Risk in Communities Hearing Pilot Study. *Am. J. Audiol.* 28, 1006–1014. doi: 10.1044/2019_AJA-19-00043

Mamo, S. K., Reed, N. S., Price, C., Occhipinti, D., and Pletnikova, A. (2018). Hearing loss treatment in older adults with cognitive impairment: a systematic review. *J. Speech Lang. Hear. Res.* 61, 2589–2603. doi: 10.1044/2018_jslhr-h-18-0077

Martinez-Amezcua, P., Powell, D., Kuo, P. L., Reed, N. S., Sullican, K. J., Palta, P., et al. (2021). Association of age-related hearing impairment with physical functioning among community-dwelling older adults in the US. *JAMA Network Open* 4:e2113742. doi: 10.1001/jamanetworkopen.2021.13742

McClannahan, K., Chiu, Y. F., Somers, M., and Peelle, J. (2021). Test-Retest reliability of audiometric assessment in individuals with mild dementia. *JAMA Otolaryngol. Head Neck Surg.* 147, 442–449. doi: 10.1001/jamaoto.2021.0012

Mener, D. J., Betz, J., Yaffe, K., Harris, T. B., Helzner, E. P., Satterfeld, S., et al. (2016). Apolipoprotein E allele and hearing thresholds in older adults. *Am. J. Alzheimer's Dis. Other Dementias* 31, 34–39. doi: 10.1177/1533317514537549

Mitchell, B. L., Thorp, J. G., Evans, D. M., Nyholt, D. R., and Martin, N. G. (2020). Exploring the genetic relationship between hearing impairment and Alzheimer's disease. *Alzheimer's Dementia* 12:e12108.

Morita, Y., Sasaki, T., Takahashi, K., Kitazawa, M., Nonomura, Y., Yagi, C., et al. (2019). Age-related hearing loss is strongly associated with cognitive decline regardless of APOE4 polymorphism. *Otol. Neurotol.* 40, 1263–1267. doi: 10.1097/mao.0000000000002415

Musiek, F., and Baran, J. (2018). *The Auditory System: Anatomy, Physiology, and Clinical Correlates*, 2nd Edn. San Diego, CA: Plural Publishing.

National Academies of Sciences, Engineering, and Medicine (2016). *Hearing Health Care for Adults: Priorities for Improving Access and Affordability.* Washington, DC: The National Academies Press, doi: 10.17226/23446

Nichols, E., Deal, J. A., Swenor, B. K., Abraham, A. G., Armstrong, N. M., Carlson, M. C., et al. (2021). Assessing bias in cognitive testing for older adults with sensory impairment: an analysis of differential item functioning in the baltimore longitudinal study on aging (BLSA) and the atherosclerosis risk in communities neurocognitive study (ARIC-NCS). *J. Int. Neuropsychol. Soc.* Online ahead of print. doi: 10.1017/S1355617721000400

Nieman, C. L., Marrone, N., Mamo, S. K., Betz, J., Choi, J. S., Contrera, K. J., et al. (2017). The Baltimore HEARS pilot study: an affordable, accessible community-delivered hearing care model. *Gerontologist* 57, 1173–1186. doi: 10.1093/geront/gnw153

Panza, F., Solfrizzi, V., Seripa, D., Imbimbo, B., Capozzo, R., et al. (2015). Age-related hearing impairment and frailty in Alzheimer's disease: interconnected associations and mechanisms. *Front. Aging Neurosci.* 7:113. doi: 10.3389/fnagi.2015.00113

Parker, T., Cash, D. M., Lane, C., Lu, K., Malone, I. B., Nicholas, J. M., et al. (2020). Pure tone audiometry and cerebral pathology in healthy older adults. *J. Neurol. Neurosurg. Psychiatry* 91, 172–176. doi: 10.1136/jnnp-2019-321897

Peelle, J. (2018). Listening effort: how the cognitive consequences of acoustic challenge are reflected in brain and behavior. *Ear Hear.* 39, 204–214. doi: 10.1097/AUD.0000000000000494

Pichora-Fuller, M. K., Kramer, S. E., Eckert, M. A., Edwards, B., Hornsby, B. W. Y., Humes, L. E., et al. (2016). Hearing impairment and cognitive energy: the Framework for Understanding Effortful Listening (FUEL). *Ear Hear.* 37, 5S–27S.

Pickles, J. O. (2013). *An Introduction to the Physiology of Hearing*, 4th Edn. Leiden: Brill.

Powell, D., Oh, E., Lin, F., and Deal, J. (2021). Hearing impairment and cognition in an aging world. *J. Assoc. Res. Otolaryngol.* 22, 387–403. doi: 10.1007/s10162-021-00799-7

Pye, A., Charalambous, A. P., Leroi, I., Thodi, C., and Dawes, P. (2017). Screening tools for the identification of dementia for adults with age-related acquired hearing or vision impairment: a scoping review. *Int. Psychogeriatr.* 29, 1771–1784. doi: 10.1017/s104161021700120x

Rabbitt, P. M. (1968). Channel-capacity, intelligibility and immediate memory. *Quar. J. Exp. Psychol.* 20, 241–248. doi: 10.1080/14640746808400158

Rafnsson, S. B., Orrell, M., d'Orsi, E., Hogervorst, E., and Steptoe, A. (2020). Loneliness, social integration, and incident dementia over 6 years: prospective findings from the English Longitudinal Study of Ageing. *J. Gerontol. Ser. B Psychol. Sci. Soc. Sci.* 75, 114–124. doi: 10.1093/geronb/gbx087

Ray, J., Popli, G., and Gell, G. (2018). Association of cognition and age-related hearing impairment in the English Longitudinal Study of Ageing. *JAMA Otolaryngol. Head Neck Surg.* 144, 876–882. doi: 10.1001/jamaoto.2018.1656

Reed, N., Altan, A., Deal, J., Yeh, C., Kravetz, A., Wallhagen, M., et al. (2019). Trends in health care costs and utilization associated with untreated hearing loss over 10 years. *JAMA Otolaryngol. Head Neck Surg.* 145, 27–34. doi: 10.1001/jamaoto.2018.2875

Reed, N. S., Garcia-Morales, E., and Willink, A. (2021). Trends in hearing aid ownership among older adults in the United States from 2011 to 2018. *JAMA Int. Med.* 181, 383–385. doi: 10.1001/jamainternmed.2020.5682

Rigters, S. C., Bos, D., Metselaar, M., Roshchupkin, G. V., Baatengurg, de Jong, R. J., et al. (2017). Hearing impairment is associated with smaller brain volume in aging. *Front. Aging Neurosci.* 9:2. doi: 10.3389/fnagi.2017.00002

Rudner, M., Seeto, M., Keidser, G., Johnson, B., and Rönnberg, J. (2019). Poorer speech reception threshold in noise is associated with lower brain volume in auditory and cognitive processing regions. *J. Speech Lang. Hear. Res.* 62, 117–1130. doi: 10.1044/2018_JSLHR-H-ASCC7-18-0142

Rutherford, B. R., Brewster, K., Golub, J. S., Kim, A. H., and Roose, S. P. (2018). Sensation and Psychiatry: linking age-related hearing loss to late-life depression and cognitive decline. *Am. J. Psychiatry* 175, 215–224. doi: 10.1176/appi.ajp.2017.17040423

Salthouse, T. (1996). The processing-speed theory of adult age differences in cognition. *Psychol. Rev.* 103, 403–428. doi: 10.1037/0033-295x.103.3.403

Sardone, R., Battista, P., Donghia, R., Lozupone, M., Tortelli, R., Guerra, V., et al. (2020). Age-related central auditory processing disorder, MCI, and dementia in an older population in southern Italy. *Otolaryngol. Head Neck Surg.* 163, 348–355. doi: 10.1177/0194599820913635

Sardone, R., Battista, P., Panza, F., Lozupone, M., Griseta, C., Castellana, F., et al. (2019). The age-related central auditory processing disorder: silent impairment of the cognitive ear. *Front. Neurosci.* 13:619. doi: 10.3389/fnins.2019.00619

Schneider, B. A., Daneman, M., and Pichora-Fuller, M. K. (2002). Listening in aging adults: from discourse comprehension to psychoacoustics. *Can. J. Exp. Pscyhol.* 56, 139–152. doi: 10.1037/h0087392

Sharma, A., and Glick, H. (2017). Cross-modal plasticity in developmental and age-related hearing loss: clinical implications. *Hear. Res.* 343, 191–201. doi: 10.1016/j.heares.2016.08.012

Sharma, R. K., Chern, A., and Golub, J. S. (2021). Age-related hearing loss and the development of cognitive impairment and late-life depression: a scoping overview. *Sem. Hear.* 41, 10–25. doi: 10.1055/s-0041-1725997

Shukla, A., Harper, M., Pedersen, E., Goman, A., Suen, J. J., Price, C., et al. (2020). Hearing loss, loneliness, and social isolation: a systematic review. *Otolaryngol. Head Neck Surg.* 5, 622–633. doi: 10.1177/0194599820910377

Shuster, B., Depireux, D., Mong, J., and Hertzano, R. (2019). Sex differences in hearing: probing the role of estrogen signaling. *J. Acoust. Soc. Am.* 145, 3656–3663. doi: 10.1121/1.5111870

Sinha, U. K., Hollen, K. M., Rodriguez, R., and Miller, C. A. (1993). Auditory system degeneration in Alzheimer's disease. *Neurology* 43, 779–785. doi: 10.1212/wnl.43.4.779

Snyder, P. J., Hohnson, L. N., Lim, Y. Y., Santos, C. Y., Alber, J., and Maruff, P. (2016). Nonvascular retinal imaging markers of preclinical Alzheimer's disease. *Alzheimer's Dementia: Diag. Assess. Dis. Monitor.* 4, 169–178. doi: 10.1016/j.dadm.2016.09.001

Sperling, R. A., Aisen, P. S., Beckett, L. A., Bennett, D. A., Craft, S., Fagan, A. M., et al. (2011). Toward defining the preclinical stages of Alzheimer's disease: recommendations from the National Institute on Aging and the Alzheimer's association workgroup. *Alzheimer's Dementia* 7, 280–292. doi: 10.1016/j.jalz.2011.03.003

Surprenant, A. M., and Neath, I. (2006). "Cognitive aging," in *Gerontology: Perspectives and Issues*, eds J. A. Wilmoth and K. Ferraro (New York NY: Springer).

Taubman, L. B., Palmer, C. V., Durrant, J. D., and Pratt, S. (1999). Accuracy of hearing aid use time as reported by experienced hearing aid wearers. *Ear Hear.* 20, 299–305. doi: 10.1097/00003446-199908000-00003

Thomson, R. S., Auduong, P., Miller, A. T., and Gurgel, R. K. (2017). Hearing loss as a risk factor for dementia: a systematic review. *Laryngoscope Investigat. Otolaryngol.* 2, 69–79. doi: 10.1002/lio2.65

Tun, P. A., McCoy, A., and Wingfield, A. (2009). Aging, hearing acuity, and the attentional costs of effortful listening. *Psychol. Aging* 24, 761–766. doi: 10.1037/a0014802

Tun, P. A., Willaims, V. A., Small, B. J., and Hafter, E. R. (2012). The effects of aging on auditory processing and cognition. *Am. J. Audiol.* 21, 344–350. doi: 10.1044/1059-0889(2012/12-0030)

Tuwaig, M., Savard, M., Jutras, B., Poirier, J., Louis Collins, D., Rosa-Neto, P., et al. (2017). Deficit in central auditory processing as a biomarker of pre-clinical Alzheimer's disease. *J. Alzheimer's Dis.* 60, 1589–1600. doi: 10.3233/JAD-170545

Uhlmann, R. F., Larson, E. B., Rees, R. S., Koepsell, T. D., and Duckert, L. G. (1989). Relationship of hearing impairment to dementia and cognitive dysfunction in older adults. *J. Am. Med. Assoc.* 261, 1916–1919. doi: 10.1001/jama.261.13.1916

Villeneuve, A., Hommet, C., Aussedat, C., Lescanne, E., Reffet, K., and Bakhos, D. (2017). Audiometric evaluation in patients with Alzheimer's diseae. *Eur. Arch. Otorhinolaryngol.* 274, 151–157. doi: 10.1007/s00405-016-4257-1

Wayne, R. V., and Johnsrude, I. S. (2015). A review of causal mechanisms underlying the link between age-related hearing loss and cognitive decline. *Ageing Res. Rev.* 23, 154–166. doi: 10.1016/j.arr.2015.06.002

Wells, H., Freidin, M., Zainul Abidin, F., Payton, A., Dawes, P., Munro, K. J., et al. (2019). GWAS identifies 44 independent associated genomic loci for self-reported adult hearing difficulty in UK biobank. *Am. J. Hum. Genet.* 105, 788–802. doi: 10.1016/j.ajhg.2019.09.008

Whalley, L. J., Deary, I. J., Appleton, C. L., and Starr, J. M. (2004). Cognitive reserve and the neurobiology of cognitive aging. *Ageing Res. Rev.* 3, 369–382.

Whitson, H. E., Cronin-Golomb, A., Cruickshanks, K. J., Gilmore, G. C., and Owsley, C. (2018). American geriatrics society and national institute on aging bench-to-bedside conference: sensory impairment and cognitive decline in older adults. *J. Am. Geriatr. Soc.* 66, 2052–2058. doi: 10.1111/jgs.15506

Wingfield, A., and Peelle, J. E. (2015). The effects of hearing loss on neural plasticity and processing. *Front. Systems Neurosci.* 9:35. doi: 10.3389/fnsys.2015.00035

Wingfield, A., Tun, P. A., and McCoy, S. L. (2005). Hearing loss in older adulthood-what it is and how it interacts with cognitive performance. *Curr. Direct. Psychol. Sci.* 14, 144–148.

World Report on Hearing (2021). *Licence: CC BY-NC-SA 3.0 IGO*. Geneva: World Health Organization.

Yuan, J., Sun, Y., Sang, S., Huynh Pham, J., and Kon, W. (2018). The risk of cognitive impairment associated with hearing function in older adults: a pooled analysis of data from eleven studies. *Sci. Rep.* 8:2137. doi: 10.1038/s41598-018-20496-w

Zhang, Y., Wang, Y., Shi, C., Shen, M., and Lu, F. (2021). Advances in retina imaging as potential biomarkers for early diagnosis of Alzheimer's disease. *Transl. Neurodegenerat.* 10:6.

Zissimopoulos, J. (2014). The value of delaying Alzheimer's disease onset. *Forum Health Econom. Policy* 18, 25–39. doi: 10.1515/fhep-2014-0013

Permissions

All chapters in this book were first published by Frontiers; hereby published with permission under the Creative Commons Attribution License or equivalent. Every chapter published in this book has been scrutinized by our experts. Their significance has been extensively debated. The topics covered herein carry significant findings which will fuel the growth of the discipline. They may even be implemented as practical applications or may be referred to as a beginning point for another development.

The contributors of this book come from diverse backgrounds, making this book a truly international effort. This book will bring forth new frontiers with its revolutionizing research information and detailed analysis of the nascent developments around the world.

We would like to thank all the contributing authors for lending their expertise to make the book truly unique. They have played a crucial role in the development of this book. Without their invaluable contributions this book wouldn't have been possible. They have made vital efforts to compile up to date information on the varied aspects of this subject to make this book a valuable addition to the collection of many professionals and students.

This book was conceptualized with the vision of imparting up-to-date information and advanced data in this field. To ensure the same, a matchless editorial board was set up. Every individual on the board went through rigorous rounds of assessment to prove their worth. After which they invested a large part of their time researching and compiling the most relevant data for our readers.

The editorial board has been involved in producing this book since its inception. They have spent rigorous hours researching and exploring the diverse topics which have resulted in the successful publishing of this book. They have passed on their knowledge of decades through this book. To expedite this challenging task, the publisher supported the team at every step. A small team of assistant editors was also appointed to further simplify the editing procedure and attain best results for the readers.

Apart from the editorial board, the designing team has also invested a significant amount of their time in understanding the subject and creating the most relevant covers. They scrutinized every image to scout for the most suitable representation of the subject and create an appropriate cover for the book.

The publishing team has been an ardent support to the editorial, designing and production team. Their endless efforts to recruit the best for this project, has resulted in the accomplishment of this book. They are a veteran in the field of academics and their pool of knowledge is as vast as their experience in printing. Their expertise and guidance has proved useful at every step. Their uncompromising quality standards have made this book an exceptional effort. Their encouragement from time to time has been an inspiration for everyone.

The publisher and the editorial board hope that this book will prove to be a valuable piece of knowledge for researchers, students, practitioners and scholars across the globe.

List of Contributors

Tingting Dong, Xuejie Zhang, Fengqiu Chen, Lulu Pan, Shaoru Hu and Min Wang
Biobank of Ninth People's Hospital, Shanghai Jiao Tong University School of Medicine, Shanghai, China

Yiqing Liu
Shanghai Ninth People's Hospital, Shanghai Jiao Tong University School of Medicine, Shanghai, China

Shan Xu and Haishuang Chang
Shanghai Ninth People's Hospital, Shanghai Institute of Precision Medicine, Shanghai Jiao Tong University School of Medicine, Shanghai, China

Min Lu
Shanghai Key Laboratory for Prevention and Treatment of Bone and Joint Diseases, Department of Orthopaedics, Ruijin Hospital, Shanghai Institute of Traumatology and Orthopaedics, Shanghai Jiao Tong University School of Medicine, Shanghai, China

Dongxiu Chen, Yanjing Luo, Jing Pan, Anning Chen, Muqing Xu and Hongzheng Zhang
Department of Otolaryngology Head and Neck Surgery, Zhujiang Hospital, Southern Medical University, Guangzhou, China
Hearing Research Center, Southern Medical University, Guangzhou, China

Dong Ma
Key Laboratory of Biomaterials of Guangdong Higher Education Institutes, Department of Biomedical Engineering, Jinan University, Guangzhou, China

Jie Tang
Hearing Research Center, Southern Medical University, Guangzhou, China
Department of Physiology, School of Basic Medical Sciences, Southern Medical University, Guangzhou, China
Key Laboratory of Mental Health of the Ministry of Education, Southern Medical University, Guangzhou, China

Wei Ren, Cong Xu, Fan-jun Zheng, Yue Zhang, Wei-wei Guo, Hui Zhao and Shi-ming Yang
College of Otolaryngology Head and Neck Surgery, Chinese PLA General Hospital, Beijing, China
National Clinical Research Center for Otolaryngologic Diseases, Beijing, China
Key Lab of Hearing Science, Ministry of Education, Beijing, China
Beijing Key Lab of Hearing Impairment for Prevention and Treatment, Beijing, China

Ting-ting Lin, Chuan-hong Liu, Xiao-yang Zhou, Lu-lu Wang and Yong Wang
Department of Laboratory Animal Science, College of Basic Medical Science, Army Medical University, Chongqing, China

Peng Jin
Department of Human Genetics, Emory University School of Medicine, Atlanta, GA, United States

Hailong Tu, Aizhen Zhang, Xiaolong Fu and Jiangang Gao
School of Life Sciences, Shandong Provincial ENT Hospital, Shandong University, Jinan, China

Shiqi Xu
University of Edinburgh Institute, Zhejiang University School of Medicine, Zhejiang University, Haining, China

Xiaohui Bai
Otolaryngology-Head and Neck Surgery, Shandong Provincial ENT Hospital, Jinan, China

Haibo Wang
School of Life Sciences, Shandong Provincial ENT Hospital, Shandong University, Jinan, China
Otolaryngology-Head and Neck Surgery, Shandong Provincial ENT Hospital, Jinan, China
Shandong Provincial ENT Hospital, Cheeloo College of Medicine, Shandong University, Jinan, China

Kefeng Ma, Xiaojun She, Honglian Yang, Kun Wang, Yingwen Zhu and Xiujie Gao
Tianjin Institute of Environmental and Operational Medicine, Tianjin, China

Anran Zhang and Bo Cui
Tianjin Institute of Environmental and Operational Medicine, Tianjin, China
Shandong Academy of Occupational Health and Occupational Medicine, Shandong First Medical University & Shandong Academy of Medical Sciences, Jinan, China

Haibo Du, Hao Zhou, Yixiao Sun, Xiaoyan Zhai and Yanfei Wang
Shandong Provincial Key Laboratory of Animal Cell and Developmental Biology, School of Life Sciences, Shandong University, Qingdao, China

Zhengjun Chen
State Key Laboratory of Cell Biology, Center for Excellence in Molecular Cell Science, Shanghai Institute of Biochemistry and Cell Biology, Chinese Academy of Sciences, Shanghai, China
School of Life Sciences and Technology, Shanghai Tech University, Shanghai, China

Zhigang Xu
Shandong Provincial Key Laboratory of Animal Cell and Developmental Biology, School of Life Sciences, Shandong University, Qingdao, China
Shandong Provincial Collaborative Innovation Center of Cell Biology, Shandong Normal University, Jinan, China

Dalian Ding, Haiyan Jiang, Senthilvelan Manohar, Xiaopeng Liu, Li Li, Guang-Di Chen and Richard Salvi
Center for Hearing and Deafness, University at Buffalo, Buffalo, NY, United States

Mingxuan Wu, Mingyu Xia and Wenyan Li
ENT Institute and Department of Otorhinolaryngology, Eye and ENT Hospital, State Key Laboratory of Medical Neurobiology and MOE Frontiers Center for Brain Science, Fudan University, Shanghai, China

Huawei Li
ENT Institute and Department of Otorhinolaryngology, Eye and ENT Hospital, State Key Laboratory of Medical Neurobiology and MOE Frontiers Center for Brain Science, Fudan University, Shanghai, China
Institutes of Biomedical Sciences, Fudan University, Shanghai, China
NHC Key Laboratory of Hearing Medicine, Fudan University, Shanghai, China
The Institutes of Brain Science and The Collaborative Innovation Center for Brain Science, Fudan University, Shanghai, China

Jian-Ping Wu
Academy of Advanced Interdisciplinary Studies, Southern University of Science and Technology, Shenzhen, China
Department of Biomedical Engineering, Southern University of Science and Technology, Shenzhen, China

Xiaojie Yang
Department of Biomedical Engineering, Southern University of Science and Technology, Shenzhen, China

Yilin Wang
Core Research Facilities, Southern University of Science and Technology, Shenzhen, China

Ben Swift
College of Computing, Australian National University, Canberra, ACT, Australia

Robert Adamson
School of Biomedical Engineering, Electrical and Computer Engineering, Dalhousie University, Halifax, NS, Canada

Yongchang Zheng
Peking Union Medical College Hospital, Chinese Academy of Medical Sciences and Peking Union Medical College, Beijing, China

Rongli Zhang
Guangdong Provincial People's Hospital, Guangdong Academy of Medical Science, School of Medicine, South China University of Technology, Guangzhou, China

Wen Zhon
School of Mechanical Engineering and Automation, Xihua University, Chengdu, China

Fangyi Chen
Department of Biomedical Engineering, Southern University of Science and Technology, Shenzhen, China
Department of Biology, Brain Research Centre, Southern University of Science and Technology, Shenzhen, China

Wenjia Wang, Jin Li, Fen Xiong and Hongyang Wang
College of Otolaryngology, Head and Neck Surgery, Institute of Otolaryngology, Chinese PLA General Hospital, Beijing, China
National Clinical Research Center for Otolaryngologic Diseases, Beijing, China

Fei Sun, Ke-yong Tian, Xin-yu Zhang, Wei Liu, Jian-hua Qiu and Ding-jun Zha
Department of Otolaryngology-Head and Neck Surgery, Xijing Hospital, Fourth Military Medical University, Xi'an, China

Ke Zhou
Department of Laboratory Medicine, Institute of Clinical Laboratory Medicine of PLA, Xijing Hospital, Fourth Military Medical University, Xi'an, China

Jie Wang
Department of Otolaryngology-Head and Neck Surgery, The Affiliated Children Hospital of Xi'an Jiaotong University, Xi'an, China

Cui-ping Zhon
Department of Otolaryngology-Head and Neck Surgery, The 940th Hospital of Joint Logistics Support Force of PLA, Lanzhou, China

Arthur Benjamin Kwesi
Department of Otorhinolaryngology, Union Hospital, Tongji Medical College, Huazhong University of Science and Technology, Wuhan, China
Hearing and Speech Rehabilitation Institute, Zhejiang Chinese Medical University, Hangzhou, China

Jintao Yu and Yu Sun
Department of Otorhinolaryngology, Union Hospital, Tongji Medical College, Huazhong University of Science and Technology, Wuhan, China

Chenlu Wang, Fengyi Chuang and Wendi Shi
Hangzhou Ren-ai Hearing Rehabilitation Research Centre, Hangzhou, China

Yonghua Wang and Xiaohui Yan
Hearing and Speech Rehabilitation Institute, Zhejiang Chinese Medical University, Hangzhou, China

Yi-Ming Zhu
Department of Otolaryngology-Head and Neck Surgery, Nanfang Hospital, Southern Medical University, Guangzhou, China
Department of Otolaryngology-Head and Neck Surgery, Lanzhou University Second Hospital, Lanzhou, China

Qi Li, Yan-Fei Li, You-Li Liu and Xiang-Ping Li
Department of Otolaryngology-Head and Neck Surgery, Nanfang Hospital, Southern Medical University, Guangzhou, China

Xue Gao
Department of Otolaryngology, PLA Rocket Force Characteristic Medical Center, Beijing, China

Pu Dai
Department of Otolaryngology-Head and Neck Surgery, Nanfang Hospital, Southern Medical University, Guangzhou, China
Department of Otolaryngology-Head and Neck Surgery, Chinese PLA General Hospital, Beijing, China

Hongyang Wang
College of Otolaryngology, Head and Neck Surgery, Chinese People's Liberation Army (PLA) Institute of Otolaryngology, Chinese People's Liberation Army (PLA) General Hospital, Beijing, China

Yun Gao, Jing Guan, Lan Lan, Ju Yang, Wenping Xiong, Cui Zhao, Linyi Xie, Lan Yu, Dayong Wang and Qiuju Wang
College of Otolaryngology, Head and Neck Surgery, Chinese People's Liberation Army (PLA) Institute of Otolaryngology, Chinese People's Liberation Army (PLA) General Hospital, Beijing, China
National Clinical Research Center for Otolaryngologic Diseases, Beijing, China
Key Lab of Hearing Impairment Science of Ministry of Education, Beijing, China
Key Lab of Hearing Impairment Prevention and Treatment of Beijing, Beijing, China

Lili Xiao, Chengqi Liu, Zhong Zheng, Ying Shen, Liang Xia, Guang Yang and Yanmei Feng
Department of Otolaryngology-Head and Neck Surgery, Shanghai Jiao Tong University Affiliated Sixth People's Hospital, Shanghai, China
Otolaryngology Institute of Shanghai Jiao Tong University, Shanghai, China
Shanghai Key Laboratory of Sleep Disordered Breathing, Shanghai, China

Yan Sun
Zhangjiagang TCM Hospital Affiliated to Nanjing University of Chinese Medicine, Zhangjiagang, China

Hongchao Liu, Longhao Wang, Pengcheng Xu, Zhaoyan Wang, Huihui Liu and Hao Wu
Department of Otolaryngology-Head and Neck Surgery, Shanghai Ninth People's Hospital, Shanghai Jiao Tong University School of Medicine, Shanghai, China
Ear Institute, Shanghai Jiao Tong University School of Medicine, Shanghai, China
Shanghai Key Laboratory of Translational Medicine on Ear and Nose Diseases, Shanghai, China

Hu Peng
Department of Otolaryngology-Head and Neck Surgery, Changzheng Hospital, Second Military Medical University, Shanghai, China

Jie Gong, Peipei Qian, Yuebo Hu, Chao Guo, Guanyun Wei, Cheng Wang, Chengyun Cai and Dong Liu
Nantong Laboratory of Development and Diseases, School of Life Sciences, Co-innovation Center of Neuroregeneration, Key Laboratory of Neuroregeneration of Jiangsu and MOE, Nantong University, Nantong, China

Danielle S. Powell
Department of Health Policy and Management, Johns Hopkins Bloomberg School of Public Health, Baltimore, MD, United States
Cochlear Center for Hearing and Public Health, Johns Hopkins Bloomberg School of Public Health, Baltimore, MD, United States

Esther S. Oh
Cochlear Center for Hearing and Public Health, Johns Hopkins Bloomberg School of Public Health, Baltimore, MD, United States
Division of Geriatric Medicine and Gerontology, Johns Hopkins University School of Medicine, Baltimore, MD, United States

Nicholas S. Reed, Frank R. Lin and Jennifer A. Deal
Cochlear Center for Hearing and Public Health, Johns Hopkins Bloomberg School of Public Health, Baltimore, MD, United States
Department of Epidemiology, Johns Hopkins Bloomberg School of Public Health, Baltimore, MD, United States
Department of Otolaryngology, Johns Hopkins University School of Medicine, Baltimore, MD, United States

Index